The
COMPENDIUM
COLLECTION

RADIOLOGY

IN PRACTICE

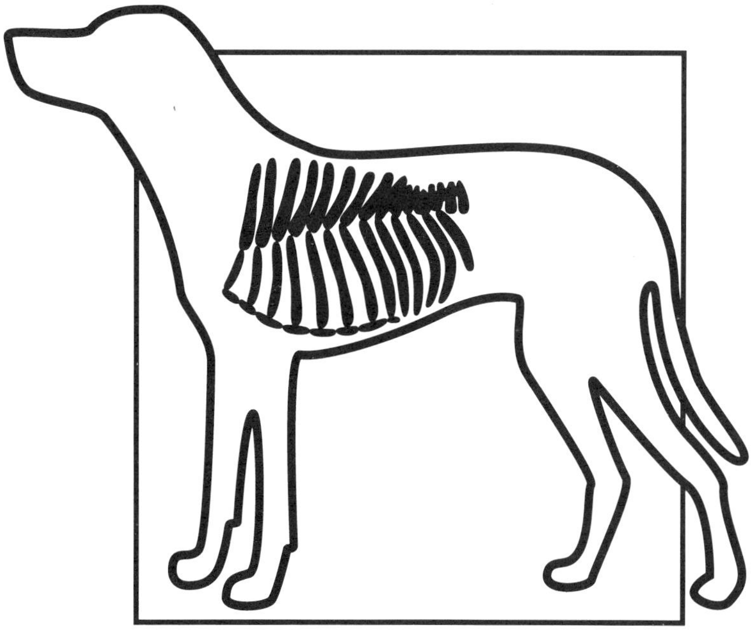

Published by Veterinary Learning Systems
Trenton, New Jersey

ISBN 1-884254-16-0

PREFACE

The use of veterinary radiology has expanded tremendously in the last two decades, primarily because of increased availability of and expertise in alternative imaging techniques. Ultrasound, echocardiography, computed tomography, magnetic resonance imaging, and nuclear scanning are now used routinely in veterinary teaching hospitals, and have greatly advanced noninvasive diagnostic capabilities.

Although there are many advantages to using alternative imaging techniques as opposed to conventional radiography, there are some disadvantages as well. Conventional radiography and alternative imaging techniques should be considered complementary procedures. Nevertheless, conventional radiographic procedures remain the first, and sometimes only, imaging techniques necessary, and are the focus of this Collection.

Although some of the articles contained in this text are several years old, the principles of radiographic interpretation have not undergone major changes and the information presented remains pertinent. It should be remembered, however, that alternative imaging techniques were not routinely used when some of these articles were published, and are not mentioned as adjunct procedures. For example, echocardiography has replaced cardiac catheterization to a great extent in the diagnosis of heart disease.

Techniques and interpretation of radiographic contrast procedures are covered in several articles. Intravenous urography, cystography, and upper gastrointestinal series are included. Even though endoscopy has reduced the need for many upper and lower gastrointestinal series, the procedure remains valuable in many situations and correct technique is essential. The same is true for cystography and intravenous urography; while abdominal ultrasound is invaluable in visualization of the kidneys, bladder, and prostate, contrast studies are necessary to determine qualitative renal function and to visualize the ureters and urethra. The articles on interpretation of avian radiographs are very helpful and are important because of the increasing number of avian patients seen both in private and referral practices.

The basics of radiology—including X-ray physics, radiation safety, and film processing—are described in several articles. The topic of radiation safety remains especially pertinent, as every effort should be made to minimize exposure for both personnel and patients. Many practices now have automatic film processors, but hand tanks are still in use, and correct techniques and maintenance are essential in the production of quality radiographs.

Finally, two articles on radiation therapy are included. This therapeutic modality is primarily available only at major veterinary institutions, but the information presented in these articles is useful to practitioners who may wish to refer patients for treatment.

The compilation is not meant to be an exhaustive volume on diagnostic radiology. Rather this text was organized to present a good overview of radiographic techniques and interpretation and serve as an excellent source of information for the veterinarian.

Martha Moon, DVM, MS
Diplomate, ACVR

CONTENTS

THORACIC RADIOLOGY

8 **Common Pitfalls in Radiographic Interpretation of the Thorax**
Cynthia P. Godshalk

15 **Radiologic Aspects of Thoracic Trauma in the Dog and Cat: Part I**
Lawrence J. Kleine

20 **Radiologic Aspects of Thoracic Trauma in the Dog and Cat: Part II**
Lawrence J. Kleine

24 **Radiographic Signs of Pulmonary Infiltration**
John W. Watters

31 **Radiographic Diagnosis of Metastatic Pulmonary Neoplasia**
Donald E. Thrall

41 **Bronchoesophageal Fistula in the Dog: Literature Survey, Case Presentations, and Radiographic Manifestations**
Richard D. Park

CARDIAC RADIOLOGY

48 **The Radiographic Diagnosis of Canine and Feline Heart Disease**
Peter F. Suter

62 **Evaluating Canine Cardiovascular Silhouettes: Radiographic Methods and Normal Radiographic Anatomy**
James P. Toombs, William R. Widmer, and Phillip N. Ogburn

ABDOMINAL RADIOLOGY

71 **Radiology of Acute Abdominal Disorders in the Dog and Cat: Part I**
Lawrence J. Kleine

76 **Radiology of Acute Abdominal Disorders in the Dog and Cat: Part II**
Lawrence J. Kleine

86 **The Role of Radiography in the Diagnosis of Intestinal Obstruction in Dogs and Cats**
Lawrence J. Kleine

UROGENITAL RADIOLOGY

94 **The Excretory Urogram: Part I—Techniques, Normal Radiographic Appearance, and Misinterpretation**
Donald A. Feeney, D.L. Barber, Gary R. Johnston, and Carl A. Osborne

100 **The Excretory Urogram: Part II—Interpretation of Abnormal Findings**
Donald A. Feeney, D.L. Barber, Gary R. Johnston, and Carl A. Osborne

109 **Retrograde Vaginocystography: A Contrast Study for Evaluation of Bitches with Urinary Incontinence**
Renee Leveille and Matthew A.O. Atilola

115 **Radiographic Aspects of Prostatic Disease in the Dog**
Donald E. Thrall

122 **Urethrography and Cystography in Cats: Part I—Techniques, Normal Radiographic Anatomy, and Artifacts**
Gary R. Johnston, Daniel A. Feeney, and Carl A. Osborne

135 **Urethrography and Cystography in Cats: Part II—Abnormal Radiographic Anatomy and Complications**
Gary R. Johnston, Daniel A. Feeney, and Carl A. Osborne

ORTHOPEDIC RADIOLOGY

151 **Diagnosis and Surgical Management of Osteochondritis Dissecans of the Elbow Joint**
J.L. Berzon

155 **Diagnosis of Common Developmental Orthopedic Conditions in Canine Pediatric Patients**
Daniel D. Lewis, Robert J. McCarthy, and Robert D. Pechman

166 **Canine Lumbosacral Diseases: Definitive Diagnosis, Treatment, and Prognosis**
Ross H. Palmer and Jonathan N. Chambers

176 **Acquired Dysplasias of the Canine Radius and Ulna**
Colin B. Carrig and Jeffrey A. Wortman

184 **Radiographic Diagnosis of Long Bone Neoplasms in the Dog**
Richard D. Park

AVIAN RADIOLOGY

190 **Radiographic Diagnosis of Avian Abdominal Disorders**
Marjorie C. McMillan

205 **Radiology of Avian Respiratory Diseases**
Marjorie C. McMillan

213 **Avian Gastrointestinal Radiography**
Marjorie C. McMillan

RADIATION THERAPY

219 **Recent Advances in Radiation Oncology**
Susan M. LaRue and Edward L. Gillette

226 **Veterinary Radiation Therapy**
W.M. Adams

TECHNIQUE, SAFETY, AND INTERPRETATION

237 **Radiation Biology and Radiation Safety**
William R. Widmer, H. Dan Cantwell, Stanley M. Shaw, Kimberly M. Vogel, Cheryl D. Hurd, Connie M. Han, and William E. Blevins

248 **Radiation Protection in Veterinary Hospitals**
John W. Watters

252 **X-ray Production**
John W. Watters

257 **The Radiographic Darkroom and Film Processing**
John W. Watters

264 **An Approach to Interpretation of Radiographs**
Sydney M. Evans

269 **Problems in Radiographic Interpretation: An Exercise Using Cases with Multiple Diagnoses**
Michael R. Metcalf and S.K. Kneller

277 **The Radiology of Aging: Its Clinical Applications**
C.S. Farrow

Common Pitfalls in Radiographic Interpretation of the Thorax

KEY FACTS

- Dorsal and rightward deviations of the trachea are often found in chondrodystrophic breeds when radiographs of the thorax are made with the neck of the patient in a flexed position.
- Older cats often appear to have a tortuous aorta and a heart with a more horizontally directed long axis on lateral radiographs.
- Barium may be used to help distinguish a nipple from a nodule on radiographs of the thorax.
- Pulmonary osteomas (small calcified opacities commonly seen in the pulmonary parenchyma of older dogs) may be mistaken for metastatic neoplastic nodules.
- The end-on view of the normal right pulmonary artery, seen in some radiographs of laterally recumbent dogs, may be confused with hilar lymphadenopathy.

North Carolina State University
Cynthia P. Godshalk, DVM, MS

Many common mistakes, or traps, are made during radiograph interpretation. A trap may be general, such as the tendency to look at only parts of the film that are considered pertinent to the animal's history, while an incidental but important abnormality on another area of the film is overlooked. During these situations, the viewer has a preconception of what to expect and stops evaluating the film once the sought-after lesion is discovered. Other traps are more specific, such as misdiagnosis of a favorite disease or misinterpretation of certain normal structures as abnormal due to breed or physiologic variation.

This article presents examples of normal variations in radiographs of the thorax mistakenly believed to represent disease. The reader can assume that the films are of diagnostic quality. Processing errors and radiographic artifacts are not discussed.

DORSAL AND RIGHTWARD DEVIATION OF THE CRANIAL THORACIC TRACHEA

There is some redundancy in the trachea of normal dogs that allows for flexibility when the neck is extended and flexed. If the head and neck of a dog are flexed during a lateral radiograph, the trachea tends to deviate dorsally in the cranial thorax, creating a bowed appearance[1] (Figure 1*A*). This deviation is often misinterpreted as being indicative of a mass in the cranioventral mediastinum[2,3] or a heart-base tumor. Dorsal deviation of the trachea due to mediastinal masses or tumors of the base of the heart is typically accompanied by increased soft-tissue opacity ventral to the trachea. If increased soft-tissue opacity is not visible, dorsal deviation of the trachea is assumed to be normal. In addition, repeating the radiograph with correct positioning of the head and neck should alleviate the dorsal tracheal deviation in normal dogs (Figure 1*B*).

The trachea may also deviate toward the right side of the cranial thorax at the thoracic inlet on a ventrodorsal radiograph of a normal animal,[3] particularly in brachycephalic and chondrodystrophic breeds[4] (Figure 2); leftward

Originally published in Volume 16, Number 6, June 1994

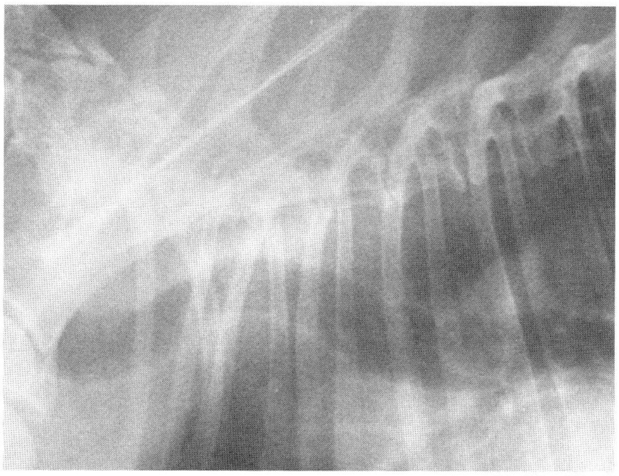

Figure 1A

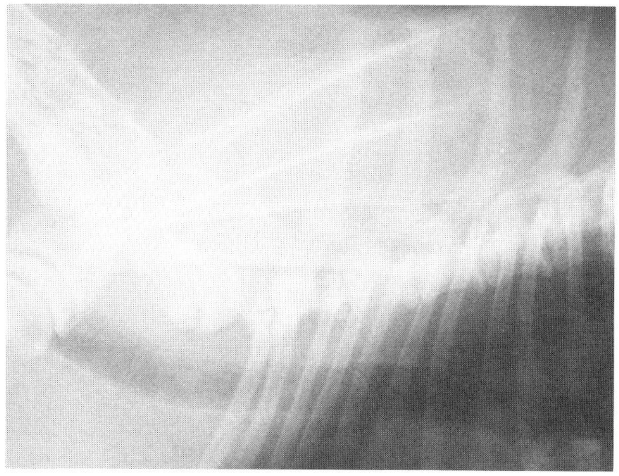

Figure 1B

Figure 1—Lateral radiograph of a toy poodle. (**A**) The head and neck are flexed, resulting in dorsal bowing of the intrathoracic trachea. (**B**) The same dog with head and neck extended; dorsal bowing of the trachea is no longer present.

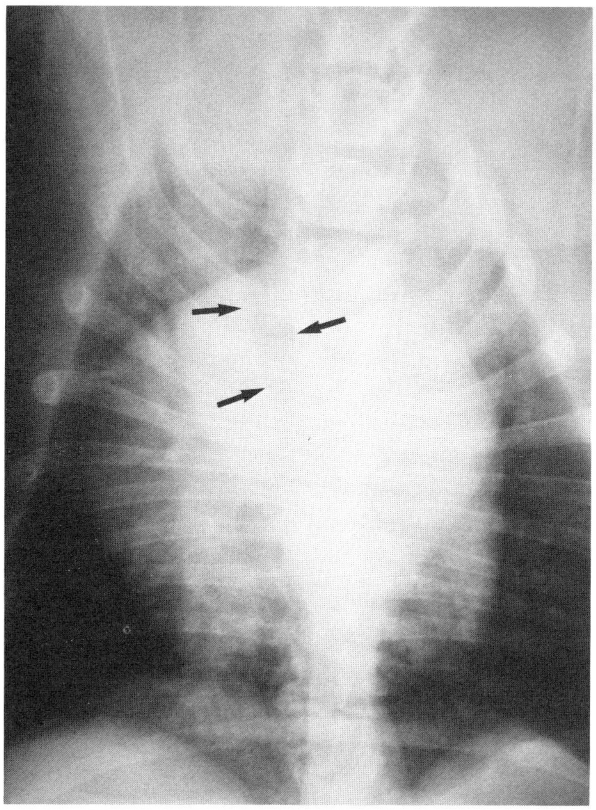

Figure 2—Ventrodorsal radiograph of a brachycephalic dog showing rightward displacement of the trachea *(arrows).*

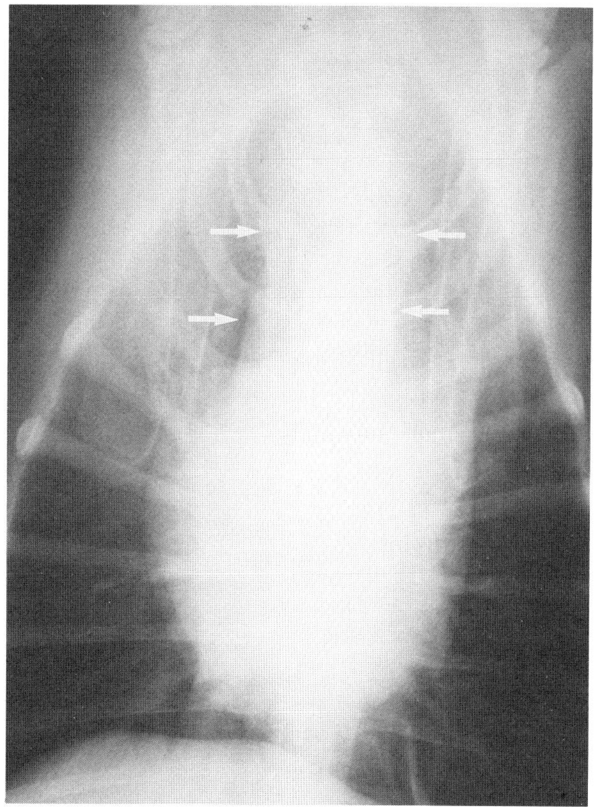

Figure 3—Ventrodorsal radiograph of an obese dog with apparent cardiomegaly and a widened mediastinum caused by fat *(arrows).*

deviation is typically prevented by the aortic arch.[3] Rightward deviation of the trachea is also affected by the position of the neck[1] and by the presence of fat within the mediastinum. There typically is not enough fat to delineate the soft-tissue structures normally present in the cranial mediastinum, even in obese dogs. Therefore, the radiopacities of fat and soft-tissue structures appear the same,[4] thereby making it difficult to tell whether rightward deviation of the trachea in obese patients is caused by a mediastinal mass or fat. In addition to causing tracheal deviation, fat will result in a widened cranial mediastinum (Figure 3), which is sometimes mistaken for an abnormality (e.g., enlarged mediastinal lymph nodes).

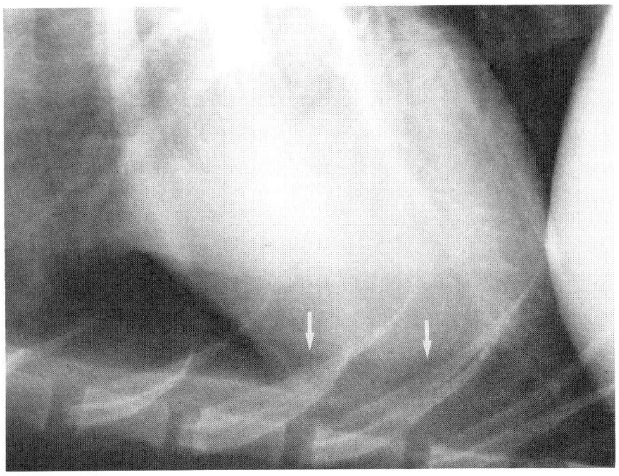

Figure 4A

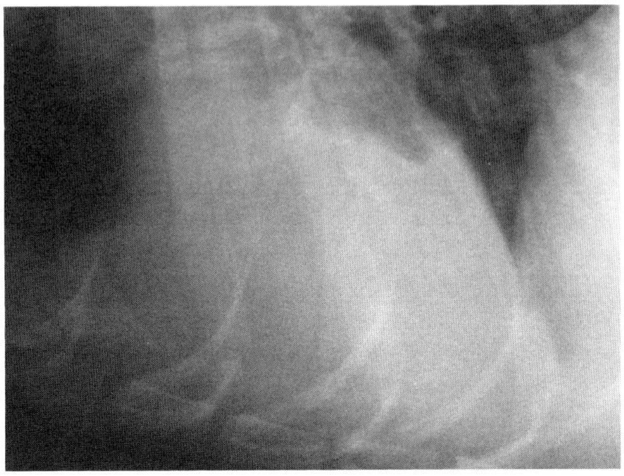

Figure 4B

Figure 4—Lateral radiographs of two dogs. (**A**) The same dog as in Figure 3 with pleural fat delineating the ventral heart border *(arrows)*. (**B**) A dog with pleural effusion obscuring the ventral heart border. The curved contour that mimics the cranial heart margin represents the ventral aspect of the lung which is less dense than the surrounding pleural fluid.

Fat, however, typically results in uniform widening of the mediastinum, whereas mediastinal masses often result in asymmetric mediastinal enlargement.

CARDIOMEGALY VERSUS OBESITY

The silhouette of the heart visible on a radiograph includes the pericardium and the major vessels of the heart.[3] Because obese animals tend to have fat in many body cavities, including the mediastinum and pericardium, fat within the sternopericardiac ligament may be visualized ventral to the heart and dorsal to the sternum on a lateral-view radiograph.[3] On a ventrodorsal or dorsoventral view, however, the fat in the sternopericardiac ligament, in addition to that in the pericardium and mediastinum, is difficult to distinguish from the heart itself. It is easy, therefore, to misdiagnose cardiomegaly in an obese animal (Figure 3). The lateral-view radiograph may be helpful in assessing the amount of fat present ventral to the heart (Figure 4*A*); however, an accurate evaluation of cardiac size may require an echocardiogram.

PLEURAL "FLUID" IN OBESE DOGS

Obese dogs also tend to have fat in the subpleural space lining the thoracic wall,[3] which causes retraction of lung lobes and a scalloped appearance of ventral lung borders, similar to that seen with pleural fluid. As mentioned previously, a large, sternal fat pad may also be visible dorsal to the sternum on a lateral- view radiograph.[3] This suprasternal fat appears ventrally to the ventral borders of the lungs[3] and can be distinguished from fluid by close evaluation of the interface with the heart. If fat is present, the radiopaque ventral heart border should be visible (Figure 4*A*). If fluid is present in the pleural cavity, the ventral heart border will silhouette with the fluid. It will not be visible because the soft-tissue ventral heart border and fluid are of equal radiopacities (Figure 4*B*). On a ventrodorsal radiograph, the sternal fat pad may also be misinterpreted as pleural effusion or alveolar lung disease affecting the right middle lobe in dogs and cats.[3]

PROLONGED RECUMBENCY VERSUS LUNG DISEASE

Prolonged lateral recumbency typically results in hypostatic congestion of the dependent lung. This condition is common in animals that are old or infirm and occurs almost immediately after they are placed under general anesthesia.[3,4] Radiographs of the thorax made while animals are under general anesthesia result in the appearance of a generalized, unstructured interstitial or alveolar pattern that is more severe in the dependent lung (Figure 5*A* and *B*). If animals are not anesthetized (Figure 5*C* and *D*), the impression may not appear. This is true regardless of the length of time under anesthesia, but the changes seem to become more severe as time increases. In addition to creating a pathologic appearance, the increased opacity in the lung may mask actual pathologic changes.[5] For these reasons, sedation is preferable to general anesthesia for thoracic radiography of animals. If general anesthesia is required, the lungs of the patient should be inflated several times before exposures are taken.[5]

LAZY HEARTS AND TORTUOUS AORTAS IN OLDER CATS

For reasons not clearly understood, the heart of an aging cat commonly assumes a more horizontal position on lateral radiographs. In addition, the aorta

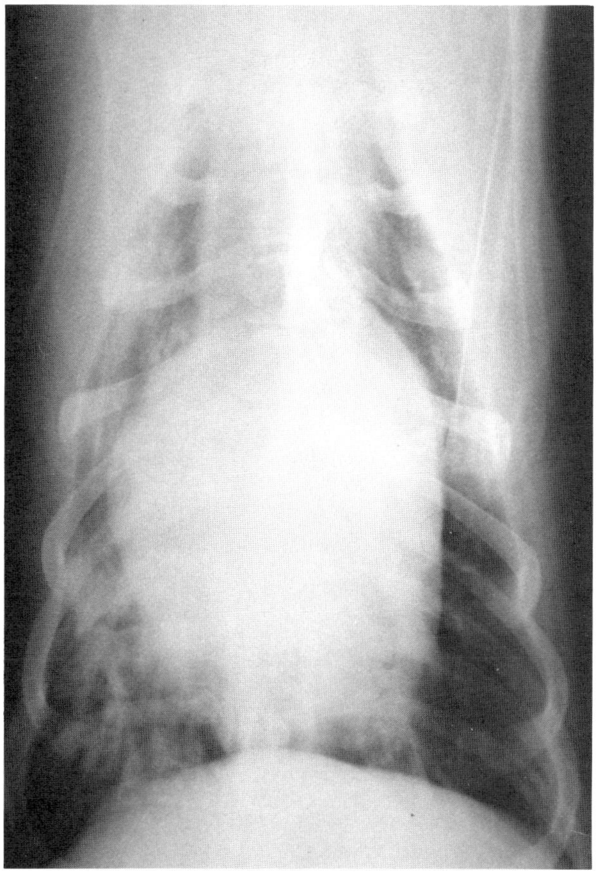

Figure 5A

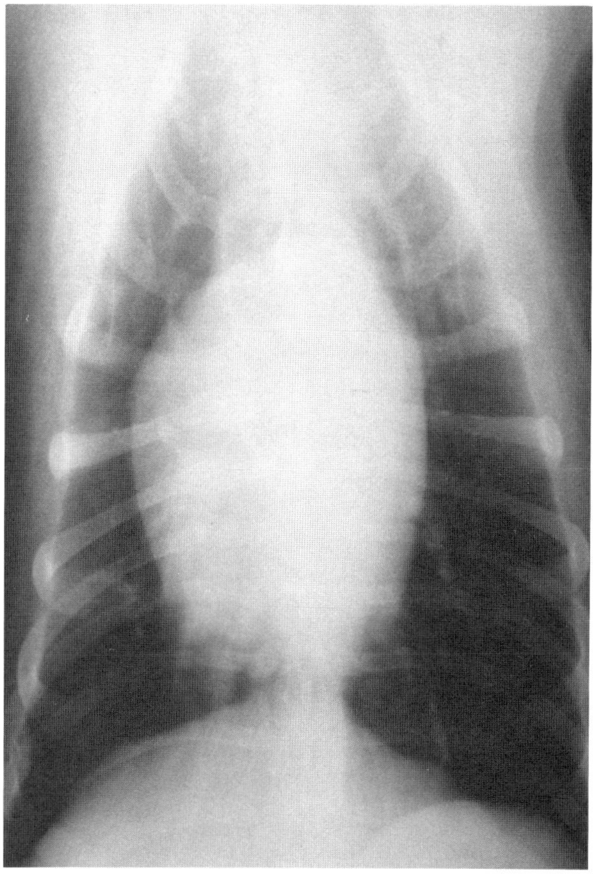

Figure 5C

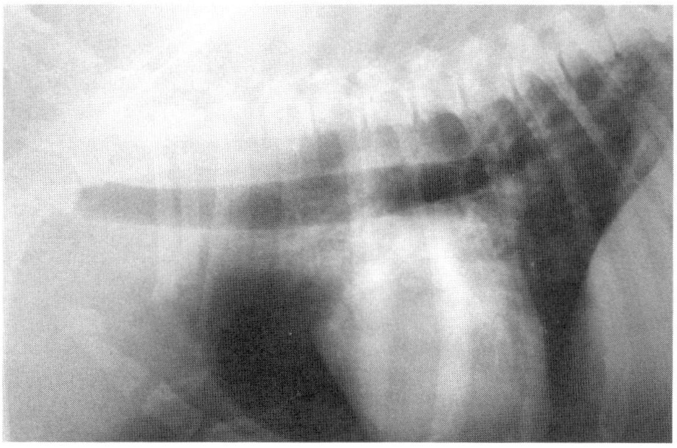

Figure 5B

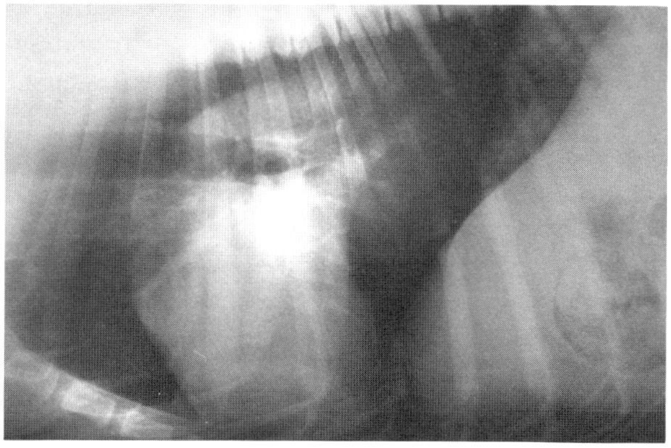

Figure 5D

Figure 5—(**A**) Ventrodorsal and (**B**) lateral radiographs made of an anesthetized dog showing patchy areas of alveolar lung disease in the right lung lobes. (**C**) Ventrodorsal and (**D**) lateral radiographs made of the same dog the day after it was anesthetized. Healing fractures of the proximal aspects of the right 5th, 6th, and 7th ribs as well as the distal aspect of the right 8th rib are visualized. The cardiac silhouette is slightly larger than in *A* and *B* because of resolution of prior hypotension.

may appear very tortuous with a prominent ventral deviation in the mid-thorax (Figure 6*A*). The combination of these two images gives the appearance of a prominent aortic knob on the ventrodorsal radiograph, which may mistakenly be interpreted as abnormal (Figure 6*B*).

NIPPLES OR NODULES?

Nipples may be misdiagnosed as masses in the lung parenchyma, appearing as dense, well-circumscribed nodules that mimic metastatic tumor nodules. Nipples, however, are more often bilaterally symmetric. Misinterpretation of nipples as abnormal structures

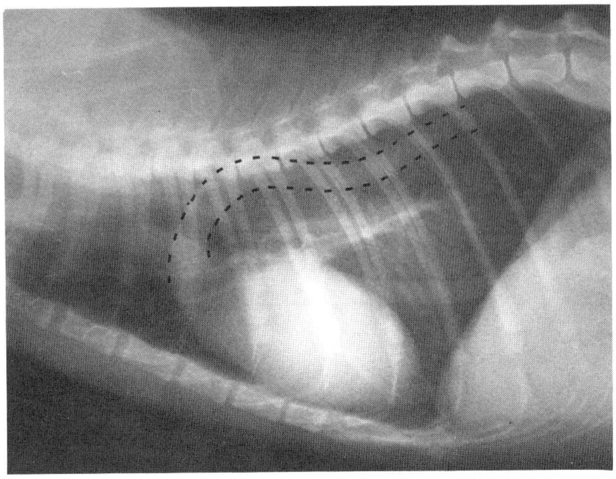

Figure 6A

Figure 6—(**A**) Lateral radiograph of a 17-year-old cat showing a near-horizontal cardiac long axis and a tortuous aorta *(dashed lines).* (**B**) Ventrodorsal radiograph of the same cat showing an aortic knob *(arrows).*

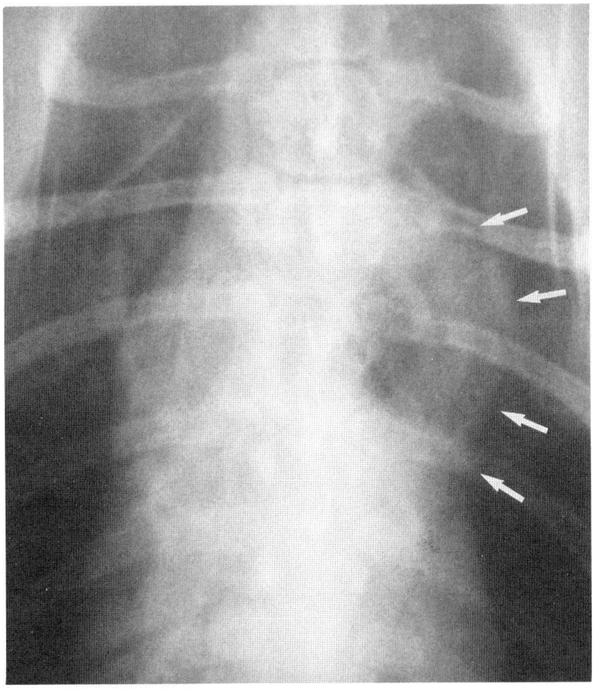

Figure 6B

readily occurs if they are unusually shaped or pendulous. Nipples that are often misdiagnosed as nodules seem to appear in the lung on ventrodorsal radiographs (Figure 7*A*) and on the ventral skin surface on lateral radiographs (Figure 7*B*). To avoid misdiagnosis, a comparison can be made between the location of the mass in question on the radiograph and the location of the nipples on the patient. If results are inconclusive, a small amount of barium may be applied to any nipple in the region of the suspected "nodule" (Figure 7*C*). Subsequent radiographs may then be used to compare the location of the barium-coated nipples to the questionable "nodule."

PULMONARY OSTEOMAS

Multiple, small (2 to 3 mm), irregularly shaped bone radiopacities in lung parenchyma called pulmonary osteomas are often seen in normal, older dogs[6] (Figure 8). The cause of pulmonary osteomas is unknown.[3] Although such osteomas may be seen in any breed, they are most prominent in collies. Pulmonary osteomas may be confused with metastatic neoplastic disease; however, metastatic neoplastic nodules are typically more circumscribed, more variably sized, and generally of soft-tissue rather than bone opacity. Pulmonary osteomas may also mimic the appearance of calcified nodules associated with a previously healed pulmonary fungal infection.[3]

HILAR LYMPHADENOPATHY OR RIGHT MAIN PULMONARY ARTERY?

Radiographs of the thorax made with animals in right lateral recumbency sometimes contain an end-on view of the right pulmonary artery that appears as a round or oval soft-tissue structure ventral to the carina[3] (Figure 9*A*). This structure is normal and is sometimes confused with hilar lymphadenopathy. Enlarged hilar lymph nodes that result from pulmonary or pleural infection or neoplasia generally appear on radiographs as an ill-defined increased opacity, primarily dorsal to the carina and ventrally depressing the caudal trachea (Figure 9*B*). The normal, right pulmonary artery, however, appears well defined as a result of its interface with the surrounding air-filled lung.

CONCLUSION

Perhaps the most important goal of this review is not to list common mistakes, but to aid the practitioner in recognizing when a mistake is being made. The following guidelines may be helpful to determine whether a structure on a radiograph of the thorax is a normal anatomic variant or a true lesion.

1. Attempt to locate the suspected abnormality on more than one view. Accomplishing this may require additional radiographs with the animal in opposite lateral recumbency. In addition, a dorsoventral and a ventrodorsal radiograph may determine whether the abnormality in question appears more than once. The use of a horizontally rather than a vertically directed x-ray beam may also be useful to determine whether the sus-

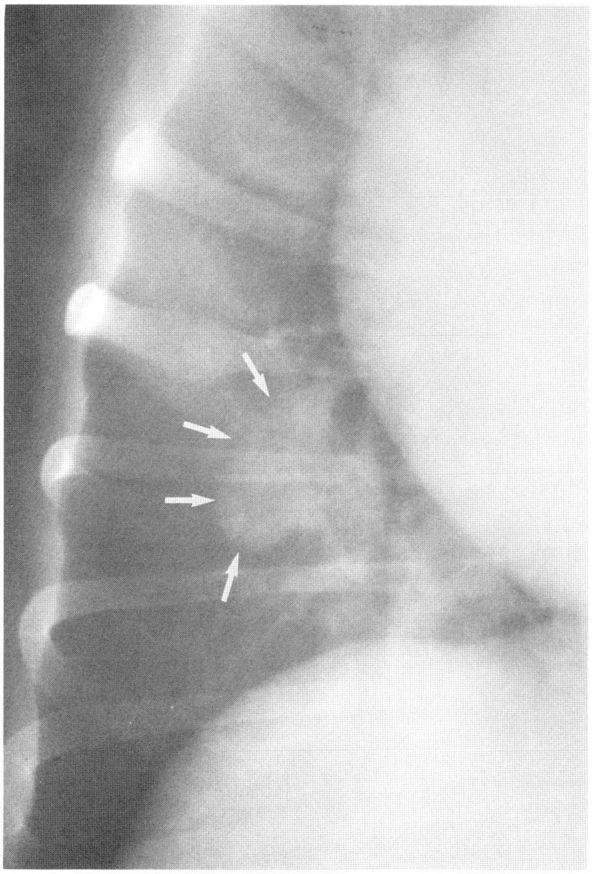

Figure 7A

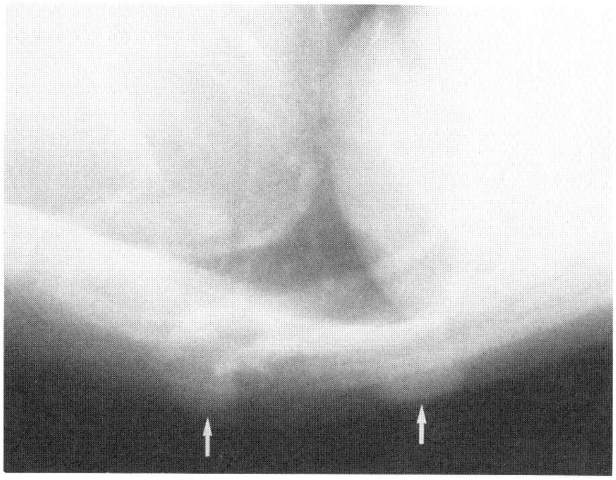

Figure 7B

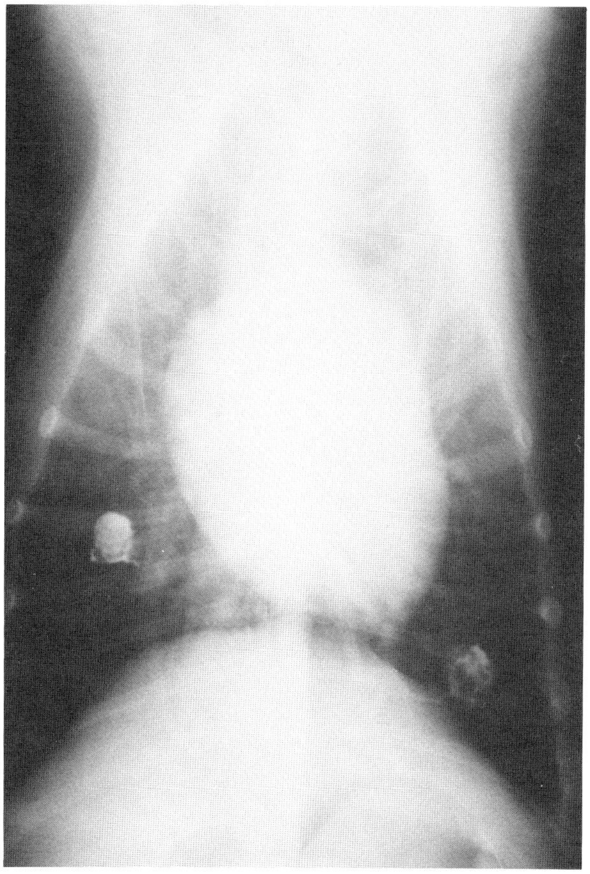

Figure 7C

Figure 7—(**A**) Ventrodorsal radiograph of a dog with a prominent nipple *(arrows)* superimposed over the lung. A healing fracture of the right 6th rib is an incidental finding. (**B**) Lateral radiograph of the same dog showing nipples on the ventral skin surface *(arrows)*. (**C**) Ventrodorsal radiograph of the same dog after barium was applied to the surface of the nipple shown in Figure 7*A*.

pected abnormality responds to the effects of gravity.

2. Compare the radiograph of the questionable abnormality with a radiograph of the same area made on another animal or to a picture of a similar radiograph in a reference text.[7] If the structure in question appears on similar radiographs of other normal animals, it is probably normal.
3. Determine the composition of the questionable structure by comparing its radiopacity to known structures in the same area on the film. Structures are visible on radiographs because of interfaces between the five basic radiopacities: metal, bone, soft tissue and fluid, fat, and air. The cranial surface of the diaphragm is visible because it is a soft-tissue structure adjacent to an air-filled lung. The caudal diaphragmatic surface cannot be seen because it is silhouetted against the liver, which is also soft-tissue radiopaque. Determining the radiopacity of the unknown structure is essential for its identification.
4. Try to trace all radiographic borders of the structure in question to determine whether it is an artifact created by overlapping of normal structures.
5. If all other methods of analysis are exhausted and the origin or existence of the structure is still unknown, wait a period and repeat the radiographic

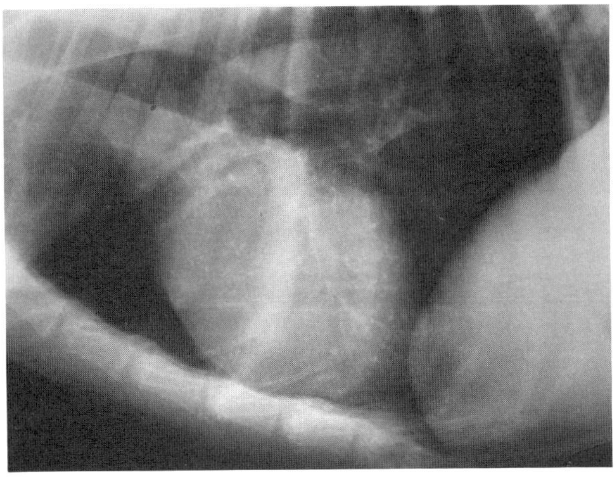

Figure 8A

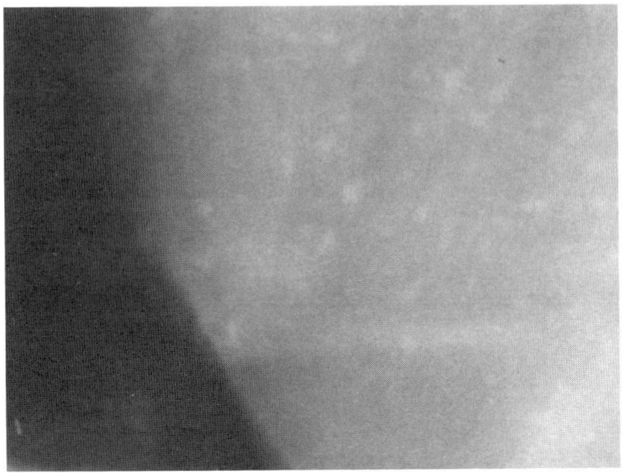

Figure 8B

Figure 8—(**A**) Lateral and (**B**) same-view closeup radiograph of a Great Dane with multiple calcified nodules in the pulmonary parenchyma that are typical of pulmonary osteomas.

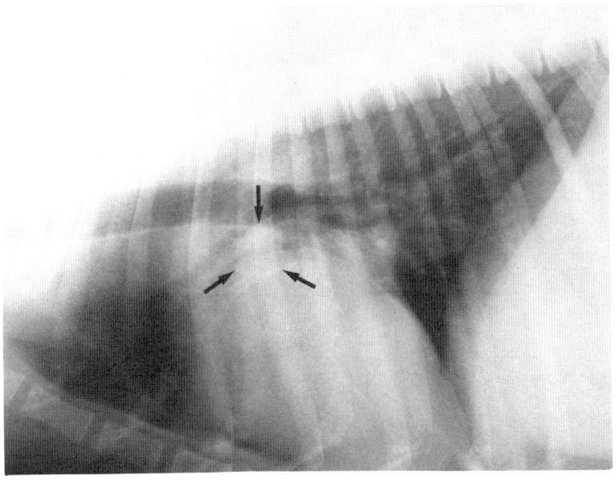

Figure 9A

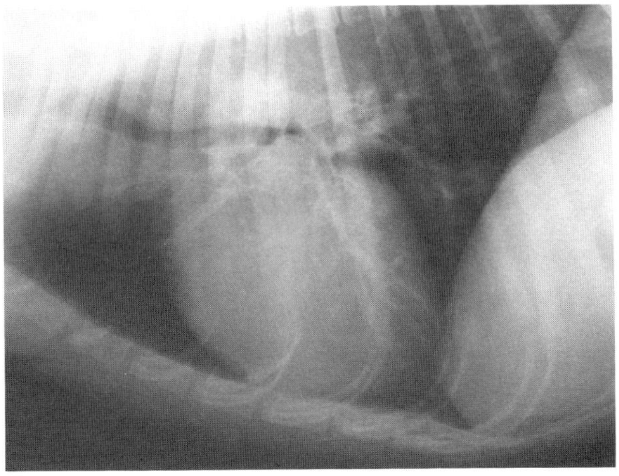

Figure 9B

Figure 9—(**A**) Right lateral recumbent radiograph of a normal English setter showing an end-on view of the right pulmonary artery *(arrows)*. (**B**) Left lateral recumbent radiograph of an English setter with hilar lymphadenopathy showing an increased soft-tissue radiopacity dorsal to the carina as well as ventral depression and compression of the trachea.

procedures. Abnormal or clinically significant structures will often change appearance in time.

ACKNOWLEDGMENT

The author thanks Mr. Dave Adams for production of the figures.

About the Author

When this article was submitted, Dr. Godshalk, who is a Diplomate of the American College of Veterinary Radiology, was affiliated with the Department of Veterinary Clinical Sciences, College of Veterinary Medicine, Kansas State University, Manhattan, Kansas. She is presently affiliated with the Department of Anatomy, Physiological Science, and Radiology, College of Veterinary Medicine, North Carolina State University, Raleigh, North Carolina.

REFERENCES

1. Burk RL, Ackerman N: *Small Animal Radiology: A Diagnostic Atlas and Text.* New York, Churchill Livingston, 1986.
2. Kneller SK: The larynx, pharynx, and trachea, in Thrall DE (ed): *Textbook of Veterinary Diagnostic Radiology.* Philadelphia, WB Saunders Co, 1986, pp 210–216.
3. Suter PF: *Thoracic Radiography: A Text Atlas of Thoracic Diseases of the Dog and Cat.* Wettswil, Switzerland, PF Suter, 1984.
4. Mitten RW: Radiology of mediastinal diseases. *Vet Clin North Am Small Anim Prac* 12(2):193–212, 1982.
5. Watters JW: The lungs, in Thrall DE (ed): *Textbook of Veterinary Diagnostic Radiology.* Philadelphia, WB Saunders Co, 1986, pp 306–317.
6. Reif JS, Rhodes WH: The lungs of aged dogs: A radiographic-morphologic correlation. *J Am Vet Rad Soc* 7:5–11, 1966.
7. Schebitz H, Wilkens H: *Atlas of Radiographic Anatomy of the Dog and Cat.* Philadelphia, WB Saunders Co, 1978.

Radiologic Aspects of Thoracic Trauma in the Dog and Cat (Part I)

Lawrence J. Kleine, DVM, MS
Associate Professor and Head, Radiology
Tufts University
School of Veterinary Medicine
North Grafton, Massachusetts

Radiology is an important diagnostic tool in the evaluation of thoracic trauma in dogs and cats. It is rapid, nontraumatic and usually easily interpreted. Furthermore, the radiographs form a permanent record which may be used as a basis for checking progress.

Each year about 400 cases of thoracic trauma (1% of all admissions) are seen in our urban practice. Ten percent of these cases die or are euthanatized because of their injuries. Often other major injuries, such as fractures, accompany thoracic trauma. The relative importance of each of the multiple injuries of each individual is determined by an intelligent clinical appraisal, solving the most urgent problem first, followed by the others in a logical sequence. Treatment of life-threatening conditions must take precedence over any diagnostic test. However, treatment can often be undertaken simultaneously with radiography, physical examination and laboratory tests. Gentleness and efficiency are essential in making an accurate and rapid diagnosis.

The basic roentgen signs of thoracic trauma are alterations in density, size, location, shape, and the margin of structures normally located in the thorax, as well as the presence of structures in the thorax which are normally located elsewhere. Decreased radiographic opacity occurs secondary to the presence of air in the subcutaneous tissues or in the pleural, pericardial, or mediastinal spaces. Abnormal soft tissue opacity may occur in the subcutaneous tissues, pleural cavity, or mediastinum due to fluid accumulation.

Atelectasis, edema, or hemorrhage causes increased lung opacity. Intrapericardial fluid will produce a large cardiac silhouette, while the size of the heart may be smaller when there is reduced circulating blood volume. Pulmonary arteries may increase in size proximal to an area of arterial embolism or thrombosis but are generally less prominent in shock.

Technique—Conventional survey radiographs made in the lateral and ventrodorsal or dorsoventral positions are frequently the most accurate and useful diagnostic procedures in thoracic trauma. The standard KVP and MAS x-ray settings for thoracic radiography are used in the initial examination. If a small amount of fluid is present in the lung or pleural cavity, a second radiograph at twice the usual MAS

Originally published in Volume 1, Number 3, March 1979

will provide better visualization of thoracic morphology. If a significant amount of the pleural cavity is obliterated by fluid, thoracocentesis should be performed before repeating the radiographs. Better visualization of pneumothorax can be achieved by reducing the MAS to half its usual value. The exposure time of thoracic radiographs should not exceed 1/30th of a second to eliminate unsharpness resulting from cardiac and respiratory motion. Ventrodorsal oblique radiographs demonstrate some rib fractures and esophageal perforations better than conventionally positioned films (Fig 1).

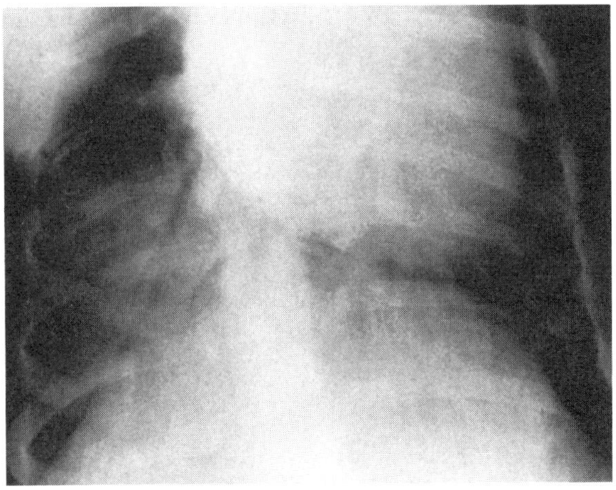

Fig 1—Ventrodorsal oblique radiographs are useful in demonstrating rib fractures because the fractures are displayed over the less dense peripheral lung fields. Fractures of the 7th through 10th right ribs are seen in this dog.

In addition to survey radiographs made with a vertical x-ray beam, certain radiographic aids are available. These include horizontal beam radiography, pleurography and fistulography. Horizontal beam radiography with changes in the animal's posture may be useful in demonstrating whether a density is liquid or solid. For instance, a dog or cat might be placed in sternal, then dorsal recumbency position using a horizontal x-ray beam to make radiographs in each position. Fluid in the pleural cavity is seen in the ventral portion of the thorax in the sternal position and in the dorsal thorax in dorsal recumbency. This technique can also be used to detect small amounts of gas in the pleural cavity. Free gas will always rise to the highest part of the cavity and free fluid will fall to the lowest part. When effusion fills more than about 25% of the pleural cavity, horizontal beam radiography, following withdrawal of fluid, will usually permit better visualization of thoracic viscera.

Contrast Pleurography—Contrast pleurography is not often needed but may occasionally be helpful in delineating pleural and diaphragmatic silhouettes when a diaphragmatic hernia is suspected but cannot be confirmed by noncontrast radiography. A local anesthetic is instilled into the dorsal part of the 7th or 8th interspace, and a short needle is used to enter the pleural space. The needle is aspirated to be sure lung parenchyma has not been punctured. (This test is difficult to evaluate if pneumothorax is present, as air can be aspirated from the pleural space as well as from lung parenchyma.) About one ml of aqueous contrast medium per kg of body weight is instilled (a concentration of about 300 mg of iodine per ml of solution is satisfactory). The animal is then rotated 360° several times to distribute the contrast medium throughout the pleural space. Conventional ventrodorsal and lateral radiographs are made. The coating produced by the procedure outlines the pleural space, defining the otherwise homogenous abdominal viscera which may have herniated into the thoracic cavity. In some cases the contrast medium also enters the abdominal cavity through the diaphragmatic opening.

Fistulography—Fistulography is performed to locate the origin of sinus tracts and to visualize nonopaque foreign bodies which have produced fistulae to the skin. A flexible end-hole catheter whose diameter is large enough to occlude the external opening of the fistula is selected. The catheter is inserted deeply into the tract and viscous contrast medium is injected.[a] Ventrodorsal and lateral radiographs are made as soon as backflow of contrast medium out of the tract is seen. The procedure is not generally useful if there are multiple, large skin openings which cannot be occluded, but discrete tracts which lead to a definitive focus can be effectively outlined.

Esophagram—If an esophagram is needed to evaluate potential perforation, an oily contrast medium intended for bronchographic use is preferred. This medium is considered safer than either barium or the water soluble organic iodides intended for gastrointestinal use, in the event that an esophageal pulmonary fistula is present.[1,4] Water soluble organic iodides are not used because they do not provide satisfactory mucosal coating. Recognition of erosions and ulcerations of the mucosa is important in rendering an accurate prognosis when an esophageal foreign body or other type of perforation is present.

Thoracic Cage—Lesions of the bone and soft tissue of the thoracic cage are usually easily seen and interpreted. However, attention may be drawn to the intrathoracic injury, and damage to the supporting structure may be overlooked. A careful, systematic observation is needed in every case to avoid this common error (Fig 2).

Fractures and dislocations of ribs, and fractures of dorsal spinous processes and scapulae without displacement, can often be treated conservatively, however they should be recognized as significant injuries and a source of pain to the animal. Rib fracture fragments sometimes penetrate either the lung or subcutaneous tissues and skin of the

[a]Author's note: Aqueous iodide media can be mixed with KY jelly. However, preferred products are Hypaque 90 (Winthrop Laboratories, New York, NY) or Dionosil (Glaxo).

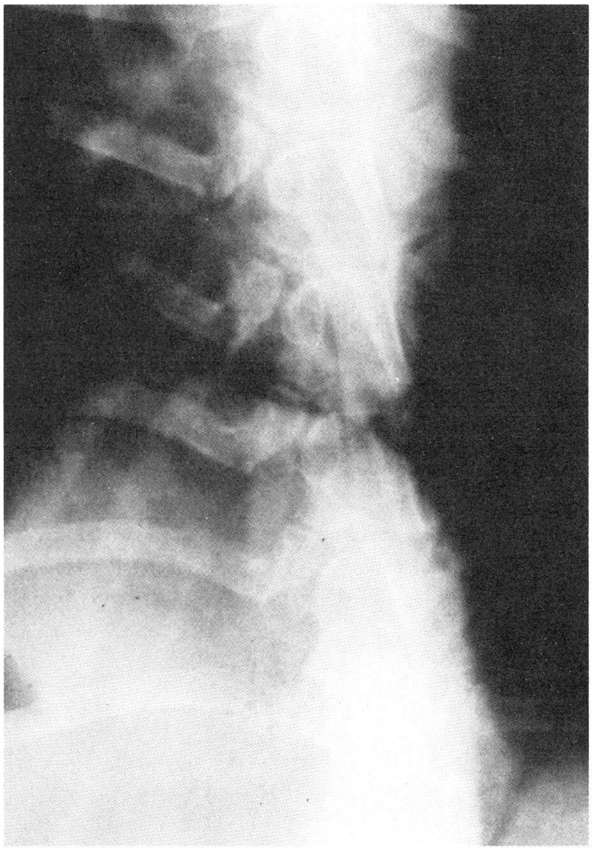

Fig 2—A ventrodorsal radiograph was taken of this dog because the clinician suspected spinal trauma. Fractures of the 7th through 11th right ribs are seen near the costo-vertebral articulation.

thorax resulting in hemo-pneumothorax which must be treated surgically.

When there are multiple segmental rib fractures, a flail chest may develop.[b] This injury is usually a surgical emergency because of the serious degree of pulmonary insufficiency which results. Fractures of the scapulae are seldom seen clearly in thoracic radiographs but are easily diagnosed by a combination of palpation and radiography of the specific area. Sternebrae and vertebral bodies can be dislocated as well as fractured. Pain and swelling are usually the only clinical signs associated with sternebral dislocation; however, sternebral fractures or dislocations may be displaced with enough violence to rupture the internal thoracic vessels causing substantial hemorrhage (Fig 3).

Fractures and dislocations of the thoracic vertebrae are significant findings indicating the need for thorough and sometimes repeated neurologic examination. An accurate prognosis can seldom be based on the radiographic findings alone. Neurological data are generally much more valuable.

[b]Editor's note: A flail chest develops when the chest wall is so mobile because of rib fractures, that it moves in a paradoxical fashion on respiration, i.e. the mobile segment moves in on inspiration.

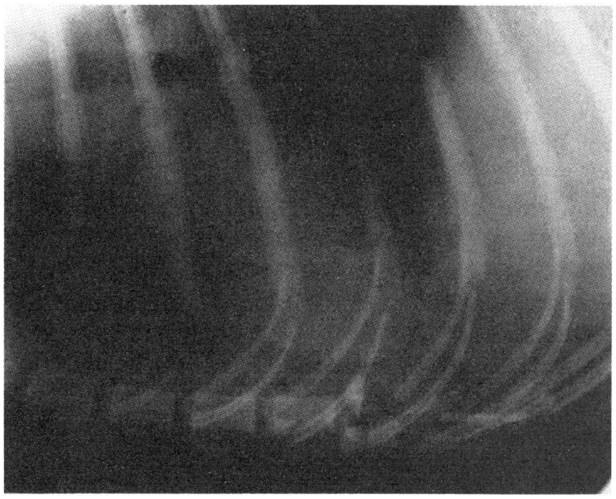

Fig 3—This dog had sternal pain after a fall of 15 feet. There is ventral displacement and fragmentation of the 7th sternebra. Density in the ventral caudal thorax is due to pleural hemorrhage.

The subcutaneous tissues of the thorax should be scrutinized for evidence of changes in opacity. In the case of breaks in the skin, air may be seen at the site of the puncture, and small amounts of air are often inadvertently introduced by subcutaneous fluid administration. When the cervical trachea is perforated or a large penetrating wound is created in the loose cervical soft tissues, dissecting emphysema may extend into the mediastinum and over the entire body (Fig 4).

Subcutaneous hemorrhage is recognizable as a swelling which has the radiographic opacity of soft tissue, and is most often associated with rib fractures. Teeth, knife fragments, and shotgun pellets are some of the opaque foreign bodies which can be seen in the thoracic cavity or soft tissues surrounding the thorax. Foreign bodies such as wood splinters or plastic which are usually radiolucent can sometimes be seen if they are surrounded by air. More often, however, fistulography is needed.

Intercostal hernia often appears as a uniform soft tissue density outside of and parallel to the rib cage, because the herniated viscus is usually omental or mesenteric fat. If the hernia contains small intestine or colon gas shadows should be seen.

Thoracic Cavity—Radiographic signs of thoracic trauma may be reflected in the pleural cavity by air or fluid accumulation in the pleural or mediastinal spaces. Pneumothorax is commonly seen following thoracic trauma and is often accompanied by pulmonary and pleural hemorrhage. Radiographic recognition of pneumothorax is easiest in the conventional lateral view. When the dog or cat lies on its side, air in the thoracic cavity rises to the highest point. In so doing, the heart and unexpanded lungs are displaced downward. This phenomenon separates the heart from the sternum so that air is seen ventral to the cardiac silhouette.

In the ventrodorsal view small amounts of air will rise to occupy the retrosternal area without

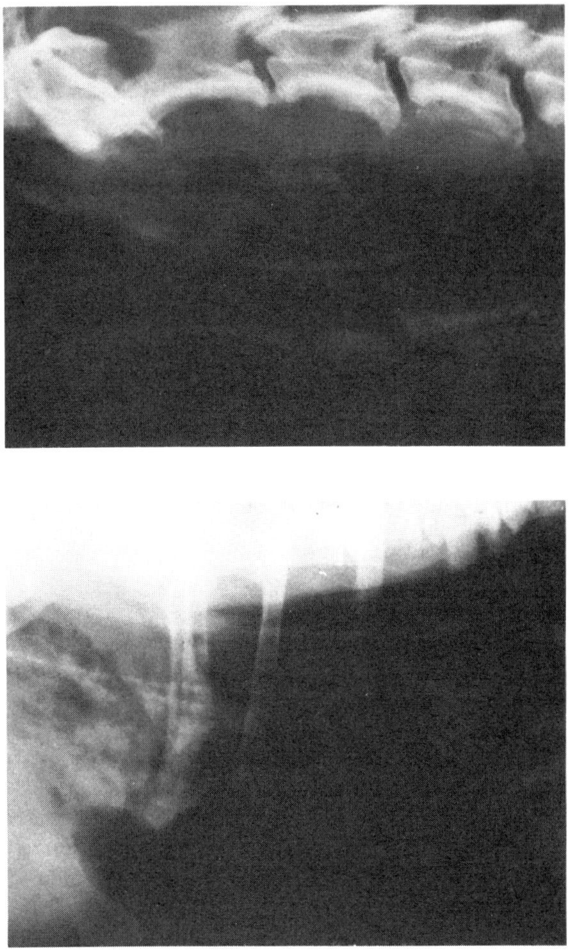

Fig 4A, B—The ventral trachea was torn by a bite wound resulting in separation of the tracheal rings and extensive subcutaneous and mediastinal emphysema in this dog.

being seen in the peripheral lung fields. In the horizontal beam lateral view air rises to the dorsal part of the thoracic cavity depressing the dorsal portion of the lungs. When a small amount of pneumothorax is suspected, a high intensity light may be useful to examine the areas of the lung for peripheral pulmonary vessels. If vessels can be identified in the peripheral lung fields, and the lungs are normally expanded, pneumothorax is probably not present. When the lungs are atelectatic because of elevated intrathoracic pressure, the visceral pleural surfaces are often seen more clearly than usual because of the air surrounding the lung and the outlining of the pleura which results.

Generally pneumothorax is a self-limiting process. The elevated intrathoracic pressure produces a tamponade effect. When the air leak has sealed, pneumothorax is dramatically reduced within 72 hours. The source of pneumothorax is seldom identifiable at the time of injury. Ordinarily the mediastinum in the dog and cat does not prevent the free passage of air from one side of the thorax to the other; therefore, unilateral pneumothorax is rarely seen.

Pneumomediastinum—Pneumomediastinum can occur secondary to a penetrating wound at the thoracic inlet, tracheal penetration due to trauma, (Fig 5) or instrumentation or dissection of air through the anatomical openings in the diaphragm, when extensive pneumoretroperitoneum is present[1]. Pneumomediastinum is recognized radiographically by clear outlining of mediastinal structures which are not usually seen, such as the esophagus, brachiocephalic, left subclavian and azygos vessels. Pneumomediastinum is seldom associated with any clinical signs and when the air leak is eliminated, the lesion usually resolves in 48 to 72 hours.

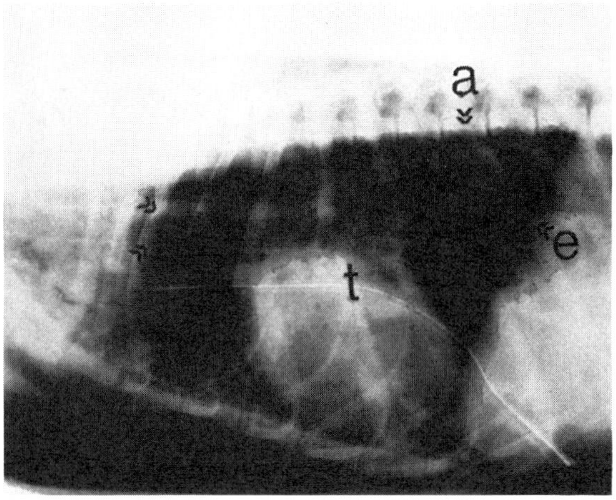

Fig 5—The recognition of pneumomediastinum depends upon visualization of both walls of the trachea (arrows), the aorta (A), and the esophagus (E). Occasionally the azygos vein is also seen. A thoracic drain tube (T) has been used to remove pleural hemorrhage.

Pleural effusion, regardless of its cause, is recognized radiographically by increased opacity and widening of the pleural space. When the effusion is slight, the only radiographic signs may be increased visualization of interlobar fissures and the rounding of the lung margin in the costophrenic angle in the ventrodorsal view. These minor changes are best seen when the radiograph is exposed on expiration. In the conventional lateral thoracic radiograph, fluid will flow to the lowest part of the thorax, obscuring the lung fields in this area.

The fluid will generally be seen dorsal to the caudal lung lobes in this view. When an x-ray film is exposed with the horizontal beam, the dorsal margin of the fluid level generally has a scalloped appearance unless pneumothorax is also present, in which case the fluid level will be horizontal and even. Plueral blood, bile, transudate and exudate can usually not be distinguished from one another on the basis of their radiographic appearance.

Cranial mediastinal hemorrhage often occurs

[1] Editor's note: Two additional causes of pneumomediastinum are perforation of the esophagus and the escape of intrapulmonary air dissecting along bronchi into the mediastinum.

along with pulmonary and pleural hemorrhage. Occasionally, however, hemorrhage or effusion is the only indication of thoracic injury and may be due to either blunt trauma or penetration of the esophagus near the heart base. Radiographic findings in either case are widening and increased density in the cranial mediastinum, blending with and obsuring the cranial aspect of the cardiac silhouette. Both pleural and mediastinal hemorrhage may mimic masses and other effusions. Therefore, thoracocentesis is often needed for definitive diagnosis.

REFERENCES

1. Chiu, C.L. and Gambach, R.R.: Hypaque Pulmonary Edema: A case report. Radiology, 111 (1974); 91-92.
2. Genereux, G.P.: The End-Stage Lung. Radiology, 116 (1975): 279-289.
3. Lord, P.F., Greiner, T.P., Greene, R.W. and DeHoff, W.D.: Lung Lobe Torsion in the Dog. JAAHA, 9 (1973): 473-482.
4. Reich, S.B.: Production of Pulmonary Edema by Aspiration of Water-Soluble Nonabsorbable Contrast Media. Radiology, 92 (1969): 367-370.

Radiologic Aspects of Thoracic Trauma in the Dog and Cat (Part II)

Lawrence J. Kleine, DVM, MS
Associate Professor and Head, Radiology
Tufts University
School of Veterinary Medicine
North Grafton, Massachusetts

Upper Airway—Occasionally, respiratory distress is associated with upper airway trauma. The degree of respiratory difficulty associated with tracheal or bronchial obstruction is directly related to the degree and level of obstruction. Complete obstruction of the trachea will result in death within minutes while partial bronchial obstruction may produce no clinical or radiographic signs.

Radiographic evidence of obstruction is primarily interruption of the air density in the trachea or major bronchi. Foreign bodies (Fig 6) and blood are common causes of airway obstruction. Foreign bodies such as plastic, which are normally radiolucent, may be seen because of the contrast provided by the surrounding air. Tracheal stenosis following tracheal injury is an infrequent cause of airway obstruction (Fig 7). Traumatic tracheal stenosis can result from overinflation of the cuff of an endotracheal tube with secondary vascular compromise, necrosis and scar tissue formation.

Lung—Some pulmonary abnormalities associated with trauma are intrapulmonary hemorrhage, pulmonary collapse, lung lobe torsion, electric shock and formation of tracheoesophageal fistulae. Trauma to the lung can range from a small localized contusion without clinical signs to massive laceration which produces rapid atelectasis and exsanguination due to pneumothorax and hemorrhage.

Pulmonary Hemorrhage—Pulmonary hemorrhage is the most common radiologic diagnosis following thoracic trauma. Radiographically, it appears as a focal increase in opacity of lung parenchyma with the presence of air bronchograms.

Since the radiographic changes are due to fluid accumulation within the air spaces, they cannot be radiographically distinguished from inflammatory lung disease. In single acute episodes of hemorrhage, the radiographic abnormalities usually resolve in 48 to 72 hours. Persistence of the radiographic changes for a longer period of time indicates continued bleeding or superimposition of inflammatory lung disease.

Lobar Collapse—Lobar collapse most often occurs as the result of the presence of space occupying material (air, fluid, mass) in the pleural space, but may also result from bronchial obstruction due to blood accumulation or foreign material within a bronchus, or lung torsion.

Originally published in Volume 1, Number 4, April 1979

Lobar Torsion—Lung lobe torsion usually occurs in deep-chested dogs, but can occur in any dog or cat.[3] The left and right cranial and right middle lobes are most frequently involved. There is often a history of trauma or a long-standing pleural effusion. The clinical signs are ambiguous and may not be severe enough to cause the owner to seek veterinary aid until the lesion has been present for several days or weeks. Lung torsion is nearly always accompanied by trapped clotted blood in the pleural space. The twisted lung lobe is usually totally consolidated and increased in size. Air bronchograms are usually not seen within the affected lobe.

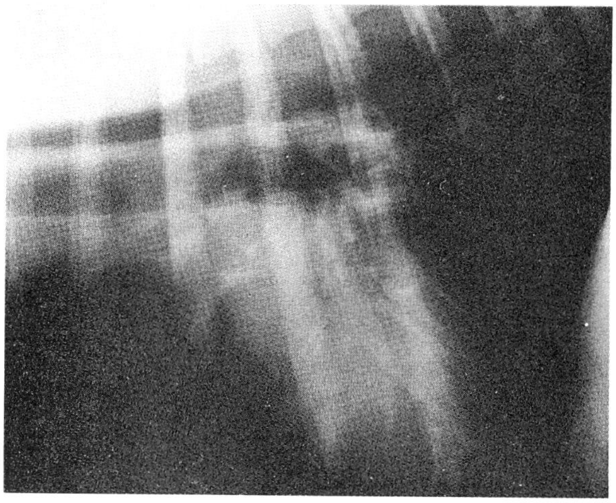

Fig 6—An oval density lies dorsal to the left atrium interrupting the air pattern of the distal trachea. Moderate dyspnea and coughing were prominent clinical signs in this dog. The oval density was an acorn.

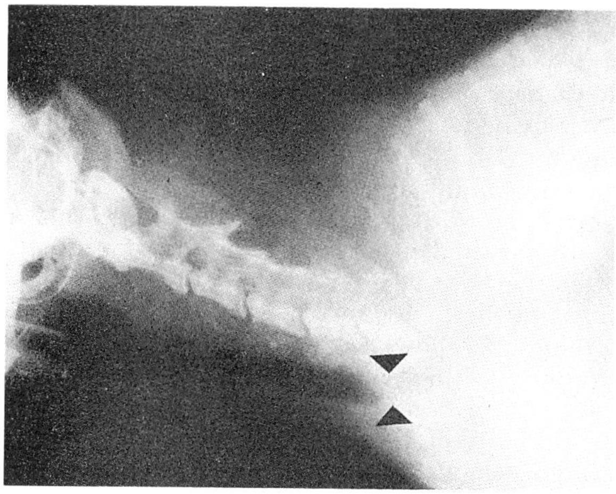

Fig 7—This radiograph was made two weeks following an episode of pneumomediastinum which had resolved. At the time of this radiograph the cat was mildly dyspneic. The arrows outline a stenotic area of the trachea which was presumed to be the site of the previous tracheal rupture which had lead to pneumomediastinum.

Electric Shock—Severe electric shock produces pulmonary edema which is frequently confined to the caudal lung lobes. Within 48 to 72 hours the lungs will become normal unless secondary infection occurs.

Tracheo-esophageal Fistulae—Tracheo-esophageal fistulae are rare. They may be congenital or acquired. Acquired trancheo-esophageal fistulae may be associated with external trauma, or more likely, chronic esophageal inflammation secondary to penetration by an esophageal foreign body. Contrast esophagraphy is necessary to confirm the diagnosis. In doing so, one must be aware that both the barium and aqueous iodide contrast agents can produce serious lung damage. Therefore a medium which is intended for bronchographic use should be employed.

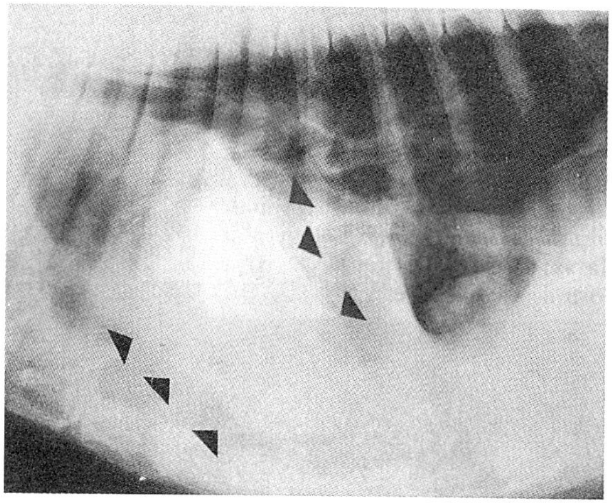

Fig 8—Lung lobe torsion usually produces pleural effusion and consolidation of the affected lobe. In this case, the left cranial middle lobe was involved. (arrows)

Inhalation Injuries—In addition to external trauma, the lung can be injured by inhalation of noxious gases or aspiration of foreign material. The quantity of material inhaled or aspirated, its irritative properties, and the presence of concomitant disease determine the severity of the radiographic signs (Fig 9). Both the physical character and the force of inhalation determine the location of the inhaled substance in the airways. Generally the dependent portions of the caudal and middle lung lobes are most severely affected.

While inhalation of solid or liquid can occur secondary to vomiting due to any cause, it is most often associated with esophageal paralysis, cricopharyngeal achalasia, or a persistent vascular ring at the heart base causing esophageal dilation. Occasionally solid or liquid medication or food is inhaled because of struggling during misguided efforts to force feed a dog or cat.

Smoke or hydrocarbon inhalation may not produce any radiographic signs in spite of clinical evidence of moderate dyspnea. Early radiographic changes are usually confined to the bronchial tree. Later, interstitial opacities may be prominent and, in severe cases, pulmonary edema may follow.

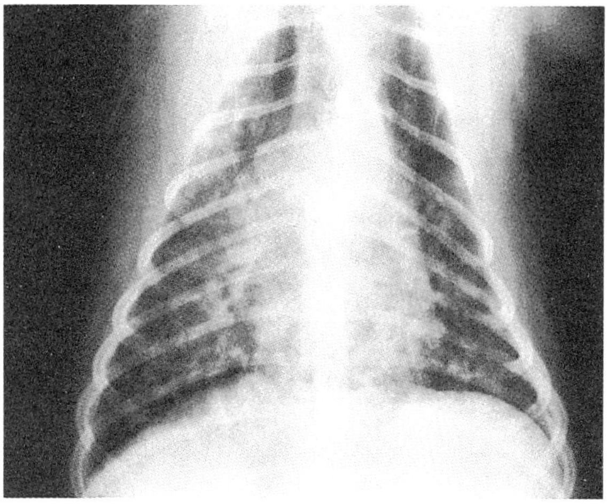

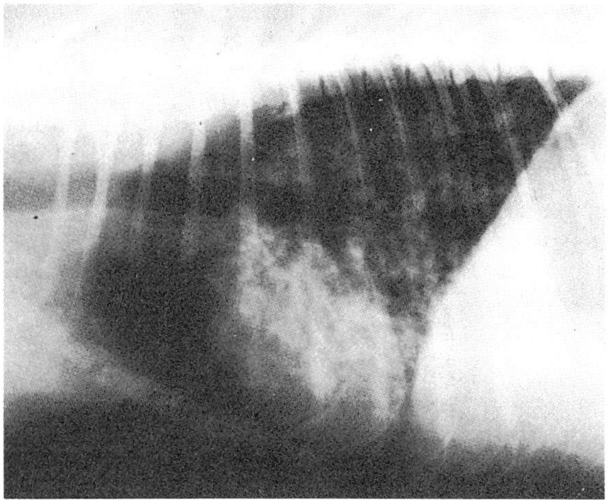

Fig 9A and B—Uniform linear densities producing pulmonary consolidation were seen in this four-year-old dog after it inhaled a saturated salt solution. The owner administered the solution to induce vomiting in the dog because of possible toxin ingestion.

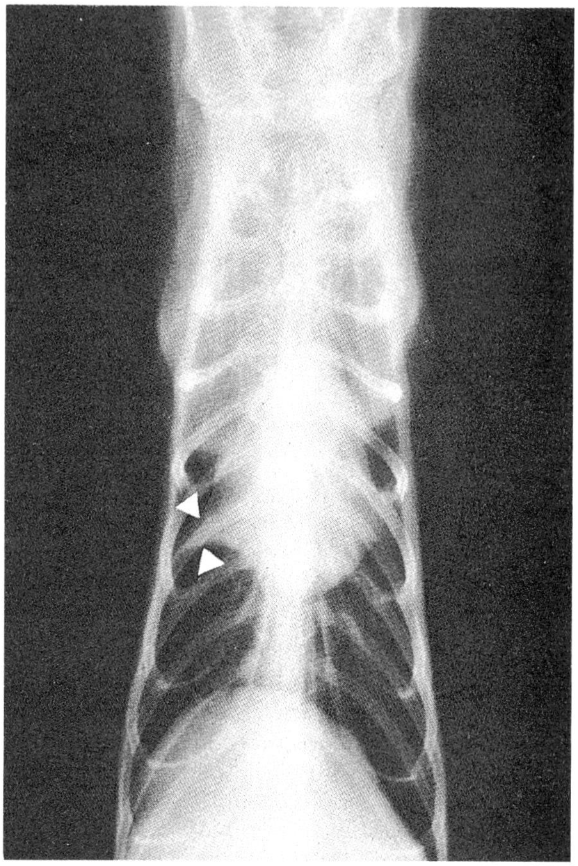

Fig 10—The triangular opacity (arrows) at the level of the right middle lung lobe is the result of atelectasis and pleural adhesions. These lesions were secondary to pleural and pulmonary hemorrhage three weeks earlier. (Editor's note: Without confirming evidence, this radiographic appearance is consistent with collapse of the right middle lung lobe, as well as the diagnosis of pleural adhesions.)

Esophagus—Blunt thoracic trauma rarely causes esophageal injury. The most common type of esophageal trauma is secondary to foreign body ingestion. Foreign bodies which are radiolucent may be seen if they are surrounded by intraesophageal air. Esophageal foreign bodies usually cause the clinical signs of salivation, dysphagia, and regurgitation, but occasionally the only clinical sign is anorexia, and the clinician does not suspect the foreign body which is found incidentally by thoracic radiography.

Esophageal perforation results in esophageal contents entering the mediastinum or pleural space. Fluid in the pleural space leads to opacification of the interlobar fissures and blunting of the costophrenic angles.

Both of these phenomena are best seen in the ventrodorsal projection. Mediastinitis, pyothorax, and septicemia may occur soon after esophageal perforation. Esophageal scarring with subsequent stenosis may occur after esophageal surgery or endoscopic removal of a foreign body.

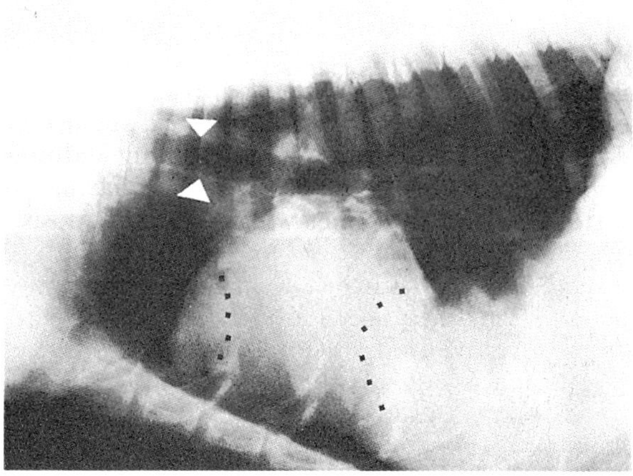

Fig. 11—Pneumomediastinum (arrows) and a wide, lobular ventral cardiac silhouette were the radiographic abnormalities in this seven-year-old spayed German Shepherd dog. The lobular appearance was due to the spleen which had passed through a diaphragmatic rupture and enveloped the heart (dotted lines).

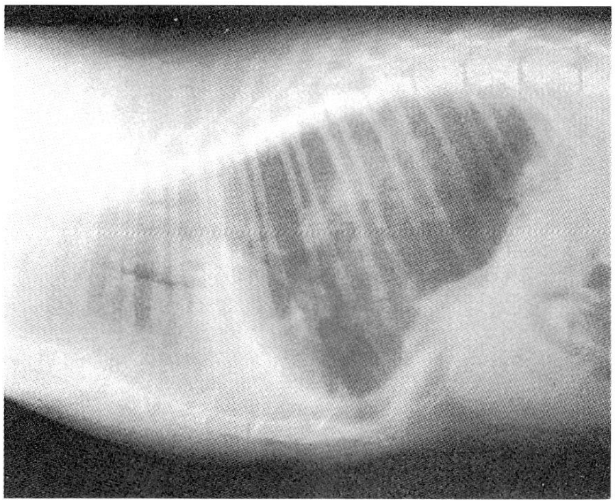

Fig 12—A large gas shadow cranial to the level of the diaphragm obliterates the heart in this five-month-old female cat. The gas is contained in a distended stomach which has passed through a ruptured diaphragm. The degree of distension suggests obstruction of the pylorus or proximal small intestine.

Diaphragm—Diaphragmatic hernia is probably the most common thoracic injury which requires surgical correction. The tear in the diaphragm may be so small as to be an incidental finding at necropsy, or so large as to permit passage of nearly all the freely movable abdominal viscera into the thoracic cavity.

Diagnosis of a diaphragmatic hernia may be easily made radiographically due to the presence of abdominal viscera in the pleural space. However, if incarceration of an organ such as omentum or liver occurs, secondary pleural effusion may obliterate the herniated organs. For this reason, repeat radiography of the thorax after thoracocentesis may be helpful if pleural effusion is significant. If sufficient fluid cannot be withdrawn to permit visualization of the caudal mediastinum and ventral diaphragm, horizontal beam radiography with the patient in dorsal recumbency may allow better visualization of the area in question. In instances where effusion is not present, but an irregularity of the diaphragm is seen, pleurography may outline the thoracic surface of the diaphragm along with any protruding abdominal viscera. Barium in the stomach and intestines will aid the diagnosis if they are herniated.

Identification of the displaced organs may give the surgeon an estimate of the size of the diaphragmatic tear (Fig 11). Also, some diaphragmatic hernias are surgical emergencies (Fig 12). For instance, if the stomach or intestine is incarcerated in the thoracic cavity and greatly distended, the abdominal viscus may become infarcted and perforate. Also the distended stomach or intestine may produce pulmonary insufficiency due to encroachment upon the lung.

Heart and Thoracic Vessels—Myocardial contusions, infarctions and a small volume of intrapericardial fluid do not result in detectable radiographic changes. Except in extreme instances, cardiac and great vessel trauma is difficult to recognize on survey radiographs. Exceptions include large volume pericardial effusion, pneumopericardium, rupture of a cardiac chamber, and aneurysm.

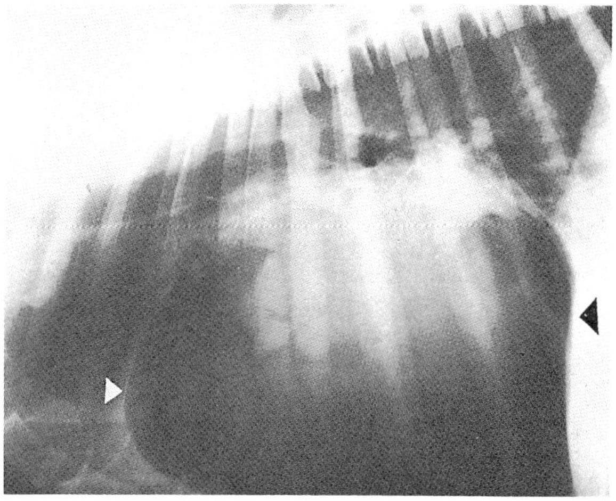

Fig 13—This three-year-old male Beagle developed severe cough with hemoptysis after a day of hunting. Hemorrhagic pericardial effusion was withdrawn and these radiographs were made. The arrows point to the margins of the air distended pericardium. A stick had been inhaled, penetrated the left mainstem bronchus and the left auricular appendage producing the hemorrhagic pericardial effusion. The hole in the left auricular appendage had sealed but when the effusion was relieved, air filled the pericardium through the bronchial-pericardial fistula.

Hemopericardium can result from rupture of a cardiac chamber due to blunt trauma, instrumentation, chronic mitral regurgitation, or rupture of blood vessels in the epicardium or pericardium. The heart generally assumes a spherical configuration in these cases. If there is a single episode of bleeding which is arrested, considerable reduction in the size of the cardiac silhouette occurs in 48 to 72 hours. Massive hemopericardium can result in cardiac failure and death due to tamponade.

Pneumopericardium is the result of communication between the pericardium and a positive pressure air sources, such as a bronchial-pericardial fistula or introduction of air during pericardiocentesis (Fig 13).

REFERENCES

1. Chiu, C.L. and Gambach, R.R.: Hypaque Pulmonary Edema: A case report. Radiology, 111, (1974):91-92.
2. Genereux, G.P.: The End-Stage Lung. Radiology, 116, (1975):225-289.
3. Lord, P.F., Greiner, T.P., Greene, R.W. and DeHoff, W.D.: Lung Lobe Torsion in the Dog. JAAHA, 9, (1973):473-482.
4. Reich, S.B.: Production of Pulmonary Edema by Aspiration of Water-Soluble Nonabsorable Contrast Media. Radiology, 92, (1969):367-370.

Radiographic Signs of Pulmonary Infiltration

John W. Watters, DVM, MS
Associate Professor of Radiology
School of Veterinary Medicine
Louisiana State University
Baton Rouge, Louisiana

Categorization of radiographic pulmonary changes into specific patterns allows the establishment of differential diagnoses from which a more precise final diagnosis can be derived. Pattern recognition of pulmonary diseases permits the ruling out of several etiologic factors which might be confusing if a systematic approach were not used. It is important in treatment planning and prognostication to be able to determine if the radiographic signs are caused by bacterial, viral or mycotic infection as opposed to trauma, neoplasia and cardiological diseases.

This pattern recognition of pulmonary diseases should be established, rather than trying to associate the radiograph with one which represents a given condition in a textbook. It is also stressed that the radiographic signs must be used in conjunction with the physical findings, history and laboratory results.

It is not always a simple task to reduce the list of differential diagnoses to a definitive diagnosis based solely on the radiographic findings because of the limited manner in which the lungs can respond, and the stage of the disease, or the past history of respiratory disease, is not always known. The lung has a long memory; it can show the scars of past problems and these may not be a part of the present problem. Pulmonary patterns are similar to road signs from which general information can be gained from the geometric configuration even if the words on the signs are not visible.

If the systematic approach to identifying pulmonary changes according to patterns and types of infiltrates is used, it will not be so easy to fall into the trap of making snap judgements based on the overall appearance of the thorax. It must be stated at the beginning that proper exposure factors and good processing techniques must be used if the minor lung changes are to be seen. It is also important that the lung tissue not be a criterion for evaluation of the exposure technique because it is an *unknown* factor. After all, the lung density is judged as a relative density compared to the less variable surrounding soft tissue and bony structures. It is important to remember that pulmonary infiltrates usually do not occur as separate entities but are frequently seen as combinations and admixtures. An attempt will be made to point out some common complicating factors.

Lung Model

A lung model was made with one air-filled soda straw and one water-filled straw inserted in holes made in a synthetic sponge in an attempt to illustrate the pulmonary patterns that will be discussed. The sponge in Fig 1A represents a normal lung with a vessel and a bronchus seen in longitudinal projection. The sponge in Fig 1B illustrates enhancement of the interstitial tissue by the simple means of soaking the sponge in water. The overall radiographic opacity of the sponge is increased as compared to normal and the vascular and bronchial margins appear irregular due to the superimposed interstitial pattern.

Originally published in Volume 1, Number 9, September 1979

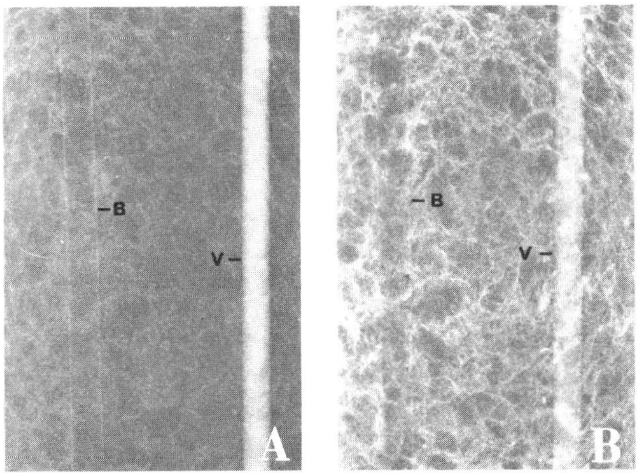

Fig 1A—The lung model illustrating a normal lung with one vessel (**v**) and one bronchus (**b**). *B*—The lung model representative of a lung with an interstitial pattern.

Specific types of interstitial patterns are perivascular (**v**) and peribronchial (**b**) as illustrated in Fig 2. Therefore, the types of interstitial patterns which one should look for are generalized, perivascular and peribronchial.

Many of the holes in the sponge are now filled with water to represent filling of alveoli to produce an alveolar pattern (Fig 3). The air-filled straw (the bronchus) is now seen very clearly because of the alveolar filling around the bronchus.

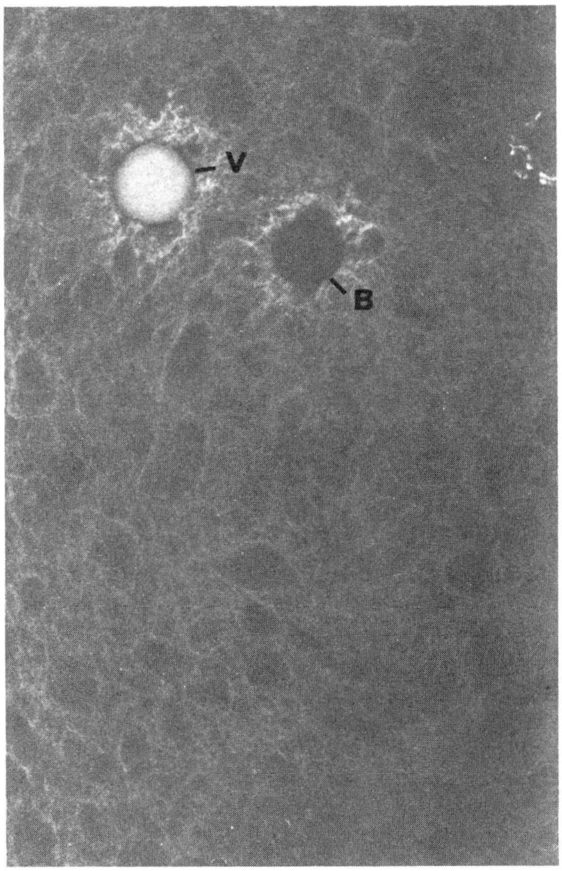

Fig 2—A cross section of the lung model illustrating perivascular (**v**) and peribronchial (**b**) interstitial patterns.

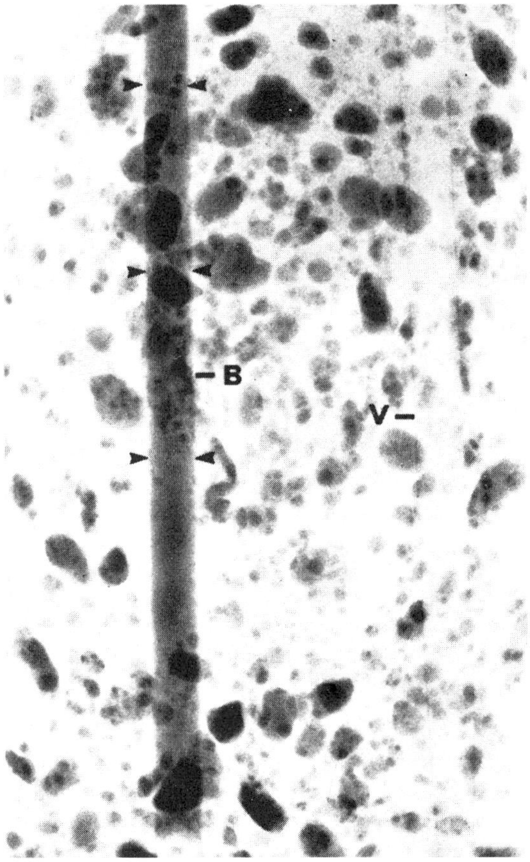

Fig 3—The lung model representation of an alveolar pattern that produces an air-bronchogram (*arrows*).

However, the water-filled straw (the vessel) is not clearly seen because the blood in the vessel has the same density as the surrounding interstitial infiltrate.

Pulmonary Patterns

Categorization of pulmonary disease into patterns is based upon radiographic signs associated with the components of the lungs. Radiographic signs are defined as changes in size, shape, location and density. Therefore, it is obvious that the normal ranges of such variables must be known before pathologic changes can be recognized. Pulmonary patterns are classified into alveolar, interstitial, vascular, bronchial, and mixed types.

Alveolar Patterns

These are produced when the lumina of alveoli become filled with fluid or cellular debris as shown in Fig 3. Air-bronchograms are seen when alveoli surrounding bronchi or bronchioles are infiltrated with any type of transudate or exudate. The air-bronchograms appear as radiolucent branching structures surrounded by radiopaque areas. Alveolar disease may affect small regions or may involve one or more entire lung lobes. *Patchy* areas with irregular fluffy margins can occur without the appearance of air-bronchograms, if only small portions of the alveoli are involved. These are usually representative of early alveolar disease. Thickening of bronchial walls and peribronchial infiltration will make the bronchi stand out more prominently; however, this should not be confused with an alveolar pattern.

Some of the causes of alveolar disease are inflammation

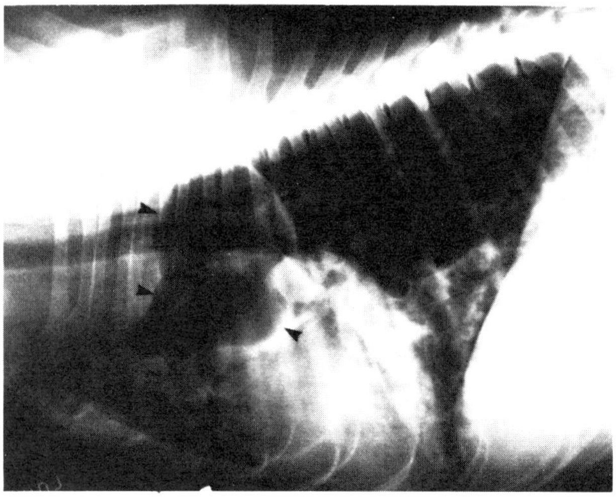

Fig 4—Two large air-filled pulmonary spaces that consist of dilated bronchi and emphysematous lung tissue are visible (*arrows*). These air-filled spaces are representative of decreased pulmonary radiopacity. The diagnosis was bronchiectasis with pulmonary emphysema.

(bronchopneumonia), pulmonary edema, contusion or hemorrhage, atelectasis (often associated with pneumothorax), neoplasia, granulomas and infarction (associated with embolism).

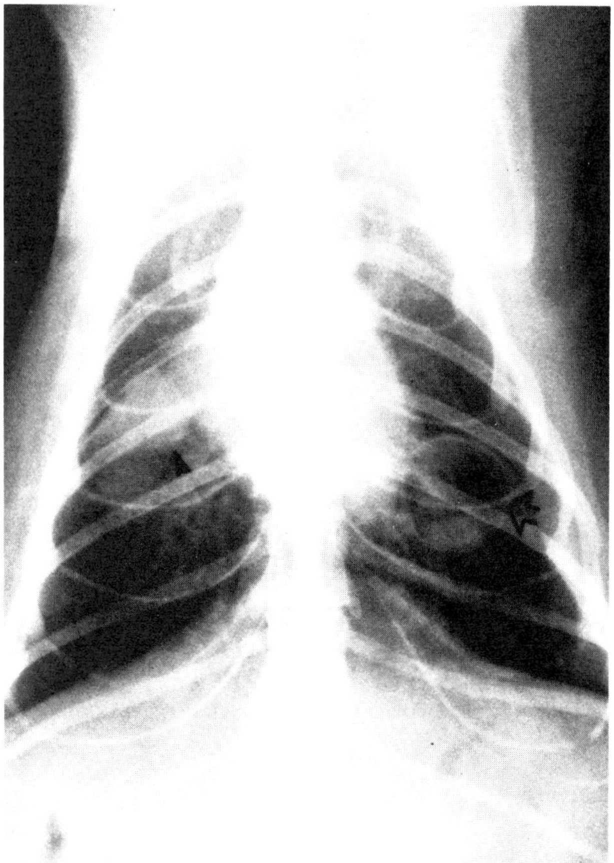

Fig 5—A well-defined circular radiopacity is present in the right lung (*closed arrow*) and a cavitated circular radiolucent lesion is depicted in the left lung (*open arrow*). These represent interstitial densities, one of which is cavitated. The diagnosis was interstitial granulomas due to Paragonimus infection.

Interstitial Patterns

These patterns are produced when the interstitial tissues become inflamed or infiltrated from any cause. The only radiographic change observed in early interstitial disease is an overall increase in the *background* radiopacity of the lung fields; the lungs appear to be more gray than normal when compared to the surrounding soft tissue and bone. This is one of the more difficult patterns to evaluate because the same appearance can be seen in a radiograph taken on expiration or partial inspiration. This overall gray radiographic appearance will also be seen in obese animals because of scattered radiation and other factors. Linear or nodular densities become more apparent as the interstitial infiltrate worsens. The pattern can be generalized or it may be localized around vessels (perivascular) or bronchi (peribronchial), as illustrated in Fig 2.

Neoplastic disease usually occurs within the interstitial tissue and can be seen as ranging from solitary lesions to diffuse miliary nodules. The interstitial pattern will not be visible if the interstitial disease worsens to the point of alveolar filling. Some causes of interstitial disease are inflammatory infiltrates (usually viral), edema (cardiac, noncardiac, iatrogenic), neoplasia, granuloma, hemorrhage and fibrosis.

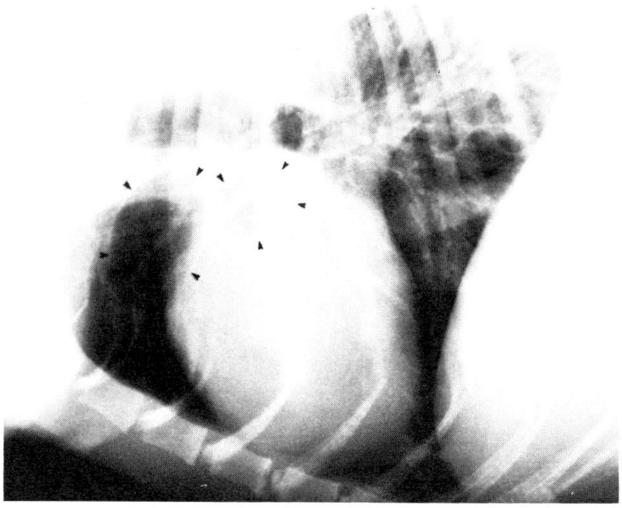

Fig 6—Several areas of increased radiolucency are seen distributed throughout the lung fields, 2 of them are marked with arrows. These are representative of localized circular increased pulmonary radiolucencies. The diagnosis was bullous emphysema.

Vascular Patterns

This pattern refers to an increase or decrease in the size of the pulmonary vasculature, either arteries or veins. An attempt should be made to identify if the change is involving the arteries, veins or both as this will help to differentiate disease entities. The determination of changes in vascular size can be subjective and is based on relative size as compared to normal. Some quantitative data has been obtained and this can be used to determine what is *normal* for each patient.[1] A rule of thumb is that the pulmonary artery should not be greater than 60% of an adjacent rib as seen on the dorsoventral view.

Causes of pulmonary hypervascularity are congestion, left-to-right shunts and dirofilariasis. Causes of pulmonary

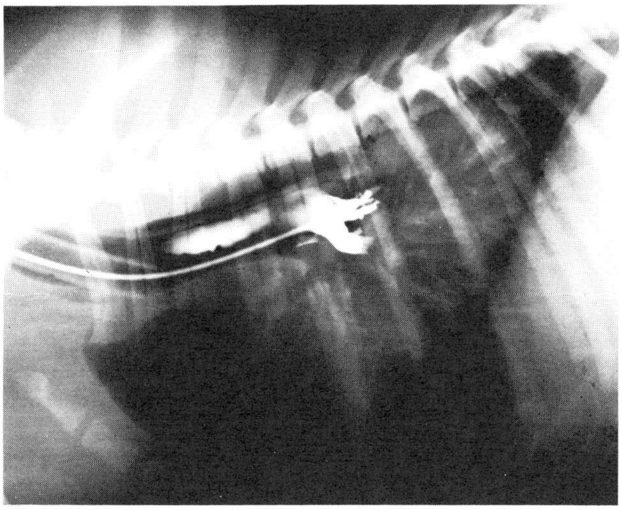

Fig 7—A large solitary area of increased radiopacity is seen in the caudal lung (*arrows*). The contrast filled bronchi are seen to be severely compressed and obstructed. The diagnosis was made at surgery and was a large abscess.

hypovascularity are hypovolemia, pulmonic stenosis and tetralogy of Fallot, emphysema and Addison's disease.

Bronchial Patterns

The bronchial tree, except for the main stem bronchi, is usually not seen in normal dogs. The bronchial pattern is produced as a result of peribronchial infiltration, thickening of the walls, calcification of the cartilage, changes in diameter of the bronchi or filling of the lumina. It is common to see the bronchial pattern in aged patients and this is considered to be normal and part of the aging process. Although bronchiectasis is uncommon, it may be recognized as tubular or saccular distension of the bronchi. Bronchography is usually necessary for the diagnosis of bronchiectasis. One of the easiest radiographic signs for recognition of a bronchial pattern is the appearance of a *doughnut*, and this represents a thickened bronchial wall viewed end-on. The bronchi can be confused with vessels in cases where the bronchial lumina are filled with fluid, but this will only be so if the surrounding alveoli are clear. Some of the causes of bronchial patterns are chronic bronchitis, aging, allergy, toxic fumes and as the result of previous inflammatory or other pulmonary disease.

Pulmonary Densities

Changes in pulmonary densities are seen that cannot be characterized in the previous patterns. Pulmonary densities can be classified either as increased or decreased radiolucencies or radiopacities. It is also important to note the location, shape, margination and distribution of the disease process.

The terms used to describe increased pulmonary radiopacities (masses) include: *diffuse* (linear), *diffuse* (nodular), *solitary, smooth margins, irregular margins, solid, cavitating,* and *localized.* The terms commonly used to describe areas of decreased radiopacity (or increased radiolucency) are: *localized, diffuse, circular* and *tubular.*

Radiographic Examples

Radiographs have been selected to illustrate some of the patterns and pulmonary conditions that have been discussed. Most of the radiographs illustrate more than one condition and it is recommended that each figure be closely

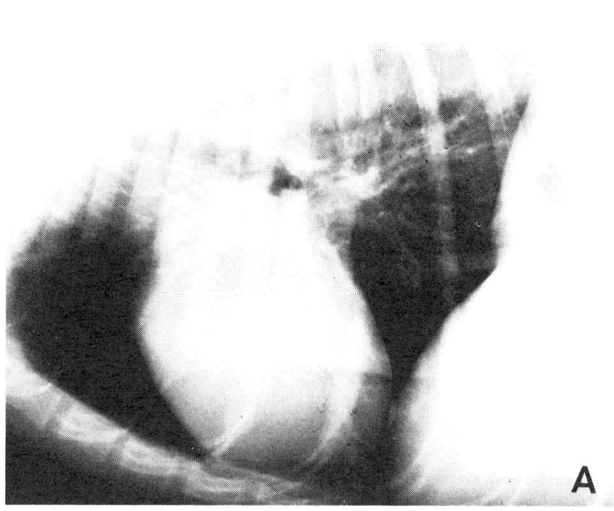

Fig 8A—A dog prior to heartworm treatment.

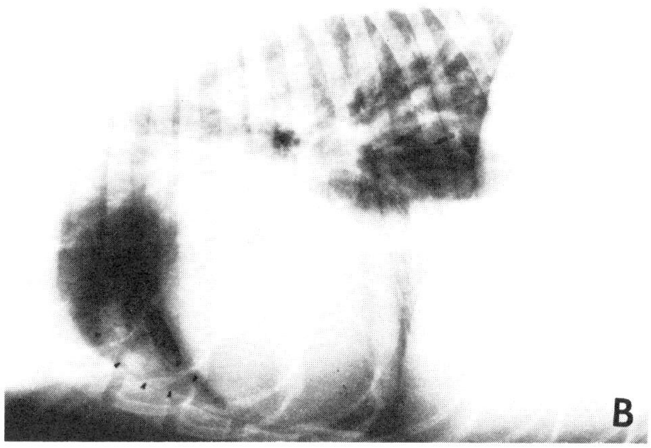

Fig 8B—The same dog 7 days post treatment. The second radiograph illustrates generalized interstitial disease in the caudal lung area (*single arrow*) and an area of alveolar disease (*small arrows*) in the ventral portion of the cranial lung field. The diagnosis was post-therapeutic embolic infarction following heartworm treatment.

examined to see how many of the patterns can be recognized.

In Fig 4, large radiolucent areas in the cranial and caudal lung lobes can be seen. The two major areas of decreased radiopacity are due to dilatation of the bronchi. There are many smaller areas that are due to rupture of adjacent alveoli which have merged to form the mottled appearance of pulmonary emphysema. A bronchial pattern is present in the ventral aspect of the caudal lobes due to bronchial wall thickening and peribronchial infiltration. Air-bronchograms are seen in the ventral portion of the cranial lobes, representing alveolar disease.

In Fig 5, a smoothly marginated, round interstitial opacity in the right middle lung lobe, and a round cavitated radiolucent lesion in the left caudal lobe can be seen. The diagnosis was interstitial granulomas due to Paragonimus infection. The diagnosis was suggested using the radiographic signs, but was confirmed by a positive fecal examination. The list of differential diagnoses includes the formation of an abscess from other inflammatory diseases or trauma and cavitating neoplasia.

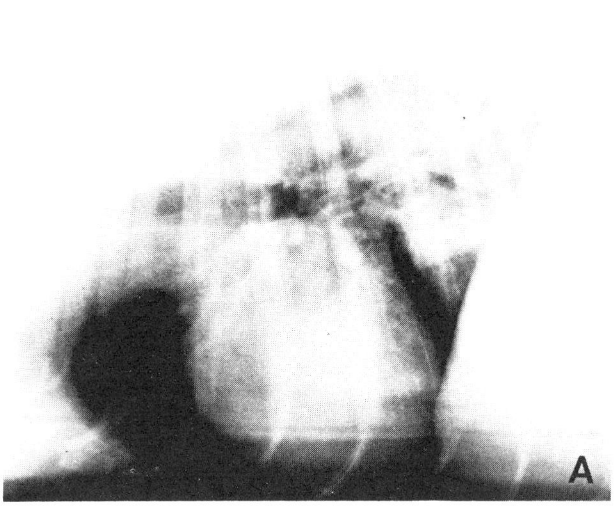

Fig 9A—Alveolar disease in the caudal lung. An air-bronchogram is seen.

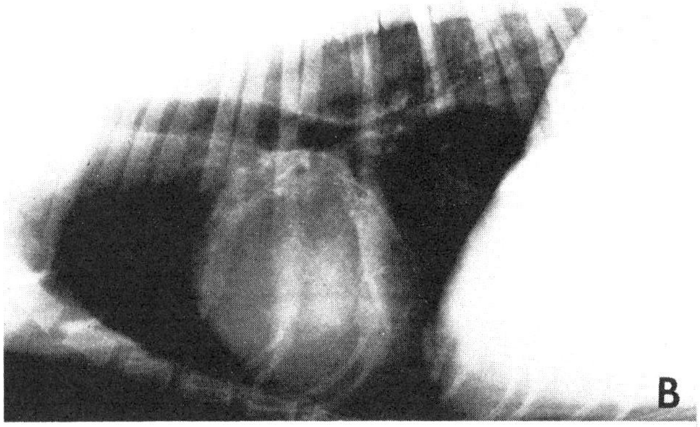

Fig 9B—A radiograph made 48 hours after the first radiograph (Fig 9A). The diagnosis was post-traumatic pulmonary hemorrhage (hit by car).

In Fig 6, areas of increased pulmonary radiolucency with circular well-defined margins can be seen. This pattern of increased radiolucency is referred to as bullous emphysema, pneumatocysts and pneumatoceles. The walls of the bronchi are very prominent indicating bronchial thickening, consistent with bullous emphysema.

A large, fairly well marginated interstitial mass in the caudal lung field is seen in Fig 7. The contrast filled bronchi are obstructed by the mass. The differential diagnosis includes neoplasia, granuloma and abscessation. The mass was found to be a large abscess at surgery.

Fig 8A represents a radiograph taken prior to heartworm therapy. A generalized abnormal interstitial pattern is seen in the caudal lung in addition to a prominent peribronchial pattern. Right heart enlargement and distended pulmonary arteries are consistent with heartworm disease. In Fig 8B, the appearance of the thorax is seen 7 days following heartworm therapy. The generalized interstitial pattern is greatly enhanced and several areas of peribronchial infiltration (*doughnuts*) are seen in the caudal lung (*single arrow*). An area of alveolar disease is seen in the ventral cranial lung lobes (*arrows*). There are small linear lucencies transversing the increased pulmonary opacities. These lucencies are representative of alveolar disease associated with post-therapeutic embolic infarctions. A differential diagnosis includes bronchopneumonia, chronic bronchitis, aspiration pneumonia, and pulmonary changes secondary to severe heartworm disease.

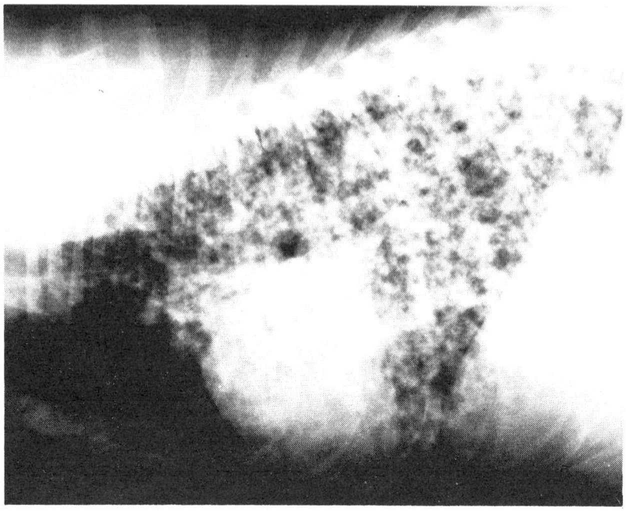

Fig 10—This case is representative of diffuse, nodular interstitial disease. The diagnosis of fungal infection (blastomycosis) was based on laboratory findings.

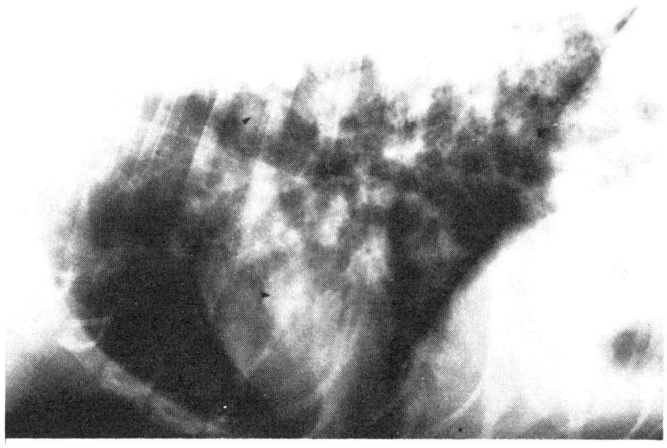

Fig 11—Extensive peribronchial infiltration is seen throughout all lung lobes. There are also some areas of alveolar disease (*arrows*). The diagnosis was bronchopneumonia secondary to aspiration of an agricultural pesticide.

Fig 9A illustrates generalized increased radiopacity in the caudal lung field of a dog that had been hit by a car a few hours prior to radiography. Several linear radiolucencies representing an air-bronchogram are present in the area of increased radiopacity which is indicative of an alveolar pattern. The margins of the lesions are fluffy and not well-defined. The diagnosis, based on history, physical examination and radiographic signs was pulmonary contusion with hemorrhage into the alveoli. There also must be interstitial bleeding; however, this pattern is obscured by the alveolar pattern.

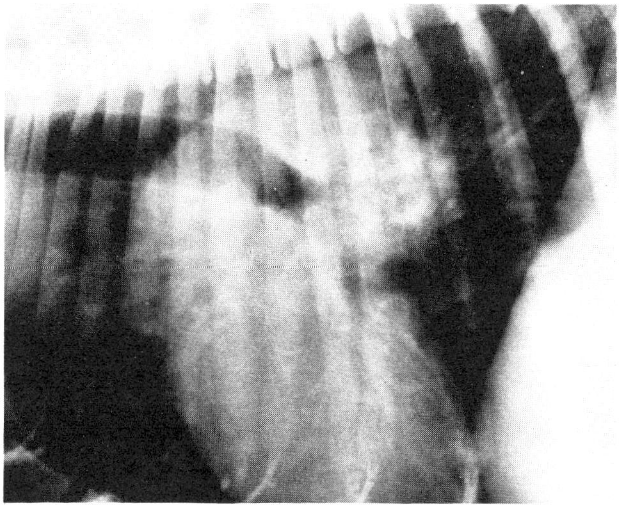

Fig 12—Enlargement of the hilar lymph nodes with a radiating interstitial pattern representing distended lymphatics in the lung fields is seen. The diagnosis was lymphadenopathy with lymphatic distention.

Fig 9B is a radiograph made 48 hours after the first radiographs were taken. All the alveolar pattern has resolved and an interstitial pattern is now visible. Several end-on bronchi with peribronchial infiltration are seen in the caudal lobes. Longitudinal sections of thickened bronchi are also observed in the caudal area.

Fig 10 illustrates a diffuse nodular interstitial pattern that is present in all areas of the lungs. There are also many bronchi which are seen to have severe peribronchial infiltration. The diagnosis was blastomycosis. If this case of pulmonary blastomycosis is compared with Fig 13, which represents diffuse metastatic neoplasia, a great deal of similarity is found.

Fig 11 illustrates predominently a peribronchial pattern which is characterized by circular radiolucent areas with surrounding tissue radiopacity. There are also some small patchy areas of increased radiopacity with small linear lucencies (bronchioles). The patchy areas are representative of alveolar infiltration. The diagnosis of bronchopneumonia was made because of the very heavy peribronchial and alveolar patterns. This condition was caused by the aspiration of an agricultural pesticide.

Fig 12 illustrates an increased radiopacity in the hilar region with radiating lines of density toward the lung margins. This is an interstitial pattern which has signs of peribronchial and perivascular infiltration. The diagnosis of lymphadenopathy with lymphatic infiltration was based on the radiographic signs and laboratory findings. A differential diagnosis would include interstitial edema.

A diffuse, nodular interstitial pattern representing metastatic neoplasia is illustrated in Fig 13. Mycotic infection, such as seen in Fig 10, must be included in the list of differential diagnoses for this type of pulmonary pattern.

Fig 14 illustrates multiple, nodular interstitial radiopacities throughout the majority of the lung fields. Consolidation of most of the left caudal lobe is observed with

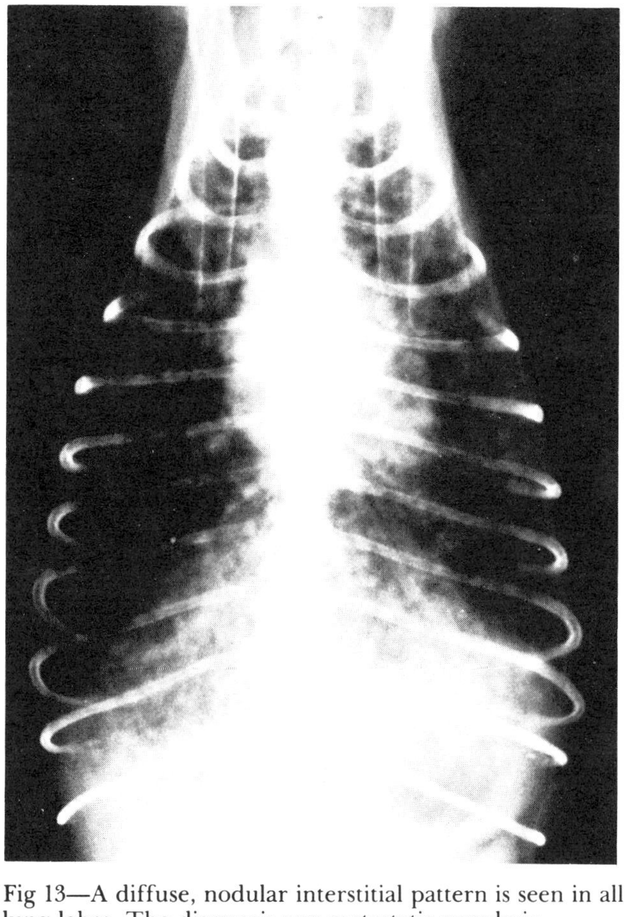

Fig 13—A diffuse, nodular interstitial pattern is seen in all lung lobes. The diagnosis was metastatic neoplasia.

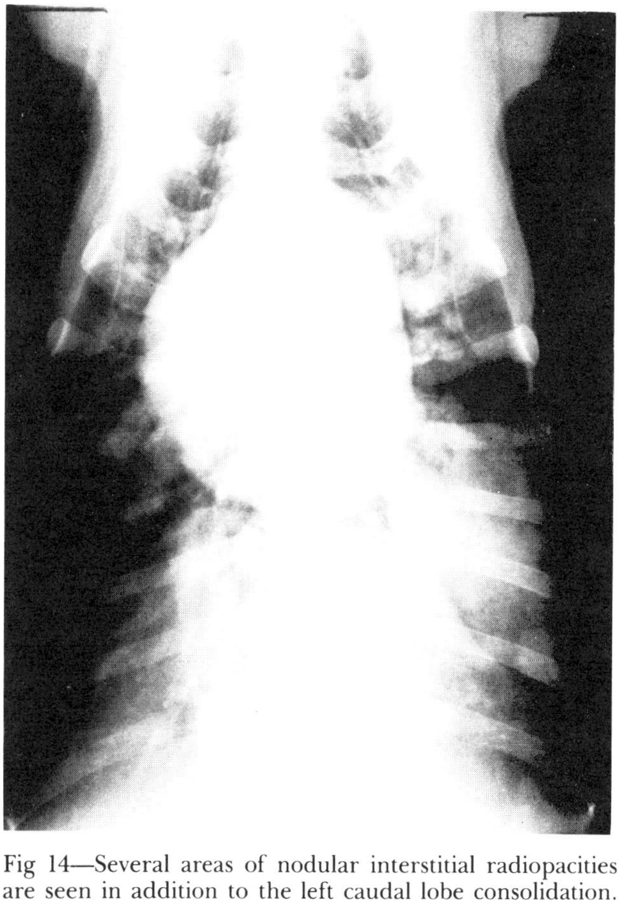

Fig 14—Several areas of nodular interstitial radiopacities are seen in addition to the left caudal lobe consolidation. The diagnosis was bronchiogenic carcinoma.

the bronchi in this area being very prominent. The alveolar pattern was produced by a bronchiogenic carcinoma. The differential diagnoses include abscessation, lobar pneumonia and neoplasia.

REFERENCE

1. Thrall DE, Losonsky JM: A method for evaluating canine pulmonary circulatory dynamics from survey radiographs. *JAAHA* 12: 457-462, 1976.

Radiographic Diagnosis of Metastatic Pulmonary Neoplasia

Donald E. Thrall, DVM, PhD
Assistant Professor of Radiology
School of Veterinary Medicine
Assistant Professor of Radiation Therapy
School of Medicine, University of Pennsylvania
Philadelphia, Pennsylvania

Radiography of the chest is an important part of the evaluation of patients *known* to have a malignant neoplasm as well as patients *suspected* of having a malignant neoplasm. In order to assure that the correct form of therapy is instituted and to avoid the unnecessary utilization of invasive techniques, chest radiography should be performed early in the patient evaluation process.

The detection of pulmonary metastatic neoplasia need not be a sentence of immediate death for the patient. Some patients with metastatic lung neoplasia live comfortably for many months. Also, with the continued development of chemotherapy in veterinary oncology the comfortable life of some of these patients can be extended even further.

Pulmonary metastases seldom produce clinical signs. Even in advance cases, the clinical behavior of the patient and pulmonary auscultation may be normal. This is due to the fact that most metastatic lung tumors are a form of interstitial rather than alveolar lung disease. When clinical signs do result from pulmonary metastases, dyspnea is most frequently encountered. Coughing and hemoptysis are rare. Dyspnea may be due to hypoxemia associated with increased intrapulmonary tissue mass, interstitial pulmonary edema secondary to lymphatic occlusion or the development of pulmonary collapse secondary to tumor induced pleural effusion.

Radiographic Technique—The diagnostic accuracy of interpreting chest radiographs is directly linked to the technique utilized in exposing and processing the radiograph. Guides are available[1,5] and only a summary will be presented here.

The anatomical configuration of the chest is such that radiographs of the chest tend to be of high contrast. This is due to the large amount of air present in the lungs. In a high contrast radiograph, small pulmonary lesions may be overlooked. Therefore, technical factors which reduce subject contrast should be chosen. This can be achieved through low mas, high kVp techniques. Typically, the mas value for most chest radiographs should be in the range of 1.0 to 2.0. This low mas value will necessitate the use of a relatively high kVp value to produce sufficient film density (blackness). As a result, the contrast of the radiograph will be lessened and the diagnostic quality increased.

Originally published in Volume 1, Number 2, February 1979

Another advantage of using low mas values is that the exposure time can be kept to a minimum. The radiographic exposure should be made at the height of inspiration so that the margin of pulmonary lesions is sharply outlined by air filled alveoli. The entire chest must be included in the radiograph. The film must then be meticuously processed and thoroughly dried prior to final viewing.

False Negative Radiograph—The finding of no abnormalities on a chest radiograph does not mean that the patient is free of pulmonary metastases. In man it has been estimated that the smallest radiographically detectable pulmonary neoplasm is in the last one-third of its growth cycle.[2,3] Also, it is impossible to detect solitary pulmonary nodules less than 6mm in diameter by conventional radiographic techniques.[3] Therefore, a patient may have extensive pulmonary metastases and yet have a normal chest radiograph (Fig 1).

Another complicating factor is that pulmonary metastatic lesions may be overlooked because of

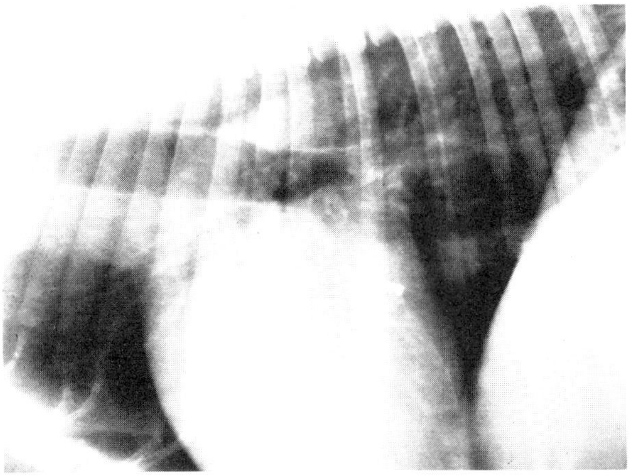

Fig 1A—Lateral chest radiograph of a patient presented for therapy of a malignant melanoma of the mandibular gingiva. The radiograph was considered to be within normal limits and a course of radiation therapy of the oral tumor was begun.

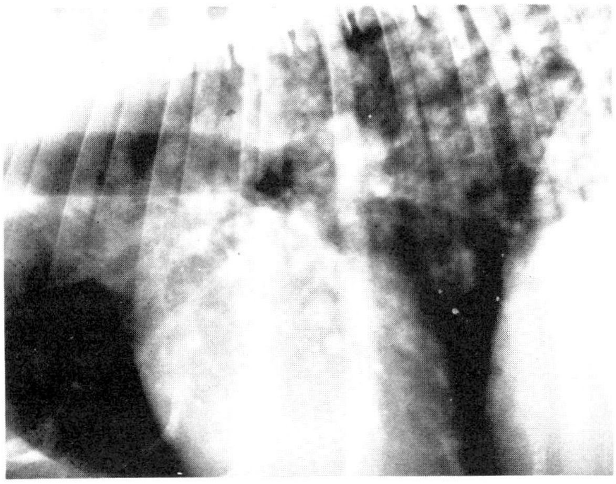

Fig 1B—Lateral chest radiograph made 4 weeks following the radiograph seen in Fig 1A. Numerous interstitial nodules are visible. There is little doubt that metastatic pulmonary disease was present when the radiograph seen in Fig 1A was made.

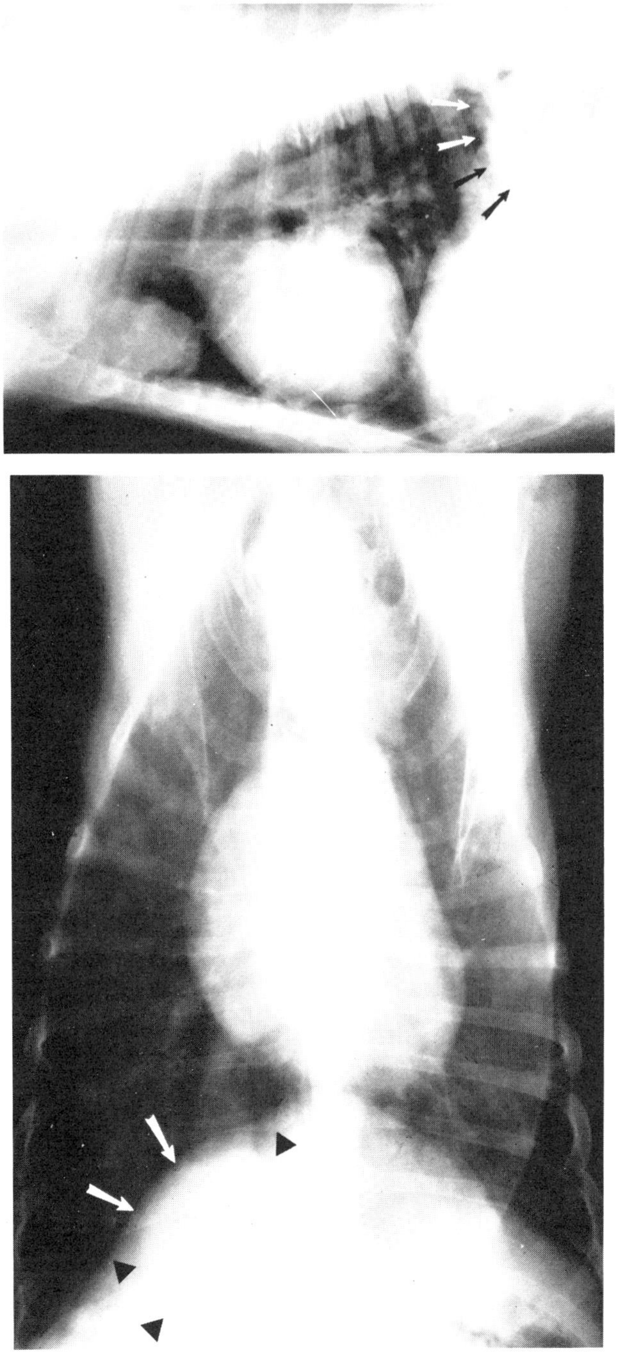

Fig 2—Lateral (A) and ventrodorsal (B) chest radiographs of a patient with metastatic mixed mammary tumor. The sternal lymph node is significantly enlarged. In addition, there is a large circular pulmonary metastatic mass in the caudodorsomedial portion of the right caudal lung lobe (arrows). This metastatic mass is superimposed on the diaphragm in both projections. Parenchymal lesions in this position in the lung are frequently over-looked due to the fact that they overlap the diaphragm.

their position within the thoracic cavity (Fig 2). Chest radiographs require rigorous scrutinization before being interpreted as normal.

False Positive Radiograph—Incorrectly identifying a radiograph as being positive for pulmonary metastatic lesions can have devastating consquences for the patient. False positive interpretations result from identifying incorrectly summation shadows, pulmonary vessels projected in cross section, chest wall masses, heterotopic bone or various pulmonary parenchymal lesions.

Summation shadows are areas of increased radio-opacity produced when portions of two separate and distinct anatomical structures are superimposed. The summation shadows produced by superimposition of a caudal lobar pulmonary artery and a rib are often misinterpreted as metastatic nodules (Fig 3), especially when the arteries are enlarged or the artery happens to be superimposed on a right and left rib simultaneously. When a pulmonary nodule is identified, the observer must take precaution that the opacity is not continuous with a vessel or a rib.

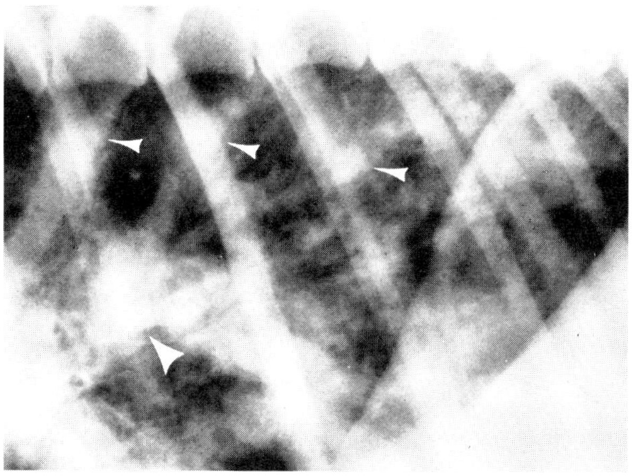

Fig 3—Lateral chest radiograph of a dog with dirofilariasis. The parenchymal pulmonary arteries are enlarged. The summation shadows (arrows) produced by superimposition of these enlarged pulmonary arteries and ribs are frequently mistaken for metastatic pulmonary disease. When a pulmonary nodule is identified, the observer must take precaution that the opacity is not continuous with a vessel or a rib.

Normal and abnormal large and small pulmonary vessels, when projected by the x-ray beam in cross section, are frequently misinterpreted as pulmonary metastases (Fig 4). These circular opacities are seen more frequently in the ventrodorsal projection than in the lateral projection. In many instances they are situated adjacent to a bronchus. The peripherally tapering architecture of the pulmonary vascular network causes the opacities situated more peripherally in the pulmonary parenchyma to be smaller in diameter than the opacities situated nearer the hilus. The marginal sharpness and degree of whiteness (radio-opacity) of these opacities are both greater than would be expected to be produced by absorption of x-rays in a spherical soft tissue mass of the same diameter. This relates to the cylindrical nature of a vessel as opposed to the spherical nature of a pulmonary metastatic lesion.

Soft tissue masses of the chest wall are frequently misinterpreted as pulmonary metastases. This is particularly true in patients with large nipples (Fig 5). This pseudonodule will be seen on the ventrodorsal projection approximately one-half the distance between the spine and the lateral margin of the chest. These pseudonodules may be either single or multiple. In order to prove whether an external mass is responsible for a possible metastatic nodule one needs only to apply a small amount of barium sulfate paste to the surface of the mass to serve as a marker.

Heterotopic bone refers to small (1-2mm) subpleural and parenchymal foci of bone found in many older dogs.[4] These osseous foci are observed more frequently in urban dogs than in rural dogs and are considered to have no clinical significance. The mineralization of these masses makes it possible to detect them radiographically at a much smaller size than if they were not mineralized. They are most easily seen in the cranial lobes on a lateral projection of the chest (Fig 6). These opacities should not be confused with pulmonary metastases. Pulmonary metastases rarely mineralize, particularly when the diameter of the mass is in the 1 to 2mm range.

The pulmonary parenchymal diseases that are occasionally misinterpreted as pulmonary metastases will be covered in association with the appearance of metastasis they most closely resemble.

True Positive Radiograph—Pulmonary parencymal lesions can be categorized into interstitial, alveolar, bronchial and mixed patterns.[5] Pulmonary metastasis usually results in the production of an interstitial type of lung disease. On other occasions, however, alveolar, bronchial or mixed patterns may result. This is related to the histologic type of the tumor, degree of aggressiveness of the tumor, immunologic competence of the patient and other factors such as the presence or absence of infection or bleeding disorders (D.I.C.).

Interstitial Lung Patterns in Metastasis—Interstitial lung disease can be divided into the types listed in Table I.

A. Solitary cavitary or non-cavitary interstitial masses (>4cm diameter) (Fig 7), interstitial nodules (2-4cm diameter) or interstitial miliary masses (<2cm diameter) rarely are representative of pulmonary metastases. In man, pulmonary metastatic masses, nodules or miliary masses are solitary in 25% of the cases.[6] Although an in-depth study of the frequency of occurrence of solitary pulmonary metastases has not been done in the dog or cat, one intuitively would expect the fraction to be lower than one out of four cases, based strictly on the rare finding of a solitary pulmonary mass in the dog or cat.

The apparent decreased frequency of solitary pulmonary metastases in the dog and cat may be related to the decreased frequency of occurrence (carcinoma of the colon, kidney, testicle) or different biologic behavior (malignant melanoma, osteosarcoma, carcinoma of the breast) of those tumors which in man frequently produce solitary pulmonary metastatic lesions. More likely consid-

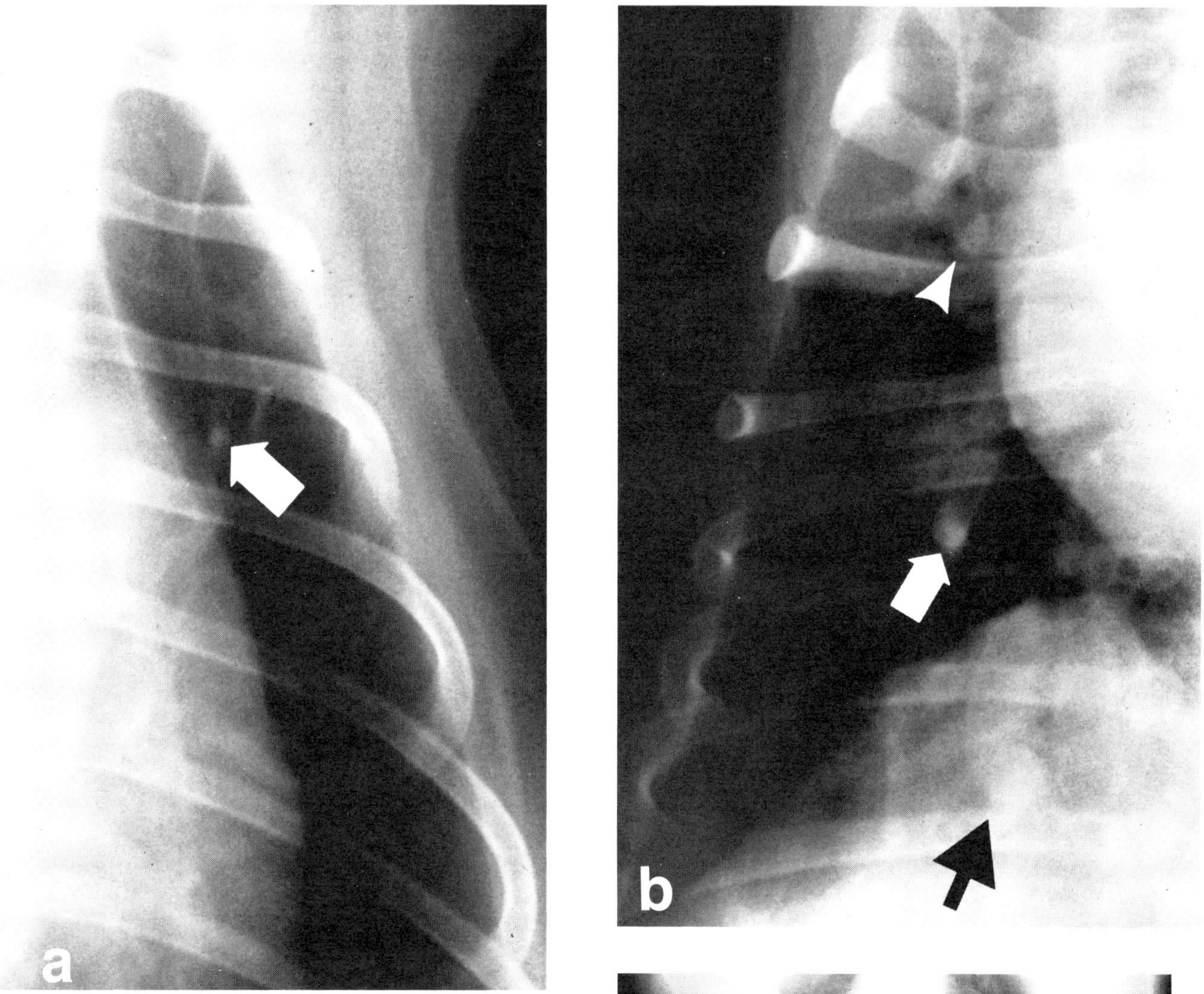

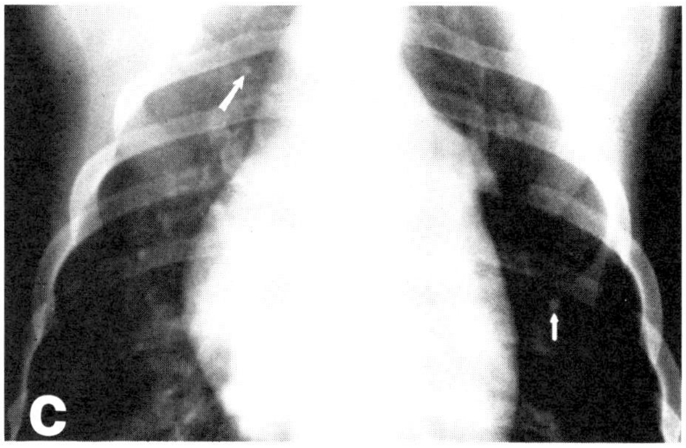

Fig 4—Ventrodorsal chest radiographs from 3 different dogs demonstrating the soft tissue opacity produced when a pulmonary artery is projected in cross section (arrows). These circular opacities are seen more frequently in the ventrodorsal projection and in many instances, are situated adjacent to a bronchus. This is apparent in each figure. Frequently, the circular opacity can be noted to be continuous with a parenchymal pulmonary artery (4B). The marginal sharpness and degree of whiteness of these opacities are both greater than would be expected to be produced by absorption of x-rays in a spherical metastatic nodule of the same diameter.

erations for solitary pulmonary masses, nodules or miliary masses, either cavitary or non-cavitary include primary tumor, abscess, granuloma or bulla.

B. The most common radiographic appearance of pulmonary metastasis in the dog and cat is multiple non-cavitary pulmonary masses (Fig 8), nodules (Fig 9) or miliary masses (Fig 10). Pulmonary metastases must be the number one consideration when these radiographic changes are observed. Other likely considerations include multicentric primary lung tumor and granulomatous disease. The radiographic appearance of the pulmonary metastatic lesions is somewhat a function of the cell type of the primary tumor. As a general rule, the mesenchymal malignancies, which metastasize primarily via the hematogenous route, produce a relatively low number of large smooth bordered pulmonary nodules while the epithelial malignancies, which metastasize primarily by the lymphatic route, produce a relatively large number of small miliary nodules with less distinct borders.

A notable exception is the hemangiosarcoma where the metastatic pulmonary lesions more closely resemble those associated with epithelial tumors (Fig 10). Mineralization occurs in these metastatic lesions only rarely, even if the primary

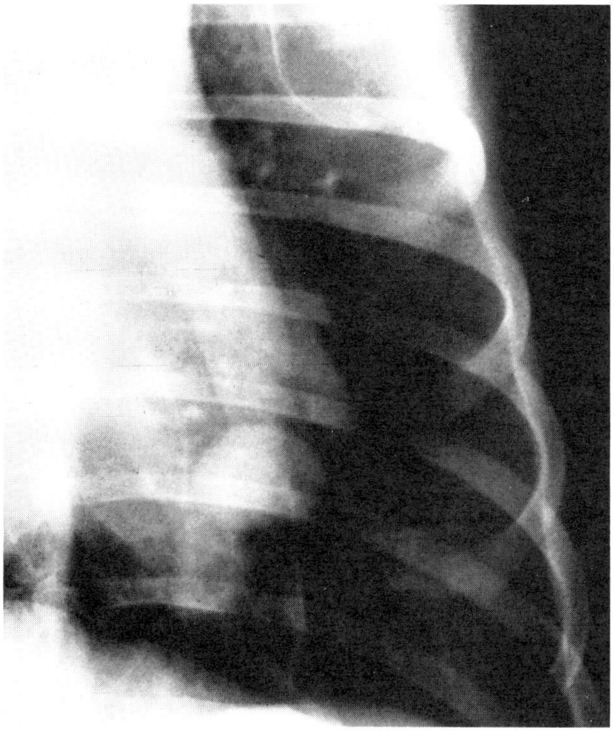

Fig 5—Ventrodorsal chest radiographs of a dog in which a large soft tissue opacity appears to be located in the left caudal lobe. This opacity is due to a large nipple. This apparent lesion would not be seen within the left caudal lobe on the lateral projection. Careful physical examination of the patient is necessary in order not to confuse such chest wall masses with pulmonary metastasis. In order to prove whether an external mass is responsible for a possible metastatic nodule, one needs only to apply a small amount of barium sulfate paste to the surface of the mass to serve as a marker.

TABLE I
Types of Interstitial Lung Disease

- MASS (>4 cm diameter)
  - Solitary
    - Cavitary
    - Non-cavitary
  - Multiple
    - Cavitary
    - Non-cavitary
- NODULE (2-4 cm diameter)
  - Solitary
    - Cavitary
    - Non-cavitary
  - Multiple
    - Cavitary
    - Non-cavitary
- MILIARY MASS (<2 cm diameter)
  - Solitary
    - Cavitary
    - Non-cavitary
  - Multiple
    - Cavitary
    - Non-cavitary
- UNSTRUCTURED LINEAR

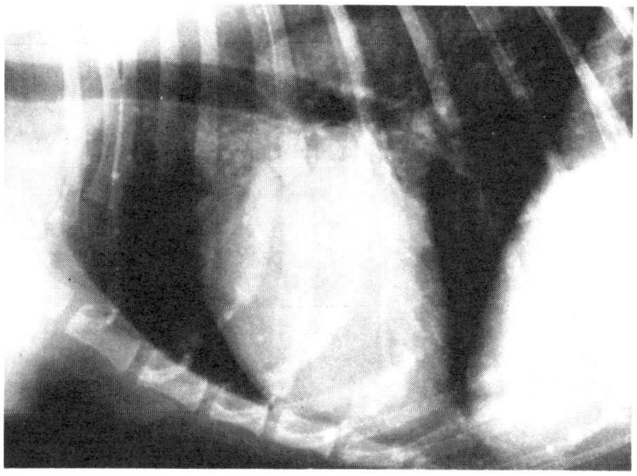

Fig 6—Lateral chest radiograph of a dog with pulmonary heterotopic bone. Numerous mineralized opacities are present in all lung lobes. These opacities should not be confused with pulmonary metastases. Pulmonary metastases rarely mineralize, particularly when the diameter of the mass is in the 1-2mm range.

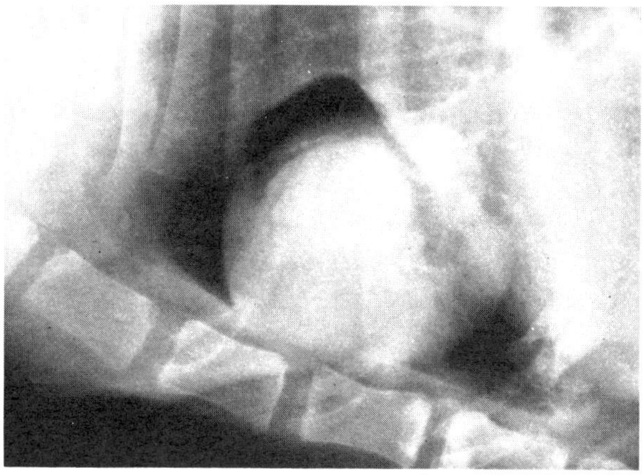

Fig 7—Close-up view of the cranial ventral lung field from a dog presented with a gingival fibrosarcoma. A large circular solitary interstitial mass is visible. No other pulmonary masses were noted. Solitary masses, nodules or miliary masses are rarely representative of pulmonary metastases. Histologic examination of this mass indicated that it was a bronchoalveolar carcinoma.

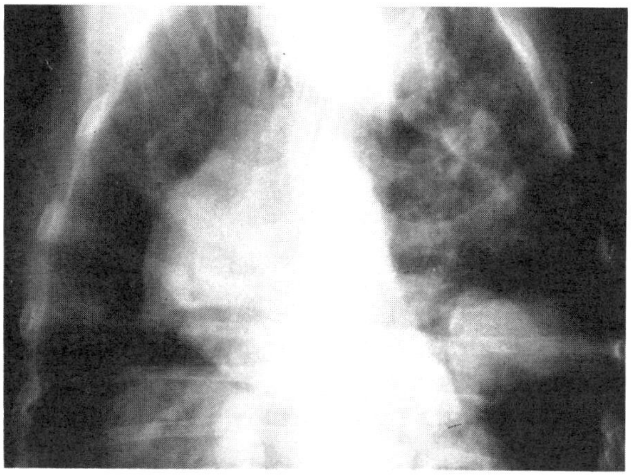

Fig 8—Ventrodorsal chest radiograph of a dog in which multiple non-cavitary pulmonary masses can be seen. This radiographic pattern is most consistent with a diagnosis of pulmonary metastases. In this case, however, the diagnosis was primary multicentric pulmonary adenocarcinoma.

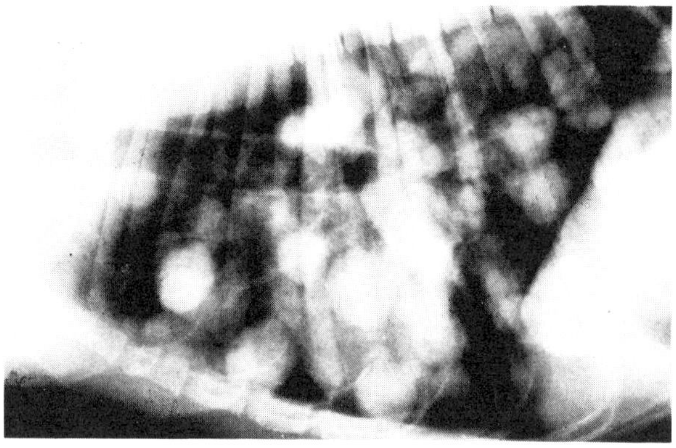

Fig 9—Lateral chest radiograph of a dog in which multiple non-cavitary pulmonary nodules can be seen. This radiographic presentation is most consistent with a diagnosis of pulmonary metastases. The diagnosis in this patient was metastatic juvenile alveolar rhabdomyosarcoma.

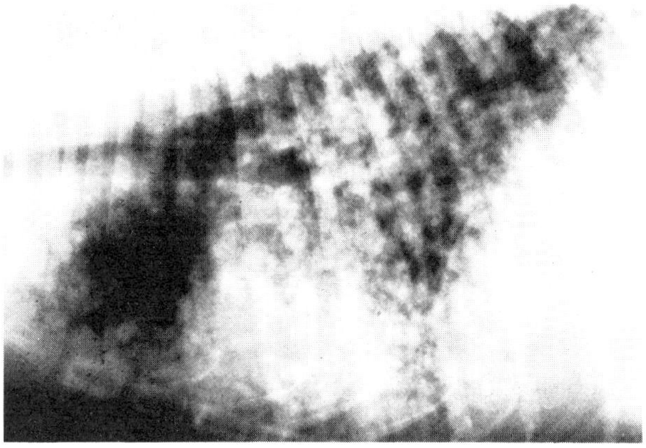

Fig 10—Lateral chest radiograph of a dog in which multiple non-cavitary pulmonary miliary masses can be seen. Pulmonary metastases must be the number one consideration when these radiographic changes are observed. Low-grade pulmonary inflammatory conditions can produce this same radiographic appearance. The diagnosis in this patient was metastatic atrial hemangiosarcoma.

tumor was an osteogenic or chondrogenic tumor. Mineralization of interstitial nodules or miliary masses occurs much more frequently when they have resulted from inflammatory causes (Fig 11). When pulmonary metastatic nodules result in the formation of pleural fluid, their detection will be more difficult because of the pulmonary collapse associated with the pleural fluid (Fig 12).

C. Pulmonary metastases must also be included in the differential diagnosis when multiple cavitary pulmonary masses, nodules (Fig 13) or miliary masses (Fig 14) are recognized. In man cavitation of metastatic lesions is not as common as with primary bronchogenic carcinoma.[7] This finding is supported by an examination of the canine and feline patients radiographed at the University of Pennsylvania. In man, cavitation occurs most often in metastatic squamous epithelial tumors where the primary tumor is most frequently located in the head and neck in men and in the genitalia in women[7].

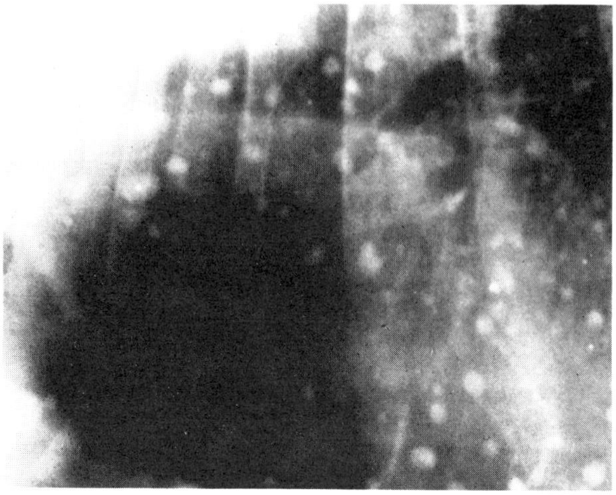

Fig 11—Close-up view of the cranial lung field of a dog in which multiple mineralized interstitial miliary masses can be seen. Mineralization of interstitial masses is usually associated with inflammatory rather than neoplastic lung disease. The radiographic pattern seen in this figure should not be confused with heterotopic bone due to the relatively large size of these lesions. The diagnosis in this patient was chronic histoplasmosis.

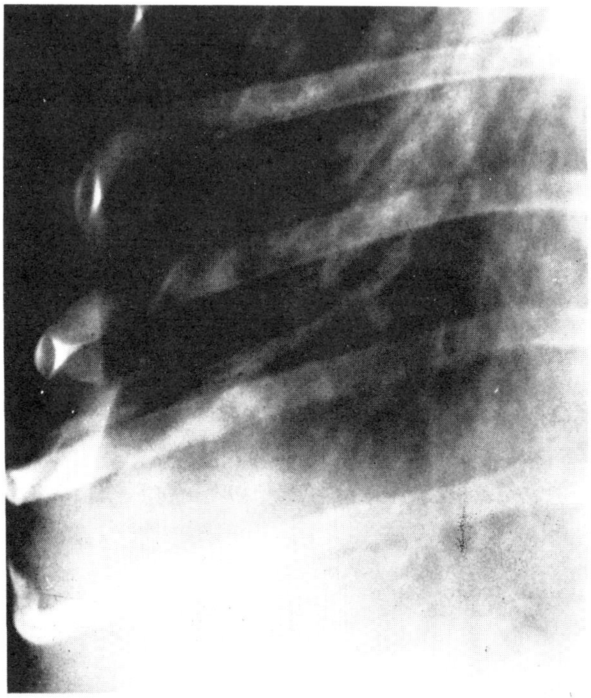

Fig 12—Close-up view of the caudal aspect of the right caudal lung lobe region of a dog. The retraction of the lung lobes away from the chest wall and the distinct visualization of interlobar fissures indicate the presence of fluid in the pleural space. Close observation of the pulmonary parenchyma also reveals the presence of small interstitial miliary masses. The detection of pulmonary metastases is more difficult when fluid is present in the pleural space because of the pulmonary collapse associated with the pleural fluid. Diagnosis: metastatic hemangiosarcoma.

The character of the wall of the cavity may be helpful in narrowing the list of differential diagnoses of multiple cavitary masses. These include multicentric cavitary primary lung tumor, paragonimiasis (Fig 15), traumatic lung bullae (Fig 16) and abscesses (Fig 17). A nodular wall, multiple holes and eccentric excavation suggest malignant tumor but none of these signs is consistently reliable[8] (Figs 13, 15, 17). Infarction, infection necrosis, autophagia and sebaceous or serous secretions by the tumor are all possible mechanisms for the development of cavitation.

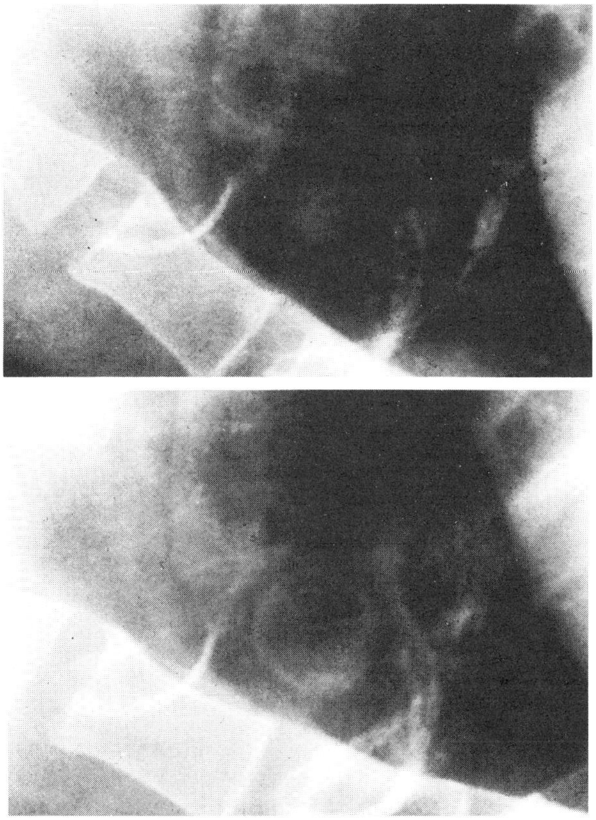

Fig 13—(A) A close-up view of the cranioventral portion of the chest of a dog in which a solid interstitial nodule, due to metastasis of a mammary carcinoma, can be seen. Other interstitial nodules were present throughout the lungs. (B) Follow-up radiograph made 2 months after that seen in (A). The nodule has increased significantly in size and it is now cavitary. During this interval, the patient had been receiving chemotherapy. Possibly the cavitation is due to necrosis associated with chemotherapy or may be spontaneous.

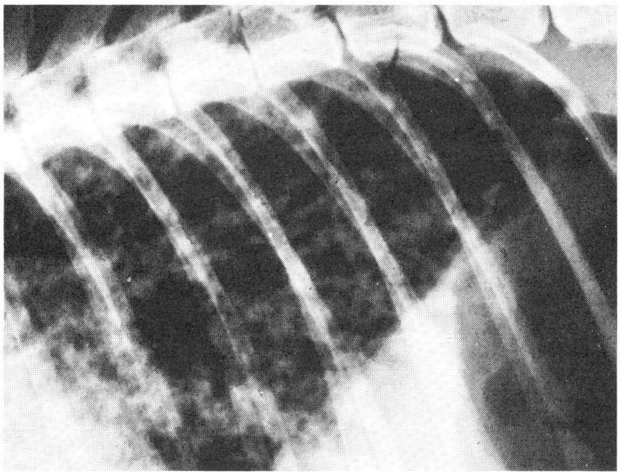

Fig 14—Close-up view of the dorsocaudal lung field of a cat. Multiple cavitary interstitial miliary masses are visible. This radiographic pattern is most consistent with a diagnosis of pulmonary metastases, however inflammatory lung disease cannot be totally ruled out. The diagnosis in this patient was metastatic adenocarcinoma with cavitation.

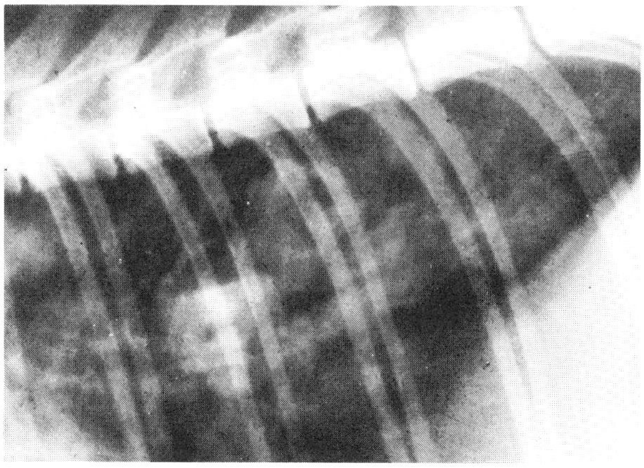

Fig 15—Close-up of the dorsal lung field of a cat. Multiple interstitial nodules with cavitation can be seen. Although metastatic neoplasia must be considered in the differential diagnosis, a more likely consideration is pulmonary infestation by the lung fluke Paragonimus.

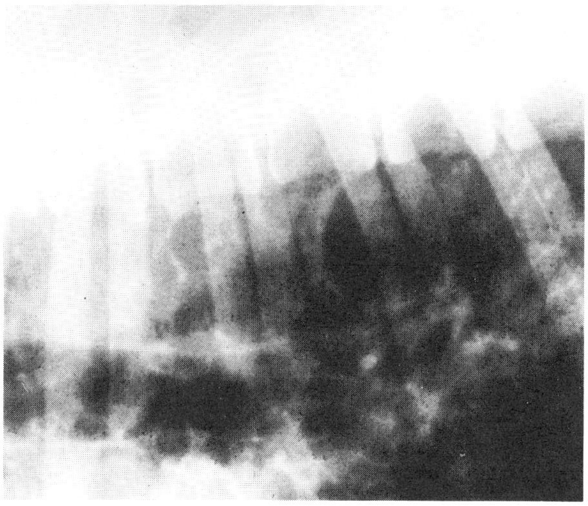

Fig 16—Close-up of the mid dorsal lung region of a dog. Three distinct circumscribed cavitary interstitial nodules are present. This dog had been struck by a car approximately one year prior to the time that this radiograph was made. Most likely these cavitary lesions represent traumatic lung bullae. However, the diagnosis of cavitary pulmonary metastases cannot be totally eliminated radiographically.

D. In a small number of instances the radiographic pattern produced in the lung by metastatic tumor will be an unstructured linear pattern (Figs 18, 19). In the human medical literature, many publications have referred to this condition as *pulmonary lymphangitic metastasis*. The name implies

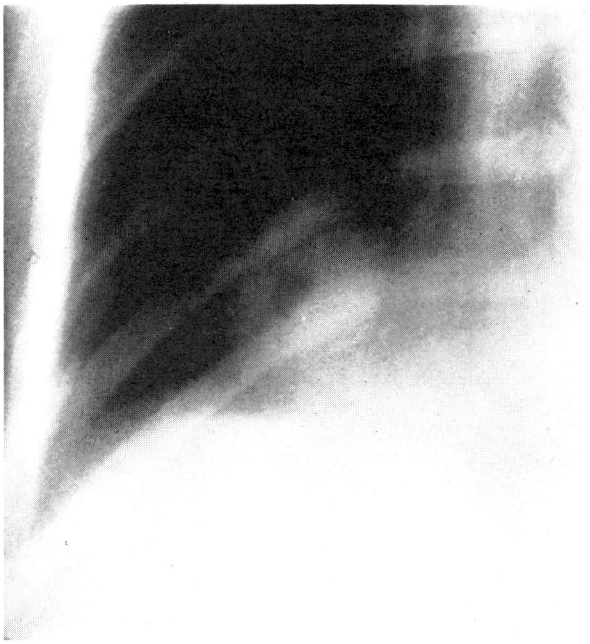

Fig 17—Tomogram of the caudal aspect of the right caudal lobe of a dog. An interstitial nodule with eccentric cavitation is apparent. The histologic diagnosis of this nodule was pulmonary abscess.

that the radiographic pattern of linear interstitial opacities seen in this condition is due to neoplastic infiltration of pulmonary lymphatics. It was thought that the tumor cells progressed in a retrograde fashion into pulmonary lymphatics from the hilar lymph nodes. It is difficult to accept this as fact since, in man, the hilar lymph nodes are not neoplastic in every instance. Also, migration of tumor cells against the flow of lymph is unlikely[9].

A more reasonable consideration is that the linear interstitial opacities observed radiographically result from disseminated intravascular tumor embolization. The tumor cells which are

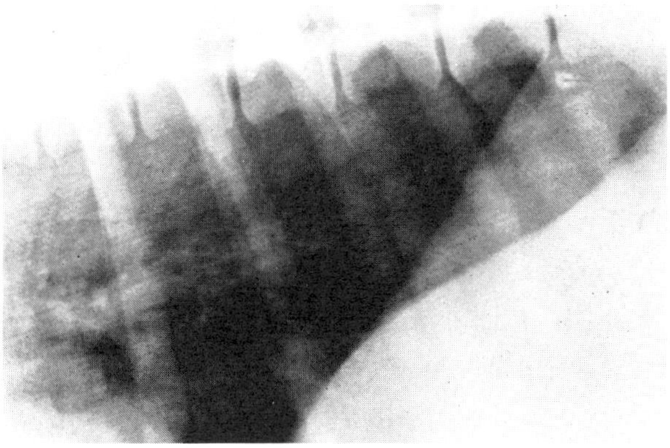

Fig 18—Close-up of the dorsal caudal lung field of a dog. A diffuse linear pulmonary interstitial opacity is apparent. This is an atypical pulmonary manifestation of metastatic neoplasia. The primary tumor in this patient was a schirrous mammary adenocarcinoma. (Reprinted, with permission of the editor, from the Journal of the American Veterinary Radiological Society, 19: 161-167, 1978).

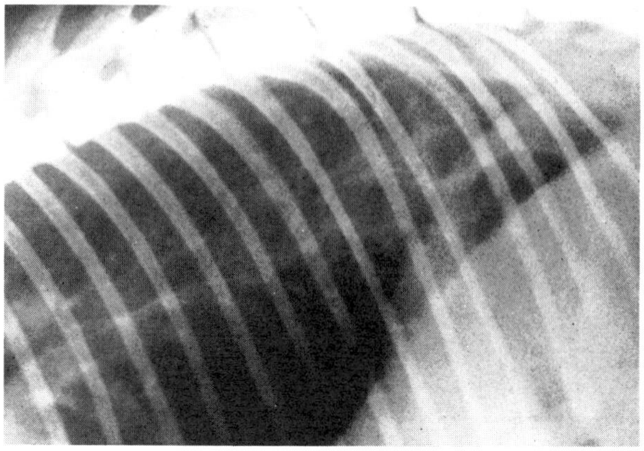

Fig 19—Close-up of the dorsocaudal lung field of a cat. An ill-defined area of increased linear interstitial opacity is noted just cranial to the left diaphragmatic crus. This is an atypical form of pulmonary metastatic neoplasia. The primary tumor in this patient was a mammary adenocarcinoma.

noted histologically to be intralymphatic probably were taken up from the interstitium following capillary extravasation.[10] A review of the pathonogenesis of this type of metastasis in the dog, along with four case reports, has recently been published.[11] In man carcinoma of the breast is the most common primary neoplasm producing this type of metastasis.[10] It appears the same is true in the dog and the cat.

Alveolar and Bronchial Lung Disease in Metastasis—The radiographic signs of alveolar and bronchial lung diseases are well known.[5] Rarely, pulmonary metastases produce alveolar or bronchial lung patterns.

A. When pulmonary metastatic lung disease results in the production of an alveolar pattern, the alveolar opacity may be either localized or generalized. This radiographic pattern may be due to complicating factors such as pulmonary infection or pulmonary hemorrhage which typically result in

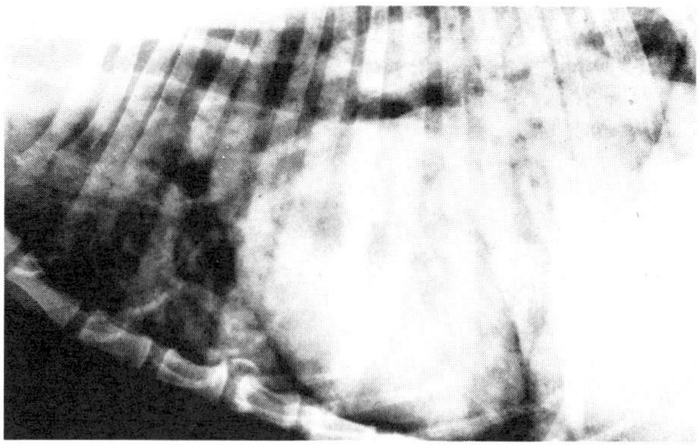

Fig 20—In this lateral chest radiograph of a dog, a diffuse increase in pulmonary opacity is present. The pulmonary opacity is predominantly alveolar in nature. Interstitial nodules are visible superimposed over the cardiac apex. This is a most unusual radiographic appearance of metastatic pulmonary neoplasia. The diagnosis was metastatic adrenal adenocarcinoma. The alveolar pulmonary opacity is due to extravasation of tumor cells from the capillaries into the alveolar spaces.

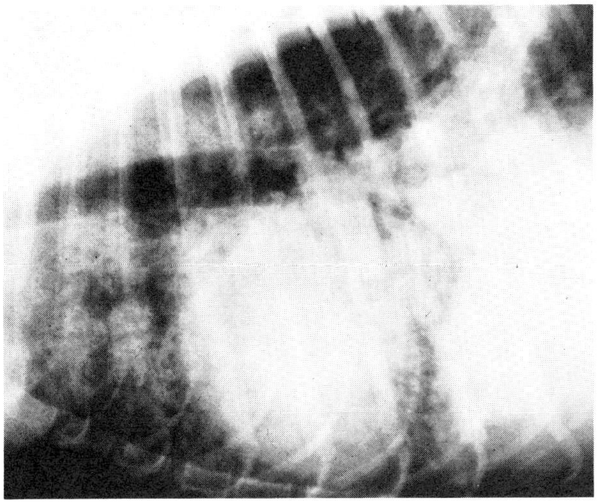

Fig 21—Lateral chest radiograph of a dog in which a diffuse increase in pulmonary opacity is apparent. The pulmonary opacity is predominantly alveolar in nature, although some nodularity is suggested. Note the similarity to Fig 20. The diagnosis in this patient was pulmonary edema secondary to acute left heart failure.

the filling of the alveolar spaces with exudate or blood respectively.

On the other hand, the alveolar opacity produced may be due to extension of the metastatic tumor cells from the pulmonary interstitium into the alveolar spaces. In such instances, an alveolar pattern will be apparent radiographically (Fig 20), and the overall appearance of the lung may not be significantly different than in other alveolar diseases of non-neoplastic origin (Fig 21). When an alveolar process is observed radiographically, the diseases considered as likely causes usually include inflammatory lung disease, intrapulmonary hemorrhage and pulmonary edema. However, in some cases, the underlying cause will be neoplastic, either primary or secondary, and this possibility must always be considered in the differential diagnosis.

B. The production of a bronchial type of pulmonary opacity in association with pulmonary metastatic lung disease is very rare. This pattern of metastases may be a form of disseminated intravascular tumor embolization,[11] or peribronchial spread of metastatic disease originating from interstitial, vascular or endobronchial metastases. In most patients the recognition of abnormal bronchial opacities will be indicative of chronic bronchial inflammatory disease. In some cases, however, the underlying cause will be a tumor (Fig 22).

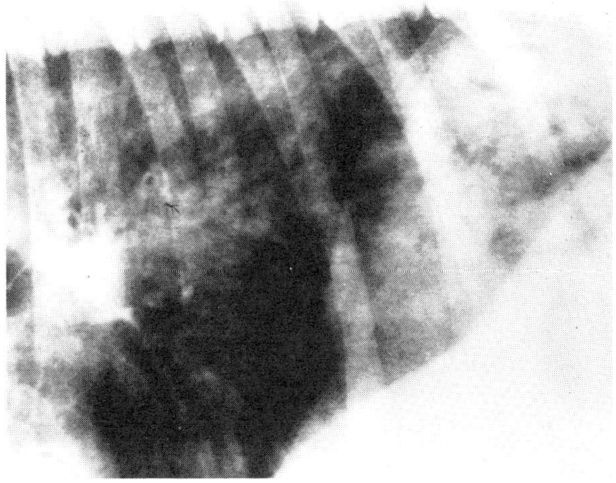

Fig 22—Close-up of the dorsocaudal lung field of a dog in which a diffuse increase in pulmonary opacity is noted. The opacity is predominantly bronchial and interstitial in nature. This radiographic appearance is most consistent with inflammatory lung disease, however metastatic tumor must also be considered. The histologic diagnosis in this patient was metastatic mammary adenocarcinoma. (Reprinted, with permission of the editor, from the Journal of the American Veterinary Radiological Society, 19: 161-67, 1978).

REFERENCES

1. Biery, D.N.: Differentiation of Lung Diseases of Inflammatory or Neoplastic Origin from Lung Disease in Heart Failure. Vet Clin N Am, 4, (1974): 711-721.
2. Spratt, J.S., Jr., Ter-Pogossian, M., and Long, R.T.: The Detection and Growth of Intrathoracic Neoplasms: the Lower Limits of Radiographic Distinction of the Antemortem Size, the Duration and the Pattern of Growth as Determined by Direct Mensuration of Tumor Diameter from Random Thoracic Roentgenograms. Arch Surg, 86, (1963): 283-288.
3. Weiss, W., Boucot, K.P. and Cooper, D.A.: The Survival of Men with Measurable Proved Lung Cancer in Relation to Growth Rate. Am J Roentgen Rad Ther Nucl Med, 98, (1966): 404-415.
4. Reif, J.S. and Rhodes, W.H.: The Lungs of Aged Dogs: a Radiographic Morphologic Correlation. J Am Vet Radiol Soc, 7, (1966): 5-11.
5. Suter, P.F. and Lord, P.F.: Radiographic Differentiation of Disseminated Pulmonary Parenchymal Diseases in Dogs and Cats. Vet Clin N Am., 4, (1974): 687-710.
6. Paglicci, A.: Metastatic Tumours of the Lung: A Study of 152 Cases. Radiol Med (Tor), 42, (1956): 184-192.
7. Fraser, R.G. and Pare, J.A.P.: *Diagnosis of Diseases of the Chest*, W.B. Saunders, Co., Philadelphia, 1973, pg. 801.
8. Felson, B.: *Chest Roentgenology*, W. B. Saunders, Philadelphia, PA, (1973): 319.
9. Heitzman, E.R.: *The Lung: Radiologic Pathologic Correlations*, C.V. Mosby, St. Louis, (1973): 329.
10. Fichera, G. and Hagerstrand, J.: The Small Lymph Vessels of the Lungs in Lymphangiosa Carcinomatosa. Act Path Microbiol Scand, 65, (1967): 505-513.
11. Adams, W.M. and Dubeilzig, R.: Diffuse Pulmonary Alveolar Septal Metastasis from Mammary Carcinoma in the Dog. J Am Vet Radiol Soc, 19, (1978): 161-167.

UPDATE

The review of metastatic pulmonary neoplasia presented in this paper remains correct. Radiographic technique is the only area that deserves comment. In the paper, specific recommendations for radiographic positioning were not made. Since this paper was published, studies have shown that lung masses in the dependent lung can be more difficult to visualize than lesions in the nondependent lung.[1,2] This is a result of the dependent lung being less aerated, and therefore reduced in volume, because of the effects of gravity. The decreased volume of the dependent lobe increases opacity, and the more opaque lung will have a tendency to silhouette, making detection of soft tissue lesions more difficult. It is therefore suggested that both right and left lateral views, in addition to either the dorsoventral or ventrodorsal view, be routinely made to optimize the chance of identifying pulmonary mass lesions.

This principle has been recently challenged. A study of various radiographic protocols for detecting pulmonary metastases concluded that both lateral views are not necessary when routinely screening dogs with cancer for pulmonary metastasis.[3] The tumor burden in dogs in that study was not apparent from the paper. When multiple nodules are present, some will very likely be seen when only one lateral view is made; however, in those patients in which only one or a few small lung nodules are present, it seems reasonable that making both lateral views will enhance the likelihood of a mass being detected. Because the size and number of lung nodules cannot be determined before radiography, the routine use of both lateral views in addition to the ventrodorsal or dorsoventral view is, in my opinion, still justified.

REFERENCES

1. Pechman RD: Effect of dependency versus nondependency on lung lesion visualization. *Vet Radiol* 28:185–190, 1987.
2. Spencer CP, Ackerman N, Burt JK: The canine lateral thoracic radiograph. *Vet Radiol* 22:262–266, 1981.
3. Barthez PY, Hornof WJ, Théon AP, et al: Receiver operating characteristic curve analysis of the performance of various radiographic protocols when screening dogs for pulmonary metastases. *JAVMA* 204:237–240, 1994.

Bronchoesophageal Fistula in the Dog: Literature Survey, Case Presentations, and Radiographic Manifestations

Richard D. Park, DVM, PhD
Department of Radiology
and Radiation Biology
Colorado State University
Fort Collins, Colorado

A bronchoesophageal fistula is a patent communication between the esophagus and bronchus. When such a fistula is present, ingested material can pass into the bronchi and lungs, and pulmonary secretions can pass into the digestive tract. Bronchoesophageal fistulas have been reported only rarely in the dog.[1-5] A bronchoesophageal fistula in the cat[6] and tracheoesophageal fistulas in the dog and cat[7-11] have been reported, but these appear to occur less frequently than bronchoesophageal fistulas do in dogs.

Because of its chronic nature and insidious onset and the nonspecificity of the clinical signs of a bronchoesophageal fistula, the disease may go undiagnosed. The radiographic manifestations of the disease can be rather distinct, and confirmation of the disease with an esophagram can be most rewarding.

In this article, previously reported cases of bronchoesophageal fistula are reviewed, and three additional cases seen at the Colorado State University Veterinary Teaching Hospital (VTH) from 1976 to 1982 are presented. The causes, pathogenesis, clinical and radiographic manifestations, and possible treatment of the disease are reviewed and discussed.

Methods

Eight cases of bronchoesophageal fistula in the dog were found in the literature with a computer search[12] of English language reports from 1966 through 1982. (Bibliographies of these papers were checked for earlier reports.) The clinical and radiographic manifestations of these cases plus those of three cases reported from the Colorado State University VTH are summarized in Tables I and II. Diagnostic documentation of the cases required either an esophagram, a combination of bronchoscopy and esophagoscopy, surgical observation, necropsy, or any combinatior of these techniques.

Case Reports

Case 1

A seven-year-old female Pekapoo was presented to the Colorado State University VTH with a chronic cough of one year's duration. The dog

Originally published in Volume 6, Number 7, July 1984

had coughing episodes at two- to three-week intervals. Treatment by a veterinarian included broad-spectrum antibiotics and steroids. The cough was alleviated only during treatment.

On physical examination, the body temperature and respiration were normal. Harsh bronchial lung sounds were heard on auscultation over the right and left caudal thorax. The dog was observed to cough immediately after drinking water.

Survey thoracic radiographs revealed a bronchial pattern in the caudal lung lobes and an abnormal radiopaque segmental bronchus outlined on the lateral view. A small amount of pleural fluid and lung opacity were also present (Figure 1).

An esophagram was made with an oral iodinated contrast agent (Gastrografin®—E.R. Squibb & Sons). An esophageal traction diverticulum was identified in the caudal esophagus, along with opacification of the intermediate lung lobe bronchus (Figure 2). Under fluoroscopy with image intensification, the contrast material was noted to remain only momentarily in the bronchus before the animal would cough and expel it into the esophagus. The cough prevented good bronchial opacification with the contrast material.

Surgery was performed and the fistula was successfully identified and closed, as demonstrated with a follow-up esophagram four days postsurgery. The dog was released to the owner and was not returned for further follow-up.

Case 2

A two-year-old, spayed female poodle-terrier crossbreed was presented to the Colorado State University VTH with a chronic cough of eight months' duration. The cough was noted most after exercise or after drinking water. A veterinarian had treated it with broad-spectrum antibiotics, which relieved the cough while the dog was on treatment. The dog would have two- to three-day intervals of lethargy and anorexia, after which it would consume large quantities of food.

On physical examination, the dog was alert and appeared normal with the exception of a productive cough. Body temperature was normal, and no abnormal lung sounds were heard on thoracic auscultation. The

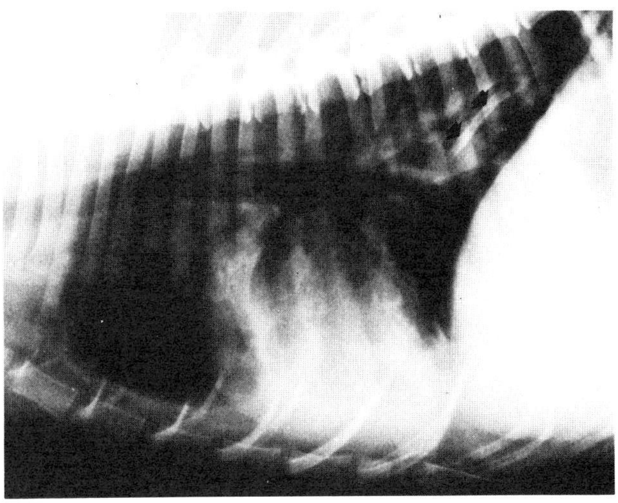

Figure 1—A lateral survey thoracic radiograph of Case 1. An abnormal increased bronchial pattern is present in the caudal dorsal lung field with a radiopaque segmental bronchus (*arrows*). Pleural fluid and mild lung changes project as an increased radiopacity over the ventral aspect of the heart.

TABLE I

Clinical Manifestations of Bronchoesophageal Fistula

Case[a]	*Age (yr)*	*Breed*	*Sex*	*Clinical Signs*
1	7	Pekapoo	Female	Coughing after drinking liquids
2	2	Poodle-terrier cross	Female (spayed)	Coughing after drinking liquids, anorexia, pyrexia
3	½	Lhasa apso	Female	Regurgitation for 5 days
4[1]	3½	Miniature poodle	Female	Coughing after eating and drinking, anorexia, pyrexia
5[3]	NR[b]	NR	NR	Gagging, anorexia, pyrexia
6[2]	2	Terrier cross	Female (spayed)	Coughing, pyrexia, depression, lameness (hypertrophic pulmonary osteopathy)
7[1]	6	Jack Russell terrier	Male	Coughing, anorexia, pyrexia, regurgitation, dyspnea
8[4]	2	Cairn terrier	Female	Coughing, retching
9[4]	5	Miniature dachshund	Female	Coughing, anorexia, regurgitation
10[1]	4	Cairn terrier	Male	Coughing, anorexia, dyspnea
11[5]	5	Miniature poodle	Female (spayed)	Coughing after drinking liquids, gagging, retching

[a]Cases 1 through 3 were reported by the Colorado State University Veterinary Teaching Hospital. Reference sources for other cases are given following the case numbers.
[b]NR = not reported.

TABLE II
Radiographic Manifestations of Bronchoesophageal Fistula

	Survey Radiographs				*Esophagram*	
Case[a]	*Lung Density Alveolar, Bronchial, and/or Interstitial*	*Lung Density Location*	*Radiopaque Esophageal Foreign Body*	*Pleural Fluid*	*Esophageal Diverticulum*	*Contrast Opacification of Bronchus*
1	+	Right caudal and left caudal	-	+	+	+
2	+	Right caudal and intermediate	-	-	+	+
3	+	Right caudal	+	-	+	+
4[1]	+	Right caudal	-	+	+	+
5[3]	+	Right caudal	+	-	NR[b]	NR
6[2]	+	Right caudal and intermediate; left caudal cyst	+	-	+	+
7[1]	+	Right caudal	-	-	+	+
8[1]	+	Right caudal	+	-	+	NR
9[1]	+	Right caudal	+	-	+	+
10[1]	+	Right caudal	+	+	+	NR
11[5]	-	-	+	-	-	+

[a]Cases 1 through 3 were reported by the Colorado State University Veterinary Teaching Hospital. Reference sources for the other cases are given following the case numbers.
[b]NR = not reported.

white blood cell count and serum chemistry profile were normal.

An abnormal, focal interstitial lung density in the intermediate and right caudal lung lobe areas was observed on survey thoracic radiographs (Figure 3).

An esophagram was made with liquid consistency (30% weight/volume) barium sulfate. Barium outlined an esophageal traction diverticulum and filled the right

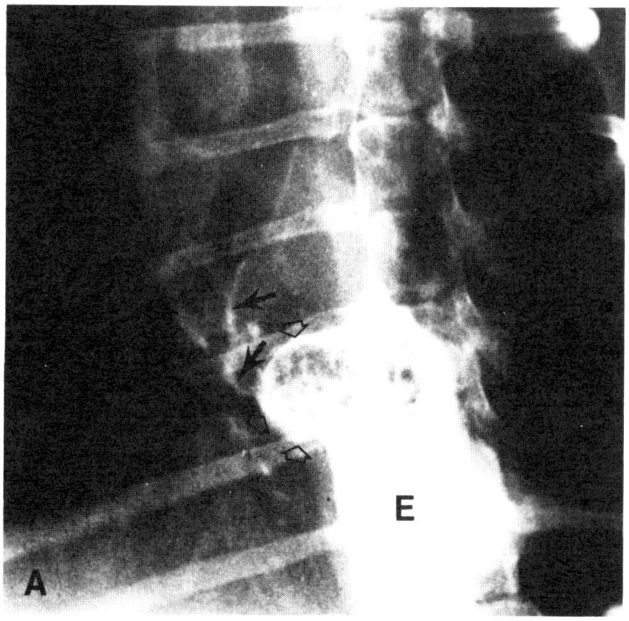

Figure 2A

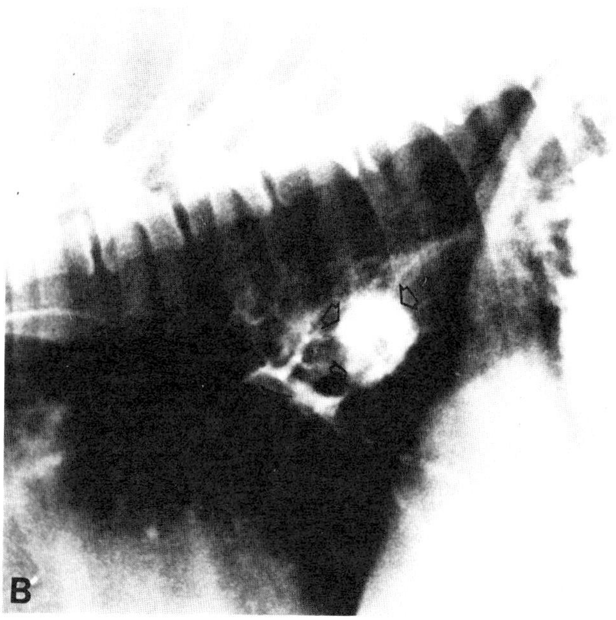

Figure 2B

Figure 2—Ventrodorsal (**A**) and lateral (**B**) 70-mm spot film radiographs of an esophagram. The esophagus (*E*) and a traction diverticulum (*open arrows*) are filled with iodinated contrast material. Bronchi to the right caudal and intermediate lung lobes are faintly seen on the ventrodorsal view and are seen with good opacification of the intermediate bronchus on the lateral view (*solid arrows*).

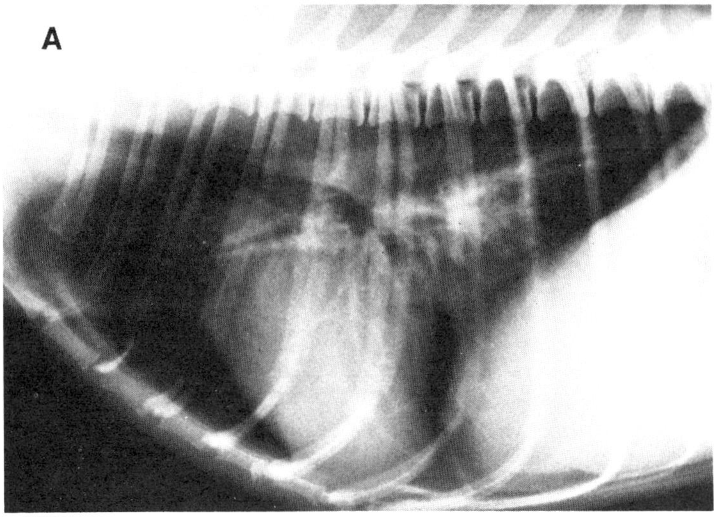

Figure 3A

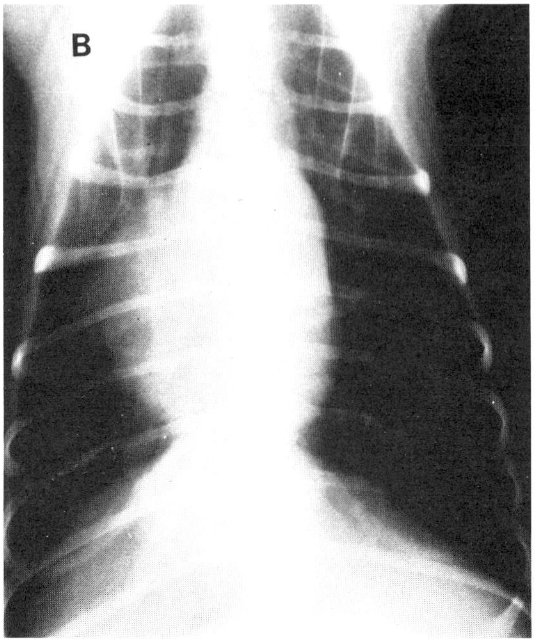

Figure 3B

Figure 3—Lateral (**A**) and ventrodorsal (**B**) survey thoracic radiographs of Case 2. There is an abnormal focal interstitial lung pattern in the caudal lungs between the heart and diaphragm on the lateral view. The lung density is not as easily seen on the ventrodorsal view but is situated to the right of the midline in the caudal thorax.

main-stem bronchus through a fistula connecting the right main-stem bronchus and the traction diverticulum (Figure 4).

Surgery was not performed, and the dog was lost to further follow-up.

Case 3

A six-month-old female lhasa apso was presented to the Colorado State University VTH because for the previous five days it had regurgitated immediately after eating.

On physical examination, the dog appeared to be depressed but otherwise normal. The white blood cell count and serum chemistry profile were normal.

On a survey thoracic radiograph, an opaque foreign body was observed in the area of the caudal esophagus (Figure 5). Esophageal endoscopy was performed and a foreign body consisting of bone was pushed into the stomach.

Four days following esophageal endoscopy, a barium esophagram was made to check esophageal function. During the examination, barium was observed opacifying right caudal and intermediate lung lobe bronchi (Figure 6).

At surgery, a fibrotic area approximately 0.25 cm in diameter was observed between the esophagus and right lung lobe pleura. This area was ligated and transected. No complications or other esophageal problems were observed on a follow-up esophagram three days after surgery. The dog had no further complications and was discharged to the owner.

Causes and Pathogenesis

Both congenital and acquired bronchoesophageal fistulas have been reported in the dog.[1-5] Most cases reported have been acquired; however, three cases appeared to be congenital.[2,4]

Congenital bronchoesophageal fistulas result from an incomplete separation of the tracheobronchial tree from the digestive tract, from which it is formed embryologically.[13]

Criteria previously proposed to differentiate congenital from acquired fistulas are based on histologic eval-

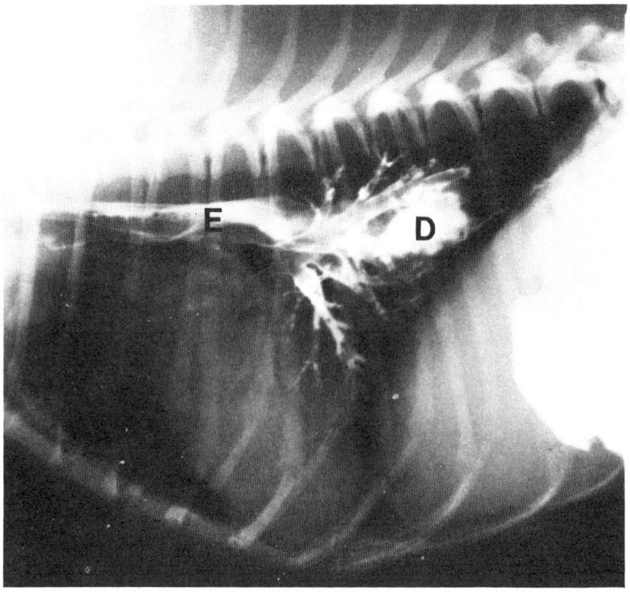

Figure 4—A lateral thoracic radiograph with a barium esophagram. Barium is present in the esophagus (*E*) and fills a traction diverticulum seen on end (*D*). The right caudal and intermediate lung lobe bronchi are opacified with barium.

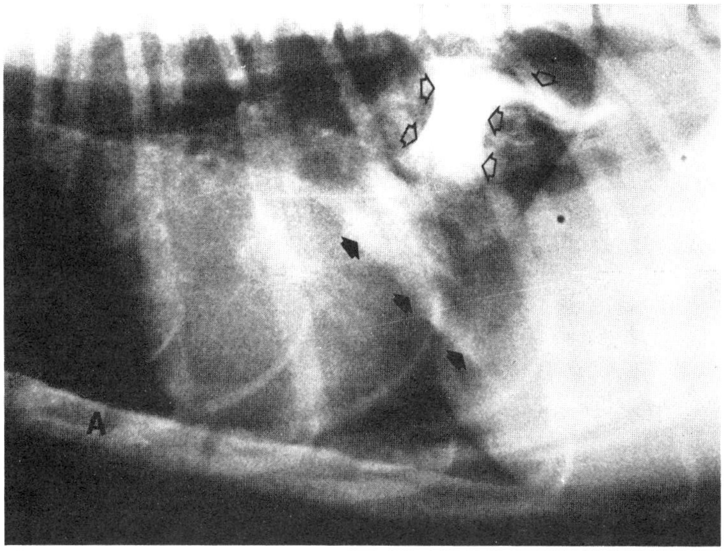

Figure 5A

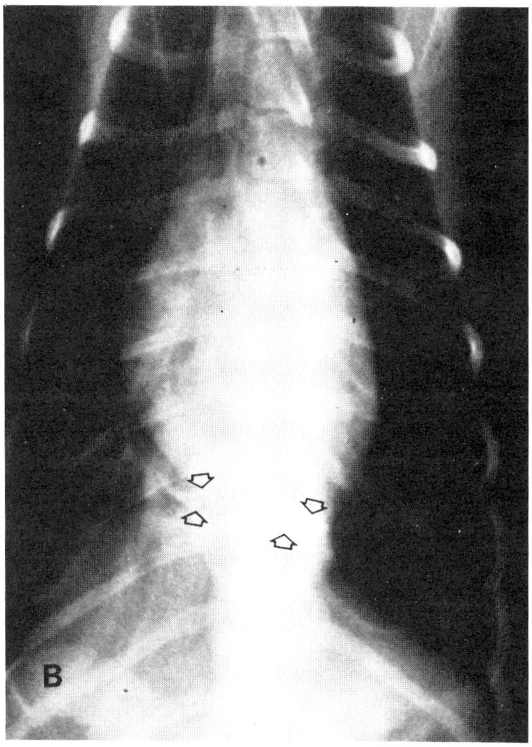

Figure 5B

Figure 5—Lateral (**A**) and ventrodorsal (**B**) thoracic radiographs of Case 3. An esophageal foreign body consisting of bone is present in the caudal esophagus (*open arrows*). A mixed alveolar-interstitial lung pattern is present in the right caudal lung lobe. The cranial border of the right caudal lung lobe is evident on the lateral view (*solid arrows*) because of fluid accumulation within the lung. These changes are compatible with a localized pneumonia secondary to the bronchoesophageal fistula.

uation.[13,14] The following have been proposed in humans as criteria defining a congenital fistula: (1) The fistula is lined with squamous epithelium or columnar epithelium, ciliated or nonciliated; (2) no inflammatory reaction is present around the fistula.

Congenital fistulas reported in the dog have had epithelial lining as described above but have also had inflammatory reaction surrounding them.[2,4]

Acquired bronchoesophageal fistulas in humans have been reported to result from malignancies, infection, and trauma.[15-18] The infections causing fistulas are generally pulmonary with secondary invasion into the

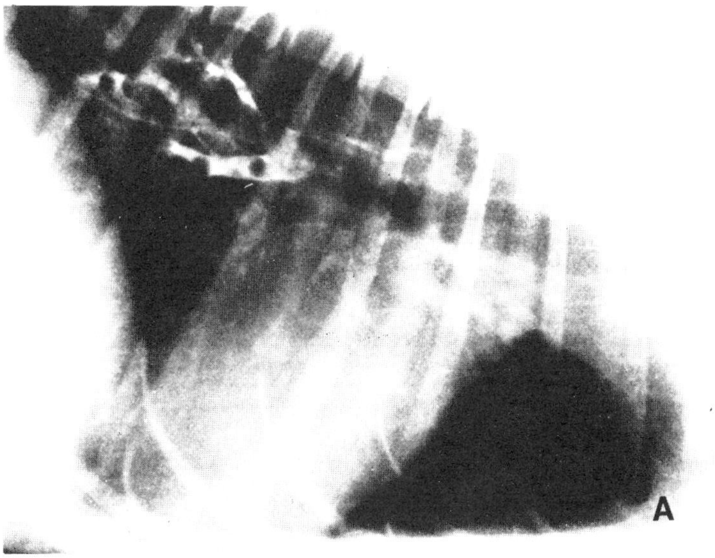

Figure 6A

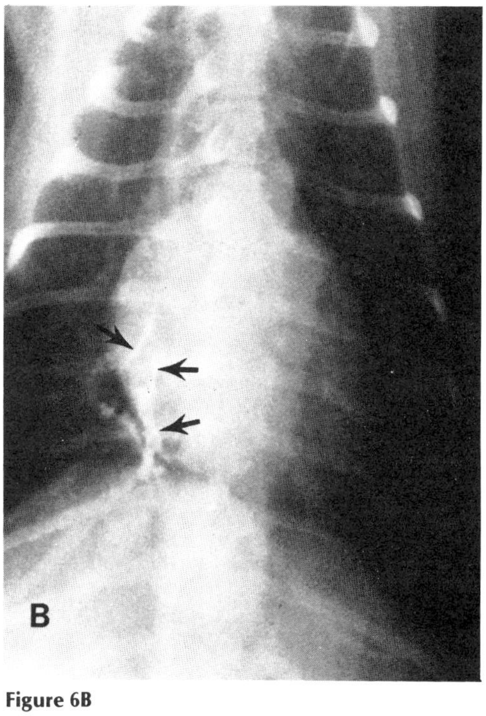

Figure 6B

Figure 6—Lateral (**A**) and ventrodorsal (**B**) thoracic radiographs made immediately after oral administration of barium sulfate. The bronchi to the right caudal and intermediate lung lobes are opacified with barium.

esophagus. The trauma may be external, the result of crushing or shearing injuries, or internal, caused by esophageal foreign bodies, caustic chemical ingestion, or tracheal intubations. In humans, malignancy-caused fistulas are four to five times more common than those produced by trauma.[19] In the dog, trauma associated with esophageal foreign bodies seems to be the most prevalent cause of bronchoesophageal fistulas. Most bronchoesophageal fistulas in the dog resulting from esophageal foreign bodies connect the esophagus with either the bronchus to the right caudal lung lobe or the bronchus to the intermediate lung lobe (Table II). Esophageal foreign bodies frequently localize in the caudal esophagus. The close anatomic proximity of the caudal esophagus and bronchi may be an important factor contributing to the high incidence of fistulas in this location.[1]

An esophageal foreign body and diverticulum are present in most cases of bronchoesophageal fistula in the dog. The pathogenesis of acquired bronchoesophageal fistulas is questionable and may not be the same for all cases. It is believed that the most common sequence of events leading to the creation of a bronchoesophageal fistula begins with an esophageal foreign body that causes esophageal wall necrosis. The necrotic reaction progresses to form a bronchoesophageal fistula, and an esophageal traction diverticulum results from the inflammatory reaction between the esophagus and bronchi. This sequence of events may be completed within a few days. It is also possible that an esophageal diverticulum, either congenital or acquired, may be already present before the acquired bronchoesophageal fistula forms. An esophageal diverticulum could result in a foreign body accumulation within the diverticulum, which would progress to cause esophageal wall necrosis and a bronchoesophageal fistula.

With congenital fistulas, the esophageal diverticulum can result from the fistula, and foreign material may then accumulate in the diverticulum.

Secondary complications that may occur with bronchoesophageal fistulas are localized pneumonias, pulmonary abscesses, and pleuritis. The severity of the secondary complications usually depends on duration and size of the fistula.

Manifestations

Clinical and radiographic signs of bronchoesophageal fistulas must be recognized and considered together to arrive at a provisional diagnosis. An esophagram should be used to confirm or reject the provisional diagnosis.

The clinical manifestations and characteristics of bronchoesophageal fistulas are listed in Table I.

All dogs reported to have a bronchoesophageal fistula were of small or miniature breeds between six months and seven years of age. No distinction based on age could be made between congenital and acquired cases. This finding corresponds to findings in humans where congenital fistulas are usually not apparent until the second decade of life.[19]

Eight affected dogs were female, two were male, and the sex of one was not reported. Although it appears that bronchoesophageal fistulas are most common in females, more documented cases would be necessary to confirm this finding.

The most common clinical signs observed with bronchoesophageal fistulas were coughing, regurgitation, lethargy, anorexia, pyrexia, dyspnea, and weight loss—with coughing the predominant sign. Although several cases of coughing immediately after drinking liquids were reported, this sign was not present in all cases. The presence of a cough after drinking liquids may depend on such factors as the size, location, and direction of the fistula. Large fistulas directed caudally and/or ventrally from the esophagus produce a more consistent cough than small fistulas directed cranially and/or dorsally.

Regurgitation occurred in some cases with an esophageal foreign body, but this sign was not observed consistently in all cases.

Anorexia, lethargy, and pyrexia were seen frequently and probably resulted from the secondary pulmonary and pleural changes.

The radiographic manifestations of bronchoesophageal fistulas on survey films consisted of localized alveolar, bronchial, and/or interstitial lung patterns, radiopaque esophageal foreign bodies, and pleural fluid (Table II).

A localized alveolar, bronchial, and/or interstitial lung pattern was observed in 10 of 11 cases. All of these cases had involvement in the right caudal and/or intermediate lung lobes, with two cases having additional changes in the left caudal lung lobes. One case with left caudal lung lobe involvement was reported as a congenital fistula,[2] and the other appeared to be an extension of a pneumonic process from the right caudal and intermediate lung lobes.

At least one radiopaque caudal esophageal foreign body was present in 7 of 11 cases; there was no apparent difference in frequency between these foreign-body occurrences in acquired and congenital fistulas.

Pleural fluid was present in 3 of 11 cases and may have been present secondary to the localized pulmonary infectious conditions or as an extension of the inflammatory reaction around the fistula.

After observing the above clinical and survey radiographic signs, an esophagram should be made to confirm or refute the suspected diagnosis. An esophagram has been shown to be the most reliable method for diagnosing bronchoesophageal fistulas in humans.[16,18,20] An esophagram demonstrated a fistula in eight cases covered in this report. In the remaining three cases, an esophagram was not done or the results were not reported.

An esophagram should be made with a thin mixture of barium sulfate (20 to 30% weight/volume). The thin consistency of the contrast medium facilitates filling of small fistulas better than barium of thick consistency or barium mixed with food could. Oral iodinated contrast agents should not be used to demonstrate a suspected fistula because they are hypertonic and can produce a localized pulmonary edema if they enter the lung. Oral iodinated contrast agents are also more irritating to bronchi and might elicit a cough, which would result in poor opacification of the fistula and/or bronchi.

Large fistulas are easily demonstrated because contrast material readily enters a bronchus from the esophagus.

Small fistulas are more difficult to demonstrate. Fluoroscopy with some form of video recording is helpful in diagnosing small fistulas or fistulas directed cranially and/or dorsally from the esophagus. In these cases, contrast medium may only momentarily fill the bronchus. In some cases with a small fistula, it may be necessary to get the esophagram with the animal in different recumbent positions to facilitate gravitation of the contrast medium into or through the fistula.

An esophagram produced with fluoroscopy also facilitates differentiating a fistula from contrast material that may have been aspirated as a result of improper administration of barium or as a result of various pharyngeal dysphagias.

A traction esophageal diverticulum was present in 9 of 10 cases; there was no record of an esophagram in the remaining case. Because of the consistent association of caudal esophageal diverticuli and bronchoesophageal fistulas, an esophagram should be thoroughly investigated to rule out a bronchoesophageal fistula when a caudal esophageal diverticulum is present.

In summary, when the appropriate clinical and radiographic signs are present, an esophagram should be made to demonstrate or rule out a bronchoesophageal fistula.

Treatment

Surgical repair is the most successful treatment for bronchoesophageal fistulas. The prognosis may be guarded to poor if secondary complications, such as pneumonia, pulmonary abscesses, or large quantities of pleural fluid, are present. Where such secondary complications are mild or not present, the prognosis should be good.

REFERENCES

1. Thrall DE: Esophagobronchial fistula in a dog. *J Am Vet Radiol Soc* 14:22-25, 1973.
2. Foor JC: A congenital bronchoesophageal fistula in a dog. *Minnesota Vet* 14:9-11, 1974.
3. Kleine LJ: Radiologic examination of the esophagus in dogs and cats. *Vet Clin North Am* 4:663, 1974.
4. Pearson H, Gibbs C, Kelly DF: Oesophageal diverticulum formation in the dog. *J Small Anim Pract* 19:341-355, 1978.
5. Caywood DD, Feeney DA: Acquired esophagobronchial fistula in a dog. *JAAHA* 18:590-594, 1982.
6. Reif JS: Solitary pulmonary lesions in small animals. *JAVMA* 15:717, 1969.
7. Tesic D, Dimitrijevic B: Osophagotracheal fistula in a dog and a cat. *Acta Vet (Belgrade)* 5:101-106, 1955.
8. Beitzel C, Brinker WO: Surgical removal of an esophageal foreign body which had penetrated the trachea. *JAVMA* 129:241-242, 1956.
9. Schebitz H: Rontgenbefund einer oesophago-trachealfistel nach fremdkorperperforation beim hund. *Tierärztliche Umschau* 15:87, 1960.
10. Pearson H: Symposium on conditions of the canine oesophagus—I. Foreign bodies of the oesophagus. *J Small Anim Pract* 7:107-116, 1966.
11. Dodman NH, Baker GJ: Tracheo-oesophageal fistula as a complication of an oesophageal foreign body in the dog — A case report. *J Small Anim Pract* 19:291-296, 1978.
12. Medlars II, *National Interactive Retrieval Services*, U.S. National Library of Medicine, Bethesda, MD.
13. Smith DC: A congenital broncho-oesophageal fistula presenting in adult life without pulmonary infection. *Br J Surg* 57:398, 1970.
14. Braimbridge MV, Keith HI: Oesophagobronchial fistula in the adult. *Thorax* 20:226, 1965.
15. Gonzalez LL, Duffy PH: Bronchoesophageal fistula secondary to Hodgkin's disease. *JAMA* 197:205, 1966.
16. Wychulis AR, Ellis FH, Anderson HA: Acquired nonmalignant esophagotracheo-bronchial fistula. *JAMA* 196:117, 1966.
17. Lajam FE, Sakurai H, McElhinney AJ: Esophago-bronchial fistula—8 years after blunt trauma. *J Trauma* 19:123-125, 1979.
18. Spalding AR, Burney DP, Richie RE: Acquired benign bronchoesophageal fistulas in the adult. *Ann Thorac Surg* 28:378-383, 1979.
19. Nelson RJ, Benfield JR: Benign esophagobronchial fistula: A curable cause of adult pulmonary suppuration. *Arch Surg* 100:685, 1970.
20. Sacks RP, DuBoois JJ, et al: The esophagobronchial fistula: Case report and review of the literature. *Am J Roentgenol, Rad Ther, Nuclear Med* 99:204, 1967.

The Radiographic Diagnosis of Canine and Feline Heart Disease

University of Zurich
Peter F. Suter, Dr.med.vet.

The management of heart failure and heart disease depends to a great degree on the proper interpretation of the radiographs. Radiographs, however, show only indirect signs and do not depict the causes of heart disease. Therefore, it is essential to thoroughly understand the correlation that exists between the compensatory and pathophysiologic mechanisms of heart disease and heart failure and their respective radiographic manifestations. The radiographic interpretation should be done stepwise. First and foremost, it is essential to adhere to a systematic review of the radiographs; second, the radiographic findings should be categorized into diseases with similar etiology and pathophysiology; and third, the final diagnosis should be arrived at by correlating the radiographic findings with the clinical history, the physical findings, and the electrocardiogram. This discussion focuses on the correlation of radiographic abnormalities with the pathophysiological and morphological changes in acquired and some congenital heart diseases of dogs and cats.

The advent of echocardiography has had a great impact on the diagnosis of heart disease. Echocardiography reveals abnormalities in internal cardiac dimensions and morphologic detail and allows detection of functional changes of blood flow and myocardial function; however, radiographic examination of the thorax remains an important tool for complete evaluation of the cardiovascular system. Several review articles and textbooks have dealt with the radiographic interpretation of cardiac anatomy and its correlation with heart disease.[1–9] Radiographic examination plays a major role in obtaining an overview of the entire thorax, in recognizing cardiomegaly and changes in cardiac position and shape, in determining the presence and degree of left heart failure, and in differentiating cardiac from noncardiac thoracic diseases.

The objectives of radiographic examination in dogs and cats with heart disease are (1) to detect abnormalities of size, shape, position, and density of the heart, (2) to recognize extracardiac abnormalities that indicate heart fail-

Originally published in Volume 3, Number 5, May 1981

ure, and (3) to combine the cardiac and extracardiac findings with clinical information to arrive at a diagnosis. Radiography can only provide indirect evidence for the underlying disease.[3] Abnormalities of cardiac size and shape, however, permit the grouping of cardiac diseases into right, left, or general heart disease, according to the chamber or chambers most severely involved. Abnormalities of cardiac size are highly sensitive indicators of heart disease, but they are not specific for a particular heart disease. Abnormalities of cardiac shape, on the other hand, have greater specificity in the identification of a particular type of disease, but they are often difficult to interpret because of the wide variation of normal hearts.

Positional abnormalities of the heart, in particular of the cardiac apex on dorsoventral or ventrodorsal radiographs, are ancillary findings which are rarely significant when encountered as isolated abnormalities. Density changes of the cardiac silhouette from homogeneous to heterogeneous are highly specific abnormalities that signal the presence of an abnormal pericardial content, such as abdominal organs or omental fat as in peritoneopericardial hernia.

The radiograph, rather than depicting the immediate cause of cardiac disease, reveals changes that have taken place as a result of existing cardiac abnormalities. Most radiographic changes either represent sequelae to compensatory mechanisms of the heart induced by an added demand, namely, increased volume load, cardiac output, or pressure load, or they depict changes that occur as a result of heart failure.

The heart has only a limited number of ways to respond to the stresses of disease; consequently, several diseases cause similar morphologic and/or functional cardiac abnormalities. The radiographic abnormalities in cardiac size and shape that can be recognized represent variable combinations of (1) changes of blood volume in the cardiac chambers at end systole or diastole (dilatation, eccentric hypertrophy), (2) changes of muscle mass of the cardiac chambers (hypertrophy), (3) changes of epicardial and pericardial fat, and (4) abnormal pericardial fluid content. An increase in pericardial fluid content is the only abnormality that may be directly related to the cause of heart failure, and only a few of the many functional abnormalities that result from heart disease are recognizable on survey radiographs. Tachycardia or arrhythmia, for example, is not visible. The redistribution of fluid and blood that occurs as a consequence of heart failure is seen, however, and is among the most characteristic changes that can be revealed radiographically.

The successful use of thoracic radiographs in the clinical workup of heart disease in dogs and cats is facilitated by a systematic review of the cardiac silhouette for size and shape, followed by a search for extracardiac changes indicative of heart failure. Such a review can be organized by asking the following basic questions: Does the cardiac apex point to the right or left? Is the cardiac silhouette larger or smaller than normal? Is the cardiac shape abnormal, and which chambers are most severely altered in size and configuration? Are there abnormalities in size, position, or shape of the major cardiac pulmonary or intrathoracic vessels? Are there signs of pleural fluid accumulation compatible with congestive right heart failure? Are there signs of pulmonary fluid retention compatible with congestive left heart failure? Can the abnormalities be explained by heart disease alone, or are concurrent related or unrelated diseases present?

By answering these questions, one or more of the following conclusions will be reached: (1) the radiographs are compatible with heart disease, (2) the radiographs indicate heart failure, (3) it is unlikely that the observed clinical signs are due to heart disease, (4) concurrence of heart disease with another disease is likely, or (5) the findings are equivocal and additional studies, radiographic or otherwise, are needed to arrive at a diagnosis.

POSITIONAL ABNORMALITIES

Any lasting change in the position of the heart which exceeds its normal variation is called *malposition.* Malposition of the cardiac apex to the right of midline instead of to the left is called *dextroposition* and is usually the result of physical displacement induced by uneven lung inflation, thoracic conformation (wide, shallow thorax), or cardiomegaly. Dextroposition is of little or no clinical significance. A congenital malposition of the heart is called *primary dextrocardia* or *intrinsic malposition of the heart* and may be associated with other congenital abnormalities such as abnormal position of the abdominal viscera (situs inversus), chronic bronchitis and sinusitis (Kartagener's syndrome), or rare, severe cardiac malformations.[10]

Malposition of the heart is an important modifying factor in the evaluation of cardiac size and shape. A shifting of the cardiac apex to the left is common in generalized and right-sided cardiomegaly of dogs and can be misread as left heart enlargement.

Placement of the cardiac apex in the midline or to the right of midline is fairly common in normal cats and in cats with left heart enlargement. Variability in apex position makes the interpretation of radiographs more difficult.

CARDIOMEGALY AND REDUCED CARDIAC SIZE

Cardiomegaly is the term used for an enlarged heart. *Microcardia* is sometimes used to designate a reduced

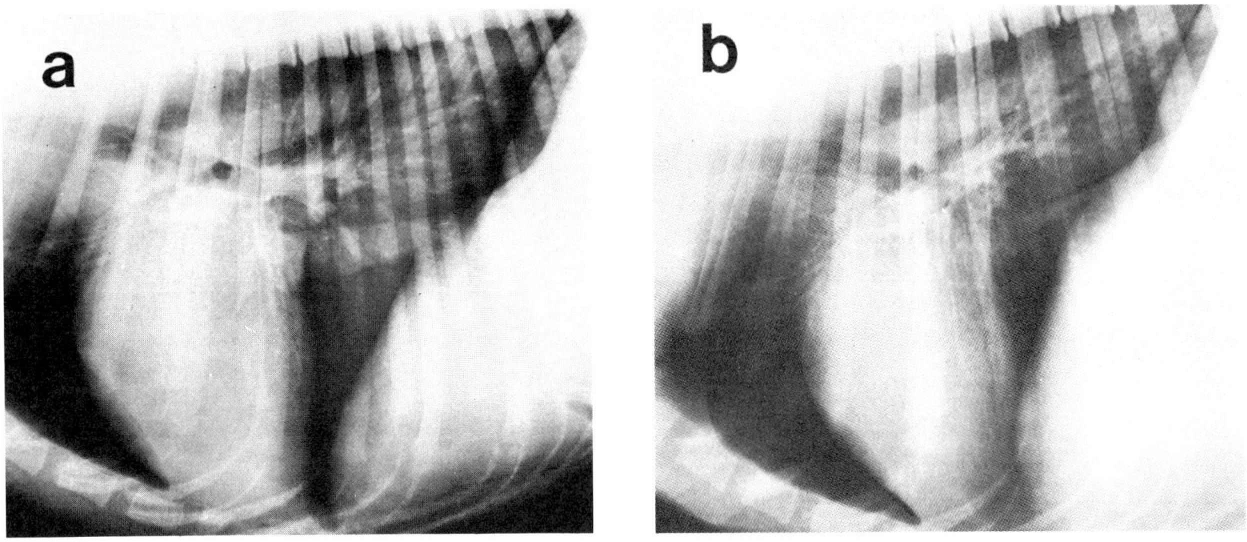

Figure 1—These radiographs illustrate the value of being able to compare radiographs of the same animal taken before and after the onset of disease. (**A**) This two-year-ole male Irish setter was radiographed because of renal disease. Seven months later the dog ran away and returned with signs of shock and respiratory difficulty. (**B**) The effects of severe hypovolemia or shock can be seen, namely, small caudal vena cava, small and pointed heart, easily visible, spidery lung vessels, and a small aorta.

heart size. *Cardiac silhouette* refers to the shadow seen on a radiographic image of the heart. This image includes the pericardium, the pericardial content, and the origin of the major vessels such as the aorta and the pulmonary artery. It sometimes includes adjacent extracardiac shadows such as fat in the sternopericardiac ligament or fluid layering around the heart in pleural effusion (pseudocardiomegaly).

In dogs, cardiomegaly is the most consistent sign of heart disease with or without heart failure. In cats, cardiomegaly is a less consistent feature of heart disease because of the occurrence of such diseases as hypertrophic cardiomyopathy, which may present with little or no cardiomegaly. Cardiomegaly is the single most important anomaly for the differential diagnosis of cardiogenic and noncardiogenic pulmonary edema and pleural disease. Changes in cardiac size also provide critical information in estimating the severity and prognosis of heart disease and heart failure and assist in the evaluation of therapy.

Cardiac diseases in individuals with a normal heart size are not unusual. Examples include mild valvular disease, arrhythmia, cardiac infarct, shock heart, traumatic and acute myocardiopathy, myocarditis and endocarditis, constrictive pericarditis, and many mild congenital heart diseases, particularly those conditions associated with concentric hypertrophy such as mild aortic or pulmonic stenosis.

Moderate or severe cardiomegaly is most often caused by dilatation of the atria and ventricles or a combination of dilatation and hypertrophy of the ventricles (eccentric hypertrophy). Eccentric hypertrophy and dilatation cannot be distinguished on survey radiographs. Pericardial effusion and peritoneopericardial hernia are less common causes of enlargement of the cardiac silhouette. Concentric hypertrophy often develops at the expense of ventricular volume, and the resulting degree of enlargement is small and often difficult to assess on survey radiographs. Even severe hypertrophy causes only a moderate degree of cardiac enlargement confined to one ventricle. Such a unilateral ventricular enlargement, however, can be easily recognized because of the change in cardiac shape.

Dilatation is a normal adaptive mechanism which enables the heart to accept an increased venous return or to cope with a leaky valve such as in mitral valve insufficiency. Dilatation also occurs as a result of reduced myocardial contractility, such as in congestive cardiomyopathy. Hypertrophy is also a compensatory mechanism which enables the heart to respond to increased wall stress. Hypertrophy can be pressure-induced, as in pulmonic or aortic stenosis, or it can be induced by an increased volume load and ejection tension, as in a leaky valve. In the latter case, hypertrophy allows an increase in cardiac output, which assists the heart in maintaining an adequate cardiac output into the aorta or pulmonary artery, despite backflow into the left or right atrium, respectively.

Cardiomegaly can be quantitated (1) empirically or by subjective grading, (2) comparatively, and (3) by measuring cardiac dimensions and comparing them to other thoracic structures (cardiac mensuration). Cardiac mensuration is time consuming and offers

TABLE I
Radiographic Features Used in Defining Cardiomegaly

Apicobasilar distance (apex to carina)
Angle of trachea with thoracic spine
Transverse diameter of heart
Extent of contact of right heart border with sternum
Distance of caudal heart border from diaphragm or overlap of caudal heart border and diaphragm
Distance of right heart border from right chest wall
Distance of left heart border from left chest wall
Position of cardiac apex
Ratio of overall cardiac size to thoracic size

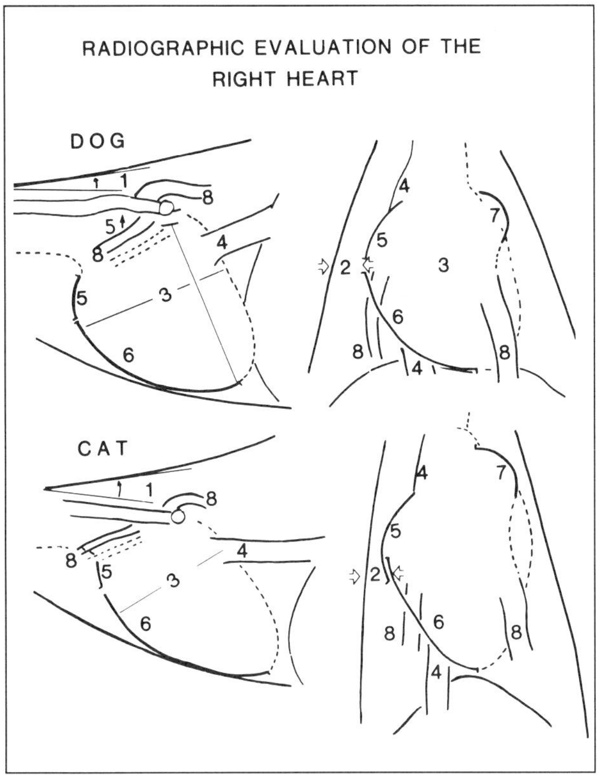

Figure 2—Evaluation of cardiac size and shape requires a systematic review. The angle of the trachea with the thoracic spine *(1)* is used in conjunction with the distance between tracheal bifurcation and cardiac apex (apicobasilar distance) and the transverse diameter of the heart *(3)* to provide reliable information on cardiac enlargement. In addition, the distance between the right thoracic wall and the farthest rightward extension of the right heart *(2)* may be used to check whether the right heart is involved. When a line between carina and apex divides the transverse diameter of the heart in dogs at a ratio greater than 2:1, right heart enlargement probably exists. For a systematic review of changes indicating right cardiac chamber or large vessel enlargement, follow the numbers 4 to 8. In the direction of blood flow, the structures are *(4)* the caudal vena cava, *(5)* the right atrium, *(6)* the right ventricular border, *(7)* the pulmonary artery segment or main pulmonary artery border, and *(8)* the main pulmonary arteries.

only minimal advantages.[6] The *comparative method* uses chest radiographs of the same or a similar sized dog or cat taken at different times to determine change in cardiac size. When the technique for obtaining the comparison radiographs is kept constant, the comparative method is effective, simple, and almost free of subjective error (Figure 1). The *subjective grading method* consists of comparing the heart size with what the observer conceives of as normal, based on past experience. Subjective grading is subject to interindividual and intraindividual inconsistencies, particularly for mild degree of cardiomegaly.

In subjective grading, the cardiomegaly should be described in the following terms: (1) mild or slight but definite enlargement, (2) moderate or obvious enlargement, and (3) gross or severe enlargement.

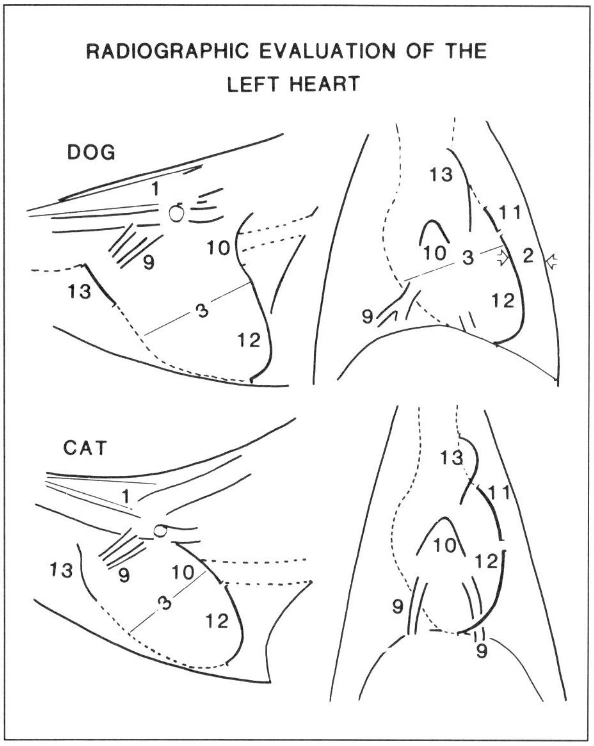

Figure 3—Evaluation of cardiac size and shape requires a systematic review. Start with the angle of the trachea with the thoracic spine *(1)* which, in conjunction with the transverse diameter of the heart *(3)*, provides reliable information on the presence of cardiac enlargement. In addition, the distance between the farthest leftward extension of the left ventricle and the left thoracic wall *(2)* may be used as a criterion for left ventricular involvement. For the continuation of the review of changes indicating left heart chamber and large vessel abnormalities, follow the numbers 9 to 13. In the direction of blood flow, the structures are *(9)* the pulmonary veins, *(10)* the left atrium, *(11)* the left auricle, *(12)* the left ventricular border, and *(13)* the aortic arch with its ascending (lateral radiograph) and descending (dorsoventral radiograph) parts.

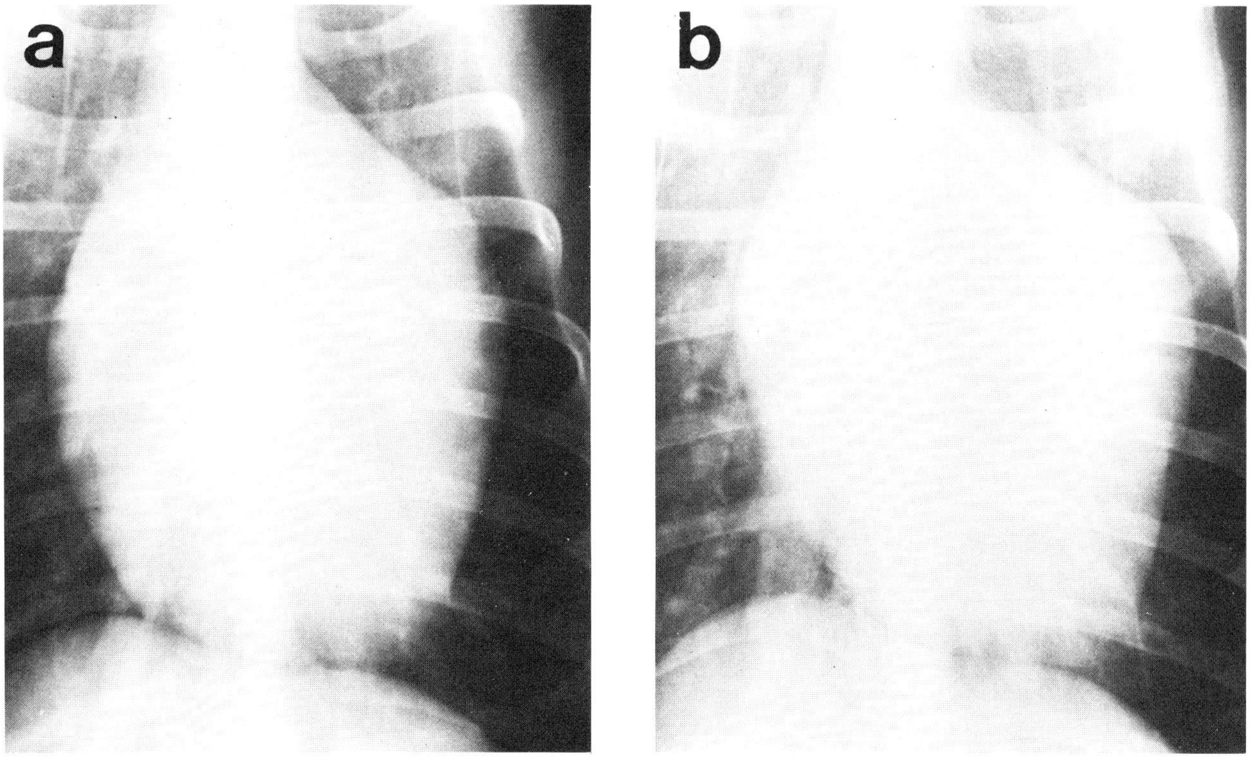

Figure 4—Both radiographs of this nine-year-old female terrier cross dog with a Phase III mitral valvular insufficiency were made within 15 minutes and in the same position. The radiographs demonstrate the differences in cardiac shape with cardiac systole and diastole. (**A**) A moderately enlarged cardiac silhouette with predominating left ventricular and left auricular enlargement. This radiograph was exposed close to ventricular diastole and shows a round widened apex (left ventricle). (**B**) A heart with a reduced cardiac diameter in the ventricular area, but with an even more prominent left auricular area when compared to **A**, indicating that the radiograph has been exposed close to ventricular end systole and maximal atrial filling (atrial diastole).

The subjective grading method is fast and convenient, and when used by experienced reviewers, the results compare favorably to those of mensuration.[6]

When grading the cardiac size of dogs or cats, it is essential to use well-defined features as a basis for rendering judgment (see Table I and Figures 2 and 3) and to consider variations induced by breed, age, special thoracic conformation, state of nourishment (obesity, emaciation), associated pulmonary and pleural disease, and radiographic technique. The effects of inspiration and expiration are particularly important considerations in small-breed dogs. It has been reported that at expiration the heart size increases absolutely and relatively to thoracic size, which can result in overdiagnosing cardiomegaly.[11] Systole and diastole also influence cardiac size if the radiographs are taken at short exposure times ($^1/_{60}$ to $^1/_{120}$ second). At end systole, ventricular size is reduced relative to end diastole, but at the same time the atria appear enlarged (Figure 4).

The use of different radiographic positions can cause artifactual changes in cardiac size and shape that may exceed the changes induced by disease. Both cardiac size and shape are substantially altered by a switch from a dorsoventral to a ventrodorsal position. A switch from right to left lateral recumbency mainly causes a change of cardiac shape. Consistency in radiographic technique is indispensable for obtaining comparable radiographs.

The accuracy of subjective grading of cardiomegaly can be enhanced by concurrent evaluation of size and shape. Only a small number of hearts maintain their normal proportions as they enlarge. Most reviewers are able to detect a small alteration in shape more easily than a mild degree of enlargement. The concurrent evaluation of cardiac size and shape is particularly critical for reliably diagnosing slight but definite enlargement in cats and in small-breed dogs that have relatively large hearts, such as Chihuahuas or toy poodles.

A reduction in cardiac size, or microcardia, is rarely a result of cardiac disease. In the majority of dogs and cats with microcardia, the reduced heart size is either artifactual or reflects an extracardiac disease. An increased, overexpanded thorax often conveys the erroneous impression of a reduced heart size. Severe weight loss in chronic diseases and malnutrition are often accompanied by a noticeable reduction in heart

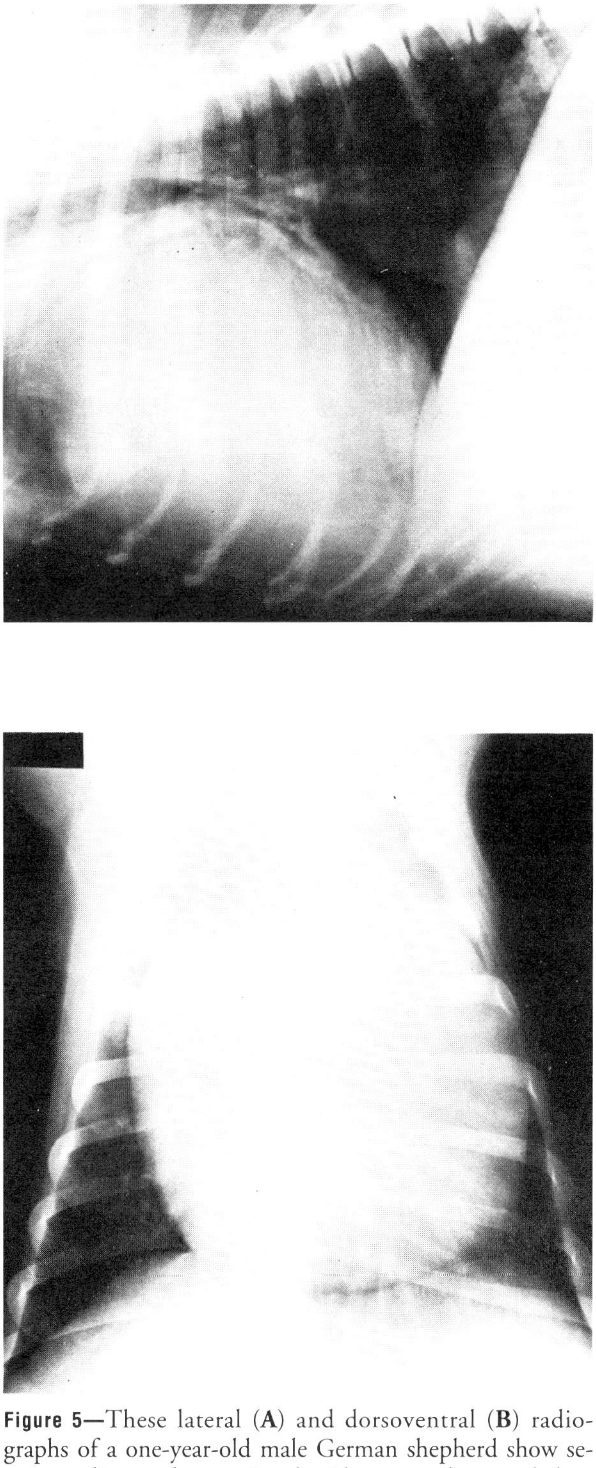

Figure 5—These lateral (**A**) and dorsoventral (**B**) radiographs of a one-year-old male German shepherd show severe cardiomegaly associated with an evenly rounded or *pumpkin-shaped* cardiac silhouette. This combination of cardiomegaly with a globular shape is typical for pericardial effusion. This dog was presented to the clinic with ascites and dyspnea. The heart sounds were muffled on both sides, the jugular veins were distended, and the abdomen was pendulous as a result of ascites. Pericardiocentesis revealed a port-wine–colored sterile fluid with no indications of malignancy. The diagnosis was idiopathic benign pericardial effusion and a pericardiectomy was performed.

size. The most common conditions that result in reduced cardiac size are hypovolemia, severe dehydration, or tension pneumothorax. In all of these conditions, the blood volume returning to the heart and ventricular filling is drastically reduced, which can be recognized radiographically as a small heart and caudal vena cava and smaller sized lung vessels (Figure 1).

A combined effect of circulatory derangement and mild myocardial atrophy accounts for the reduced heart size seen in approximately half the dogs with chronic Addison's disease.[5,12,13]

ALTERATIONS IN CARDIAC SHAPE

By considering alterations of cardiac shape, it is possible to discriminate between right, left, and general heart enlargement and to separate cardiomegaly from moderate to large pericardial effusion. Changes in cardiac shape are the result of (1) selective dilatation or hypertrophy of the cardiac chambers, (2) distention of major cardiac arteries or veins contiguous with the heart, (3) rotation or shifting of the heart on one or more of its three axes, (4) pericardial fluid accumulation, and (5) positioning of the patient. Dilatation of cardiac chambers or large vessels is sometimes inferred by changes in structures adjacent to the heart such as the trachea, pulmonary vasculature, diaphragm, or mediastinal structures.

A loss of the typical distorted oval cardiac shape, an excessive smoothing of all cardiac bumps in two projections, a caudal expansion of the caudal heart border in the lateral radiograph, and moderate to marked cardiomegaly are typical features of pericardial effusion (Figure 5) or peritoneopericardial hernia. In the latter condition, the density of the cardiac silhouette is inhomogeneous or contains loculated gas. In pericardial effusion, the cardiac silhouette takes on a homogeneous density. Small to moderate pericardial effusions are difficult to distinguish from severely dilated hearts such as those that occur in dilative cardiomyopathy in dogs and cats. Differentiating these two conditions in the absence of typical clinical and electrocardiographic signs can be a major problem requiring echocardiographic examination.

In evaluating an abnormal cardiac shape, the right and left heart structures should be treated as parts of two separate functional units. Right heart diseases are characterized by one or more changes in the right ventricle, right atrium, caudal vena cava, cranial vena cava, main pulmonary artery segment, and/or pulmonary arteries (Figure 2). Left heart diseases are characterized by one or more changes involving the left ventricle, left atrium, pulmonary veins, and/or aortic arch (Figure 3). In dogs and cats with heart failure, the respective features of right and left heart

TABLE II
Radiographic Features of Acquired and Congenital Heart Diseases

	Caudal and Cranial Vena Cava	*Right Atrium*	*Right Ventricle*	*Main Pulmonary Artery*	*Peripheral Pulmonary Arteries*	*Pleural Effusion, Ascites, Hepatomegaly (RHF)**	*Pulmonary Veins*	*Left Atrium*	*Left Ventricle*	*Ascending Aorta or Aortic Arch*	*Altered Lung Perfusion (Arteries and Veins Altered)*	*Interstitial or Alveolar Lung Density (LHF)†*	*Characteristic Features*
Tricuspid valvular insufficiency	↑–↑↑	↑–↑↑	↑–↑↑			n–↑↑					n–↓		
Tricuspid valvular dysplasia	n–↑↑	↑↑–↑↑↑	↑–↑↑↑			n–↑↑					n–↓		Globular heart
Dirofilariasis (dog)	n–↑↑	n–↑↑	↑–↑↑	↑–↑↑↑	↑–↑↑↑	n–↑↑						?	Inverted D heart
Pulmonic stenosis (rare in cat)	n–↑↑	n–↑↑	↑–↑↑	n–↑↑		n–↑↑					n–↓		RVH ‡
Tetralogy of Fallot			↑–↑↑	n–↑	↓–↓↓		↓–↓↓	n–↓	n–↓	n–↑	↓–↓↓	↓	Cyanosis
Reversed PDA§; Eisenmenger's syndrome			↑–↑↑	↑–↑↑	↑		↓	?			↓–↓↓	n–↓	Distorted lung vessels
Mitral and tricuspid valvular insufficiency (rare in cat)	↑–↑↑	↑–↑↑	↑–↑↑↑			↑–↑↑↑	n–↑	↑–↑↑↑	↑–↑↑↑			↑–↑↑↑	Bumpy heart
Congestive cardiomyopathy	↑–↑↑	↑–↑↑	↑↑–↑↑↑			↑–↑↑↑	↑–↑↑	n–↑↑	↑–↑↑			↑–↑↑↑	Round heart
Hypertrophic cardiomyopathy (cat)	?	↑–↑↑					↑–↑↑	↑–↑↑				↑–↑↑	Valentine heart
Intermediate type cardiomyopathy (has features from hypertrophic and congestive cardiomyopathies [cat])	n–↑↑	↑–↑↑	↑–↑↑			n–↑↑	↑–↑↑	↑–↑↑	↑			↑–↑↑	
Pericardial effusion	↑–↑↑	↑↑–↑↑↑	↑↑–↑↑↑			↑–↑↑↑	?		↑↑–↑↑↑			n–↑	Globular heart
Patent ductus arteriosus	?		n–↑↑	↑–↑↑	↑–↑↑		↑–↑↑	↑–↑↑↑	↑–↑↑↑	↑	↑–↑↑↑	n–↑↑↑	Aortic aneurysm
Aortic stenosis								n–↑	n–↑↑	n–↑↑↑		n–↑	LVH‖
Ventricular septal defect	?	?	n–↑↑	n–↑	n–↑		n–↑	↑–↑↑	n–↑↑		n–↑	n–↑	
Mitral valve dysplasia			n–↑				n–↑	↑↑–↑↑↑	↑–↑↑			n–↑↑	
Mitral valve insufficiency			n–↑↑				n–↑	↑–↑↑↑	↑–↑↑↑			n–↑↑↑	
Hypovolemia; Addison's disease	↓		↓		↓		↓		↓	↓	↓↓↓	↓	Microcardia

*RHF = right heart failure
†LHF = left heart failure
‡RVH = right ventricular hypertrophy
§PDA = patent ductus arteriosus
‖ LVH = left ventricular hypertrophy

Key:
↑ = mildly but definitely enlarged
↑↑ = moderately enlarged
↑↑↑ = severely enlarged
↓ = mildly reduced
↓↓ = moderately reduced
? = unpredictable
n = normal

TABLE III
Radiographic Phases of Progressive Mitral Valve Insufficiency

Phase	*Dorsoventral Projection*	*Lateral Projection*
I—Compensated mitral valve insufficiency phase	Small bulge of left auricle; unremarkable left ventricle; normal lung	Slightly enlarged left atrium; left ventricle unremarkable; clear lung
II—Prodromal phase, occasional signs of decompensation with exercise; animal comfortable at rest	Left ventricular border and apex rounder than normal; enlarged left ventricle; auricular bulge may be visible or obscured by ventricle; unremarkable lung; veins mildly enlarged and/or denser than arteries	Trachea displaced slightly dorsally; ventral deflection of trachea at carina, eliminated or reduced; left stem bronchus elevated; caudal heart border moved caudally and stretched, eliminating caudal waist; left atrium and ventricle moderately enlarged; clear lung
III—Signs of mostly left heart failure and fatigue with exercise and occasionally at night; animal appears normal at rest	Overt left ventricular and some right ventricular enlargement; left auricle bulges across a bowed out left ventricular border; apex shifted to left (or right); blunted stem bronchi angle; blurring and/or enlarged pulmonary veins; lungs congested, hazy	Trachea dorsally displaced and straight; stem bronchi split and compressed by large atrium; caudal heart border displaced caudally and stretched; increased sternal contact and rounding of right heart; craniocaudal heart diameter markedly increased; pulmonary vessels blurred in perihilar zone; congested, hazy lung; veins may be accentuated
IV—Signs of congestive left and right heart failure noticeable at rest; signs are greatly increased by physical activity and stress	Cardiac size and shape as in Phase III or more enlarged; perihilar or central lung zone with alveolar edema (air bronchograms; blotchy, confluent consolidations); visible interlobar fissures, pleural and/or pericardial effusion, ascites, hepatomegaly	Cardiac size and shape as in Phase III or more enlarged; pulmonary alveolar edema mostly perihilar and in caudal lobes; cranial lobes seemingly free; increased ventral thoracic radiodensity; pleural and/or pericardial effusion. Associated signs: large postcava, ascites, hepatomegaly

failure further support the discriminating evaluation of cardiac shape. By evaluating the right and left hearts as separate but interrelated units, one avoids attaching too much emphasis to incidental abnormalities. Table II summarizes the major radiographic features of the common canine and feline heart diseases.

Dividing heart diseases into right, left, and general heart diseases correlates well with the pathophysiologic classification into right, left, and general heart failure. This subdivision simplifies the diagnosis and markedly shortens the list of differential diagnoses by automatically excluding from consideration the diseases that do not fulfill the basic criteria of one particular group. Such subdivision does not, however, imply that right and left heart diseases occur as completely separate entities.

PLEURAL, PULMONARY, AND ABDOMINAL ABNORMALITIES THAT INDICATE HEART FAILURE

Heart failure is a clinical syndrome that results from the heart's inability to maintain circulation adequate for tissue metabolism. The radiographic diagnosis of heart failure requires familiarity with the mechanisms causing the basic circulatory imbalances. The term *heart failure* has slightly different connotations for clinicians and physiologists. The clinical classifications are based on physical and radiographic signs that are consequences of the effects of compensatory mechanisms (Table III). Compensated heart failure indicates that the animal is comfortable at rest, but that physical activity may result in fatigue, respiratory discomfort, and coughing. The resting cardiac output is preserved in compensated heart failure, but pulmonary and/or systemic venous pressure is moderately or markedly increased.[14] In decompensated heart failure, signs of congestive heart failure are present at rest. The cardiac output at rest is not commensurate with systemic metabolic requirements (perfusion insufficiency).

The radiographic diagnosis of heart failure is based on the recognition of imbalances in the blood and fluid distribution. The circulatory imbalance is the result

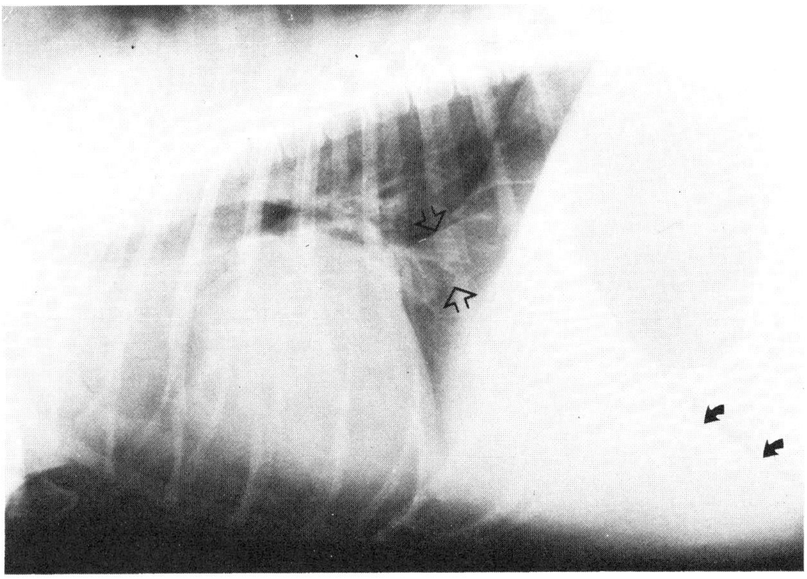

Figure 6—Right heart failure in a two-year-old female Scottish terrier caused by a congenital tricuspid valvular insufficiency. The ventral parts of the cardiac silhouette are obstructed by a hazy density representing pleural effusion. The abdomen is very radiodense and distended. Within the distended abdomen, the shadow of an enlarged liver *(arrows)* can be recognized. The liver borders are poorly seen because of ascites resulting from the increased right atrial and caudal vena cava pressure. The caudal vena cava is distended *(empty arrows)*. The elevation of the trachea indicates cardiomegaly. The left atrial area does not appear significantly enlarged and the lung field is clear; the pulmonary vessels are small and normal in size. The small size of the pulmonary vessels probably reflects a reduced right ventricular output.

of a reduced acceptance of blood by the failing ventricle (congestive heart failure) and a diminished cardiac output into the pulmonary or systemic vascular bed (perfusion insufficiency). The cardiac events set in motion a number of complex neurologic, humoral, and biochemical interactions (sympathoadrenal reaction) that have a short-term beneficial effect but which eventually contribute to the chronic state of heart failure. Depending on which side is more severely affected, blood is shifted from the systemic to the pulmonary circulation (congestive left heart failure) or from the pulmonary to the systemic circulation (congestive right heart failure). The backing up of blood into the veins upstream to the failing ventricle increases venous pressure and transudation of fluid from the capillary bed into the interstitium. The location of the veins that are subjected to an elevated hydrostatic pressure determines the location of the edema.

Radiography is best suited to detect congestive left heart failure. In many cases of congestive heart failure, cardiac output is also reduced. Radiographic features that indicate reduced cardiac output may be noticed only in the lung, where radiographs show a reduced lung perfusion with both arteries and veins being smaller than normal (Figure 1B). The pulmonary density is slightly reduced as a result of oligemia. The objectives of the radiographic examination in animals with heart failure are (1) to establish the diagnosis of congestive heart failure, (2) to determine its severity, (3) to discriminate between right, left, and general heart failure, (4) to document the course of congestive heart failure during therapy, (5) to provide clues as to the origin of the underlying heart disease, and (6) to detect complications from intercurrent diseases.

The radiographic subdivision into right heart failure, left heart failure, and general heart failure is convenient for correlating the clinical signs with the radiographic findings. This somewhat simplistic subdivision emphasizes the site of the primary impairment of cardiac function and establishes priority among clinical signs. It is apparent that in the absence of shunts or regurgitation one side cannot pump significantly more blood for any length of time than the other side. Consequently, failure of one side of the heart sooner or later impairs the performance of the other ventricle.

In *right heart failure*, an inadequate right ventricular output into the pulmonary artery exists concomitantly with a reduced acceptance of blood from the systemic veins. The blood volume and pressure in the splanchnic and systemic veins are elevated. The venous congestion causes hepatomegaly and makes the intestines look fuzzy on the radiographs (Figure 6).

Even a mild elevation of pressure in the splanchnic veins induces increasing amounts of fluid, solutes, and protein to escape from the capillary bed of the liver and intestines. When the excess fluid can no longer be accommodated by a greatly increased lymph flow, fluid spills into the serosal cavities, causing pleural effusion, ascites, and pericardial effusion. The consequences of right heart failure are not as easily seen and quantitated on radiographs as those of left heart failure. Noncardiogenic factors, such as the albumin content of blood plasma, substantially modify the quantity of fluid spilled into the serosal cavities.

Every animal with concurrent pleural and abdominal effusion should be suspected of having right heart failure or hypoalbuminemia. This elementary fact is often disregarded in the diagnosis of animals with as-

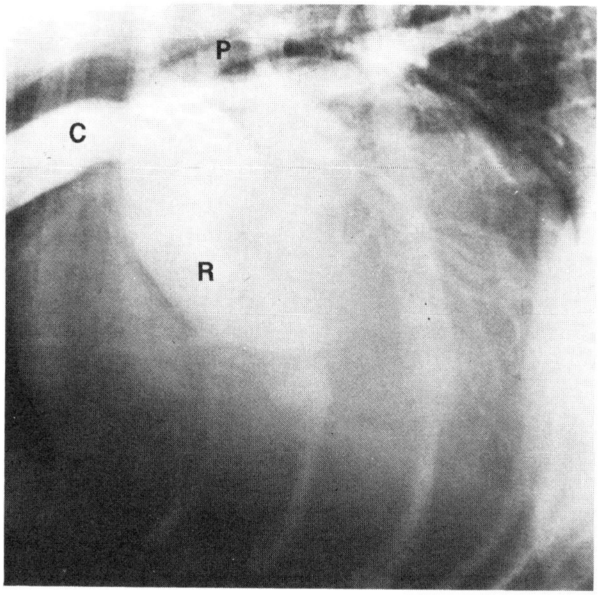

Figure 7—Nonselective angiocardiogram performed in a dog with extensive pericardial effusion causing pericardial tamponade. Contrast medium is seen in the cranial vena cava (**C**), in the right ventricular outflow tract (**R**), and in the left pulmonary artery (**P**). Notice the wide distance that separates the cranial border of the round cardiac silhouette from the border of the right ventricular outflow tract. Such a wide separation between cardiac border and ventricle is typical for an expansion of the pericardial space with fluid. In this particular case, the cardiac size is actually reduced, reflecting the inhibition of the fluid on the right heart to expand and accept the full venous return from the periphery during diastole. Notice the small diameter of the left pulmonary artery which indicates that the right ventricular output is probably reduced and unable to distend the pulmonary artery to its normal width.

cites. Instead of taking a thoracic radiograph, clinicians often subject these animals to liver biopsy and/or laparotomy. In the presence of right ventricular and atrial enlargement, dilatation of the caudal vena cava, and hepatomegaly, a diagnosis of right heart failure is inevitable. In chronic heart failure, hepatomegaly may be absent. In isolated right heart failure, which is uncommon outside of endemic heartworm areas, cardiomegaly is usually moderate and may be difficult to see because of the existing pleural effusion. Removing the pleural fluid or radiographing the animal in a ventrodorsal instead of a dorsoventral position may free the cardiac silhouette from the obscuring fluid density.

In mild right heart failure, small amounts of abdominal fluid are usually missed and small quantities of pleural fluid are only seen on dorsoventral radiographs around the caudoventral mediastinum and in the interlobar fissures. Echocardiography should be used to identify small effusions.

A severe degree of cardiomegaly with signs of right heart failure strongly suggests the presence of either an advanced congestive cardiomyopathy, pericardial effusion, or a combination of the two. When these signs occur in young dogs and cats, a tricuspid valve dysplasia should also be considered. In pericardial effusion, the accumulation of fluid within the pericardial sac causes diastolic mechanical inhibition of ventricular filling, which intervenes with the normal return of venous blood from the systemic circulation to the right ventricle. As a result of the reduced ventricular filling, blood backs up into the systemic veins, which leads to signs of right heart failure. Differentiating between moderately severe pericardial effusion and cardiomyopathy can be accomplished using echocardiography. Pericardiocentesis is best performed under echocardiographic control. If echocardiography is not available, nonselective angiocardiography can be used to confirm pericardial effusion (Figure 7). By opacifying a normal right and left ventricle within an enlarged cardiac silhouette, it is fairly easy to differentiate pericardial effusion from congestive cardiomyopathy, which is characterized by left and/or right ventricular dilatation.

Left heart failure is defined as an inadequate left ventricular output into the aorta and a diminished acceptance of blood from the pulmonary veins. It is most commonly caused by mitral valve insufficiency, myocardial insufficiency, or a combination of the two. The diminished output into the aorta cannot be assessed on survey radiographs. The backing up of blood into the left atrium and the pulmonary veins, however, is easily detected. The self-fueling process of pulmonary edema proceeds through degrees of increasing severity which can be monitored radiographically. The basically continuous process has been subdivided into three distinct phases of failure which are useful in describing the severity of left heart failure. The phases correspond well with the clinical signs.

The three phases of cardiogenic lung edema are lung congestion, interstitial lung edema, and alveolar lung edema (see Table III). In *pulmonary congestion,* which is also called the *preedema phase,* engorgement and distention of the pulmonary veins may be seen, particularly at their junction with the left atrium. The diameters of the veins may slightly exceed those of the pulmonary arteries. The pulmonary radiodensity is often unchanged. In the *interstitial lung edema phase* (Figure 8), the pulmonary density is increased and hazy. The pulmonary vasculature is still visible, but the borders of the veins and arteries appear indistinct because of the accumulation of fluid in the perivascular interstitial space. The increased interstitial pulmonary radiodensity is best seen in the central portions of the caudal lobes where it often partially obscures the left atrium. In some dogs, fluid also ac-

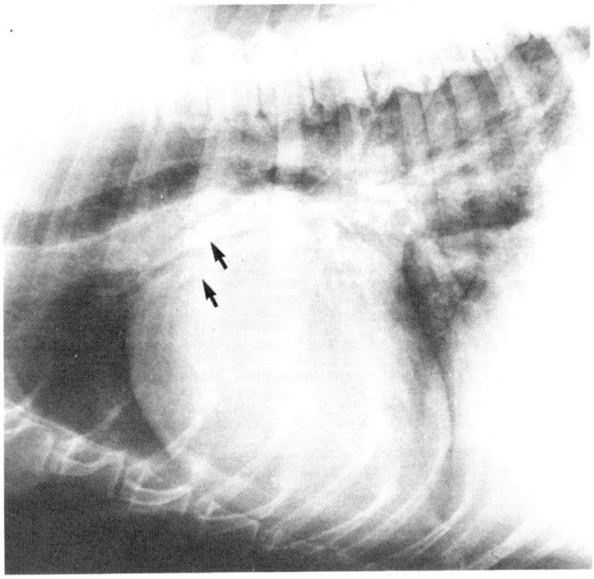

Figure 8—This radiograph shows severe generalized cardiomegaly, based on the criteria indicated in Figures 2 and 3, and a Phase III left heart failure. Notice the slight dorsal elevation of the trachea immediately cranial to the carina, which indicates right atrial enlargement. The right heart border is much fuller than normal and has increased contact with the sternum. In addition, the distance between the caudal heart border and the carina is increased, which indicates left atrial enlargement. The caudal heart border is displaced caudally and intersects with the diaphragm. The left ventricular border dorsally merges into the caudal border of the left atrium which fades caudally in the direction of the caudal lobe veins. In the caudal lung lobe, the vascular structures are partially obscured by an interstitial lung density. The increased density is greatest near the left atrium where it reaches almost alveolar quality. The vessels to the cranial lobes are congested *(arrows).*

cumulates around the larger bronchi and forms peribronchiolar cuffs or ring shadows. In the *alveolar edema phase,* fluid enters the alveoli and bronchioli and causes a diffuse, fairly homogeneous alveolar type of radiodensity which may contain air bronchograms. The alveolar radiodensity usually reaches its greatest density in the perihilar area and leaves the lung periphery seemingly unaffected. In dogs, the right caudal lobe is often more severely affected by edema than the other lobes.

In cats, pulmonary edema is usually paroxysmal in onset and fails to show a typical perihilar arrangement as that which occurs in dogs with progressive heart disease. Edema in cats may appear as noncircumscribed, cloudy single lesions or as multiple consolidations typically in the caudal lobes. In very rapidly developing pulmonary edema in dogs, large numbers of patchy or noncircumscribed, focal alveolar consolidations may be distributed all over the lung field. These focal lesions are regularly surrounded by an extensive interstitial density and may contain faint air bronchograms.

With alveolar pulmonary edema, some pleural thickening (pleural edema) and small amounts of pleural fluid may also be noticed. Large pleural fluid accumulation is indicative of right or general rather than left heart failure.

A variable degree of cardiomegaly, in particular left atrial and left ventricular enlargement, is present regularly in both dogs and cats with left heart failure (Figure 9, A and B). The severity of cardiac enlargement, however, is not always commensurate with the phase of left heart failure indicated on the radiograph. In acute heart disease, mild to moderate cardiomegaly may be associated with alveolar pulmonary edema. In chronic heart disease with severe cardiomegaly, pulmonary changes are often barely noticeable. There are several explanations for these seemingly contradictory findings. A greatly enlarged left atrium is able to accommodate backflow of blood from the ventricle across an incompetent valve without a substantial pressure increase (Figure 9C) and thus prevent pulmonary venous pressure from rising to critical levels. In an acutely developing valvular insufficiency, however, the atrium is usually small and unable to prevent the elevated pressure of the regurgitant blood flow from reaching the pulmonary veins, which rapidly leads to edema formation. In chronic heart disease, compensatory mechanisms such as neurogenic pulmonary venous constriction and a rise in the pulmonary vascular resistance partially protect the lung from edema formation. This increases right ventricular work load and can eventually induce right heart failure. Left heart failure is the most common cause for right heart failure. A failing right heart, by virtue of a diminished cardiac output, reduces pulmonary perfusion, lessens the chance of edema formation, and relieves the load on the failing left heart.

It is important to avoid making premature conclusions as to the clinical severity of heart failure based on the radiographic appearance of the lung field. On one hand, radiographs are very sensitive in providing information on early left heart failure based on venous congestion and interstitial pulmonary edema. These changes may be present before abnormal pulmonary auscultatory findings can be detected. On the other hand, the effects of compensatory mechanisms and complications which may modify the radiographic changes must be considered. A common erroneous interpretation equates the cardiac size reduction and complete disappearance of pulmonary edema following drastic diuretic therapy with the disappearance of heart failure and a compensated state, when in fact cardiac output may have been reduced to the extent that the animal is worse than before

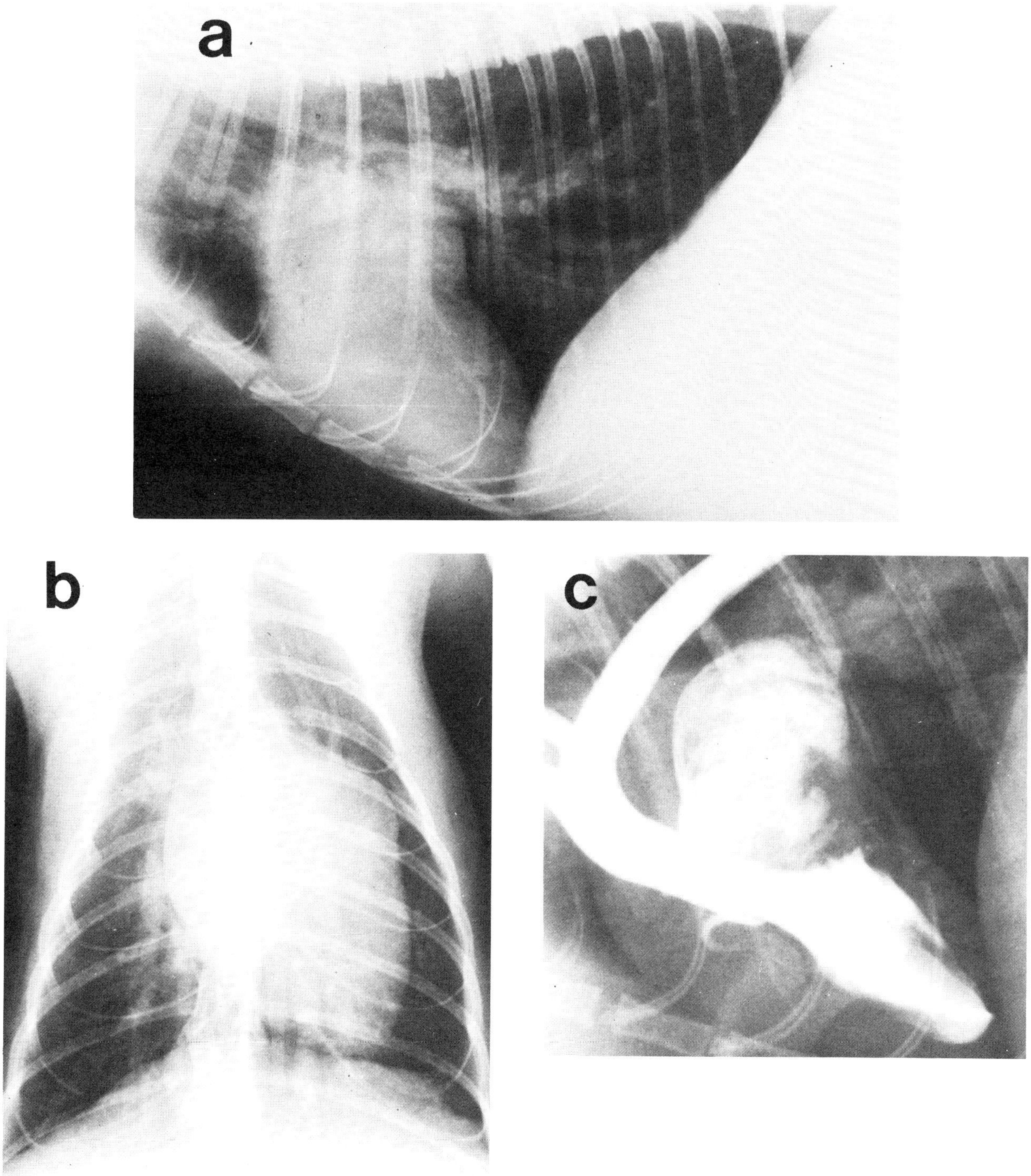

Figure 9—This series of radiographs of a three-year-old cat with cardiomyopathy and right and left heart failure illustrates the marked differences in cardiomegaly and cardiac shape in heart diseases of the cat as compared to those of the dog. (**A**) Notice that despite an elongation of the apicobasilar distance, the trachea is only mildly elevated. The caudal vena cava is clearly enlarged, indicating right heart failure. A fullness to the base of the heart is due to biatrial enlargement, which contrasts with the rather mild increase of transverse cardiac diameter and the near-normal appearing left ventricular border. The right ventricular border follows the sternum for an extended distance. The pulmonary veins are congested, but the lung field appears almost normal in radiodensity. (**B**) In the dorsoventral radiograph, the biatrial enlargement cranially and the near-normal ventricular area provide the heart with a roughly triangular shape, which is also referred to as *valentine-shaped heart.* The normal shape of the ventricular area should lead clinicians to suspect the presence of cardiomyopathy of the hypertrophic or mixed type. (**C**) A selective left ventricular angiocardiogram shows a normal sized left ventricle with a large papillary muscle causing a caudal filling defect in the contrast medium. The greatly dilated left atrium is partially filled with contrast medium that has regurgitated across an incompetent mitral valve. The caudal atrial filling defect could represent a thrombus (ball valve thrombus) in the left atrium.

Pulmonary radiodensity	=	right cardiac output, arterial perfusion (right heart failure)	+	acceptance of blood by left heart, venous perfusion (left heart failure)	–	air content (inflation)

Figure 10—Factors varying pulmonary radiodensity in heart failure.

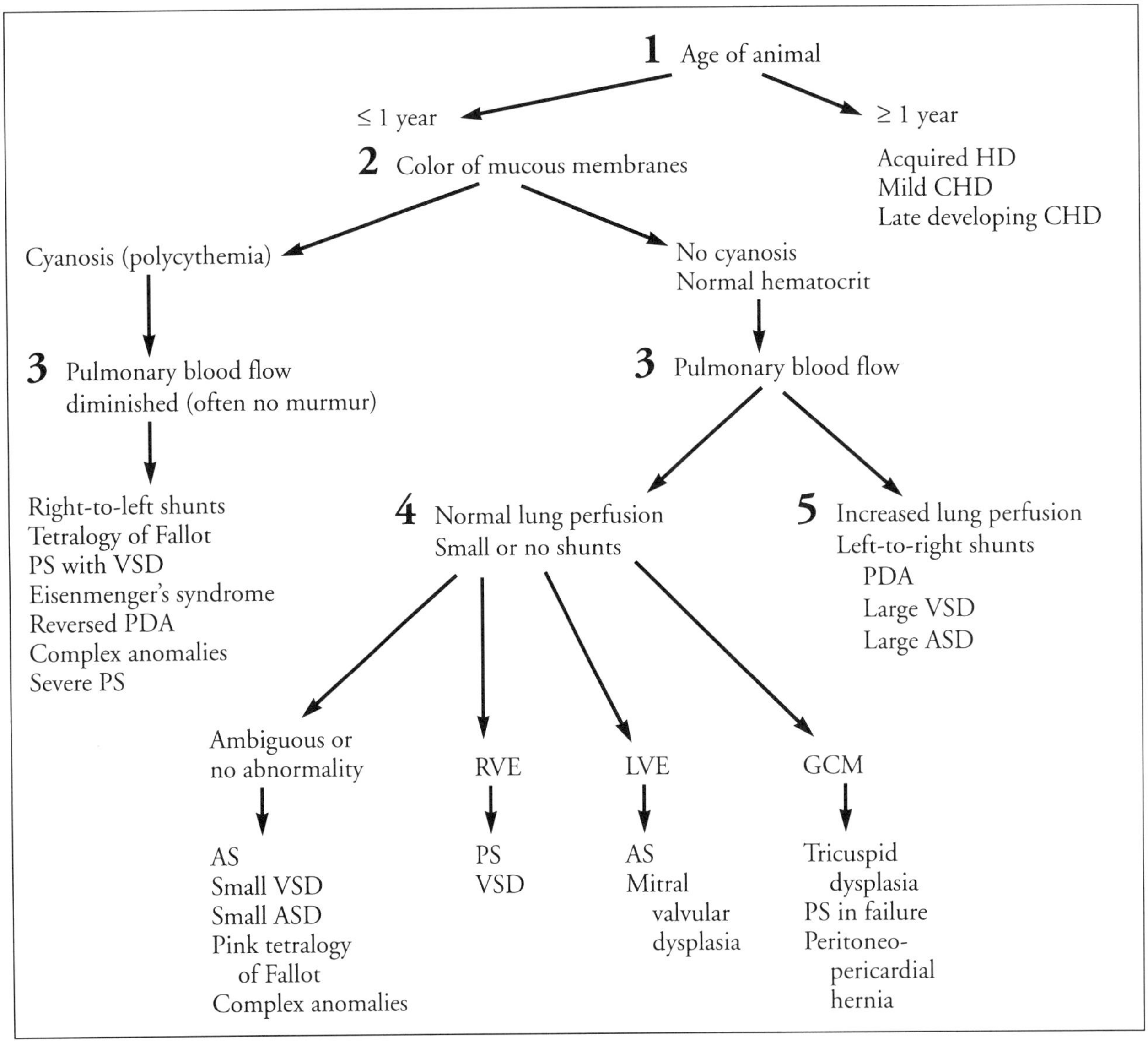

Figure 11—Diagnostic approach to congenital heart disease. *HD*, heart disease; *CHD*, congenital heart disease; *PS*, pulmonic stenosis; *VSD*, ventricular septal defect; *PDA*, patent ductus arteriosus; *AS*, aortic stenosis; *ASD*, atrial septal defect; *RVE*, right ventricular enlargement; *LVE*, left ventricular enlargement; *GCM*, general cardiomegaly.

therapy. Overaggressive diuretic therapy can be recognized by a marked reduction of the size of the pulmonary arteries and veins. The interrelation of these factors in determining final pulmonary radiodensity is summarized in Figure 10.

Figure 10 is meant to illustrate how overall pulmonary density may vary in heart failure with the sum of lung inflation and blood perfusion. Lung density can be reduced by a diminished right cardiac output (oligemia). Lung density can be increased by left heart failure. The individual factors in Figure 10 can have varied effects on the visible lung density (normal right cardiac output plus marked left heart failure, or left heart failure and increased lung inflation), or they can neutralize each other (right heart failure causing a reduced right cardiac output, which reduces the effects of left heart failure).

The radiographic visualization of pulmonary edema is often slightly out of phase with the observed clinical signs. The radiographic abnormalities are delayed both in appearance and in clearance of acute pulmonary edema when compared to the clinical signs. Substantial variations in lung density due to disease can be equalized or accentuated by altering radiographic technique. Increased density of expiratory radiographs or shallow rapid respiration can be easily mistaken for interstitial lung edema. Forceful pulmonary inflation can drastically reduce the density of pulmonary alveolar edema.

The careful scrutiny of the lung field is very important for detecting arterial abnormalities compatible with dirofilariasis or pulmonary thrombosis and for classifying congenital heart diseases. Enlargement, distortion, lack of peripheral tapering or normal branching, and abrupt narrowing of a major pulmonary artery are sensitive and specific findings for chronic heartworm disease. The pulmonary vascular changes are more specific and more sensitive than right heart and pulmonary artery enlargement, pulmonary consolidations, or pulmonary fibrosis. The so-called inverted D-shaped heart is a late and inconsistent sign of dirofilariasis.

The diagnosis of *congenital heart disease* is a logical exercise in correlating clinical history, location of punctum maximum of murmur, quality of murmur, electrocardiography, presence or absence of cyanosis, radiographic changes in cardiac shape and size, and an altered or normal lung perfusion on radiographs with circulatory pathophysiology. The radiographic interpretations can be divided into three basic groups: (1) the radiographic features are typical for a particular disease and support the tentative clinical diagnosis, (2) the radiographic changes of cardiac size and shape are ambiguous, but the state of the lung perfusion allows consideration of a left-to-right or a right-to-left shunting lesion, or (3) the radiographic findings are equivocal because of heart failure that obscures detail, normal lung perfusion, or the absence of specific signs. Congenital heart diseases of the first group, often with typical radiographic abnormalities, are pulmonic stenosis, a few cases of aortic stenosis, patent ductus arteriosus, congenital mitral or tricuspid valvular dysplasia, and peritoneopericardial hernia (for details, see Figure 11). Congenital heart diseases of the second group are patent ductus arteriosus (left-to-right and right-to-left shunting types), tetralogy of Fallot, and large ventricular and atrial septal defects. The third group of congenital heart diseases encompasses most aortic stenoses, some pulmonic stenoses and congenital heart diseases in failure, all complex anomalies and small defects, and atypical cardiac changes with otherwise typical heart diseases. Figure 11 outlines a stepwise approach to the diagnosis of congenital heart disease.

In heart diseases of the first group, it may be possible to proceed with corrective surgery or palliative therapy without delay. Heart diseases of the second and third group usually require a further workup by echocardiography, Doppler echocardiography, and/or complete cardiac catheterization and selective angiocardiography. The procedures last mentioned require referral of the patient to institutions with the necessary sophisticated equipment.

REFERENCES

1. Rhodes WH, Patterson DF, Detweiler DK: Radiographic anatomy of the canine heart. Part I. *JAVMA* 137:283–289, 1960.
2. Hamlin RL: Radiographic diagnosis of heart disease in dogs. *JAVMA* 137:458–464, 1960.
3. Hamlin RL: Prognostic value of changes in the cardiac silhouette in dogs with mitral insufficiency. *JAVMA* 153: 1436–1445, 1968.
4. Detweiler DK, Patterson DF, Luginbühl H, Rhodes WH, Buchanan JW, Knight DH, Hill JD: Diseases of the cardiovascular system, in Catcott EJ (ed): *Canine Medicine*, ed Catcott 1. Santa Barbara, CA, American Veterinary Publications, 1968, p 559.
5. Ettinger SJ, Suter PF: *Canine Cardiology*. Philadelphia, WB Saunders Co, 1970, pp 225–226.
6. Suter PF, Lord PF: A critical evaluation of the radiographic findings in canine cardiovascular diseases. *JAVMA* 158:358–371, 1971.
7. Lord PF, Zontine WJ: Radiologic examination of the feline cardiovascular system. *Vet Clin North Am* 7:291–308, 1977.
8. Harpster NK: Cardiovascular diseases of the domestic cat. *Adv Vet Sci Comp Med* 22:39–74, 1977.
9. Thrall DE, Losonsky JM: Dyspnea in the cat: Part III—Radiographic aspects of intrathoracic causes involving the heart. *Feline Pract* 9:36–49, 1979.
10. Carrig CB, Suter PF, Ewing GO, Dungworth DL: Primary dextrocardia with situs inversus, associated with sinusitis and bronchitis in a dog. *JAVMA* 164:1127–1134, 1974.
11. Silverman S, Suter PF: Influence of inspiration and expiration on canine thoracic radiographs. *JAVMA* 166:502–510, 1975.
12. Rendano VT, Alexander JE: Heart size changes in experimentally-induced adrenal insufficiency in the dog: A radiographic study. *J Am Vet Rad Soc* 17:57–66, 1976.
13. Feldman EC, Tyrell JB: Hypoadrenocorticism. *Vet Clin North Am* 7:555–581, 1977.
14. Mason DT: *Congestive Heart Failure*. New York, Yorke Medical Books, Dun-Donnelley Publishing Corp, 1976.

Evaluating Canine Cardiovascular Silhouettes: Radiographic Methods and Normal Radiographic Anatomy

James P. Toombs, DVM, MS
William R. Widmer, DVM, MS
Department of Veterinary Clinical Sciences
School of Veterinary Medicine
Purdue University
West Lafayette, Indiana

Phillip N. Ogburn, DVM, PhD
Department of Small Animal Clinical Sciences
College of Veterinary Medicine
University of Minnesota
St. Paul, Minnesota

The cardiac silhouette is the most prominent soft tissue structure of the normal thorax and incorporates the combined radiographic densities of the pericardium, the myocardium, the endocardium, the blood within the chambers, and the walls and blood of the great vessels. Routine thoracic radiography, one of several methods used to evaluate the heart, has proven to be an invaluable aid in diagnosing canine cardiac disease.[1]

Radiographic signs of heart disease consist of changes in the size, shape, and position of the cardiac silhouette and its associated major vessels; changes in other organs affected by altered circulation also are signs of disease.[2] Meaningful interpretation of these signs depends on a sound understanding of three-dimensional cardiovascular anatomy and on an awareness of the limitations imposed by the methods used to produce two-dimensional radiographic images.[3,4] The purpose of this article is to review the normal radiographic anatomy of the canine heart and to discuss how survey radiographic methods influence its interpretation.

Standard Radiographic Methods and Their Limitations

Equipment

Because the value of the information obtained from a radiograph is directly proportional to the radiograph's quality, the factors required to produce diagnostic thoracic radiographs are of prime importance. The first factor is the type of x-ray machine used. A radiographic unit must have a focal-film distance of 91 cm or greater; a moving grid or a good quality, stationary, aluminum interspaced grid (103 lines/inch); and a timer allowing for exposures of 1/60 sec or less. The unit must be capable of generating at least 100 kVp (preferably 300 kVp) at 100 mA to produce thoracic radiographs of good quality in large-breed dogs.[3,5]

A second factor to consider is standardized radiographic technique. To compare radiographs made at different stages of disease, film quality must be consistent; this depends on strict attention to standardized technique. The same type of film and screens, consistent radiographic exposure and processing techniques, and identical positioning must be used. The focal-film distance must be constant (91 cm or greater) because

Originally published in Volume 7, Number 7, July 1985

radiographic magnification and distortion of the heart are inversely proportional to this distance.[3] High-speed intensifying screens should be used to enable exposure times of 1/60 sec or less. Rare earth screens are recommended with machines that can generate only 100 kVp at 100 mA. Decreasing the exposure time minimizes the distortion of the cardiac silhouette that results from movement during the cardiac and respiratory cycles.[3]

Technique

The formulation of radiographic technique charts and rules for adapting exposures to the thoracic diameter of the patient are beyond the scope of this article but have been described in detail in the literature.[5-7] The standard exposure technique chosen should produce high-contrast, high-definition radiographs. The ribs and the spine should show good bony detail on lateral projections, and the thoracic spine should be barely visible where it overlies the image of the heart on ventrodorsal (VD) or dorsoventral (DV) projections[4] (Figures 1 and 2). The sharpness, contrast, and density of the film should be such that vascular markings are visible from the hilar region of the lungs to their periphery, the outline of the heart is clear and sharp, and the aorta and the caudal vena cava are readily visible.[4]

All exposures should be made at peak inspiration, which maximizes visualization of the pulmonary arteries and veins and minimizes the chance of interpretive error related to changes in the size, shape, and position of the cardiac silhouette attributable to the different phases of the respiratory cycle.[6,8] If follow-up radiographs are made to assess response to treatment, it is imperative that the exposure technique be identical to that used for the original films.

Positioning

Accurate and consistent patient positioning is vital to standardizing radiographic technique. Slight deviation from standard position can introduce marked deviations in the appearance of the cardiac silhouette.[3,9]

The following eight guidelines will help to standardize positioning: (1) the entire bony thorax should be included on the film[4]; (2) the front legs should be pulled forward to minimize superimposition of the scapulae and the muscles of the brachia over the lung fields[4]; (3) the caudal outline of the diaphragm should be included on the film[4]; (4) on DV and VD films, the thoracic spine should lie in the same vertical plane as the sternum, and the radiographic beam should be centered at the intersection of this plane with the fifth or sixth intercostal space (slightly caudal to the scapulae)[3]; (5) DV or VD films should be symmetrical around the spinal column—deviations greater than 5° from true vertical positioning can introduce significant distortions of the

Slight deviation from standard position can introduce marked deviations in the appearance of the cardiac silhouette.

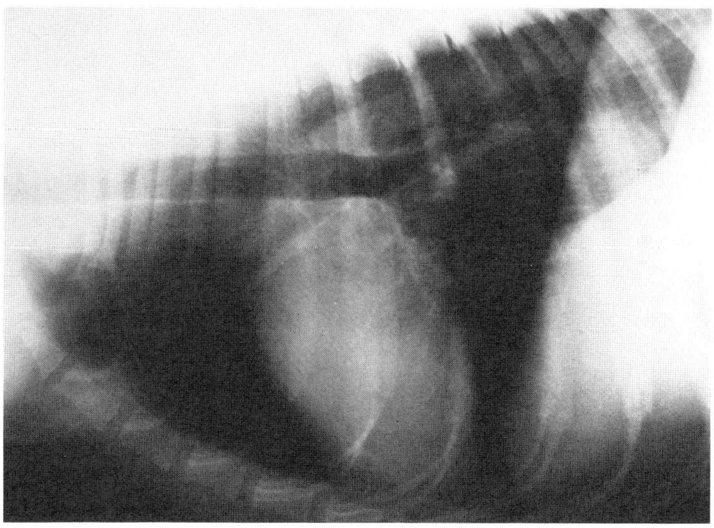

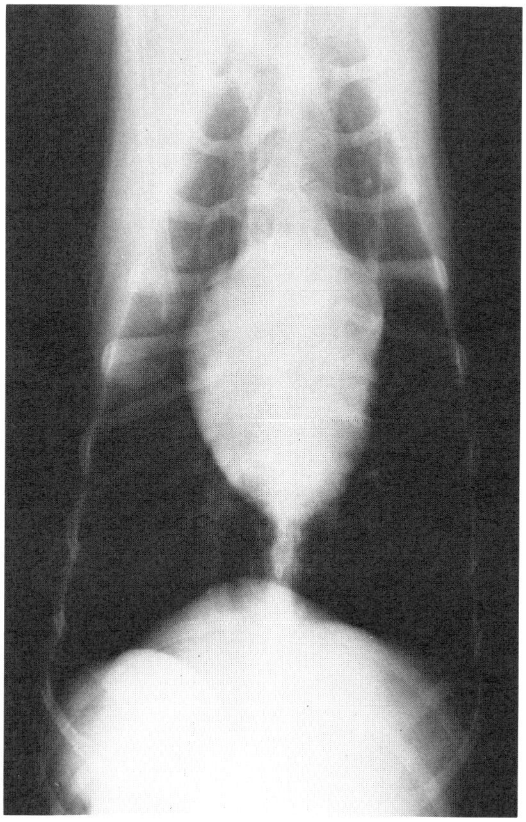

heart shadow[9]; (6) on lateral films, the costochondral junctions of both sides should be in the same plane and the ribs should not extend above the spine[3,10]; (7) films in both projections should be taken at peak inspiration to minimize contact of the heart with the diaphragm[3]; and (8) alternation between DV and VD positioning should be avoided because it introduces changes in the appearance of the cardiac silhouette.[4,11]

Normal and abnormal anatomy has been described for DV and VD vertical-beam radiographic projections.[3,12] In VD radiographs, the craniocaudal axis of the heart appears longer, the heart has a more constant position relative to the thoracic spine, and a greater length of the caudal vena cava is visible than in DV radiographs.[11] Caudal lobar pulmonary arteries are identified more easily in DV radiographs, but a larger area of the accessory lung lobe is visible in VD projections[11] (Figure 2). Differences between the appearance of the heart shadow in DV and VD films are most pronounced in large-breed dogs.[11]

It is claimed that the DV projection is superior to the VD projection for evaluating the heart shadow[4,13] because of more-constant positioning of the heart within the thorax. Selection of DV or VD radiographs should be based on (1) the dog's disposition—true VD positioning often is easier than DV positioning in the uncooperative patient in which tranquilization is contraindicated; (2) the dog's physical status—dorsal recumbency results in severe compromise of pulmonary function in some patients; (3) the position used for previous radiographs; and (4) the preference of the clinician, who might be able to interpret one projection better than another.

Physiologic Factors

Radiographic interpretation of cardiac silhouettes is imprecise, even under the following optimum conditions.

1. Standardized radiographic technique
2. Standardized patient positioning
3. Absence of noncardiogenic anatomic or pathophysiologic factors that can alter the position of the heart
    a. Intrathoracic masses, e.g., neoplastic and granulomatous
    b. Megaesophagus
    c. Pneumothorax
    d. Diaphragmatic hernia
    e. Broken ribs
    f. Abnormal conformation of the bony thorax, e.g., pectis excavatum and pectis cavinatum
    g. Lung lobe torsion (atelectasis)
4. Absence of conditions that impair visualization of the heart shadow, e.g., thoracic effusions and pulmonary neoplasia.

The cardiac silhouette is a static two-dimensional image of a contracting and expanding three-dimensional structure. Variations in the silhouette of the normal heart are to be expected in different phases of the cardiac

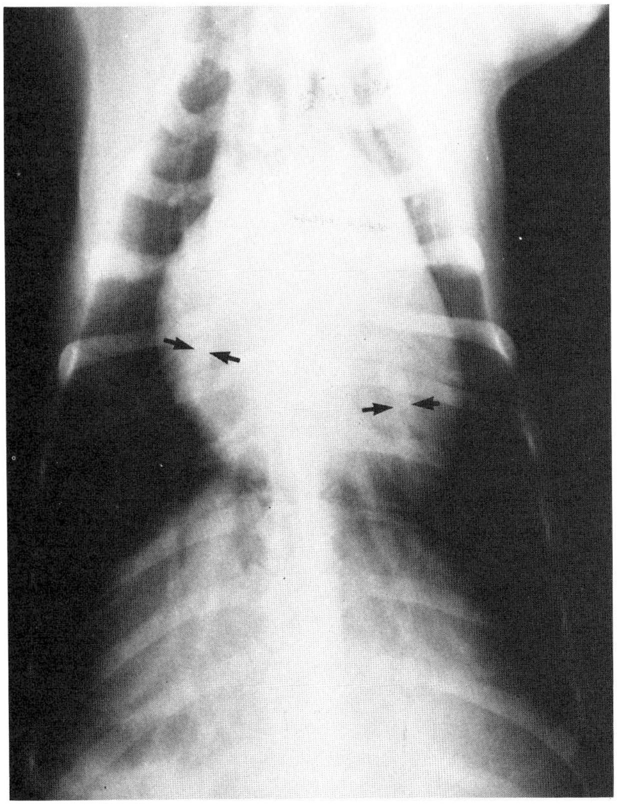

Figure 2A

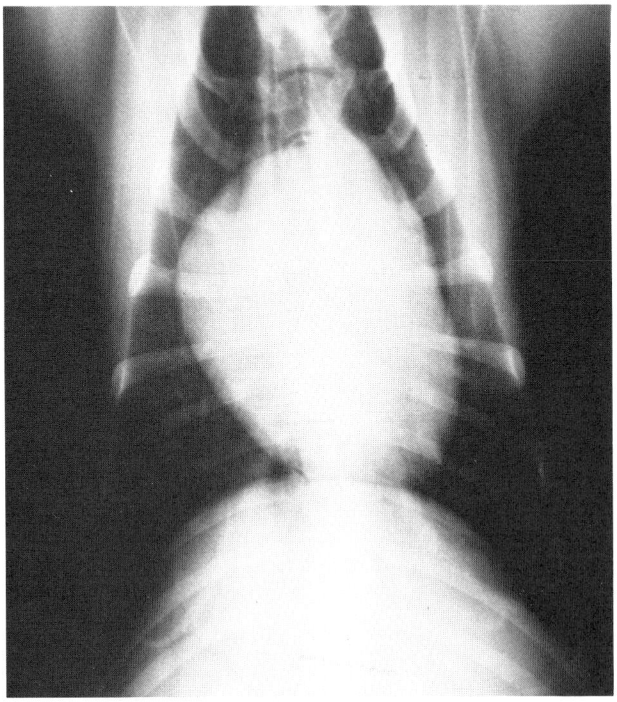

Figure 2B

Figure 2—(**A**) DV and (**B**) VD radiographic views of the heart of a normal mixed-breed dog weighing 22 kg. In the dorsoventral view, the heart appears wider and the caudal lobar pulmonary arteries (*arrows*) are more readily visualized.

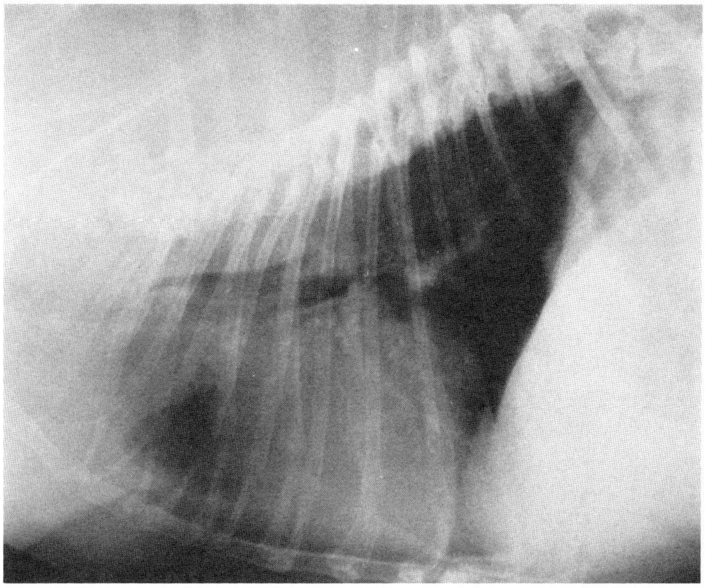

Figure 3A

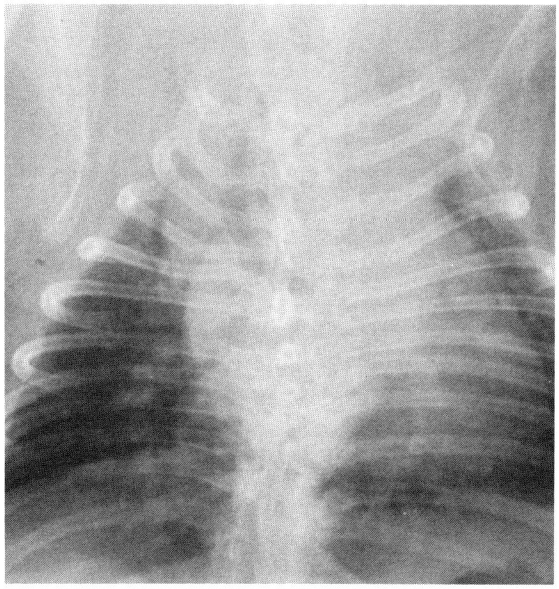

Figure 3B

Figure 3—(**A**) Lateral and (**B**) DV radiographic views of the heart of a normal French bulldog with barrel-chested conformation. Note the forward inclination of the heart shadow in the lateral view and the inclination of the apex toward the left thoracic wall in the DV view.

and respiratory cycles.[3,8] The cardiothoracic ratio (Figure 5) has been demonstrated to increase by as much as 17% during the expiratory phase of respiration in normal dogs, resulting in the perception of cardiac enlargement.[8] Additional radiographic changes associated with the expiratory phase include generalized increase in pulmonary density, decreased visualization of pulmonary arteries and veins, shifting of the apex of the heart toward the left thoracic wall, increased cardiodiaphragmatic contact, decreased clarity of the cardiac silhouette, ventral slanting and enlargement of the cranial portion of the caudal vena cava, and decreased visualization of the caudal portion of the caudal vena cava.[8]

The cardiac silhouette is smallest and most distinct when peak inspiration of the respiratory cycle coincides with end systole of the cardiac cycle.[3] In DV radiographs, the left border of the cardiac silhouette appears straighter, the main pulmonary artery segment is larger and more distinct, and the heart is slightly smaller and more distinct at end systole than in full diastole.[3]

Breed Variation

There is no well-defined configuration of the cardiac silhouette considered normal for all canine breeds.[4] In dogs with narrow, deep thoraxes, such as Afghan hounds, setters, collies, and whippets, the cardiac silhouette tends to be more upright in the lateral projection (Figure 1) than in dogs with wide, shallow thoraxes, such as English bulldogs and Boston terriers. In the latter body type, the heart appears wider and occupies a greater portion of the thorax.[3] In the DV and VD projections, a dog with a deep thoracic conformation, such as a setter, will tend to have a narrower cardiac silhouette and a cardiac axis closer to the vertical midline of the body (Figure 1) than will a dog with an average thoracic conformation, such as a German shepherd. In short dogs with barrel-chested conformation, the apex of the heart is often shifted toward the left thoracic wall and the cardiothoracic ratio tends to be greater[1] (Figure 3). These differences are magnified radiographically. At a focal-film distance of 120 cm (47 inches), radiographic enlargement of the heart of a 36-kg dog is approximately 6 mm.[14] At shorter focal-film distances, the degree of radiographic enlargement is more pronounced.

Cardiac mensuration, the use of comparative measurements to detect enlargement of the cardiac silhouette, is useful in humans.[15,16] Similar techniques have been attempted in dogs[14,17–19] (Figures 4 and 5), but the results have been equivocal because of the marked breed variations previously discussed.[2–4] The various measurements and ratios established by canine studies offer rough guidelines for assessing cardiac enlargement. Evaluating absolute cardiac dimensions and cardiothoracic ratios in dogs with an accuracy similar to that described in humans would require extensive statistical analyses of all breeds, ages, and body configurations.[18] Many veterinary radiologists believe that, with experience, the trained eye can assess heart size with an accuracy closely approximating that provided by the use of mensuration.

In the DV and VD projections, a dog with a deep thoracic conformation ... will tend to have a narrower cardiac silhouette ....

The positional relationships of the trachea to the heart and to the thoracic spine are important in evaluating the dorsal border of the cardiac silhouette.

Normal Anatomy

Lateral Projection

In a radiograph of a patient in the lateral recumbent position, the cardiac silhouette occupies the midventral portion of the thorax and has three borders.[20] The cranial border, which forms a curve extending rostrally to the level of the third rib,[21] has little or no contact with the sternum in deep-chested breeds but can contact as many as two and one-half sternebrae in barrel-chested breeds. The caudal border is straighter and usually is separate from the diaphragm during inspiration; it can extend caudally as far as the eighth costal cartilage at the apex of the heart.[3] The dorsal border is formed by the base of the heart and is contiguous with the caudoventral portion of the trachea.[22]

The positional relationships of the trachea to the heart and to the thoracic spine are important in evaluating the dorsal border of the cardiac silhouette.[3] The long axes of the trachea and the thoracic spine form a divergent angle at the thoracic inlet. This angle can be extremely small in certain miniature breeds, such as the Yorkshire terrier and the Boston terrier; slightly wider in most barrel-chested breeds; and widest in deep-chested breeds.[22] The trachea courses caudally toward the heart and then takes a slight ventral bend over the heart. This bend can be absent in puppies and in some barrel-chested breeds.[3] The trachea terminates between the fifth and sixth ribs in a bifurcation called the *carina*, which is the origin of the two mainstem bronchi.[22] The mainstem bronchi visually are inseparable in a true lateral radiograph of a normal dog.[22] The circular radiolucency seen immediately cranial to the carina is the right cranial lung lobe bronchus.[23]

The apicobasilar line (an imaginary line drawn from the apex of the heart to the tracheal carina) normally forms an angle with the sternum of 55° to 60° (Figure 6). This angle can approach 75° to 80° in deep-chested breeds; it can be as acute as 45° in barrel-chested breeds.[22] The apicobasilar line divides the cardiac silhouette into a cranial three fifths (the right atrium and the right ventricle) and a caudal two fifths (the left atrium and

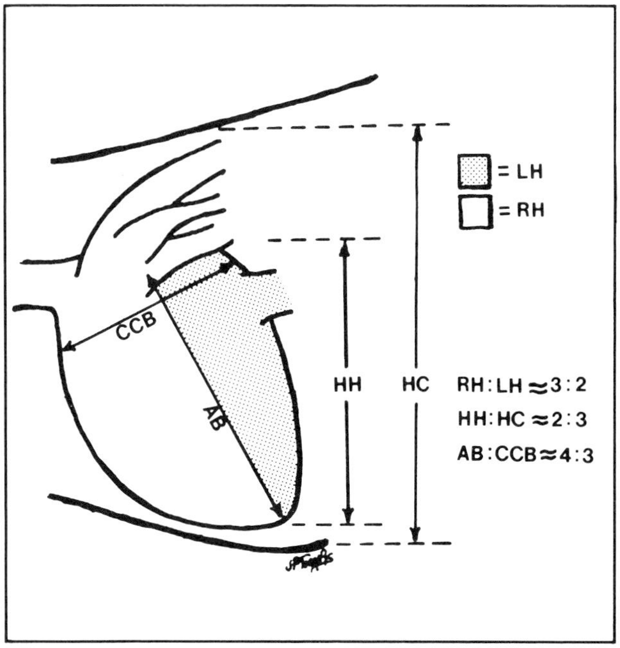

Figure 4—Comparative measurements of the lateral cardiac silhouette and normal measurement ratios. *RH* = right heart, *LH* = left heart, *HH* = height of heart, *HC* = height of chest, *AB* = apicobasilar distance (distance from cardiac apex to tracheal carina), and *CCB* = craniocaudal distance at the base of the heart. In barrel-chested breeds, HH:HC normally will be approximately 3:4.

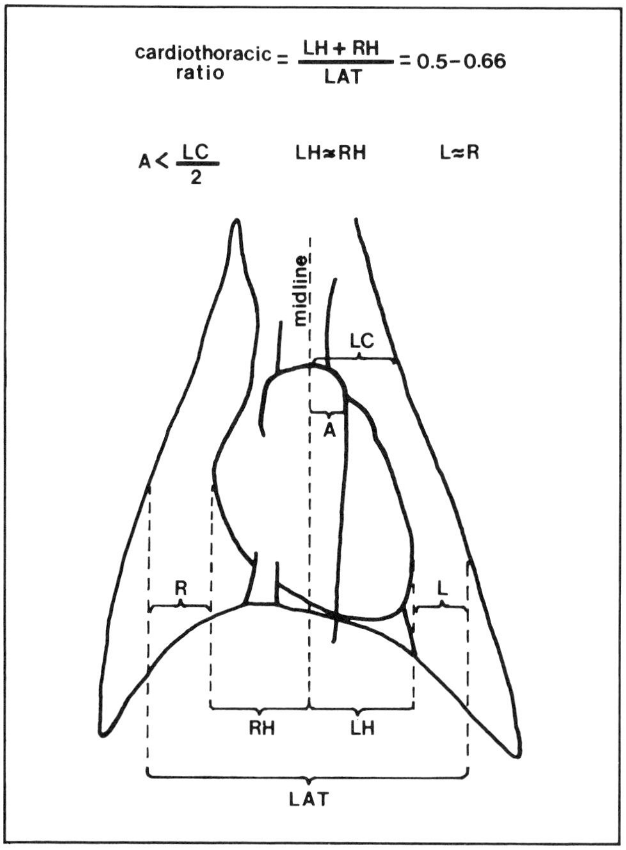

Figure 5—Cardiac mensuration scheme for DV cardiac silhouette[17] and normal measurement ratios. *R* = distance between the right ventricular free wall and the right thoracic wall, *L* = distance between the left ventricular free wall and the left thoracic wall, *RH* = distance of the rightward expanse of the right ventricle from the midsagittal axis, *LH* = distance of the leftward expanse of the left ventricle from the midsagittal axis, *LAT* = distance between the right and left thoracic walls ($R + RH + LH + L$), *LC* = distance from the intersection of the cranial cardiac contour with the midsagittal axis to the left thoracic wall, and *A* = distance from the leftward expanse of the aorta to the midsagittal axis.

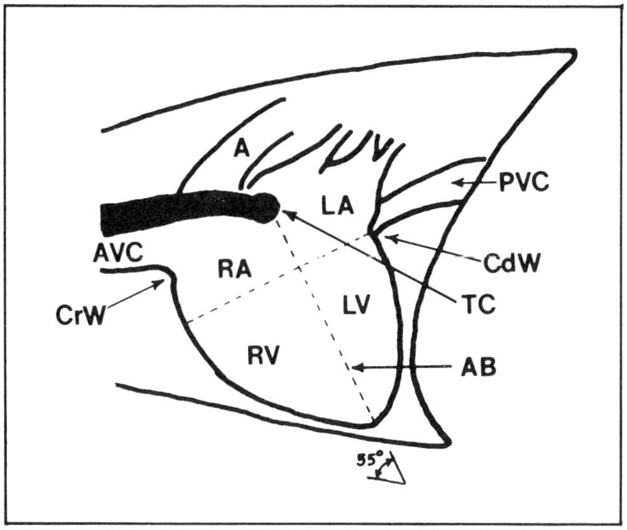

Figure 6—Basic characteristics of the lateral cardiac silhouette of a normal dog. *CrW* = cranial waist, *CdW* = caudal waist, *AVC* = anterior (cranial) vena cava, *PVC* = posterior (caudal) vena cava, *TC* = tracheal carina, *A* = aorta, *RA* = right atrium, *LA* = left atrium, *RV* = right ventricle, *LV* = left ventricle, and *AB* = apicobasilar line. Note that the apicobasilar line and the sternum form an angle of approximately 55°.

the left ventricle). A second line drawn perpendicular to the apicobasilar line and dividing the heart into a dorsal third and a ventral two thirds roughly demarcates the atrioventricular border[21] (Figure 6).

The cranial and caudal borders of the heart curve inward at the base of the heart, producing the appearance of a waist in the region of the atria (Figure 6). The

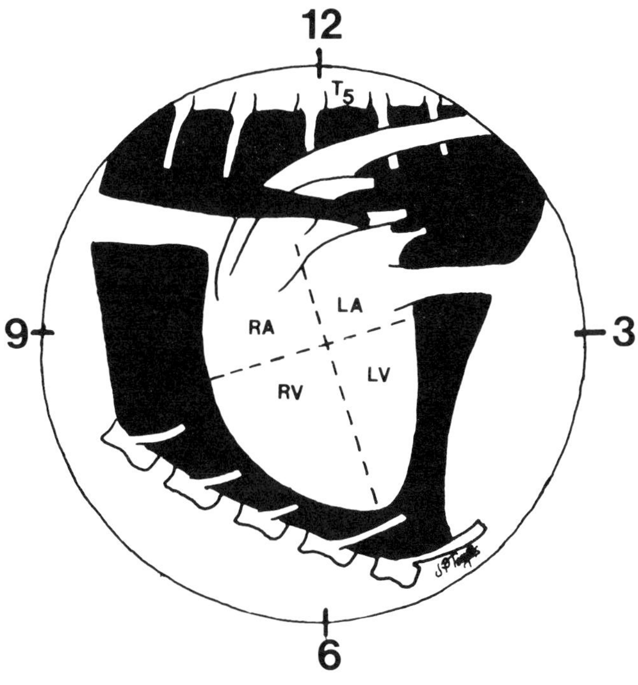

Figure 7—Lateral cardiac silhouette projected onto a clockface to describe chamber and vessel locations. T_5 = body of the fifth thoracic vertebra, *RA* = right atrium, *RV* = right ventricle, *LA* = left atrium, and *LV* = left ventricle.

. . . the cardiac apex falls away from the midline slightly in left lateral recumbency and thus offers a smaller cardiac profile to the x-ray beam.

cranial waist is formed by the junction of the dorsal wall of the right atrium with the caudoventral aspect of the cranial vena cava; this waist is more pronounced in dogs with upright hearts (deep-chested breeds).[3] The caudal waist is formed by the atrioventricular groove and is more pronounced in hearts in which the apicobasilar line has a greater forward inclination (barrel-chested breeds).[3]

In describing the borders of the lateral cardiac silhouette, a clockface analogy helps to indicate the approximate positions of the chambers and the great vessels (Figure 7). With the cranial border of the heart to the viewer's left, the contribution of the left atrium to the border of the heart shadow is visible from 11:30 to 2:00, that of the left ventricle from 2:00 to 5:30, that of the right ventricle from 5:30 to 8:30, and that of the right atrium from 8:30 to 11:30. The base of the heart extends from 9:30 to 1:30, and the aortic arch and the main pulmonary artery segment overlap the right atrial density at 9:00 to 11:30. This analogy, although helpful for descriptive purposes, does little to foster a three-dimensional understanding of cardiovascular anatomy. Figure 8 is a more precise depiction of the relative anatomic locations of these structures.

The right lateral projection is believed to provide the most accurate information for evaluating cardiac size because the cardiac apex falls away from the midline slightly in left lateral recumbency and thus offers a smaller cardiac profile to the x-ray beam.[24] Differences in the appearance of the cardiac silhouette between right lateral and left lateral radiographs, considered to be minimal, are thoroughly reviewed in the literature.[24]

Dorsoventral Projection

Many of the normal characteristics of the DV cardiac silhouette are shared by the VD projection. If both radiographic projections are viewed with the left thoracic wall positioned to the viewer's right, the anatomic relationships of the various cardiac structures are similar. Major differences in the normal appearance of the DV and VD cardiac silhouettes are discussed earlier (in the section on Standard Radiographic Methods and Their Limitations).

In the vertical-beam DV radiograph, the shape of the cardiac silhouette resembles that of a lopsided egg.[4] The silhouette extends from approximately the third to the eighth rib and has rounded cranial and right borders

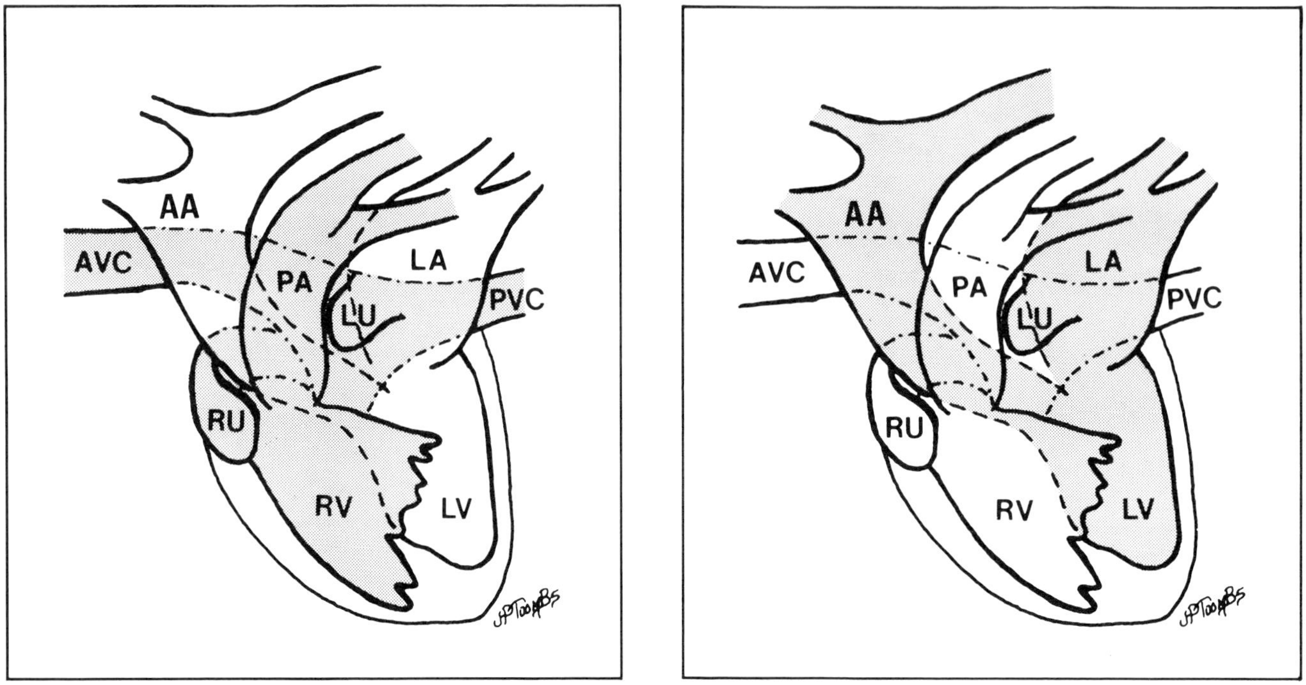

Figure 8A **Figure 8B**

Figure 8—Lateral aspect of the heart as viewed from the left side of the dog; **A** highlights the right heart structures and **B** highlights the left heart structures. In areas where structure borders overlap, those nearest to the viewer are indicated by solid lines, those slightly deeper by dashes, and those that are deepest by dashes alternating with dots. *AVC* = anterior (cranial) vena cava, *PVC* = posterior (caudal) vena cava, *RU* = right auricle, *RV* = right ventricle, *PA* = main pulmonary artery, *LA* = left atrium, *LU* = left auricle, *LV* = left ventricle, and *AA* = aortic arch.

and a nearly straight left border.[3] The base of the heart is roughly bisected by the midsagittal plane, and the apex is directed slightly to the left of the midline. In most canine breeds, the midsagittal plane and the longitudinal axis of the heart form an angle of approximately 30°.[20] In barrel-chested breeds, the apex points further to the left side than in deep-chested breeds, in which the longitudinal axis of the heart can be nearly parallel to the midsagittal plane.[3] In brachycephalic breeds, the apex of the normal heart often is visible slightly to the right of the midline.[3]

The borders of the DV cardiac silhouette are well delineated by the surrounding air density of lung tissue, with the exception of the most cranial border; here the heart is confluent with structures of the cranial mediastinum. If the lungs are well inflated, the caudal border should be visually separate from the diaphragm.[22] A thin, radiopaque line is visible running from the apex of the heart to the diaphragm, slightly to the left of the midline.

The cardiac silhouette is a static two-dimensional image of a contracting and expanding three-dimensional structure.

Although this has sometimes been incorrectly identified as the cardiophrenic ligament, the radiodense line is actually the caudoventral mediastinum and the pleura of the left caudal and accessory lung lobes.[25] The cardiophrenic ligament is not visible radiographically.

The cardiac silhouette is more complex in the DV projection than in the lateral projection because there is more superimposition of chambers and great vessels in the former.[4] In describing the location of the structures that contribute to the borders of the DV cardiac silhouette, the clockface analogy again is useful[26] (Figure 9). With the left border of the heart to the viewer's right, the contribution of the aortic arch to the border of the heart shadow is visible from 11:00 to 1:00, that of the main pulmonary artery segment from 1:00 to 2:00, that of the left ventricle from 2:00 to 5:00, and that of the right ventricle from 5:00 to 10:00. The right atrium and a portion of the caudal vena cava overlap the right ventricle along the curved right border of the heart; the right atrium contributes to the border of the silhouette from 9:00 to 11:00. The left atrium is located centrally in the caudal half of the DV cardiac silhouette and normally does not contribute to its borders. The left auricular appendage, also called the *auricle,* overlies the cranial portion of the left ventricle and makes a minor contribution to the normal heart shadow from 2:00 to 3:00. Figure 10 is a more precise depiction of the positions of the major inflow and outflow tracts relative to one another as viewed from the dorsal aspect of the heart.

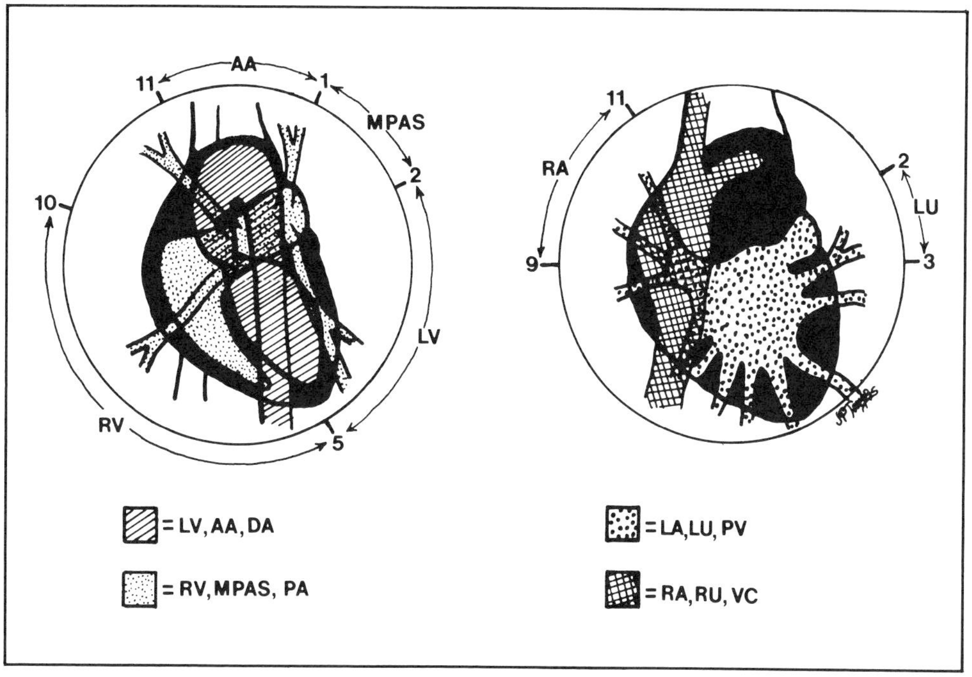

Figure 9—The clockface analogy used with DV cardiac silhouettes. The ventricles and their respective outflow tracts are illustrated at left: *LV* = left ventricle, *AA* = aortic arch, *DA* = descending aorta, *RV* = right ventricle, *MPAS* = main pulmonary artery segment, and *PA* = pulmonary arteries. The atria and the major veins emptying into them are depicted at right: *LA* = left atrium, *LU* = left auricle, *PV* = pulmonary veins, *RA* = right atrium, *RU* = right auricle, and *VC* = vena cavae.

. . . the difference between normal and abnormal in a given dog can be far less dramatic than the difference between normal heart shadows of disparate breeds.

Discussion

The normal canine cardiovascular silhouette should be conceived as a breed-dependent range of shapes with numerous basic similarities, not as a discrete entity. Attention to the patient's chest conformation is critical to accurate radiographic evaluation of the heart because the difference between normal and abnormal in a given dog can be far less dramatic than the difference between normal heart shadows of disparate breeds.

In the absence of congenital heart defects, the best criterion of normality for a particular patient is a set of thoracic radiographs taken after maturity but before the onset of cardiovascular disease. When such films are unavailable, normal radiographs of another dog of the same breed and size can be substituted for reference.

Under the best of circumstances, accurate survey radiographic evaluation of the heart can be elusive. Therefore, it is imperative that the clinician eliminate all controllable variables in order to produce radiographs of diagnostic quality; in addition, the radiographic appearance of the heart should be correlated with clinical and electrocardiographic findings.

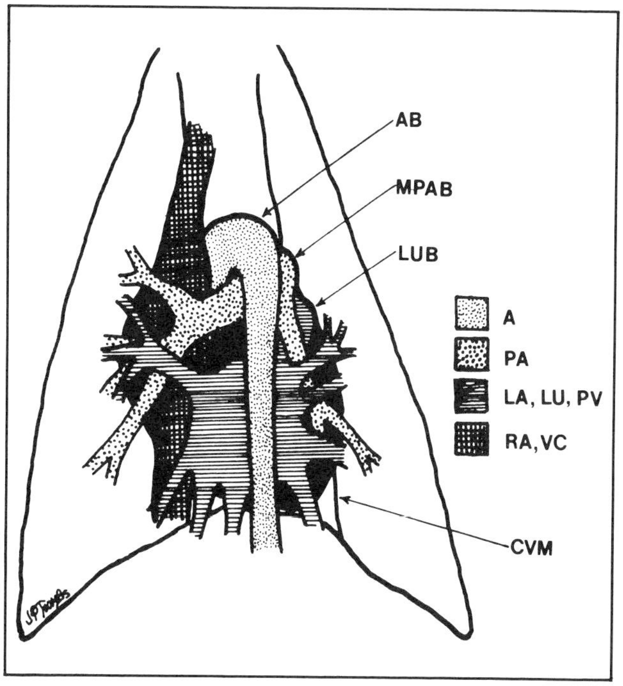

Figure 10—Relative anatomic positions of the major inflow and outflow tracts of the heart, viewed from the dorsal aspect (the left thoracic wall is to viewer's right). *AB* = aortic bulge, *MPAB* = main pulmonary artery segment bulge, *LUB* = left auricular bulge, *A* = aorta, *PA* = pulmonary arteries, *LA* = left atrium, *LU* = left auricle, *PV* = pulmonary veins, *RA* = right atrium, *VC* = vena cava, and *CVM* = caudoventral mediastinum.

REFERENCES

1. Buchanan JW: Radiography of the heart. *AAHA 39th Annu Meet Proc*: 78-86, 1972.
2. Suter PF, Lord PF: A critical evaluation of the radiographic findings in canine cardiovascular diseases. *JAVMA* 158:358-371, 1971.
3. Ettinger SJ, Suter PF: *Canine Cardiology*. Philadelphia, WB Saunders Co, 1970, pp 40-101.
4. Wyburn RS, Lawson DD: Simple radiography as an aid to the diagnosis of heart disease in the dog. *J Small Anim Pract* 8:163-170, 1967.
5. Carlson WD: *Veterinary Radiology*, ed 2. Philadelphia, Lea & Febiger, 1967, pp 57-74.
6. Douglas SW, Williamson HD: *Principles of Veterinary Radiography*. Baltimore, The Williams & Wilkins Co, 1963, pp 170-176.
7. *The Fundamentals of Radiography*, ed 11. Rochester, NY, Eastman Kodak Co, 1968.
8. Silverman S, Suter PF: Influence of inspiration and expiration on canine thoracic radiographs. *JAVMA* 166:502-510, 1975.
9. Perkins RL: Effect of radiographic positioning on the heart shadow in dogs. *Mod Vet Pract* 60:801-805, 1979.
10. Rhodes WH, Patterson DF, Detweiler DK: Radiographic anatomy of the canine heart—Part I. *JAVMA* 137:283-289, 1960.
11. Ruehl WW, Thrall DE: The effect of dorsal versus ventral recumbency on the radiographic appearance of the canine thorax. *Vet Radiol* 22:10-16, 1981.
12. Gillette EL, Thrall DE, Lebel JL: *Carlson's Veterinary Radiology*, ed 3. Philadelphia, Lea & Febiger, 1977.
13. Hamlin RL: Prognostic value of changes in the cardiac silhouette in dogs with mitral insufficiency. *JAVMA* 153:1436-1445, 1968.
14. Schulze W, Noldner H: Rontgenologische Fernaufnahme des Hundeherzens und Versuch ihrer Deutung mit Hilfe einer linearen Messmethode. *Arch Exp Veterinarmed* 11:442, 1957.
15. Friedberg CK: *Diseases of the Heart*, ed 3. Philadelphia, WB Saunders Co, 1966, pp 160-170.
16. Meschan I: *Roentgen Signs in Clinical Practice*, vol II. Philadelphia, WB Saunders Co, 1966, p 1024.
17. Hamlin RL: Analysis of the cardiac silhouette in dorsoventral radiographs from dogs with heart disease. *JAVMA* 153:1446-1449, 1968.
18. Hamlin RL: Radiographic diagnosis of heart disease in dogs. *JAVMA* 137:458-464, 1960.
19. Hamlin RL: The x-ray shadow of the normal canine heart. *Speculum* 10:6, 1957.
20. Hamlin RL: Radiographic anatomy of the heart and great vessels in healthy living dogs. *JAVMA* 136:265-273, 1960.
21. Roberts R, Banks WC: Radiographic considerations in the normal and altered cardiac silhouette of the canine patient. *Southwest Vet* 26:11-16, 1972.
22. Roberts R: Radiographic examination and heart disease. *AAHA Autotutorial Shortcourse*, 1976, pp 55-76.
23. Burk RL, Corwin LA, Bahr RJ, et al: The right cranial lung lobe bronchus of the dog: Its identification in a lateral chest radiograph. *J Am Vet Radiol Soc* 19:210-212, 1978.
24. Spencer CP, Ackerman N, Burt JK: The canine lateral thoracic radiograph. *J Am Vet Radiol Soc* 22:262-266, 1981.
25. Burk RL: Radiographic definition of the phrenicopericardiac ligament. *J Am Vet Radiol Soc* 17:216-218, 1976.
26. Suter PF, Gomez JA: *Diseases of the Thorax—Radiographic Diagnosis*. Davis, CA, Venture Press, 1981, pp 57-75.

Radiology of Acute Abdominal Disorders in the Dog and Cat (Part 1)

Lawrence J. Kleine, DVM, MS
Associate Professor and Head, Radiology
Tufts University
School of Veterinary Medicine
North Grafton, Massachusetts

Acute abdominal disorders are among the most difficult problems to diagnose in small animal practice. Even though the clinical signs are of short duration, the underlying lesion may be either acute or chronic. Since many of these disorders must be treated promptly to prevent rapid deterioration of the patient's condition, a practical approach is urged. It is suggested that an attempt be made to classify the disorder as *inflammatory, hemorrhagic, obstructive*, or *traumatic*. This initial approach may permit management decisions which will reduce morbidity without excluding other diagnoses. An exact diagnosis can often be made only during an exploratory laparotomy or after biopsy or necropsy.

The inevitable question that must be answered is, should surgery be performed? Survey radiography and specific radiographic procedures often provide crucial data which not only categorize the disorder but determine if surgery is needed. Utilization of special techniques in the diagnosis of acute abdominal disorders is limited by the animal's inability to tolerate stress. These individuals must be handled gently because of their painful and often precarious metabolic state. Yet radiographic examinations must be thorough if morbidity and mortality are to be reduced to a minimum.

Clinical Aspects and Physical Examination–First priority in caring for the dog or cat with an acute abdominal disorder is to determine the necessity for support of both the respiratory and circulatory systems. Such intervention is accomplished by administration of oxygen, colloid or crystalloid fluids, and by maintaining body temperature. After emergency care a more thorough physical examination should be carried out to estimate the need for other tests. The importance of repeating the physical examination cannot be overemphasized in reevaluating the dog or cat's condition.

Careful inspection of the animal's conformation gives an indication of the nature and presence of any abnormality. A recumbent posture may indicate weakness, spinal injury, or pain, and if there is a unilateral painful condition, the affected side is generally kept uppermost. Kyphosis may indicate back or kidney pain. Rapid shallow breathing often accompanies abdominal pain regardless of the organ involved, making a short x-ray exposure time essential. Wounds, bruising, or pain should lead to further examination for internal injuries that are not immediately apparent.

Originally published in Volume 1, Number 7, July 1979

Thorough but careful palpation of the external surface of the body and abdomen is essential for adequate diagnosis. However, routine abdominal palpation may be difficult or even impossible in the injured animal because of pain. Therefore, changing the position, such as laying the animal on its back so that it cannot tense its abdominal muscles, or the use of analgesics may aid in this critical part of the examination.[3]

Body temperature and pulse are criteria used in determining the seriousness and location of an injury. A rapid pulse rate, rising rectal temperature, and concomitant radiographic and clinical signs of obstruction are highly suggestive of small bowel infarction. Simple laboratory tests such as packed cell volume and white blood cell count are useful in determining the likely source, and sometimes the seriousness of the condition. Blood gas evaluations are needed, not only for diagnosis, but as aids in deciding the type of fluid to be administered. When peritoneal effusion is suspected, paracentesis with laboratory examination of any fluid thus obtained may be diagnostic.

General Radiographic Technique—The primary considerations in selecting x-ray exposure factors are the thickness and composition of the tissue being examined. A general technique chart will usually suffice for abdominal radiography. However, if the x-ray generator can produce a short exposure time at high milliamperage it may be desirable to produce a second chart utilizing low kilovoltage technique with a high milliampere-second setting in order to enhance patient contrast. A high milliampere-second setting is necessary to compensate for the decreased radiographic density that would otherwise result from lowering the kilovoltage. If the exposure is longer than 1/10th of a second there will be an inherent lack of sharpness due to motion of viscera during the exposure.

The primary x-ray beam should be collimated only to the area of interest. This reduces the secondary radiation exposure to personnel who restrain the animal and also increases detail on the x-ray film by reducing scatter. The most important factor in reducing scatter, and thereby increasing detail, is the use of a grid. Grids should be used when the area being radiographed is thicker than 10 cm. The grid will absorb scattered radiation that would otherwise fall on the x-ray film thereby reducing contrast and image sharpness. Either a stationary or moving (Bucky) grid can be used. The higher the grid ratio[a] the greater the amount of scatter that will be reduced. When a grid is used, the radiation necessary to produce the image must be increased to compensate for primary beam absorption.

With low output equipment compromise is necessary so that increased radiation exposure does not require a length of exposure time that increases the possibility of motion. For lower power equipment a 5 to 1 stationary table-top grid may be the best compromise, whereas with maximum power equipment a 10 to 1 high speed movable grid may be more desirable.

Both ventrodorsal and lateral projections are necessary for evaluation of the abdomen. One view or the other will not usually give a satisfactory evaluation. Gas within the gastrointestinal tract or the abdominal cavity will rise and fluid will fall; therefore, in the left lateral radiograph one would expect air to rise into the pylorus and fluid to fall into the fundus of the stomach. The reverse is true in the right lateral projection. Bearing these facts in mind, one may choose whether the right or left lateral view is more desirable under a particular set of circumstances. In some cases, both projections are needed.

The ventrodorsal view is generally preferred over the dorsoventral view because in the former the animal may be stretched somewhat thus reducing the amount of tissue to be penetrated by the x-ray beam. It is also usually easier to position the animal correctly in the ventrodorsal view because the landmarks for positioning are more readily seen. Oblique views project an image of the structures that lie at the margin of the abdomen but would be otherwise partially obliterated by overlying viscera in the standard ventrodorsal and lateral projections.

Special views such as recumbent lateral or horizontal beam radiographs are useful in determining whether a particular opacity is fluid or solid. Horizontal beam radiography is also used to demonstrate air-fluid levels in the intestine or free gas in the abdominal cavity.

Radiographic Examination of the Gastrointestinal Tract Utilizing Contrast Medium–There are several reasons why barium is the most commonly used contrast medium in the gastrointestinal tract. Not only is barium unexcelled as a coating agent of mucosal surfaces, it is readily obtainable and inexpensive. As long as it remains in the gastrointestinal tract, it is nontoxic and its transit time through the gastrointestinal tract is predictable.[8] On the other hand, the organic iodides intended for gastrointestinal use are hypertonic and have a tendency to draw fluid into the gastrointestinal tract.[11] In the case of a debilitated patient this feature is highly undesirable and may lead to increased morbidity. In addition, the transit time of organic iodides through the gastrointestinal tract is less predictable than that of barium, they are more expensive, have a bitter taste, and generally do not provide satisfactory mucosal coating.

However, since these agents are much less irritating to peritoneal and pleural surfaces than barium, it would seem that organic iodides have a place in contrast studies of the gastrointestinal tract where perforation is suspected. A caveat to consider is that these contrast agents are generally

[a]This is the ratio between the height and distance between the lead strips that form the grid.

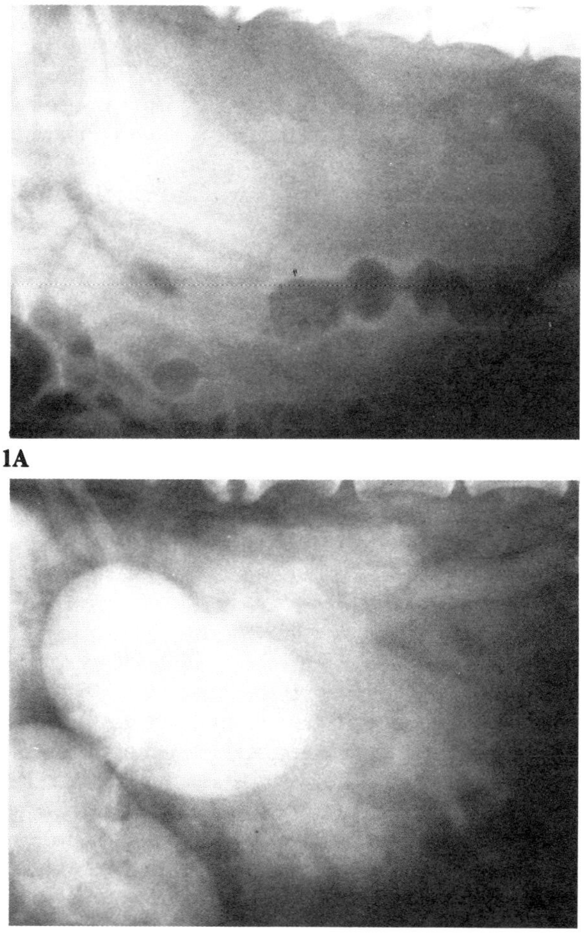

1A

1B

Fig 1–This 13-year-old Beagle had an abdominal mass and pitting rear leg edema. Since only one kidney was seen in the survey radiograph **A** an excretory urogram was performed **B.** Both kidneys were outlined and the mass contains contrast medium. A few hours later the dog suddenly became weak, pale, and died. The mass was a post caval aneurysm.

diluted by fluid that accumulates proximal to the site of obstruction or perforation, and therefore the site of perforation may not be seen radiographically. Moreover, one must recognize that these agents are rapidly absorbed from the peritoneal surface, so that if perforation is present it may not be visualized because of rapid reabsorption of the contrast medium across the peritoneal membrane.

It is *not* true that contrast visualization of the kidneys, ureters, and urinary bladder during organic iodide upper gastrointestinal examination (UGI) indicates gastrointestinal tract perforation. Occasionally the organic iodide is absorbed by the mucosa of the small intestine and excreted by the kidneys.[10] For these reasons organic iodides have a restricted role in gastrointestinal radiography of the dog and cat.

Spilling of barium into the peritoneal cavity as the result of perforation may not be as serious as once thought if lavage of peritoneal surfaces is carried out at exploratory laparotomy immediately upon recognition of such a perforation.[13] Because of the hazards of barium granulomas in the peritoneum and the possibility of not visualizing the perforation when organic iodides are used, it may be desirable to perform exploratory laparotomy based on clinical and survey radiographic findings rather than performing any type of contrast examination when perforation is suspected.

Pure USP barium sulfate is generally an unsatisfactory product for use in an UGI. Commercial barium preparations which are micropulverized and have added suspending agents are much more desirable. Their transit time through the gastrointestinal tract is more predictable and there is much less tendency for these agents to precipitate during the examination.

Barium products may be mixed by the user or may be purchased already mixed. Since the latter are uniform in consistency, they are usually the best and most convenient choice for UGI in the dog and cat. If barium is mixed manually, the manufacturer's instructions should be carefully followed. Vigorous agitation in a blender will produce the most uniform suspension. The contrast medium should be weighed and mixed with the appropriate volume of water.

Before administering any oral contrast agent for the UGI the stomach and small intestine should be free of food and the colon should not contain feces. Without proper preparation, transit of barium through the gastrointestinal tract will be impeded. Furthermore, dense ingesta may overlap and obliterate lesions so that radiographic examination is not only not useful, but possibly misleading.

However, since many patients suffering from acute abdominal conditions cannot receive enemas or laxatives because of the nature of their illness, it may be necessary to perform contrast examination without bowel preparation. Under these circumstances the radiographic study may be limited in its accuracy and if the examination is inconclusive it should be repeated later if the animal's condition will permit.

In general, it is preferable to give a large amount of barium (11 to 15 ml per kg of body weight) for the UGI. Contrast medium is administered by stomach tube to encourage passage through the gastrointestinal tract as a bolus. This permits better evaluation of the gastrointentinal tract than when barium is present in all parts of the GI tract simultaneously. A more accurate judgement of transit time is obtained if the contrast medium is deposited in the stomach quickly.

If the stomach is the primary area of interest, the UGI technique can be modified by administering a small amount of contrast medium (4 to 7 ml per kg of body weight). The animal is then rotated and radiographed in the dorsoventral, ventrodorsal, right, and left lateral projections. Ventrodorsal-oblique views may also be useful if a lesion near the cardia is suspected. After these radiographs are made, the UGI may be continued by administering another 9 to 11 ml per kg of body weight of con-

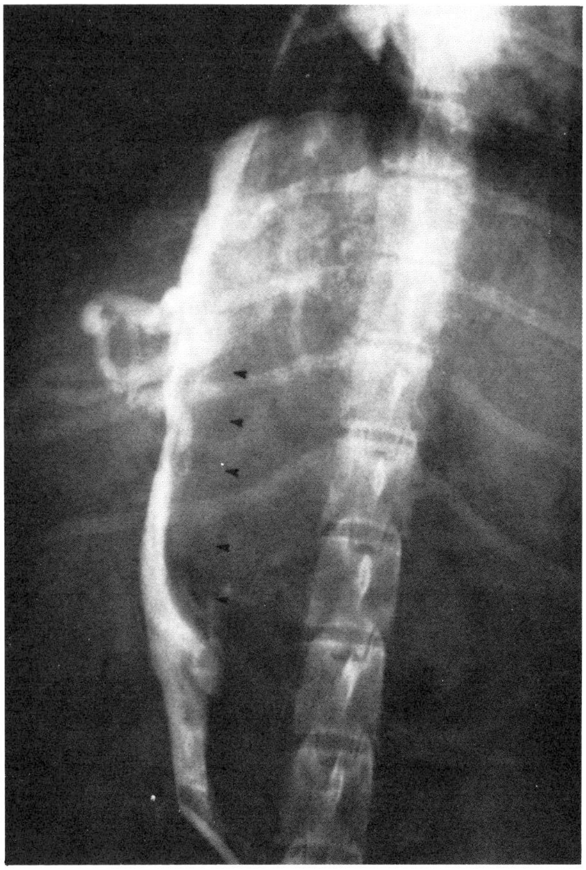

Fig 2–A 7-year-old spayed female Dachshund was examined for ascites and rear leg edema and weakness. The post-vena-cava gram indicates a large filling defect (*arrows*) due to invasion of the vena cava by an adrenal pheochromocytoma. Acute weakness was due to bleeding from the neoplasm.

trast medium by stomach tube and repeating the radiographic procedure. This technique permits evaluation of the stomach in several planes in both the distended and undistended states. Further examination of the stomach can be accomplished by instilling room air or carbon dioxide through the stomach tube or by mixing barium suspension with an effervescent agent.[b]

During the UGI examination, radiographs in both the ventrodorsal and lateral projections are generally made at each of the following times: immediately, 30 minutes, 60 minutes, 3 hours, 6 hours, and 24 hours. However, in each case the examination is tailored to the animal's needs and consideration is given to the expected pathologic change. If the passage of contrast medium is exceptionally rapid, radiographs should be taken more frequently early in the course of the examination. If transit time is slow some of the early films may be eliminated. Both ventrodorsal and lateral radiographs are essential for complete examination of the gastrointestinal tract. Some examiners choose to increase their millampere-seconds by 25% or kilovoltage by 10% to provide penetration of the barium column, permitting better evaluation of the intestinal wall during the UGI.

If the colon is the primary area of interest the best radiographic examination is a barium enema rather than the UGI. The consistency of contrast medium is not uniform when it finally reaches the colon in the UGI, so that its coating characteristics are altered, and there is a longer wait to visualize the colon when barium is given orally rather than by enema.

The barium enema procedure is generally performed under anesthesia and should not be preceded by punch biopsy of the colon or vigorous colonoscopy because the colon can be weakened, increasing the danger of perforation with subsequent spilling of barium into the peritoneum. There is no uniform opinion as to the length of time that should elapse before a barium enema can be given after these procedures, however, a delay of 7 days is preferred.

The most satisfactory barium enema technique is to use a commercially available plastic bag which contains dry barium and has plastic tubing with an attached inflatable cuff.[c] After suspending the barium in water, the tubing is inserted in the rectum so that the cuff lies just beyond the pelvic brim. The cuff is inflated to maintain the position of the tubing and to prevent leakage of barium from the patient during the examination. For small dogs or kittens a bulb syringe inserted into the rectum may serve the same purpose as an inflatable cuff, but air administration is difficult to control when the examination is performed in this manner. The barium is instilled by gravity flow, until the colon and rectum are outlined by contrast. This generally requires 22 to 33 ml of contrast medium per kg of body weight. When the colon has been filled, radiographs are made in the right and left lateral projections and the ventrodorsal and dorsoventral projections.

Barium is drained from the colon by placing the administration bag lower than the level of the dog. Gentle abdominal palpation helps to empty the colon and rectum. Usually 15 to 20 minutes is required to drain most of the contrast medium. After removing the barium, all projections are repeated. Finally the colon is insufflated with carbon dioxide or room air and the four projections are repeated again. This final procedure provides double contrast and distends the colon, providing superior mucosal detail.

Radiographic Examination of the Urogenital Tract Using Contrast Medium–Contrast radiographic examination of the urinary tract is essential in diagnosing many cases of acute abdominal disease. The male canine urethra is most clearly seen when 5 to 10 ml of a sterile aqueous iodine solution, with an iodine concentration of approximately 200 mg per ml, is administered by uri-

[b]E-Z Gas, E-Z-EM Company, Inc., Westbury, NY 11590

[c]Barium enema, E-Z-EM Company, Inc., Westbury, NY 11590

nary catheter into the distal urethra while occluding the urethral orifice. X-ray exposure is made at the conclusion of this procedure. The entire urethra and neck of the urinary bladder are outlined to show filling defects or mucosal irregularities.

The urinary bladder is drained and an attempt is made to flush out blood clots or debris with sterile saline. The bladder is then distended with either gas or organic iodine contrast medium until back pressure is exerted on the syringe by the medium, or until the volume of contrast medium administered equals the estimated capacity of the urinary bladder. The potential hazard of fatal air embolism resulting from air insufflation of the urinary bladder, particularly in patients with hematuria, must be considered. Less risk is associated with carbon dioxide insufflation of the bladder. Radiographs are made in the ventrodorsal and lateral projections. Ventrodorsal oblique views are needed if a bladder neck lesion is suspected.

Excretory urography is done to evaluate the kidneys and ureters. For this procedure, aqueous organic iodine contrast medium, at a dose of 250 to 900 mg of iodine per kg body weight, is injected rapidly intravenously. The lower dosage is suggested in giant breeds of dogs and when the pyelographic phase of the urogram is the area of primary interest. The upper dose range is utilized when working with small dogs and cats, when hypotension or uremia are present, or when the nephrographic phase of the urogram is of greatest importance.

The contrast medium can be administered through an indwelling venous catheter rather than a needle to facilitate visualization of the vascular phase of the urogram in the immediate radiographs. Ordinarily, compression techniques are not used because of the diminished visibility which results when there is overlapping of small bowel silhouettes on the kidneys, and because tranquilization is usually necessary for effective compression.

In the conventional intravenous urogram both ventrodorsal and lateral radiographs are obtained at the following times after injection of the contrast medium: immediately, 10 minutes, 30 minutes and 60 minutes. If a lesion is suspected in the trigone area, ventrodorsal oblique radiographs which include the pelvic canal should be taken in addition to the standard lateral and ventrodorsal views. The nephrographic phase is best seen in the immediate radiographs while the pyelographic phase is best seen at 10 and 30 minutes. The one hour radiograph is used to evaluate the renal silhouettes for the presence of a pyelographic phase and prolonged distortion of pelvic diverticula.

In cases of a prolonged nephrogram or pyelogram, additional radiographs are generally taken at 2 and 4 hours. A crude measure of renal function is given by the quantity and density of contrast medium in the kidneys and urinary bladder. The ureters are seldom visualized completely in a single exposure regardless of its timing because the contrast medium is carried away from the kidney in peristaltic waves.

Cholecystography—Where ultrasound is available, it has largely replaced cholecystography in gallbladder evaluation. The oral cholecystogram is generally used to evaluate dogs and cats for cholecystitis. For performing oral cholecystography, 200 mg of iopanic acid tablets[d] per kg of body weight are given per os, and radiographs are then made 10 to 14 hours later. If the gallbladder is not visualized, radiographs are repeated in 24 hours. There are many causes of nonvisualization of the gallbladder, but most can be readily eliminated on a clinical basis. Among these causes are: drug not administered, drug vomited after administration, proximal duodenal obstruction, malabsorption syndrome, insufficient liver excretion of drug, obstruction of cystic duct, absence of gallbladder, and cholecystitis.

When the gallbladder is not visualized by the oral technique, an intravenous cholecystogram using meglumine iodipapide[e] may then be performed. The contrast medium is administered intravenously at a dose rate of 0.5 ml per kg of body weight over a period of ten minutes. Radiographs are made 30, 60 and 180 minutes after injection. This procedure outlines the intrahepatic bile ducts, and may permit the examiner to determine whether or not intrahepatic bile duct obstruction is present.

Angiography–Angiography is used extensively in man to evaluate abdominal trauma.[9] However, this technique has not found wide acceptance in small animal practice because of the need for special equipment and expertise not generally available to the private practitioner. In renal infarction or rupture of the renal pedicle angiography is the preferred method of diagnosis. There are other vascular lesions that may require angiography for ante mortem diagnosis (Figs 1 and 2).

When aortic embolism is suspected the most accurate radiographic approach to the problem is to catheterize the aorta through a carotid artery approach. However, a simpler and usually satisfactory technique is to use a venous catheter inserted by means of the cephalic or jugular vein, making a rapid injection of approximately 2 ml of contrast medium per kg of body weight. Radiographs are made between 7 and 20 seconds following the administration of the medium, which will not be as dense as with the aortic approach, but usually will outline any major obstruction of the abdominal aorta.

ACKNOWLEDGMENT

The author gratefully acknowledges the help of Paula Ruel, BSN, RN, in the preparation of the manuscript.

[d]Telepaque, Winthrop Laboratories, New York, NY 10016

[e]Cholegraffin, Squibb & Sons, Princeton, NJ 08540

(continues on page 85)

Radiology of Acute Abdominal Disorders in the Dog and Cat (Part II)

Lawrence J. Kleine, DVM, MS
Associate Professor and Head, Radiology
Tufts University
School of Veterinary Medicine
North Grafton, Massachusetts

In acute abdominal disorders survey film findings are exceptionally important because contrast examinations may be impossible to perform due to the animal's poor condition or the need for a rapid diagnosis. When the radiographic findings are correlated with physical and laboratory tests a decision whether a contrast examination should be performed can be made. Survey radiographs also indicate whether the initial radiographic technique was correct and whether factors are present that will preclude a contrast examination or will prevent adequate visualization of the various abdominal structures during the contrast examination. These factors include the presence of feces or excessive gas in the intestine and the presence of gas in the intraperitoneal space.

Each examiner should develop a method of evaluating radiographs to determine whether they are of adequate technical quality and also to evaluate the films so that no abnormality will be overlooked. Clinical judgement is used to assign proper significance to any abnormalities that are found.

When examining the radiograph one should first visualize those structures external to the abdomen, including the bony portion of the spinal column, the ribs and the ilia. Next, the abdominal wall should be evaluated for any break in its integrity, changes in opacity (Fig 1) or the presence of a foreign body. The diaphragmatic silhouette should be examined and the general abdominal configuration evaluated. A search should be made for evidence of free gas or fluid within the peritoneal cavity. Free gas tends to accumulate in the subdiaphragmatic area between the liver and the diaphragm in both the ventrodorsal and lateral projections. Horizontal beam radiography in a recumbent lateral or standing position may be useful in further delineating small amounts of gas. Another manifestation of free intraperitoneal gas is the formation of small bubbles due to gas becoming trapped within the mesentery. These bubbles will tend to occupy a central position in the abdomen, may have the same stippled appearance as hemorrhage of the omentum and be difficult for the inexperienced observer to discern.

Next, the appearance of the retroperitoneum and kidneys should be evaluated for masses or uneven opacity which generally indicates extravasation of fluid. The uneven appearance does not reveal the

Originally published in Volume 1, Number 8, August 1979

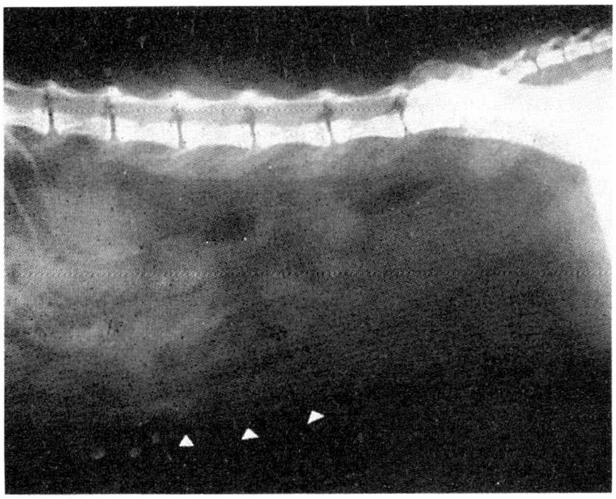

Fig 1—A one-and-a-half-year old cat experienced pain when its abdomen was touched. In abdominal radiographs an irregular opacity was present in the ventral subcutaneous soft tissues (*arrows*). The microscopic diagnosis was pansteatitis.

nature of the fluid but merely its presence. It may be hemorrhage, an exudate or a transudate. After the evaluation of the skeletal structures of the abdomen, the abdominal wall, the abdominal cavity and retroperitoneum, each abdominal viscus in turn should be examined. The entire gastrointestinal tract including the stomach, small intestine and colon should be evaluated. In addition, special attention should be paid to the liver, spleen and pancreas.

Stomach

The normal gastric silhouette lies parallel to the arch of the rib in the lateral radiograph, except in deep-chested dogs, where it is nearly perpendicular to the sternum. Hepatomegaly displaces the pyloric antrum in a dorsocaudomedial direction causing the fundic-pyloric axis to lie more parallel to the spine than usual. When gastric thickening or edema of mucosal folds is suggested, no specific conclusions can be drawn with respect to the cause. This finding is often associated with vomiting, regardless of whether the vomiting is due to pyloric or intestinal obstruction, irritation of the gastrointestinal tract, or secondary to metabolic upset such as uremia. In chronic uremia, gastric mineralization may occur.

Direct trauma to the stomach is seldom easily evaluated radiographically. Granular material within the stomach is sometimes the result of gastric hemorrhage which may be secondary to trauma, inflammatory disease or a neoplasm. In gastric perforation free air is usually released into the abdominal cavity. Volvulus of the stomach results because of rotation of the stomach around the mesenteric axis. The pylorus comes to lie in a more dorsal and cranial position than normal on the left of the midline. When this occurs neither air nor fluid can easily leave the stomach and further distension leads to toxemia and strangulation. There is reduced venous blood flow to the heart due to compression of the caudal vena cava. Gastric volvulus can be recognized by the displacement of the pylorus and by a dense line along the cranial aspect of the gastric silhouette, resulting from the folding of the pylorus upon the body of the stomach.

Diaphragmatic hernia is a very common acute abdominal injury. It is most often recognized radiographically by the presence of abdominal viscera within the thoracic cavity or by the absence of viscera which would normally be present in the abdomen. These displaced viscera usually partially obliterate the cardiac silhouette. Transudation of fluid into the pleural or intraperitoneal space occurs if there is incarceration of a viscus within the thoracic cavity. A gastric diaphragmatic hernia must be recognized as a surgical emergency because it can be rapidly fatal, leading to strangulation, toxemia, interference with lung expansion, and reduced cardiac filling.

Vomiting is the most frequent clinical sign associated with a gastric foreign body, pyloric obstruction, or mucosal irritation.

Intussusception of the stomach into the esophagus is a rare condition that can be rapidly fatal if not recognized early.

Any time shock or difficult breathing is present, the gastric silhouette may be greatly distended with air.

While neoplasms are not generally considered the cause of acute abdominal disease, if they cause obstruction, massive blood loss, or perforation, clinical signs will be acute.

The stomach may be indirectly involved in either pancreatic or hepatic masses or pancreatitis.[4] In these situations gastric displacement is a prominent finding. With a pancreatic mass or pancreatitis the pylorus may be displaced to the left. Other findings that may be associated with pancreatitis include spreading of the angle between the descending duodenum and the greater curvature of the stomach and lack of definition in the cranial abdominal quadrant due to inflammatory response of the tissues in that region[4] (Fig 2).

Small Intestine

Injury to the small intestine due to blunt trauma is not common because of its ability to be displaced. With a large perforation of the intestine free gas is found in the intraperitoneal space, whereas when small tears occur the free gas may be confined to small bubbles trapped in the mesentery and omentum.

Weeks or months following trauma, an abdominal mass may develop due to adhesions between the lacerated portion of intestine, mesentery, and omentum. Obstruction can occur because of narrowing of the lumen due to fibrosis. Bruising of the intestine may not produce any immediate radiographic abnormality except for a slight loss of contrast due to hemorrhage. An organizing intramural hematoma is capable of producing small bowel obstruction after a period of several hours.

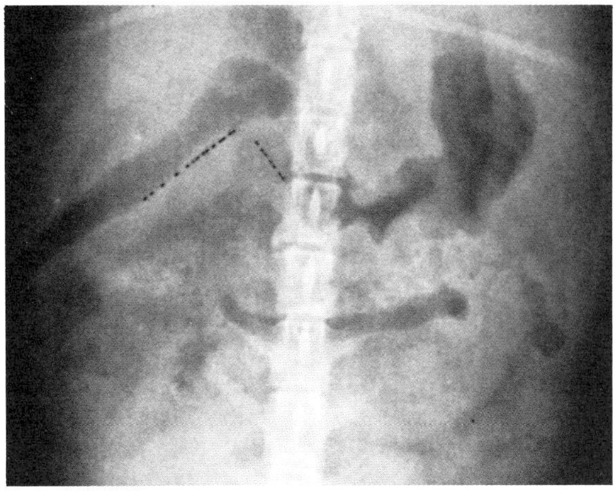

Fig 2—This 6-year-old male miniature poodle had an acute episode of hematemesis. The duodenum and stomach were both displaced caudally by the enlarged liver. In addition, the duodenal-gastric angle was widened (*dotted line*). The microscopic diagnosis was acute, necrotizing pancreatitis.

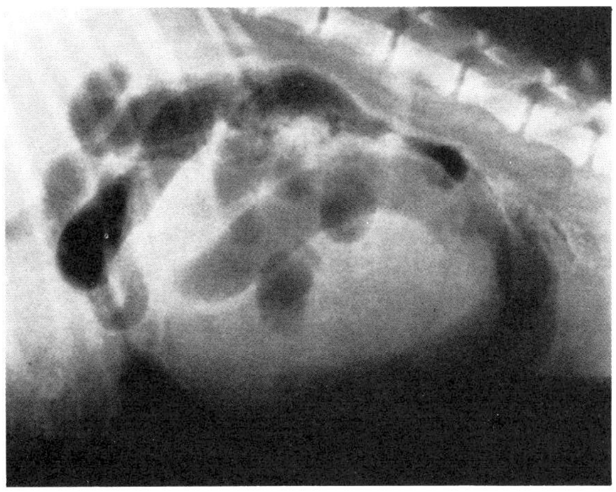

Fig 3—In this lateral abdominal radiograph of a four-year-old male miniature poodle, a large oval midabdominal mass is apparent. There is also gaseous distension of the small intestine. These findings, in the presence of clinical signs of intestinal obstruction, are highly suggestive of small bowel infarction. Surgical examination revealed an 18 cm segment of infarcted jejunum.

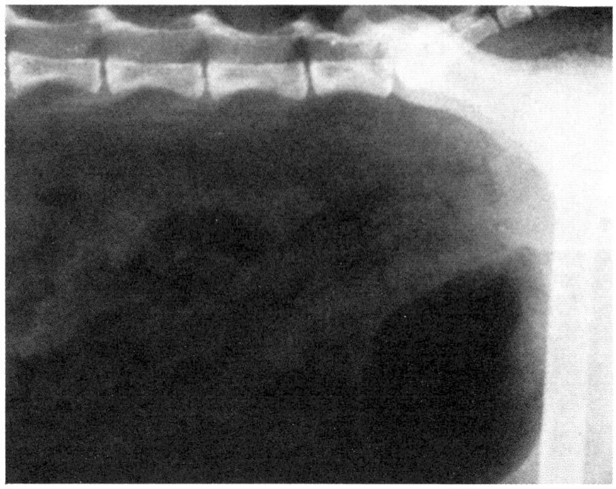

Fig 4—This 3-year-old cat presented with stranguria and ventral-caudal abdominal swelling after an automobile accident. The small intestine was displaced into a ventral hernia. A pneumocystogram demonstrated herniation of the urinary bladder also. There was rupture of the prepubic tendon.

If massive infarction of the intestine occurs one expects to find both gas and fluid distending the small intestine due to paralysis and diminished absorption of material from the infarcted segment (Fig 3).[1] Small areas of infarction may not produce any radiographic findings initially but fibrosis can cause obstruction in the subsequent days and weeks.

Small Bowel Herniation

Small bowel herniation through an opening in the diaphragm is one of the most common results of blunt abdominal trauma. Paracostal, abdominal and inguinal herniae containing small intestine are less common but the importance of finding such lesions cannot be overemphasized (Fig 6). Incarceration with or without volvulus in the hernia may result in obstruction and vascular compromise with subsequent toxemia.

Foreign Bodies and Intussusceptions

Foreign bodies and intussusceptions are also considered under the broad definition of trauma. Foreign bodies are the most common cause of intestinal obstruction in the dog and cat, and the size and nature of ingested objects defy the imagination. The most common complication of foreign body ingestion is obstruction of the intestinal lumen. The radiographic signs are those of distension with delayed transit of material through the gastrointestinal tract (Fig 5). When a linear foreign body such as a string is ingested, the small intestine becomes hyperactive and becomes *bunched* as peristalsis causes the bowel to move along the string (Fig 6). Perforation may occur soon after such hyperperistalsis is initiated.

In early intussusception, obstruction may not be complete but vascular compromise can produce infarction and necrosis. Usually a tubular structure of fluid opacity is visualized in mid abdomen, with gas accumulation proximal to the point of obstruction. A barium enema should be diagnostic in cases of cecocolic or ileocolic intussusception (Fig 7). In intussusceptions confined to the small intestine, an UGI may be necessary to reach a definitive diagnosis.

Tumors

Tumors of the small intestine cause acute or chronic clinical signs by obstruction or blood loss from an ulcerated surface. Intestinal adenocarcinoma and lymphoma are the most common

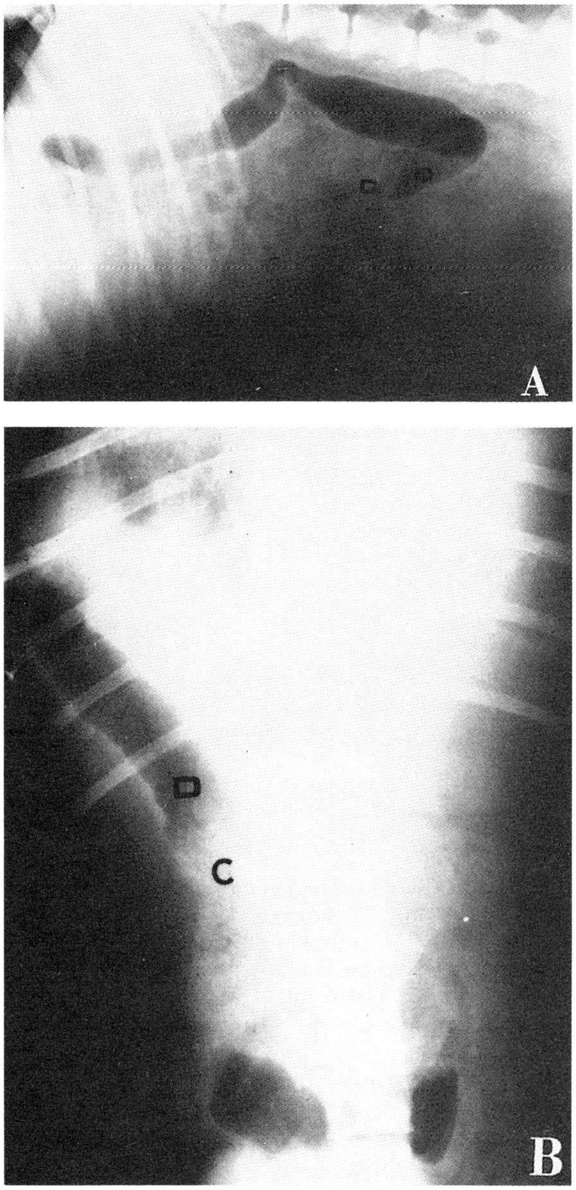

Fig 5 A and B—This 11-year-old terrier dog had an acute onset of vomiting. The gas distended duodenum (*D*) and the obstructing foreign body (*C*, corn cob) are clearly seen.

gastrointestinal neoplasms seen in this practice.

Adynamic (Paralytic) Ileus

Adynamic (paralytic) ileus occurs from peritonitis, shock, intestinal obstruction and administration of anticholinergic drugs. In paralytic ileus it may be difficult to determine whether dilated loops of intestine that contain gas are small bowel or colon. As a general rule, small bowel occupies a more central position in the abdomen while the laterally located loops are more likely to be colon.

Simple and Strangulated Obstruction

Intestinal obstruction regardless of its cause may be either simple or strangulated. In simple obstruction there is closure of a loop at a single site, whereas in strangulation there is closure of a loop at two sites resulting in interference with intestinal blood supply. When the ischemic area becomes

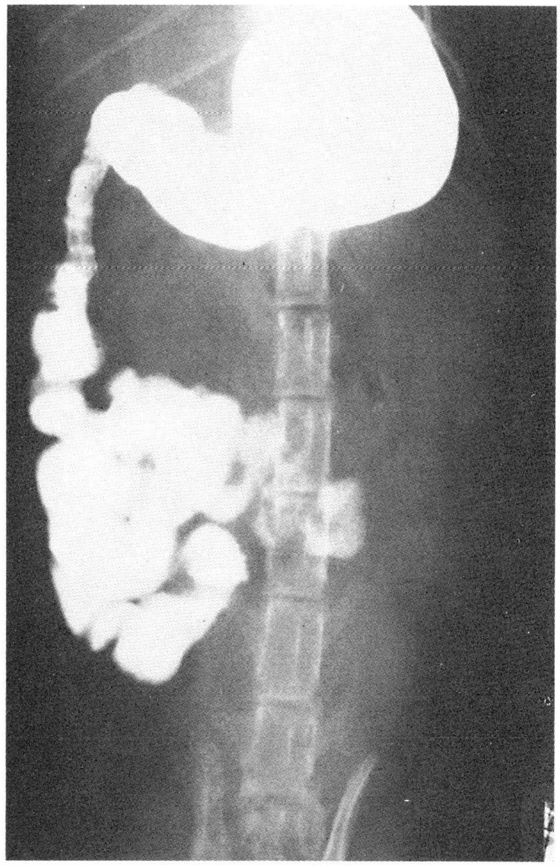

Fig 6—Acute abdominal pain and vomiting were prominent signs in a 9-month-old female cat. A 30-minute radiograph in the UGI shows convolutional plication of the proximal small intestine, highly suggestive of a linear foreign body. An 8-inch string was removed surgically.

infarcted, perforation rapidly follows.[1,7] Horizontal beam radiography may demonstrate intralumenal air-fluid levels at different heights in the same loop and can be an invaluable technique in the diagnosis of strangulation obstruction (Fig 8).[2]

Inflammatory Disease

Inflammatory disease of the small intestine is common in dogs and cats but does not always produce radiographic signs. The expected signs include thickening of intestinal walls and evidence of hyperperistalsis during contrast examination (Figs 9 and 10). Abscesses of the small intestine may protrude into the lumen and become large enough to cause obstruction.[12] Often there is resolution before obstruction develops, but fibrosis and occasionally stenosis are possible sequelae to this condition. Adhesions secondary to surgical procedures, previous inflammatory diseases, or external trauma will occasionally produce obstruction of the small intestine. Dogs can develop obstruction due to adhesions as long as three months after a traumatic incident.

Pancreatitis is capable of producing secondary changes in the intestinal tract and this assists in making the diagnosis. The duodenum may be somewhat thickened and distended and displaced to the right. An uneven granular opacity may be

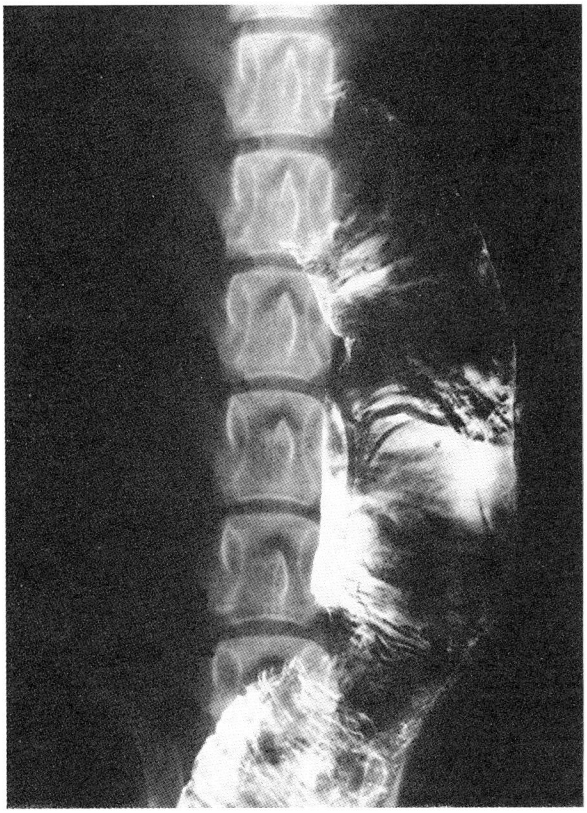

Fig 7—This 4-month-old Golden Retriever had several bouts of vomiting and diarrhea. An abdominal mass was palpated and a barium enema was performed. The multiple circumferential filling defects in the colon were caused by invagination of the small intestine into the lumen of the colon. A large percentage of the small intestine was involved in the intussusception.

present in the left cranial quadrant of the abdomen due to inflammatory disease within the peripancreatic tissues.[4]

Cecum and Colon

Blunt abdominal trauma seldom produces any radiographic changes in the cecum or colon. Penetrating foreign bodies may perforate either of these structures and produce pneumoperitoneum with associated bacterial contamination of the peritoneal cavity. Foreign bodies causing clinical signs in the cecum and colon are much less common than those in the stomach or small intestine.

Volvulus and Intussusception

Volvulus of the cecum associated with neoplasm initiates dramatic distension. Cecocolic intussusception may be a chronic disease with vague signs such as vomiting, intermittent abdominal pain and diarrhea. Cecocolic intussusception is therefore a difficult condition to diagnose clinically, but is easily recognized with a barium enema by noting a coiled filling defect in the ascending and transverse colon. Occasionally the diagnosis can be strongly suspected based on survey film findings of a soft tissue mass (invaginated cecum) in a gas filled ascending or tranverse colon (Fig 11).

Inflammatory Lesions and Tumors

Inflammatory lesions of the cecum are most often due to parasitic infestation or extension of enterocolitis.

Histiocytic colitis is expected to produce ulceration and thickening of the colon and this may be detected by barium enema. Tumors in the cecum

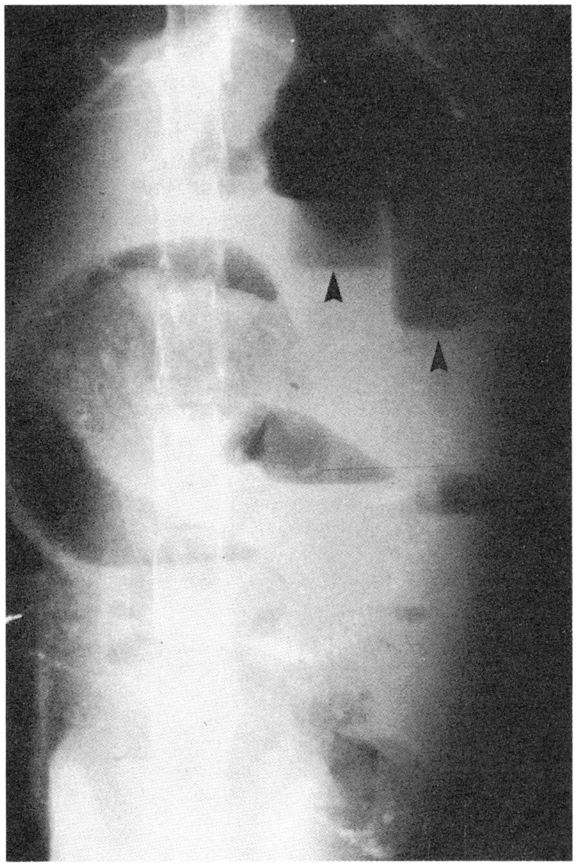

Fig 8—A 13-year-old cat had clinical signs of acute small bowel obstruction. A horizontal beam dorsoventral radiograph demonstrated multiple intralumenal air-fluid levels (*arrows*) in a loop of intestine in the left cranial abdomen. There was strangulating obstruction of the midjejunum.

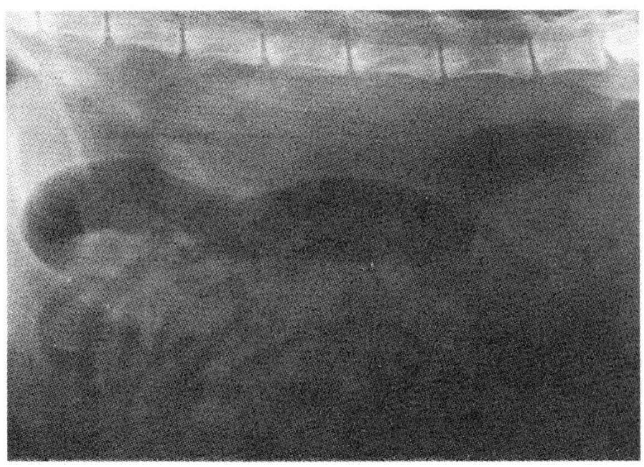

Fig 9—There was thickening of the wall of the entire small intestine with gas accumulation but no evidence of distension in this three-year-old castrated male cat. The cat had a sudden onset of vomiting and anorexia. The clinical and radiographic diagnosis was nonspecific enteritis.

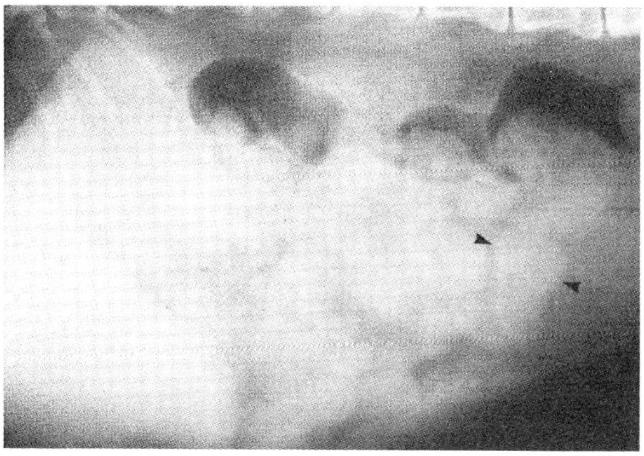

Fig 10—An 11-year-old castrated male cat was presented because of acute blood-stained diarrhea. The major radiographic abnormalities were an enlarged liver and spleen and a turgid small intestine (*arrows*). The biopsy diagnosis was eosinophilic enteritis.

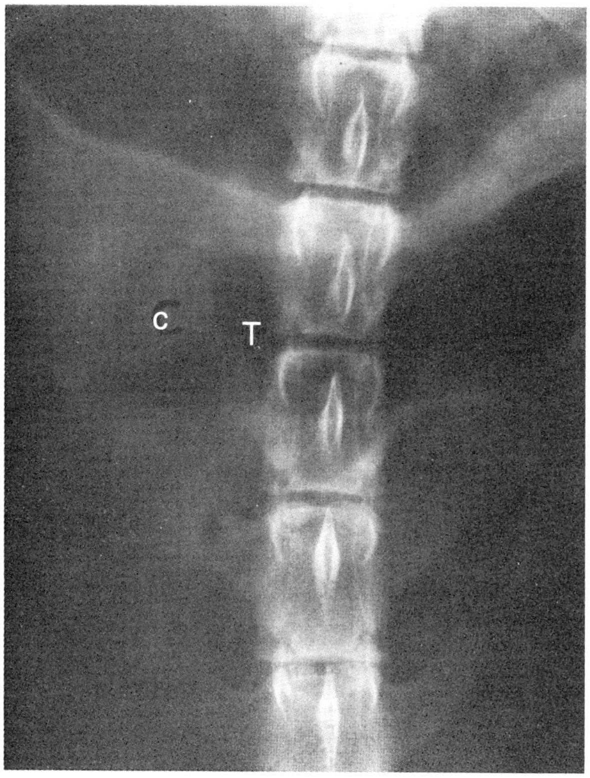

Fig 11—This 4-year-old male Labrador Retriever had several episodes of vomiting and acute abdominal pain. The filling defect (*c*) in the transverse colon (*T*) is the invaginated cecum (cecocolic intussusception).

and colon may produce acute signs of obstruction. Shock may occur due to massive bleeding secondary to ulceration of the free surface of the tumor.

Supporting Structures and Retroperitoneum

Trauma to the abdominal wall is a frequent occurrence in the dog and cat but radiographic findings are usually limited to the recognition of soft tissue swelling due to bruising, or gas accumulation secondary to laceration of the skin and subcutaneous tissue. External hernias or opaque foreign bodies are easily recognized. Increased opacity of the subcutaneous tissue may be caused by inflammatory soft tissue disease, which simulates an acute abdominal disorder (Fig 1). Fractures of the last few ribs or transverse processes of lumbar vertebrae may be associated with lacerations of the liver, spleen, or kidneys. Bleeding into the abdominal cavity has no distinct diagnostic appearance to differentiate blood from a transudate or exudate. Peritoneal effusion can be due to many abdominal disorders such as pancreatitis; rupture of prostatic abscess; mesenteric abscess; rupture of bile ducts, intestine, or uterus (Fig 12); infectious feline peritonitis; penetrating abdominal wounds; and intestinal obstruction with strangulation. Tumors and abscesses involving the omentum and mesentery are recognized by formation of a mass and stippled opacities in the mid ventral abdomen due to breakdown of fat planes which usually provide contrast between the abdominal viscera. Mesenteric and cecal node enlargement can be the cause of acute abdominal pain (Fig 13).

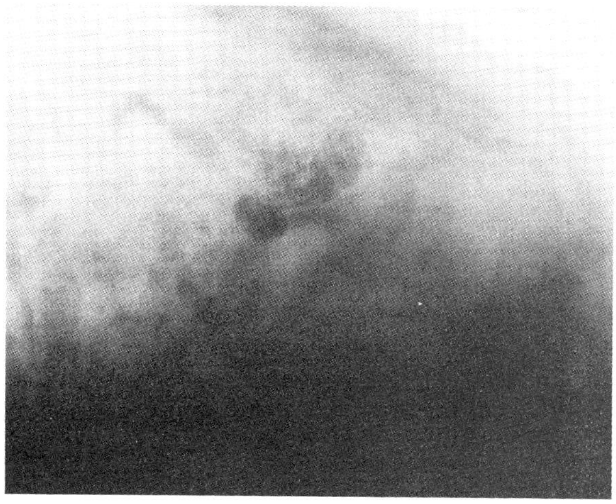

Fig 12—This 13-year-old female, shepherd-cross dog had a persistent purulent vaginal discharge for several weeks, then suddenly developed a distended abdomen and weakness. The abdomen lacked normal definition and there was a tubular, fluid-filled density in the caudal abdomen. The surgical findings were peritonitis secondary to ruptured pyometra.

Trauma to the kidneys and ureters is recognized by increased size and an uneven opacity of the retroperitoneal space. Retroperitoneal hemorrhage, without urinary tract pathology, may produce this same radiographic appearance. Such trauma is often accompanied by fractures of dorsal spinous processes or transverse processes of lumbar vertebrae and fractures of the last few ribs.[5] Retroperitoneal abscesses produce radiographic signs similar to those seen with retroperitoneal hemorrhage or tumor.

Urethra

Perineal swelling, following trauma or associated with anuria, should lead to investigation of the integrity of the urethra by means of positive con-

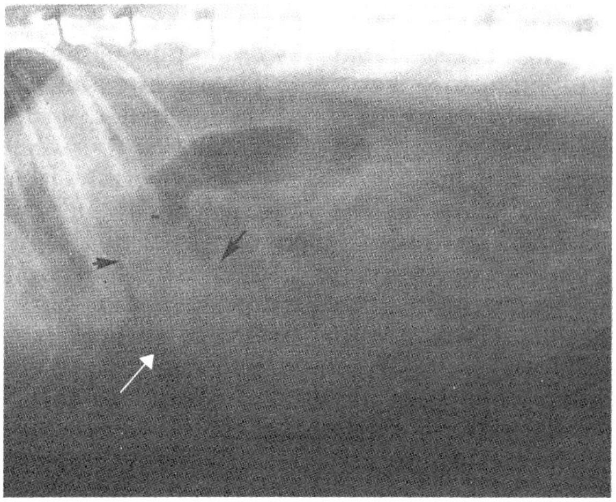

Fig 13—The arrows outline an oval abdominal mass in a 2-year-old male cat that had fever and leucocytosis. The mass was an abscessed ileocecal lymph node.

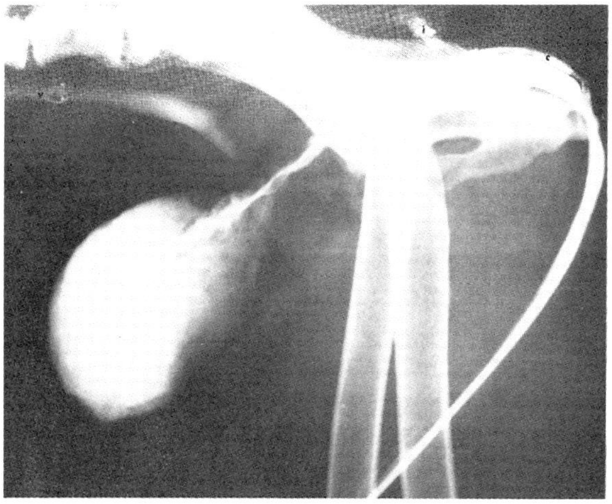

Fig 14—This 6-year-old, male retriever has extravasation of contrast medium into the corpus spongiosum penis* (*c*) The internal pudendal vein (*i*), and the caudal vena cava (*v*) are outlined. The radiographic findings are due to an injury of the urethra in the region of the ischium. Gas can also escape into the venous system when vascular areas are injured, leading to fatal air embolism. (*Editor's note: *Corpus spongiosum penis* is the term that replaces *corpus cavernosum urethrae*. Nomina Anatomica Veterinaria, 1973.)

trast urethrography (Figs 14 and 15). Negative contrast urethrography may also be useful but it carries with it the hazard of air embolism unless carbon dioxide or a soluble gas other than room air is used. In addition to trauma, acute signs may be due to obstructing calculus, urethritis, or post-operative or post-traumatic stricture. Iatrogenic injury may occur with catheters that are too large or inflexible, and occasionally results in tearing of the mucosa with subsequent stricture formation.

Prostate Gland

The prostate gland is generally well-protected by the bony pelvis and is seldom seriously injured by external force. Occasionally, however, a prostatic cyst may be ruptured by external trauma or by passage of a urinary catheter into a cyst which

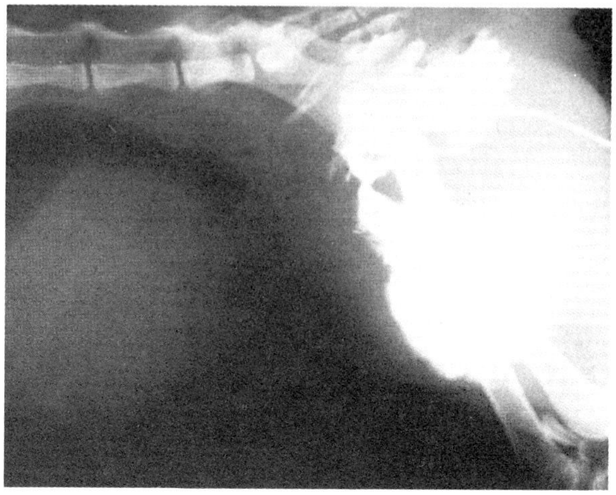

Fig 15—A 2-year-old cat was unable to urinate following an automobile accident. The right ilium and pelvic floor were fractured. The urinary bladder was distended. There was extravasation of contrast medium into an inguinal hernia because of a ruptured urethra.

communicates with the prostatic urethra. When a cyst ruptures, hemorrhage, hematoma formation and necrosis occur. Prostatitis and abscess formation may also cause acute abdominal signs due to pain, dysuria, obstruction, infection or sepsis.

The various types of prostatic enlargement can usually not be distinguished from one another by radiographic means alone. Prostatic enlargement is best recognized by abdominal survey radiography and retrograde cystourethrography. Cysts communicating with the prostatic urethra do not mean that the primary prostatic disease is cystic hyperplasia. Communicating cysts may also be present with prostatitis, abscesses or prostatic tumors. Prostatic neoplasms metastasize to the lumbar spine and pelvis and may produce acute lameness and pain.

Urinary Bladder

Blunt trauma to the urinary bladder in an automobile accident is relatively common.[5] Such lesions include lacerations, contusions, hernias and volvulus of the urinary bladder. When an inflexible catheter is inserted too deeply it can penetrate the wall of the bladder. If a flexible catheter is inserted too deeply it can be knotted. Overinflation during pneumocystography can cause local tears in the mucosa or even complete rupture of the bladder wall. The urinary bladder may be traumatized when the uterine stump is litgated during an ovariohysterectomy.

Volvulus of the urinary bladder may occur following removal of its median ligament in abdominal surgery. In acute cystitis the urinary bladder may be only minimally thickened and the signs of cystitis may be functional (straining and spasm) rather than anatomical changes of thickening and irregularity which are most often seen with chronic cystitis. Granulomas sometimes occur at the bladder neck secondary to an infected uterine stump. Tumors of the urinary bladder may cause obstruction or bleeding thereby producing acute abdominal signs.

Kidneys and Ureters

In trauma to the kidneys and ureters the primary survey radiographic signs are accumulation of fluid in the abdominal cavity or retroperitoneal space or renal enlargement or displacement. These lesions are best evaluated by survey radiography and intravenous urography (Fig 16).

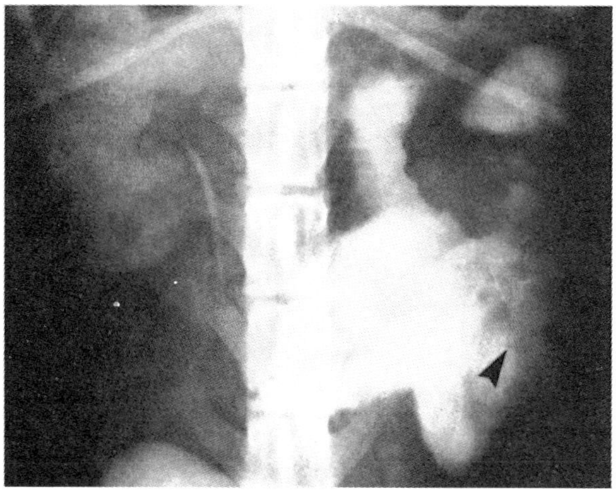

Fig 16—This 5-year-old Cocker Spaniel had been struck by a car several hours before radiographs were made, dislocating its left hip. The black arrow shows the point of rupture of the left renal pelvis in a 30-minute intravenous urogram.

Acute Inflammatory Diseases

Acute inflammatory diseases of the kidneys include pyelitis, pyelonephritis and nephritis. While pyelitis and pyelonephritis are ordinarily caused by infection, nephritis may be either infectious or toxic. The radiographic signs are usually subtle, early and are best recognized by means of intravenous urography. Later in the disease one expects to find distortion of the renal pelvis, a prolonged pyelogram, a variable degree of hydronephrosis, and blunting of the pelvic diverticula. In nephritis there may be enlargement of the parenchymal portion of the kidney with or without hydronephrosis. In some cases of acute nephritis the kidneys may appear more dense than usual.

Calculi Formation

While formation of calculi is not an acute phenomenon, the clinical signs may have a sudden onset due to passage of a renal calculus into a ureter causing obstruction and extreme abdominal pain. Nonradiopaque renal stones cannot be visualized without the aid of intravenous urography.

Tumors

If tumors of the kidneys and ureters rupture, they may cause massive bleeding and the clinical signs will be acute.

Genital Organs

Volvulus of Ovary or Testicle

Volvulus of an ovary or a retained testicle causes abdominal pain due to vascular compromise and swelling of the parenchyma of the organ (Fig 17). A retained testicle or ovary can be recognized radiographically as an oval abdominal mass in the caudal or mid abdomen.

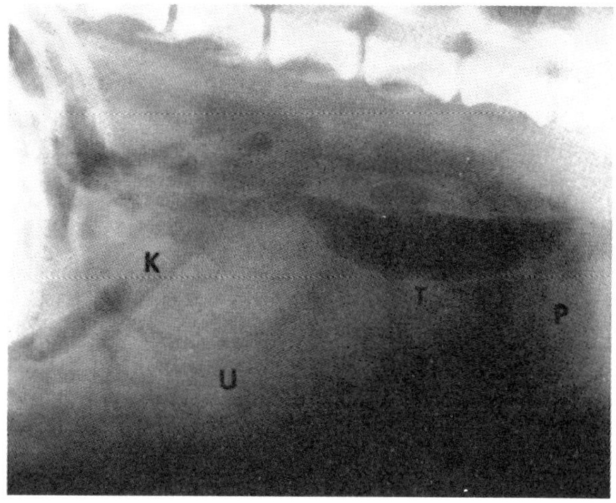

Fig 17—This 6-year-old male dog was presented in acute abdominal pain. The abdominal densities were left kidney (*K*), urinary bladder (*U*), abdominal testicle (*T*), and prostate glad (*P*). There was torsion of the testicle.

Uterus

The uterus may be traumatized directly by a blunt force such as an automobile accident, causing laceration accompanied by peritoneal bleeding with loss of abdominal contrast. Volvulus of a gravid uterus may occur with vascular compromise, particularly when it enters an inguinal or abdominal hernia. Inflammatory lesions of the uterus are common in both dogs and cats. In endometritis the uterus has a turgid, nodular appearance and is usually two to three times normal size. With pyometra, the uterus is usually not lobulated but instead has a smooth configuration, may be five to eight times its normal diameter and filled with fluid. Both conditions may cause either acute or chronic abdominal signs. Occasionally the infected uterus may rupture, producing radiographic signs of peritoneal effusion and peritonitis (Fig 12).

Dystocia

Dystocia caused by fetal head, maternal pelvis incompatibility, is easily diagnosed radiographically. Fetal death can be recognized by the presence of air within the fetus or uterus or fetal skull fractures (Fig 18).

Other Abdominal Viscera

Liver and Biliary System

Ultrasound examination of the liver and associated viscera is highly effective in evaluation of the acute abdomen. The liver, bile ducts, and gallbladder can be involved in blunt abdominal trauma although they are protected by the rib cage. Laceration and bruising of the liver is usually not clinically significant. Massive laceration with hemorrhage and rupture of the bile ducts or gallbladder results in bile peritonitis. Occasionally

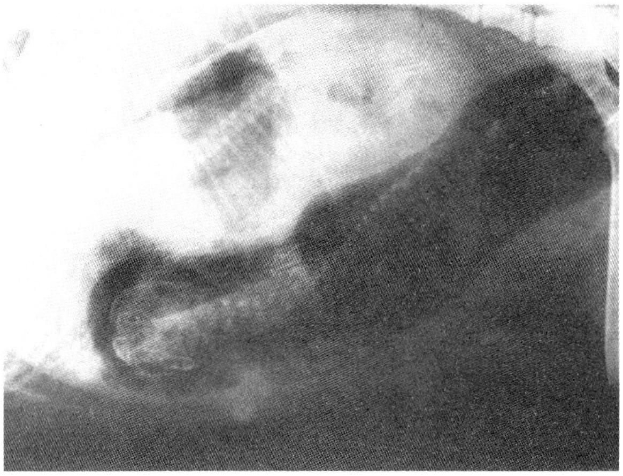

Fig 18—There were clinical signs of septicemia in this 3-year-old female Fox Terrier that had been in labor for 12 hours. Gas surrounds the fetus that is engaged in the pelvic canal in a caudal presentation. The radiographic and clinical findings are those of emphysematous metritis.

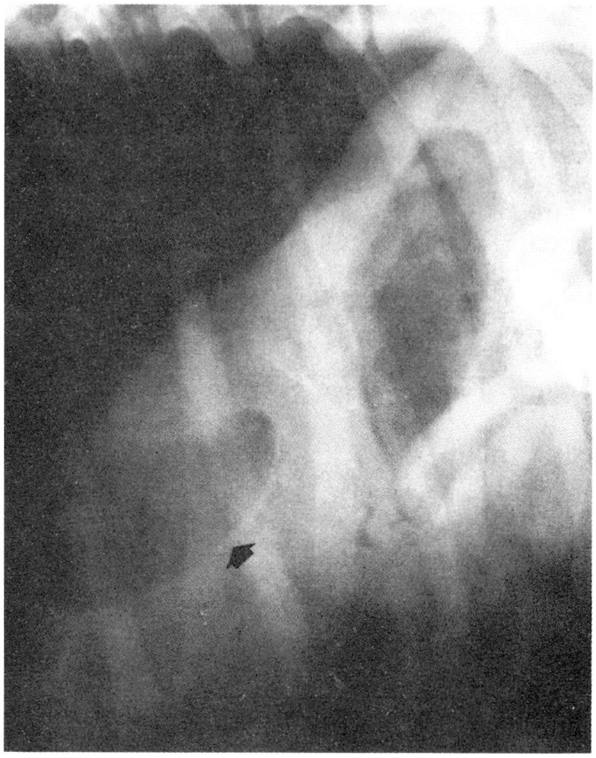

Fig 20—The arrow points to air in the wall of the gallbladder. Intralumenal air was also present in this case of emphysematous cholecystitis in a 6-year-old, male Shepherd-cross dog.

traumatic portal vein thrombosis is the cause of an acute abnormality. Hepatitis, cholecystitis, and choledochitis are difficult to diagnose clinically. Oral or intravenous cholegraphic agents may be helpful in differentiating one condition from another or in ruling out the gallbladder as the source of acute abdominal disease. Tumors of the liver, bile ducts, and gallbladder may cause acute abdominal disease by bleeding. Gallstones with bile duct obstruction produce acute abdominal pain and icterus (Fig 19). Emphysematous cholecystitis can be seen as an accompanying lesion of pancreatitis (Fig 20).

Pancreas

The pancreas is afforded protection by the ribs and associated viscera, but when traumatic pancreatitis occurs, the abdominal findings are similar to those described for acute pancreatitis.[4] Pancreatic neoplasms may produce upper gastrointestinal obstruction when they reach sufficient size or invade the duodenum. Ultrasound examination of the pancreas is often more useful than radiography.

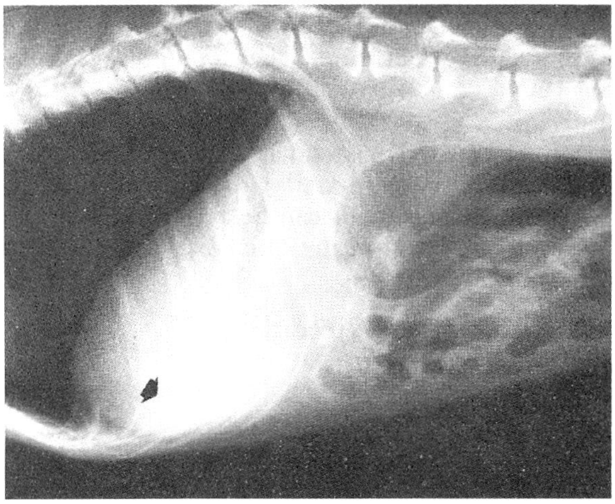

Fig 19—Choleliths are capable of causing cystic duct obstruction and signs of acute pain and jaundice. The arrow points to gallstones in this 7-year-old spayed female cat.

Spleen

The spleen is often involved in abdominal trauma. Lesions that can cause acute abdominal signs include volvulus, infarction, and laceration. Volvulus of the spleen may produce toxemia due to vascular compromise, while lacerations produce either an abdominal mass when a hematoma forms, or, free fluid in the peritoneal cavity in the case of hemorrhage. Infectious disorders of the spleen (splenitis) are an infrequent cause of abdominal pain. Tumors of the spleen may cause acute abdominal signs due to bleeding, especially following vigorous abdominal palpation.

ACKNOWLEDGEMENT

The author gratefully acknowledges the help of Paula Ruel, BSN, RN in the preparation of the manuscript

REFERENCES

1. Dixon JA, et al: Intestinal motility following luminal and vascular occlusion of the small intestine. *Gastroenterology*, 58: 673-678, 1970
2. Donahue JK, Hunter C, Balch HH: Significance of fluid levels in x-ray films of the abdomen. *New Eng J Med* 259: 13-15, 1958
3. Hornbuckle WE, Kleine LL: Obstruction of the small intes-

tine, in Kirk RW, (ed): *Current Veterinary Therapy* VI. Philadelphia, WB Saunders Co., 1977, pp. 952-958.
4. Kleine LJ, Hornbuckle WE: Acute pancreatitis: Radiographic findings in 182 dogs. *J Am Vet Rad Soc* 19: 102-106, 1978.
5. Kleine LJ: Radiographic diagnosis of urinary tract trauma in the dog and cat. *Small Animal Vet Med Update* 7: 1-6, 1978.
6. Kleine LJ: The role of radiography in the diagnosis of intestinal obstruction in dogs and cats. *Compen Contin Educ for Sm An Pract* 1: 44-51, 1979.
7. Laufman H.: Intestinal strangulation fever. *Surg Gynec Obstet* 135: 271-272, 1972.
8. Miller RE, Skucas J.(eds): *Radiographic Contrast Agents*. Baltimore University Park Press, 1977.
9. Osborn D, et al.: The role of angiography in abdominal nonrenal trauma. *Rad Clin No Am* 11: 579-592, 1973.
10. Poole CA, Rowe MI: Clinical evidence of intestinal absorption of gastrografin. *Radiology* 118: 151-153, 1976.
11. Rowe MI, et al. Gastrografin induced hypertonicity: The pathogenesis of neonatal hazard. *Am J Surg* 125: 185-188, 1973.
12. Wolfe DA, Meyer WC: Obstructing intestinal abscess in a dog. *JAVMA* 166: 518-519, 1975.
13. Zheutlin N, Lasser EC, Rigler LG: Clinical studies on effect of barium in the peritoneal cavity following rupture of the colon. *Surg* 32: 967-979, 1952.

Acute Abdominal Disorders, Part I *(continued from page 75)*

REFERENCES

1. Dixon JA, et al: Intestinal motility following vascular occlusion of small intestine. *Gastroenterology* 58: 673-678, 1970
2. Donahue JK, Hunter C and Balch HH: Significance of fluid levels in x-ray films of the abdomen. *New Eng J Med* 259: 13-15, 1958.
3. Hornbuckle WE, Kleine LJ: Obstruction of the small intestine, in *Current Veterinary Therapy VI*, Kirk R(ed): Philadelphia, WB Saunders Co, 1977, pp 952-958.
4. Kleine LJ, Hornbuckle WE: Acute pancreatitis: radiographic findings in 182 dogs. *J Am Vet Rad Soc* 19: 102-106, 1978.
5. Kleine LJ: Radiographic Diagnosis of urinary tract trauma in the dog and cat. *Sm An Vet Med Update Series* 7:2-6, 1978.
6. Kleine LJ: Radiography in the diagnosis of intestinal obstruction in dogs and cats. *Compen Contin Educ for Sm An Pract*, 1: 44-51, 1979.
7. Laufman H; Intestinal strangulation. *Surg Gynec and Obst* 135: 271-272, 1972
8. Miller RE, Skucas J: *Radiographic Contrast Agents*. Baltimore, University Park Press, 1977.
9. Osborn D, et al: Role of Angiography in abdominal nonrenal trauma. *Rad Clin N Amer* 11: 579-592, 1973.
10. Poole CA, Rowe MI: Clinical evidence of intestinal absorption of gastrograffin. *Radiology* 118: 151-153, 1976.
11. Rowe MI, et al: Gastrograffin induced hypertonicity: the pathogenesis of neonatal hazard. *Am J Surg* 125: 185-188, 1973.
12. Wolfe DA, Meyer WC: Obstructing intestinal abscess in a dog. *JAVMA* 166: 518-519, 1975.
13. Zhuetlin N, Lasser EC, Rigler LG: Clinical studies on effect of barium in the peritoneal cavity following rupture of the colon. *Surg* 32: 967-979, 1952.

The Role of Radiography in the Diagnosis of Intestinal Obstruction in Dogs and Cats

L. J. Kleine, DVM, MS
Director of Radiology
Angell Memorial Animal Hospital
Boston, Massachusetts

Obstruction of the intestinal tract is a frequent and important diagnostic problem in dogs and cats, and rapid diagnosis is essential to prevent serious complications and death. Recognition is not difficult when clinical and radiographic findings can be correlated. With a few readily available tests and careful observation, an accurate diagnosis can usually be made without expensive or time-consuming techniques.

After clinical and radiographic correlation, obstructions can be categorized as: acute or chronic, partial or complete, proximal or distal, simple or strangulating, and most importantly, mechanical or non-mechanical. Furthermore, one can often recognize the most likely source of obstruction based upon the radiographic findings. In dogs and cats, ingested foreign bodies are often the cause of obstruction. Less frequently seen causes are neoplasm, intussusception, post-traumatic adhesion or stricture, congenital malformation, intramural hemorrhage or abscess, volvulus, and internal hernia.

Clinical Features—A carefully taken accurate history can be invaluable and lead to an early diagnosis because it will direct the veterinarian to make the appropriate tests and observations. Vomiting is the most frequent sign in dogs and cats with intestinal obstruction. These factors should be considered: onset of vomiting; effort involved; description of the vomitus; retention of liquids; relationship to eating; and whether the animal's appetite remains normal. The owner should be asked about the animal's chewing habits and whether any of its toys are missing. Assessment of the animal's general condition should be followed by gentle, thorough, systematic abdominal palpation.[1] Repeated physical examination may be valuable in evaluating changes in the animal's physical status. Abdominal mass, pain, visceral displacement, abdominal fluid, or distension are physical findings which indicate the need for further investigation by means of radiography. Laboratory tests may aid in ruling out other diseases which mimic obstruction, as well as helping to assess the animal's general condition and need for specific supportive treatment.

Technique—The importance of careful radiographic technique, positioning and preparation have been emphasized by others[2,3] and will only be reviewed briefly here. Since one of the problems in interpretation of abdominal radiographs is difficulty in delineating borders of various viscera, low kilovoltage technique which enhances radiographic contrast may be useful. Radiographs may be made with as low kilovoltage as is consistent with an exposure which will prevent motion (less than 1/10 second).

Survey radiographs are essential to confirm the clinical findings in

Originally published in Volume 1, Number 1, January 1979

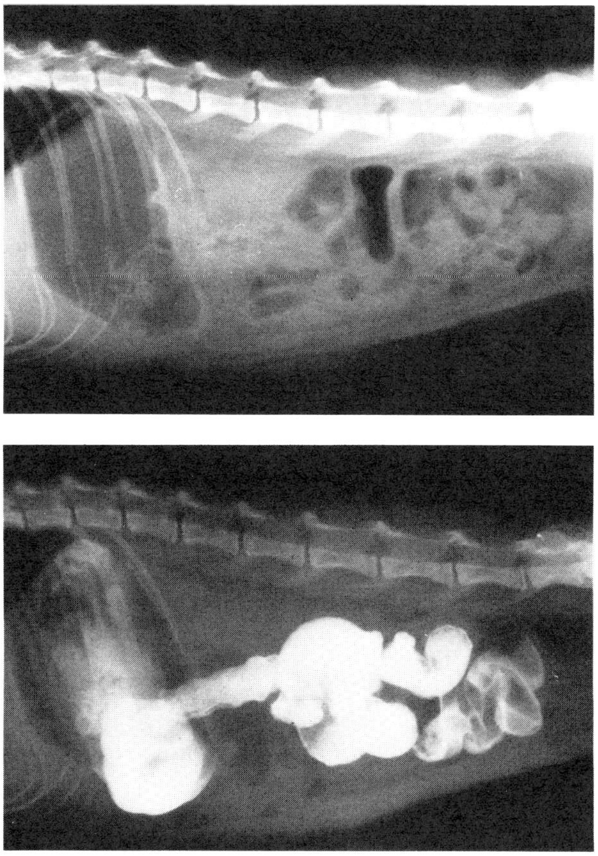

Fig 1,2—Linear foreign bodies generally produce characteristic plication in both the survey films and in the UGI. This 4-year-old cat had an acute episode of vomiting with severe retching. There was cellophane lodged in the pylorus extending into the proximal 1/3 of the small intestine.

suspected cases of intestinal obstruction and must always precede a contrast examination. Survey radiographs permit evaluation of exposure factors and visualization of opaque foreign bodies which might be obscured by contrast medium.

An additional technique which may be useful in contrast or survey radiographic examinations involves the use of the horizontal x-ray beam. The animal is restrained in either an upright ventrodorsal position, or decubital lateral position in front of an x-ray cassette which is held vertically by a cassette holder. This position will permit evaluation of air-fluid levels which may be an aid in the diagnosis of mechanical obstruction of the small intestine.

Preparation—The presence of ingesta and feces makes interpretation of radiographs more difficult. Ingesta will prevent adequate coating of the mucosa with barium, will alter the transit time of the contrast medium, and the appearance of the medium. A distended urinary bladder may significantly displace the small intestine. However, if obstruction is present, it is possible to further injure the animal by administration of laxatives or enemas. Additional fluids can lead to vomiting or rupture of organs. In most cases of acute intestinal obstruction little, if any, preparation can be done. Therefore, the type of bowel preparation to be used is based on a correlation of the preliminary radiographic findings and the available clinical data. When stool is present in the rectum, a saline enema may be the only treatment needed. If the small intestine and colon are also filled, a routine bowel preparation, consisting of a 12-hour fast, administration of a laxative, and a saline or soap-water enema is given when possible. If enough time does not elapse between the administration of the enema and radiography, the intestine will be distended with both fluid and gas making interpretation of radiographs difficult. The use of a suppository helps to eliminate residual feces and gas which remain in the terminal colon after the administration of an enema.

Procedure—The commercial brand of barium sulfate suspension used in the upper gastrointestinal examination (UGI) is subject to personal preference. The characteristics for satisfactory proprietary barium medium include the ability to coat the gastrointestinal mucosa in a predictable manner, and a reproducible transit time through the gastrointestinal tract with minimal foaming and flocculation during the examination. The medium should be easily obtainable, economical, and easily prepared and administered. USP barium sulfate without suspending agents is not a desirable product for the UGI because of its tendency to precipitate from suspension in the stomach and small intestine producing uneven mucosal coating.

Organic iodides for gastrointestinal use do not usually produce satisfactory mucosal coating. Because these products are hypertonic, they attract fluid into the small intestine. This osmotic attraction for fluid causes dilution and reduced opacity of the contrast agent. When gastrointestinal perforation is suspected, but not confirmed by correlation of clinical and plain radiographic findings with sufficient certainty to justify exploratory laparotomy, organic iodides may be used instead of barium for the contrast examination of the gastrointestinal tract. Organic iodides are less irritating to the peritoneal surface than barium. However, perforation may be present but not detected with the iodide media because of the dilution of these media in the small intestine and in peritoneal fluid, and because of the rapid absorption of these media from the peritoneum. Because of the hyperosmolar nature of the iodides, they are capable of producing dehydration.[4,5,6] This consideration is especially important in the debilitated animal or neonate.

Other contrast media that can be used in cases of suspected perforation of the stomach or intestinal tract are the water-soluble low osmolality agents with iodine concentrations of at least 200 mg iodine per ml of solution, such as iohexol and iopamidol. Since these compounds are not osmotically active, they do not draw fluid into the gas-

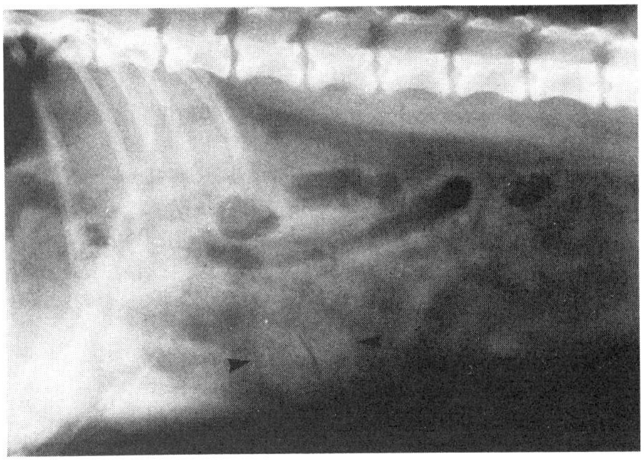

Fig 3—This 4-year-old miniature Schnauzer dog had been vomiting and inappetent for about 4 days. The foreign body is outlined by arrows. It is circular and contains air. It was an acorn.

trointestinal tract and do not have a dehydrating effect on the animal. If these media leak into the peritoneal cavity through a perforation, they are not irritating.[6a,6b] Although the low osmolality agents are not as opaque as barium, they attenuate x-rays sufficiently to be satisfactory for gastrointestinal use. The high cost of these media (approximately $1.00/ml), however, precludes their use in most cases.

When properly performed and correlated with clinical and plain radiographic findings, the UGI is an extremely accurate diagnostic technique in evaluating gastric and small intestinal morphology and some aspects of function. While the test is accurate if radiographic signs are present, a reasonably low yield of diagnoses can be expected. The method of administering contrast medium, its quantity, and timing of radiography can be varied to suit the individual case.[a] If tranquilization is necessary for restraining the animal during radiography or passing the stomach tube, care in selection of the drug is necessary to prevent interference with passage of contrast medium through the intestinal tract.[7] Acetyl promazine maleate[b] is the tranquilizing drug of choice in this hospital. In 90% of cases, no drugs should be needed.

It is preferable to administer the barium by stomach tube to dogs and cats because the medium can be deposited in the stomach in a short period of time, providing a more predictable transit time through the gastrointestinal tract and with less air in the medium. The stomach can be more effectively distended by this method, permitting better evaluation of the pliability of the stomach wall. The dosage range is 10–15 cc/kg of body weight. The lower dosage is used in larger dogs; the higher dosage is used in puppies and kittens. Radiographs are made in the ventrodorsal and lateral planes immediately upon conclusion of administration of contrast medium, at 30 minutes, 60 minutes, 3 hours, 6 hours, and 24 hours. This schedule of

[a]Editor's note: An experienced radiologist can make the decisions to vary the dose and technique. The average clinician should adopt a standard technique so that only one variable is present—the disease process.

[b]Acepromazine maleate, Wyeth-Ayerst Laboratories, Philadelphia, PA.

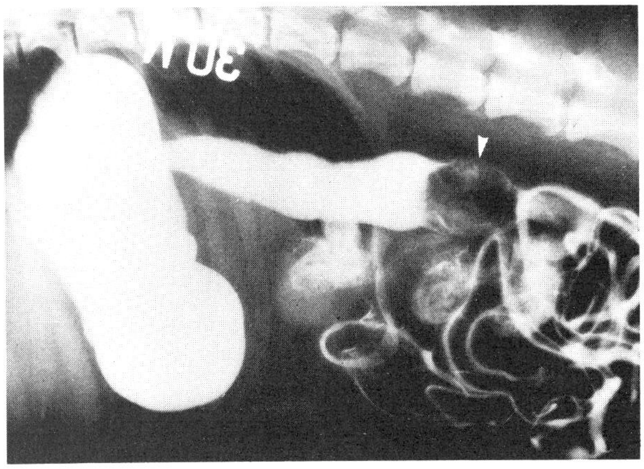

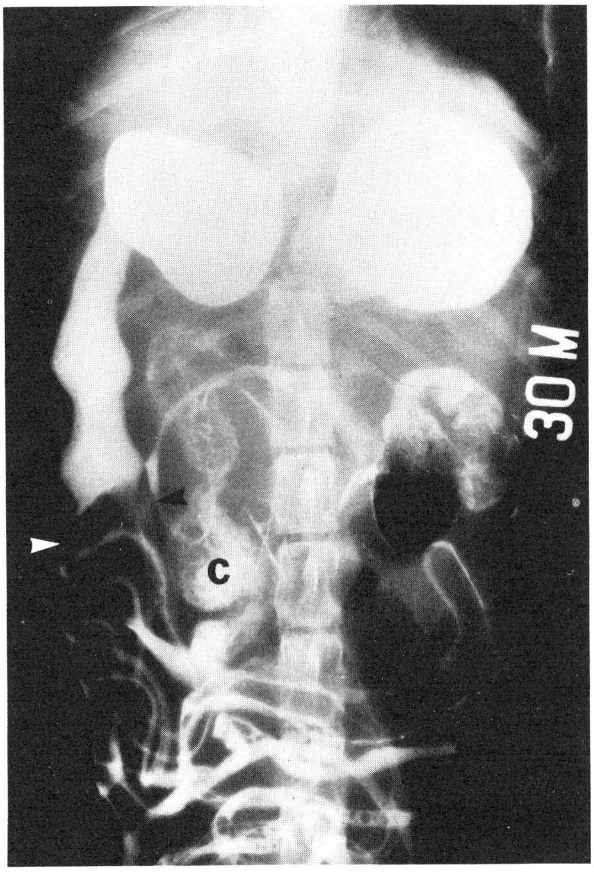

Fig 4,5—In early, partial obstruction of the small intestine, intestinal activity may be accelerated as in this 4-year-old, male Dalmatian. The dog had been hospitalized elsewhere overnight to have a front leg laceration sutured and bandaged. Shortly after coming home from the hospital it vomited twice. It was then brought to AMAH for examination. A painful abdominal mass was palpated and an UGI was performed. Barium had passed into the colon (c) 30 minutes after oral administration. An oval foreign body (arrows) was causing dilation of the proximal duodenum. The foreign body was a surgical sponge which the dog had eaten.

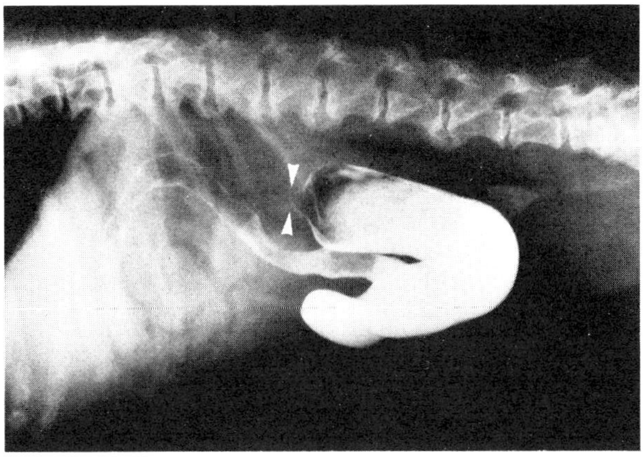

Fig 6—These radiographs were made 24 hours after the oral administration of liquid barium. The dog is a 13-year-old Boxer which had a history of vomiting for 2 months before this examination. Weakness and weight loss were apparent in the preceding 2 weeks. The dog vomited barium during the UGI. There is dilatation of the small intestine proximal to a constriction (arrows). This concentric stenotic lesion in an older dog is highly suggestive of intestinal neoplasm such as adenocarcinoma. However, any type of constricting lesion such as fibrosis could produce a similar appearance. The histologic diagnosis was intestinal adenocarcinoma.

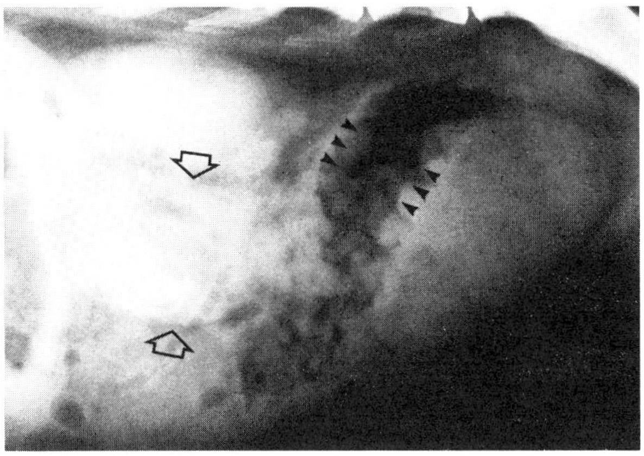

Fig 7—Occasional vomiting and chronic weight loss were the clinical signs in this 12-year-old, castrated male, Siamese cat. There is gas in the colon and this outlines the thickened wall of the colon and multiple smooth filling defects (arrows). This is an example of an infiltrative lesion in the wall of the colon. There is also an oval, well-circumscribed mid-abdominal mass (dotted lines). The colonic lesion was due to infiltration with lymphosarcoma. The mass was due to lymphosarcoma in the mesenteric lymph nodes.

filming is altered depending on the results of the recent exposures.

If the stomach is of special interest, a lower dose of barium is used and exposures in the ventrodorsal, dorsoventral, and right and left lateral positions are made.[c] These exposures will demonstrate different parts of the stomach as the gas and con-

[c]Editor's note: Again, a standard dose and technique is applicable. The stomach can be evaluated after some of the barium has left the stomach.

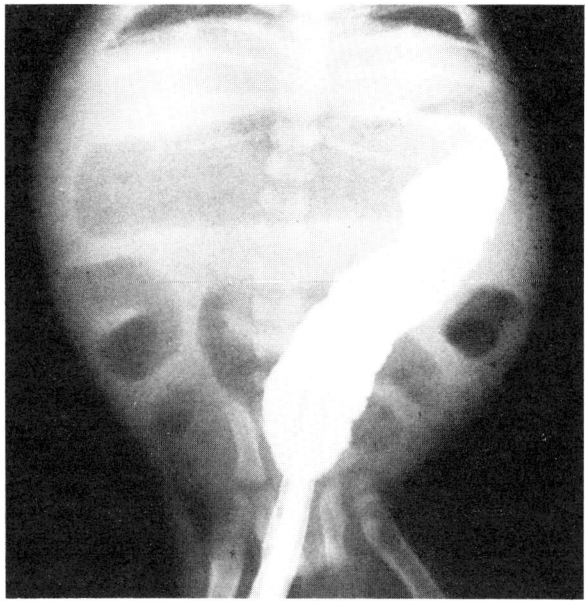

Fig 8—This 5-week-old puppy had been vomiting for 2 days and was dehydrated. An abdominal mass was palpated. The barium enema shows a large, tubular filing defect in the transverse colon caused by an ileocolic intussuception.

trast medium change position in the different postures. If a midline structure such as the cardia of the stomach is of special interest, right and left ventrodorsal oblique views should be made.

Double contrast examination of the stomach (gastrogram) can be performed by administering a small amount of barium by stomach tube, rotating the animal to distribute the barium to all areas of the stomach. The stomach can be distended by insufflation with air, carbon dioxide, or by administering a carbonated beverage, and then making the appropriate x-ray exposures. The animal will usually need to be sedated for this technique, otherwise eructation of the gas will occur too soon to permit radiography. Double contrast gastrography produces excellent visualization of the gastric mucosa and outlines filling defects.

The barium enema is an accurate and rapid method of diagnosing ileocolic and cecocolic intussusceptions as well as mucosal abnormalities and obstructive lesions in the colon. Anesthesia is usually required to administer the contrast medium. Large bore tubing with a cuff that can be inflated with air is introduced beyond the pelvic brim. The cuff is then inflated to prevent the tubing from slipping out of the anus. The barium container is elevated to permit the medium to flow into the colon by gravity until approximately 10-15 cc/kg have been given. Then the tubing is clamped.

A radiograph is made to determine if the quantity of medium is appropriate to visualize the entire colon. When the colon is filled, radiographs are exposed in the ventrodorsal, dorsoventral, and right and left lateral planes. Then the tubing is held lower than the animal, the tubing clamp is released, and the contrast medium is permitted to

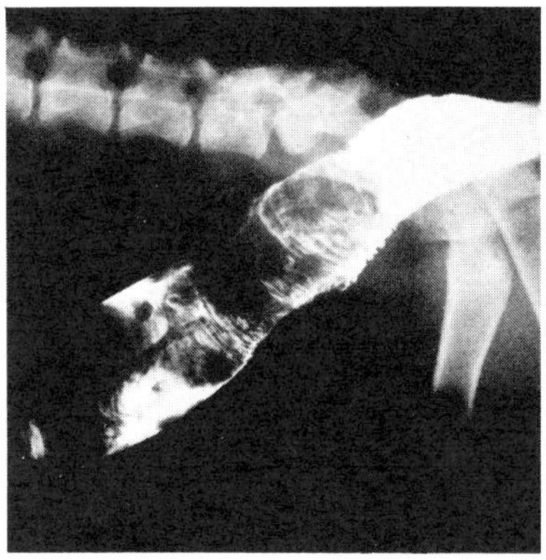

Fig 9,10—This 4-month-old, male, Golden Retriever was referred to AMAH because of tenesmus and rectal prolapse. The diagnosis was uncertain from the clinical findings. Therefore a barium enema was performed. There are multiple smooth filling defects in the descending colon and rectum. No barium passed proximal to the descending colon. The surgical finding was an intussuception which contained the entire jejuneum and ileum.

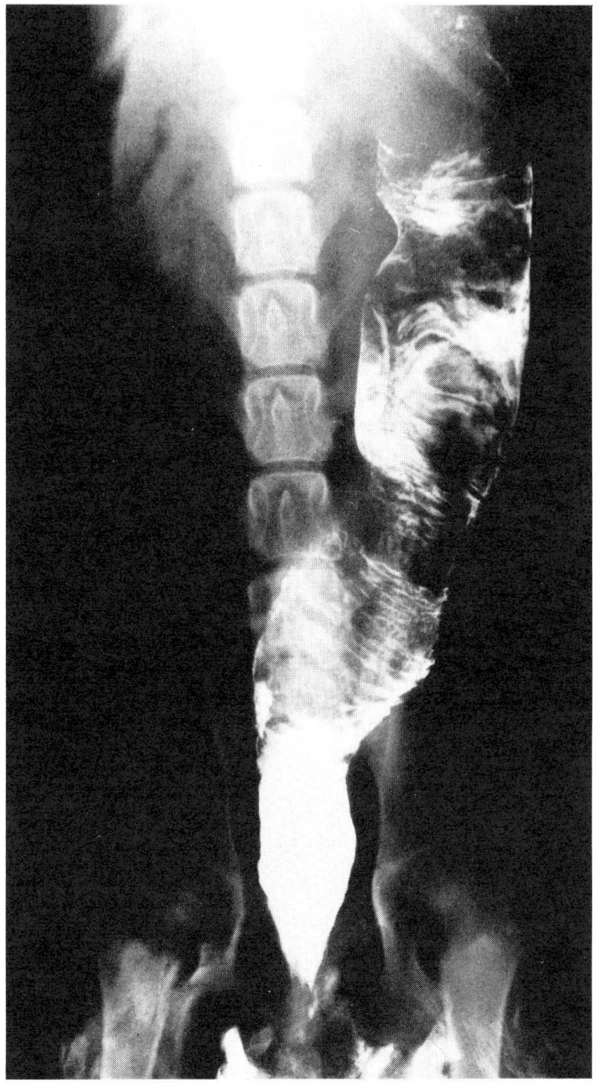

drain out of the colon while the abdomen is gently compressed. When no more contrast medium flows out (usually within 15 minutes) the same radiographic projections are repeated. One may then choose to inflate the colon with either carbon dioxide or room air to perform a double contrast examination which will give better visualization of colonic mucosa and filling defects.

Radiographic Interpretation—In evaluating radiographs of normally motile organs one must bear in mind that the radiographic exposure represents only a small sample in time of a continuously changing configuration. Therefore, reproducibility of the roentgen findings assumes great importance. One of the advantages of an UGI is to allow the veterinarian to see many different stages of gastrointestinal activity in the individual dog or cat in question. If a finding persists it is much more likely to represent a valid observation than a sign that is seen only once.

Dilatation is common and is the most easily recognized radiographic sign of intestinal obstruction. The extent, location and contents of the dilated intestine will vary with degree, duration, site, and cause of obstruction. As a rule of thumb, a complete, proximal, acute obstruction has localized and extreme gaseous distension while a partial, distal, chronic obstruction is characterized by generalized and moderate fluid distension. A progressively greater length of intestine becomes dilated as an adynamic ileus occurs.

Aerophagia secondary to respiratory disease or pain, may simulate obstruction by producing generalized intestinal dilatation. In such cases the air usually is not segmented, but instead large amounts are present in both the colon and small intestine. In cases of small intestinal obstruction, one expects to find proportionally more gas or fluid in the dilated small intestine and smaller amounts of gas in the colon and rectum.

The obstructed segment of gut may first be gas filled and later fluid filled because of continued secretion of intestinal fluid combined with inhibited transport of fluid through the tract. Infarcted intestine usually contains fluid also because of intraluminal hemorrhage.

The stomach, duodenum, cecum, and colon normally occupy a relatively constant location in the abdomen. But the normal small intestine not only propels its contents but also moves to different locations in the abdominal cavity within the limits of its mesenteric attachments. When obstruction is present, not only is transportation of intestinal contents slowed or stopped, but the intestinal tract tends to occupy the same location in sequential radiographs. This phenomenon is referred to as fixation, and is another radiographic sign of obstruction.

Delayed transit of intestinal contents is the third important sign of intestinal obstruction. One expects to find changes in the location and size of gas

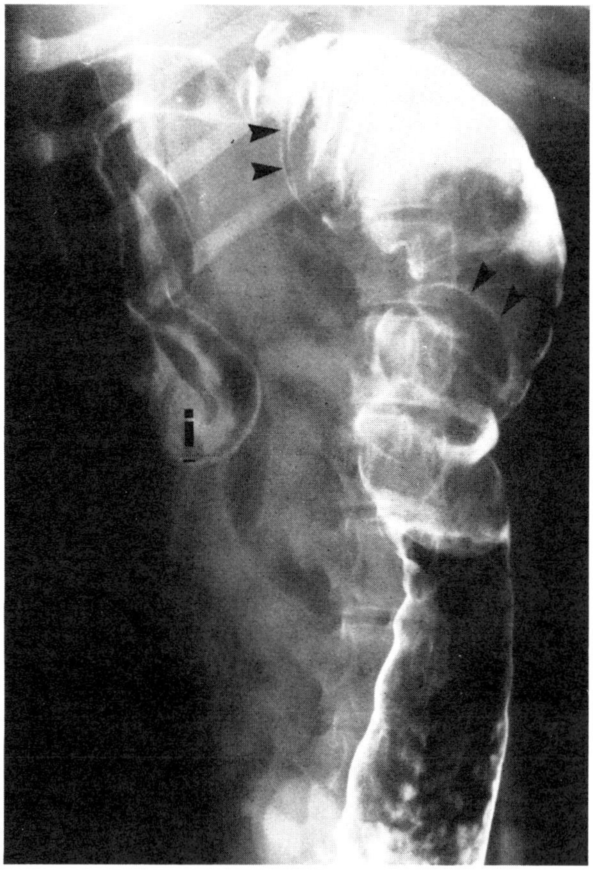

Fig 11—This 3-month-old, male, Doberman Pinscher had periodic bouts of vomiting and diarrhea over the past 3 to 4 weeks. There was a questionable mass found by abdominal palpation. The barium enema indicates a spiral filling defect in the colon (arrows). The cecum is not seen in the right side of the abdomen, but the ileum (I) contains a small amount of contrast medium. These findings are diagnostic of intussuception of the cecum into the ascending and transverse colon.

silhouettes and fluid densities in sequential abdominal radiographs. The UGI serves to identify the particular area of intestine which has diminished or absent motility. If distension is prominent, sequential survey films can be valuable in incriminating intestinal obstruction.

The size and bizarre character of foreign material ingested by dogs and cats is extremely varied. Generally foreign bodies which cause obstruction can be categorized as linear or non-linear. The linear type of foreign body causes plication of the small intestine as well as eccentric location of gas bubbles within the bowel lumen which can usually be recognized in the survey radiographs but are better seen in the UGI. Non-linear foreign bodies which are radiolucent can sometimes be seen because of the air which surrounds them. More often, a UGI is needed to recognize the nature of the obstructive lesion and the degree of obstruction which has been produced.

Neoplasms of the small intestine may cause obstruction by either filling the lumen with a growing lesion, or by narrowing the lumen by encircling the bowel. The form in which an intestinal neoplasm is seen depends on the degree of invasiveness, the shape of the tumor, and its site of origin in the intestine. The lumen is the only portion of the intestine that is generally visualized in the UGI, and the lumen must be deformed in order to detect a tumor.

Occasionally the thickness of the wall of the intestine will be visible in the radiograph. Neoplasms may also affect the intestine by infiltrative rather than discrete growth. In that case, the intestinal lumen may actually be larger than normal due to diminished motility of the area, while the wall of the intestine is thickened due to the infiltration of the tumor. Malignant lymphoma is an example of such an infiltrative growth.

Ileocolic intussuception can be tentatively diagnosed by the clinical findings of blood-stained feces

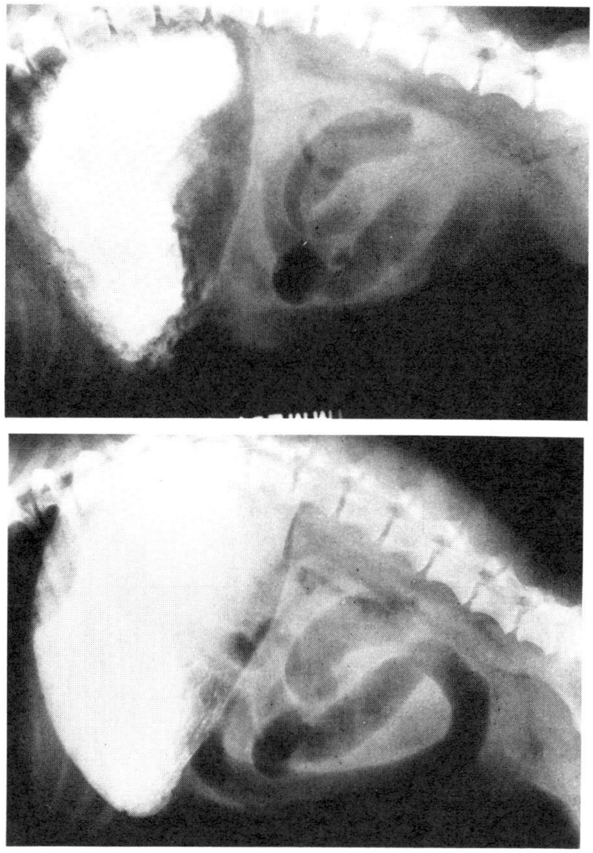

Fig 12,13—The value of sequential radiographs in evaluating the bowel for fixation is demonstrated. Figure 12 is a radiograph of a 2-year-old Dachshund which had been hit by a car 2 months before this examination. At the time of radiography, acute abdominal pain and fever were the most prominent clinical signs. There is distension of the small intestine with both fluid and air. Figure 13 is a radiograph made three hours later. In addition to delayed gastric emptying, there is no substantial change in the location of the distended loops. This fixation, distension, and delayed transit of barium indicate obstruction. The clinical signs and the loss of abdominal contrast suggest strangulation. Surgical findings were infarction of jejunum due to incarceration of bowel through an internal hernia in the mesentery. It was presumed that the mesentery had been torn in the previous automobile accident.

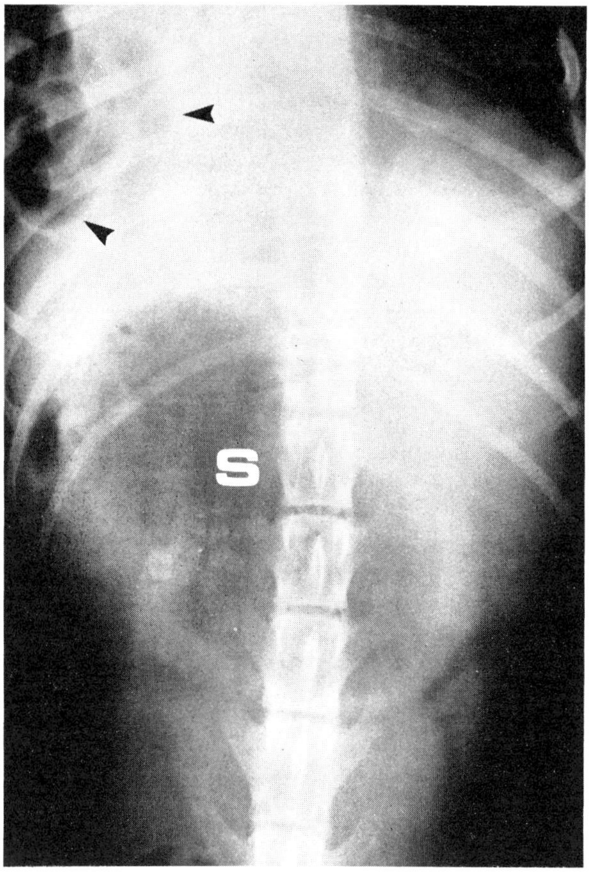

Fig 14—This dog had been hit by a car the day previous to examination. In the 8 hours preceding the examination the dog had vomited several times, was becoming more depressed, and was weak. The stomach is distended with fluid and ingesta(S). The small intestine has passed into the thoracic cavity through a tear in the right side of the diaphragm (arrows). Surgery was performed, and twisting of the mesentery of the proximal small intestine was discovered. This twisting had produced obstruction.

and a palpable, tubular, painful abdominal mass. There is radiographic evidence of distension of the small intestine with both fluid and gas if obstruction is present. The intussusception itself has a fluid density radiographically, but it is not always visualized because of overlapping gas and a fluid-filled intestine. If a UGI is performed the exact nature and site of the obstruction can be better defined. However, a barium enema provides the most clear-cut image of an ileocolic intussusception because the small intestine which lies in the area will not contain contrast medium and the point of obstruction is usually well outlined.

Cecocolic intussusception has less profound radiographic and clinical findings because the degree of obstruction is usually less than in the ileocolic variety. In some cases the cecum can be visualized within the air-filled ascending or transverse colon. The upper GI findings may be equivocal, depending on the size of the cecum and the degree of overlapping of the small intestine. The noninvasive diagnostic procedure of choice in suspected cecocolic intussusception is a barium enema. A spiral filling defect in the ascending colon and lack of visualization of normal cecum in its usual location is diagnostic. Gastroesophageal and enterogastric intussusceptions usually produce acute signs related to high grade obstruction or vascular compromise. The telescoped segment may be outlined by air in the plain radiographs. One expects to find esophageal air in these cases, indicating possible proximal gastrointestinal obstruction.

Fibrosis of the intestine with stenosis and obstruction may occur secondary to trauma, surgery, enteritis, foreign body, or peritonitis. The type and severity of signs are related to the degree and location of stenosis.

Intestinal abscesses and intramural intestinal hemorrhage are rare causes of intestinal obstruction.

An internal hernia is defined as protrusion of a viscus through a normal or abnormal aperture within the confines of the peritoneal cavity. This type of lesion is rare in the dog and cat. It can be due to trauma, congenital mesenteric anomaly, eroding neoplasm, or previous surgery. The clinical signs are usually those of acute obstruction, leading to early strangulation of the herniated segment. The radiological findings consist of distension and fixation of the intestine proximal to the point of obstruction.

A viscus may also herniate through a normal or abnormal aperture outside the confines of the peritoneal cavity. The most frequent example of this type of lesion is diaphragmatic hernia. These lesions can result in intestinal obstruction when the

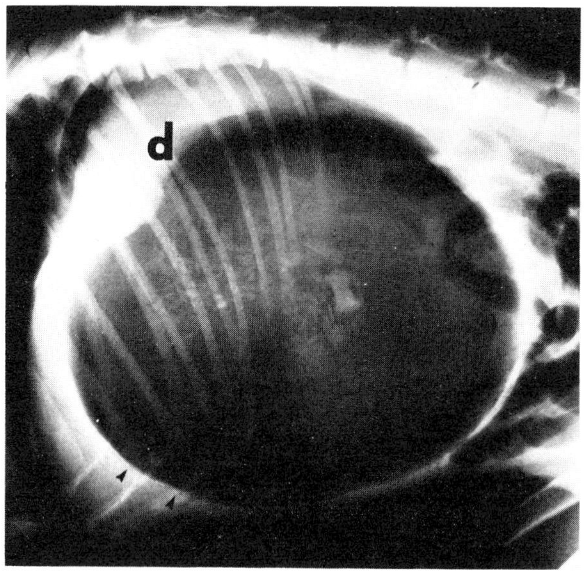

Fig 15—A 2-year-old female, Afghan Hound was presented to AMAH because of sudden onset of abdominal distension. The dog was prostate at the time of examination. There is extreme gaseous distension of the stomach. The location of the dorsal duodenum (D) and the incisure are characteristic of gastric volvulus. There is a small amount of intramural gastric air (arrows). This air has an ominous significance as it indicates that gastric perforation has occurred or is imminent.

herniated part of the intestinal tract is distended with gas and fluid and becomes incarcerated or twisted. Another mechanism of obstruction in intestinal herniation is formulation of adhesions which compress the lumen of the herniated bowel. The clinical signs of obstruction may be acute or chronic. The radiographic findings of distended abdominal viscera outside the peritoneal cavity is usually easily recognized. In some cases the administration of gastrointestinal contrast medium is useful by enhancing visualization of the intestine. If obstruction occurs in other types of hernias, it is usually due to volvulus of the herniated segment of the intestine rather than incarceration.

Volvulus refers to twisting of a part of the gastrointestinal tract around either the mesenteric or intestinal axis. Gastric volvulus is most commonly seen in deep-chested dogs following a large meal and vigorous exercise, It usually results in abdominal distension and rapid deterioration of the dog's condition. The severity of signs is related to the degree of rotation. The radiological diagnosis depends upon the identification of the pylorus to the left of the midline in the ventrodorsal view and dorsal of its normal location in the lateral radiograph. Usually the twisted body of the stomach produces a linear density which can be seen running obliquely in a dorsocranial direction through the stomach.

It is possible for gastric dilatation to produce a stomach as large as occurs with gastric volvulus. The key differential feature is the normal location of the pylorus and duodenum in gastric dilatation. Volvulus of the small intestine, cecum, and colon are much more unusual lesions. The clinical signs are acute obstruction with strangulation. Distension of the intestine proximal to the site of volvulus, fixation of the twisted segment, and peritoneal effusion are prominent radiological findings.

Distension, fixation, and delayed transit are important radiographic features of intestinal obstruction. However, these signs can also be present with other conditions. For instance, aerophagia with distension may be secondary to pain, respiratory difficulty or excitement. In suckling puppies and kittens and in brachycephalic breeds greater amounts of gas will be present in the gastrointestinal tract than in other individuals. Gas and fluid will also accumulate when gastrointestinal motility is diminished for any reason. Among conditions which may mimic obstruction are peritonitis, enteritis, pancreatitis, shock, malabsorption syndrome, spinal trauma, uremia, and anticholinergic drug administration. Correlation of clinical, radiologic, and laboratory findings is essential to differentiate these conditions from intestinal obstruction. Pseudo-obstruction will produce clinical and radiographic signs which are indistinguishable from obstruction. This condition can be differentiated from intestinal obstruction only by means of exploratory laparotomy.[8]

When the diagnosis of intestinal obstruction can be made on basis of clinical and plain radiographic findings, exploratory laparotomy is indicated. In those cases where findings are difficult to correlate, or when findings are equivocal, a UGI will usually provide the necessary information as to whether or not surgery should be performed. One must be aware that animals that are extremely weak or have uncontrollable vomiting should not have oral contrast examinations performed. There is the danger of aspiration of the contrast agent and because hypomotility will probably be present regardless of whether or not obstruction is present. Severe, even fatal, lung damage can occur with pulmonary aspiration of either the organic iodide or barium contrast agents.

Instead, the clinician should attempt to rely on survey radiographs, clinical findings, and possibly exploratory surgery for a diagnosis.

References

1. Hornbuckle, W.E. and Klein, L.J.: Obstruction of the Small Intestine. *Current Veterinary Therapy*. Ed. Kirk, R., W.B. Saunders, Philadelphia, PA (1977):952–958.
2. Root, C.R.: Interpretation of Abdominal Survey Radiographs. *Vet Clin No Amer*, **4,** (1974):763–804.
3. Ticer, J.W.: *Radiographic Technique in Small Animal Practice*. W.B. Saunders, Philadelphia, PA (1975):360–395.
4. Rowe, M.I., Seagram, G., Weinberger, M.: Gastrograffin Induced Hypertonicity: The Pathogenesis of Neonatal Hazard. *Amer Jour Surg*, **125,** (1974):185–188.
5. Rowe, M.I., et al: Neonatal Response to Gastrograffin Edema. *Pediatrics*, **48,** (1971):29–35.
6. Poole, C.A. and Rowe, M.I.: Clinical Evidence of Intestinal Absorption of Gastrograffin. *Radiology*, **118,** (1976):151–153.

6a. Cohen D.M.: Choosing Contrast Media for the Evaluation of the Gastrointestinal Tract of Neonates and Infants. *Radiology*, **162,** (1987):447–456.

6b. Ferrante S.L., Schreiman J.S., Rouse J.W., et al: Iopamidol as a Gastrointestinal Contrast Agent. *Invest Radiol*, **25,** (199):141–145.

7. Zontine, W.J.: Effect of Chemical Restraint on the Passage of Barium Sulfate Through the Stomach and Duodenum of Dogs. *JAVMA*, **162,** (1973):878–884.
8. Arrick, R.H. and Kleine, L.J.: Intestinal Pseudo-obstruction in a Dog. *JAVMA*, **172,** (1978):1201–1205.

The Excretory Urogram: Part I Techniques, Normal Radiographic Appearance, and Misinterpretation

D. A. Feeney, DVM, MS
Assistant Professor
Department of Small Animal Clinical Sciences
College of Veterinary Medicine
University of Minnesota
St. Paul, Minnesota

D. L. Barber, DVM, MS
Assistant Professor
Department of Anatomy and Radiology
College of Veterinary Medicine
University of Georgia
Athens, Georgia

G. R. Johnston, DVM, MS
Assistant Professor

C. A. Osborne, DVM, PhD
Professor and Chairman

Department of Small Animal Clinical Sciences
College of Veterinary Medicine
University of Minnesota
St. Paul, Minnesota

As excretory urography evolved in veterinary medicine over the years two major shortcomings persisted: (1) a standardized technique for excretory urography was not widely adopted, and (2) quantitation of parameters of normal excretory urography and factors affecting these parameters for each of the various techniques were not available. Comparison of results of serial studies performed in the same patient or comparison of findings of one group of investigators with those of another is significantly hindered if a standardized technique is not used. This article presents (1) a standardized method of excretory urography for use in dogs and cats, (2) the normal radiographic appearance of the canine and feline urinary tract based on this technique, and (3) radiographic findings that may be misinterpreted. Adoption of a standardized technique by the veterinary profession will facilitate recognition of disease entities and a better understanding of the pathophysiology of various disorders of the urinary system by allowing meaningful comparison of results obtained by different investigators.

Use of the excretory urogram as a diagnostic modality in small-animal practice was first documented in 1953.[1,2] Five years later, some recommendations for standardizing technique and analysis of some variables (i.e., contrast medium dose, exposure sequence, abdominal compression) affecting the appearance of the normal canine excretory urogram were reported.[3] Since that time numerous authors have described variations of the technique and interpretation of the excretory urogram in dogs and cats.[4-13]

The primary use of the excretory urogram is to evaluate portions of the urinary tract that cannot be adequately visualized by survey radiography. Evaluation of the size, shape, position, and surface contours of the kidneys, ureters, and urinary bladder plays an important role in localizing and diagnosing various disorders of the urinary tract.[4,14] Because there are many variables that affect the appearance of the excretory urogram, it should not be used as a quantitative index of renal function.

Technique

Preparation of the patient for excretory urography has been addressed

Originally published in Volume 4, Number 3, March 1982

previously.[4,5,10,12-14] In general, food should be withheld for 24 hours and cleansing enemas and/or laxatives should be administered to ensure that the gastrointestinal tract is empty. Water should be available at all times. Preliminary dehydration is not advised.[3,4,8-10,15] Sedation or anesthesia has been recommended[1,2,5,11] but should be avoided if the procedure can be performed satisfactorily without it. Commonly used sedative and anesthetic compounds may have variable effects on blood pressure and ureteral motility, and these effects may alter radiographic appearance.

Survey radiographs should always be made before contrast medium is administered. A wide range of contrast media and doses have been recommended.[1,4,5,9,13] Various methods of administration of contrast media also have been recommended, including rapid intravenous bolus injection,[9,15,16] slow intravenous injection,[1,5] and drip infusion of the diluted contrast material.[6,7,10-12] The authors' recommendation is bolus intravenous injection of 400 mg of iodine per lb (0.45 kg) of body weight.[15,16] Quantification of the normal appearance of the excretory urogram in dogs has been evaluated by the authors using this dosage.[15,16]

Recommendations for sequence of exposing radiographs following administration of contrast medium have varied widely.[1-12] Since the appearance of the normal excretory urogram varies predictably with the length of time after injection, the authors recommend a definitive filming sequence.[15,16] Table I is a general summary of the recommended technique for excretory urography in the dog and cat.

TABLE I

TECHNIQUE FOR INTRAVENOUS UROGRAPHY*

1. Routine patient preparation
   a. 24 hours without food; water ad libitum
   b. Cleansing enema at least 2 hours before radiography
2. Assess hydration status; proceed only if it is normal
3. Obtain survey radiographs
4. Infuse contrast medium intravenously via the cephalic or jugular vein as rapidly as possible (bolus injection)
   a. Dose: 400 mg of iodine/lb body weight†
   b. Contrast medium: sodium iothalamate or sodium diatrizoate
5. Make abdominal radiographs in the following sequence:
   a. Ventrodorsal views at 5 to 20 seconds, 5 minutes, 20 minutes, and 40 minutes postinjection for general assessment
   b. Lateral view at 5 minutes postinjection for general assessment
   c. Oblique views at 3 to 5 minutes postinjection for ureteral termination in urinary bladder
   d. Lateral and ventrodorsal views at 30 to 40 minutes postinjection to observe urinary bladder if retrograde cystography is contraindicated or impossible

*From Feeney DA, Barber DL, Osborne CA: Advances in canine excretory urography, in *30th Gaines Veterinary Symposium (1981)*. White Plains, NY, 1981, pp 8-22. Adapted with permission.
†If renal function is extremely poor, use 800 mg of iodine/lb body weight.

Currently available radiographic contrast media are ionic, triiodinated benzoic acid derivatives. The anionic component is usually iothalamate or diatrizoate; the cationic component is usually sodium or methylglucamine. The anionic portions of the contrast agent are excreted almost exclusively by glomerular filtration.[17] In the authors' experience, sodium compounds give a denser opacification of the renal pelves and ureters.

Abdominal compression has been recommended to improve visualization of the renal pelves and pelvic diverticula by causing temporary ureteral compression which impedes urine outflow.[1,3,5,10,12-14] Provided the ureters can be compressed, increased pressure may distend the renal pelvis and its diverticula with urine containing contrast material. The authors do not recommend this procedure because it induces unpredictable effects on glomerular filtration and often does not uniformly compress both ureters.[4,8,17] Although abdominal compression has been advocated as an important technique to detect the early stages of pyelonephritis, this disorder can be diagnosed radiographically without abdominal compression using the technique described herein.[18]

Normal Appearance

The excretory urogram has two basic phases: the nephrogram and the pyelogram. The nephrogram represents opacification of the kidney by accumulation of contrast medium in the renal vessels (vascular nephrogram), which occurs within 10 to 15 seconds after bolus intravenous injection, and/or subsequent accumulation of contrast medium within renal tubules (tubular nephrogram). During the early vascular phase, the cortex is denser than the medulla (Figure 1). Nephrographic opacity rapidly becomes uniform in normal kidneys and becomes most dense 10 to 20 seconds after injection. Renal opacity decreases progressively for one to three hours following injection of contrast medium until it is no denser than that observed on survey radiographs (Figure 1).[16]

The pyelogram represents opacification of the renal pelves, pelvic diverticula, and ureters. Opacity of the pyelogram is much greater than that of the nephrogram since contrast medium has been concentrated by obligatory and facultative resorption of water as glomerular filtrate passed through the renal tubules. The pyelogram is normally visualized one to three minutes following intravenous injection of contrast material, and it persists for several hours after injection. The pyelogram is best visualized within one hour after contrast medium injection (Figure 1).[16]

Studies of the effects of dose, time, and individual dog variations on the canine excretory urogram have been reported.[16] Quantitative parameters of canine and feline excretory urography are summarized in Table II. The radiographic appearance of the normal canine and feline excretory urograms is shown in Figures 2 and 3.

Although excretory urography is not the optimal

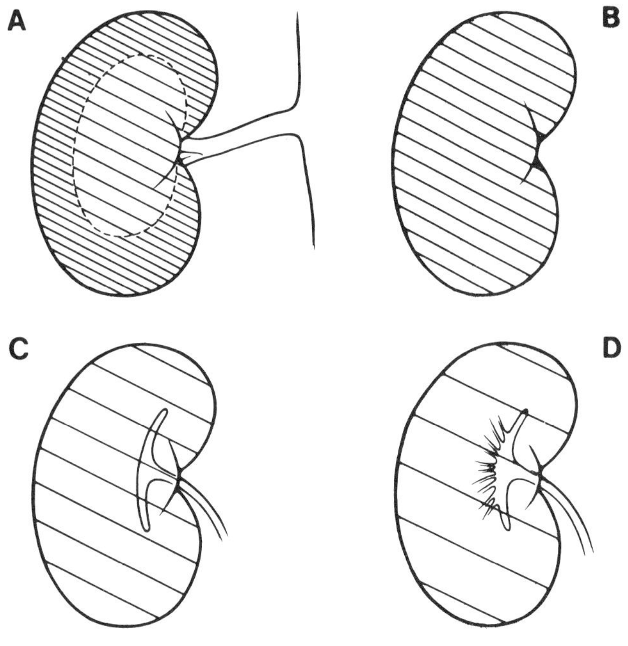

Figure 1—Diagram of a normal canine urogram. **(A)** Early vascular nephrogram; **(B)** tubular nephrogram; **(C)** 5-minute postinjection nephrogram and pyelogram; **(D)** 20- or 40-minute postinjection nephrogram and pyelogram. (From Feeney DA, Barber DL, Osborne CA: Advances in canine excretory urography, in *30th Gaines Veterinary Symposium (1981)*. White Plains, NY, Gaines Dog Research Center, 1981, pp 8-22. Reprinted with permission.)

contrast study for evaluation of the urinary bladder, it can be used for this purpose. On occasion, catheterization required for positive contrast cystography may be impossible or contraindicated. Provided renal function is adequate, satisfactory opacification and adequate distention of the urinary bladder may be obtained 30 to 40 minutes following injection of contrast medium as described for excretory urography. The urinary bladder is normally ovoid; its caudal aspect is more pointed in the region of the trigone. The mucosal surface is smooth and the bladder wall is of uniform thickness, provided nearly complete distention is achieved. The ureters commonly curve anteriorly and ventrally just prior to their entry into the trigone of the bladder.

Common Misinterpretations

The excretory urogram, as is true of any procedure performed on a living organism, has effects and variables that must be recognized to ensure accurate interpretation. For example, the end-on view of the deep circumflex iliac arteries visualized by survey radiography should not be mistaken for ureteral calculi in the caudal lumbar area of the abdomen in the lateral projection.[8] The following discussion summarizes interpretive pitfalls; the technical pitfalls have been described elsewhere in detail.[21]

The radiographic appearance of the normal pyelogram is somewhat variable. Pelvic diverticula often cannot be visualized in the normal dog without abdominal compression.[16] This is of no consequence, provided the renal pelves and proximal ureters are normal in size and the renal pelvis has a uniform shape (Figure 2). Absence of detectable pelvic diverticula following excretory urography without abdominal compression is therefore not a reliable index of early pyelonephritis if the renal pelvis is normal.

Ureters propel urine containing contrast medium from the kidney to the bladder via rhythmic peristaltic contractions. Filling defects within the ureters caused by these contraction waves should not be misinterpreted as obstructive lesions (e.g., calculi, blood clots, or strictures). Peristaltic contractions of various portions of the ureters may be readily distinguished from obstructive disorders because they do not remain at the same site on serially obtained views.

On occasion, administration of radiographic contrast media may be followed by systemic hypotension and collapse. This may result in persistence of the nephrographic opacity and delay in pyelographic opacity. This is not the normal appearance of an excretory urogram, and it should arouse suspicion of contrast medium–in-

TABLE II

QUANTITATIVE APPEARANCE OF NORMAL CANINE AND FELINE EXCRETORY UROGRAMS

Structure	*Measurement**	*Value†*	*Reference*
Kidney	Length	Dog	
		3.00 ± 0.25 × L-2	16
		2.50 to 3.50 × L-2	19
		2.25 to 3.00 vertebrae	9
		Cat	
		2.4 to 3.0 × L-2	20
		4.0 to 4.5 cm	5
	Width	Dog	
		2.00 ± 0.20 × L-2	16
		Cat	
		3.0 to 3.5 cm	5
Renal pelvis	Width	Dog	
		0.03 ± 0.017 × L-2 (generally ≤ 1.0 mm)	16
		Cat	
		Not reported	
Pelvic diverticula	Width	Dog	
		0.02 ± 0.005 × L-2 (generally ≤ 1.0 mm)	16
		Cat	
		Not reported	
Proximal ureter	Width	Dog	
		0.07 ± 0.018 × L-2 (generally ≤ 1.0 mm)	16
		Cat	
		Not reported	
Distal ureter	Width	Not reported in dogs or cats	

*Measurements apply only to the VD view.
†L-2 = the length of the body of the second lumbar vertebral body as visualized on the ventrodorsal view.

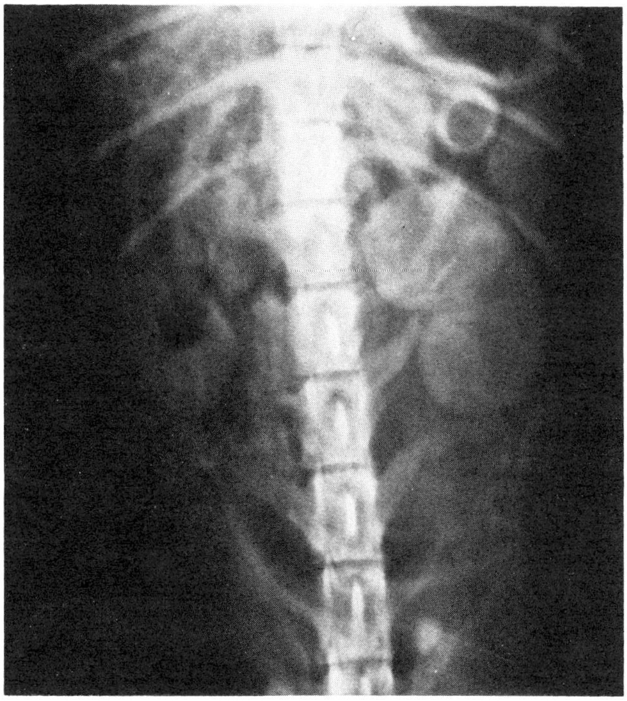

Figure 2A

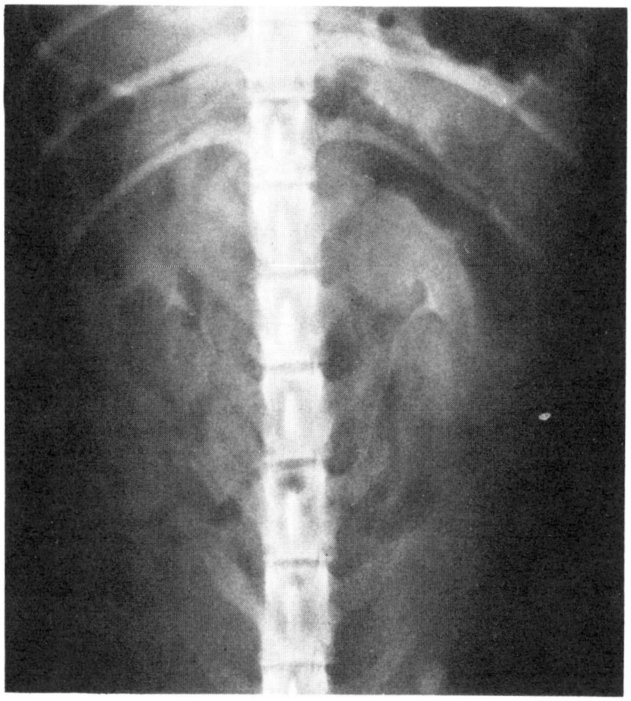

Figure 2C

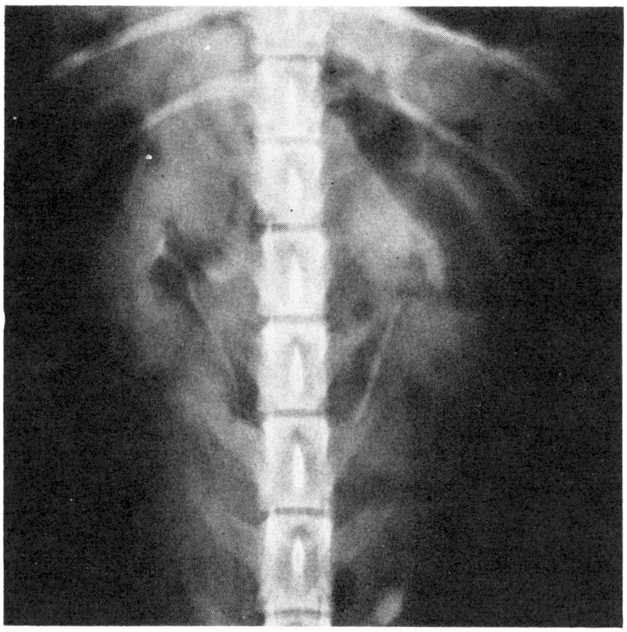

Figure 2B

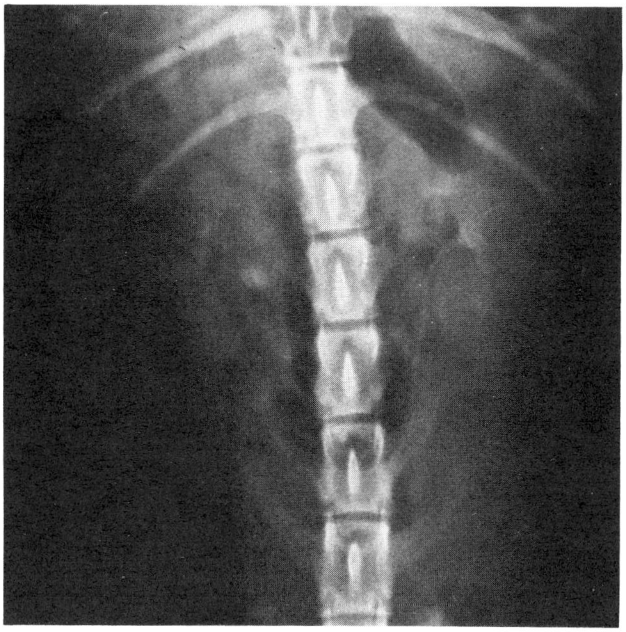

Figure 2D

Figure 2—Normal canine excretory urogram. Ventrodorsal radiographs made at **(A)** 10 seconds, **(B)** 5 minutes, **(C)** 20 minutes, and **(D)** 40 minutes following contrast medium administration.

duced systemic hypotension and should be treated in the same manner as hypovolemic shock. Intravenous administration of atropine (routine preanesthetic dose) should also be considered since parenterally administered contrast media may cause bradycardia despite systemic hypotension. A persistent nephrogram has also been associated with urine outflow obstruction, contrast medium–induced renal failure, glomerular disease, and renal tubular necrosis.[17,22]

Radiopaque contrast medium may cause a false-positive reaction for protein and alter specific gravity values determined during routine urinalyses.[23] False-positive protein reactions have most commonly been observed when sulfosalicylic acid is used. However, radiographic contrast medium does not interfere with tests that incorporate indicator dyes (bromphenol blue[a] and tetra-

[a]Albutest®, Ames Co., Elkhart, IN 46515.

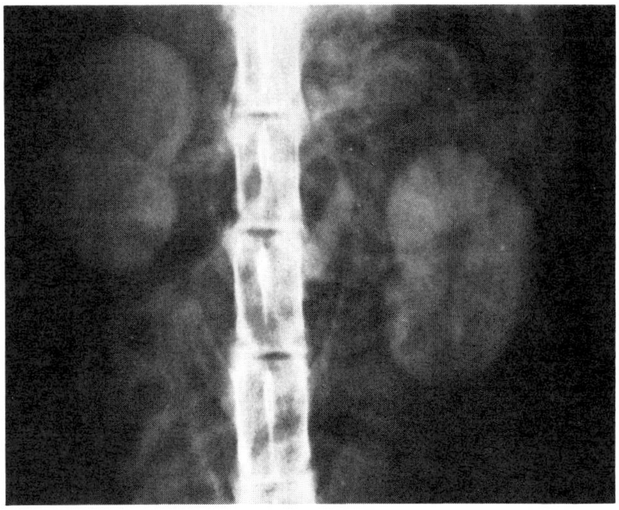

Figure 3A

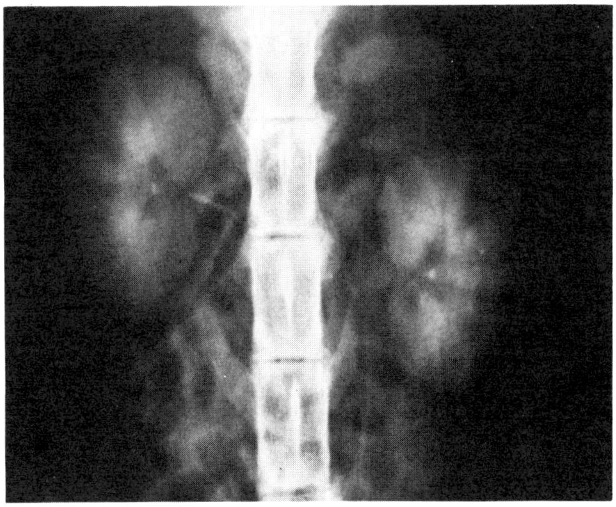

Figure 3B

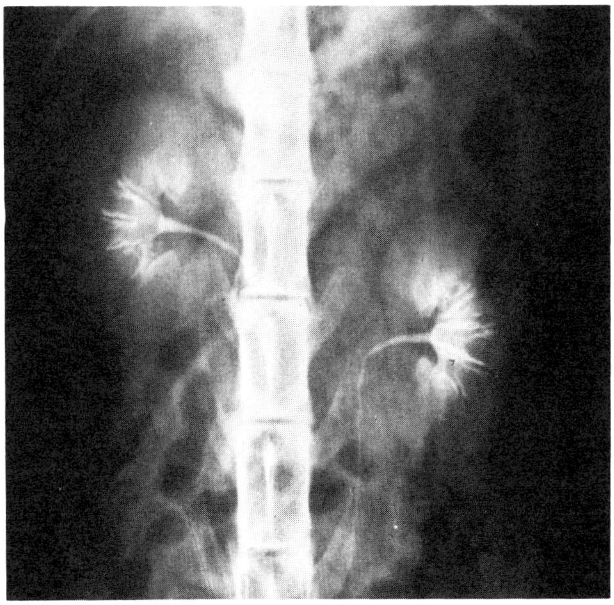

Figure 3C

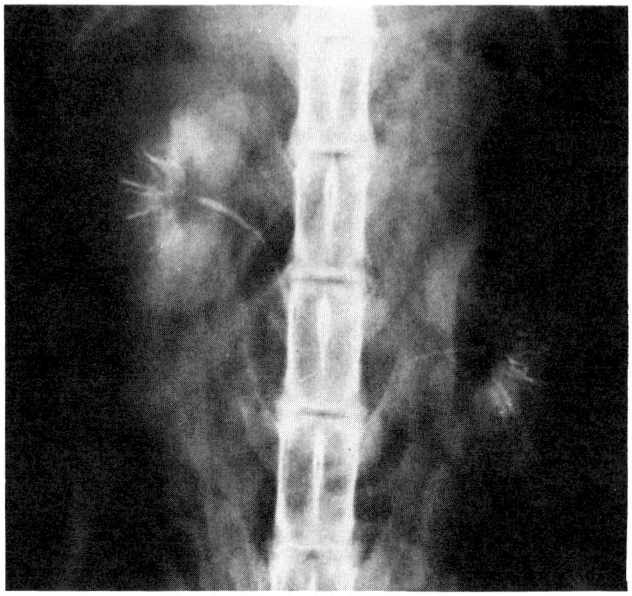

Figure 3D

Figure 3—Normal feline excretory urogram. Ventrodorsal radiographs made at **(A)** 10 seconds, **(B)** 5 minutes, **(C)** 20 minutes, and **(D)** 40 minutes following contrast medium administration.

bromphenol blue[b]).[23] Changes in urine specific gravity following excretory urography in dogs have been reported.[23] In dogs, the direction and magnitude of change in urine specific gravity are dependent on the degree of urine concentration prior to administration of the contrast agent.[23] If the urine specific gravity prior to excretory urography is below 1.040, radiographic contrast agents may cause a significant increase which is not due to renal conservation of water in excess of solute. Care should be taken not to misinterpret such findings as evidence of adequate renal function. To avoid contrast medium-induced errors in urinalysis, at least 24 hours should be allowed to elapse before samples are collected for analysis.

[b]Albustix®, Ames Co., Elkhart, IN 46515.

REFERENCES

1. Bishop EJ: A method of visualizing the urinary tract and a basis for assessing renal function in small animal radiography. *JAVMA* 123:187-192, 1953.
2. Drury F, Dyce KM: The radiography of the normal urinary tract of the dog. *Vet Rec* 65:647-649, 1953.
3. Tennile NB, Thornton GW: Intravenous urography studies in the unanesthetized dog. *Vet Med* 53:29-40, 1958.
4. Ackerman N: Intravenous pyelography. *JAAHA* 10:277-284, 1974.
5. Bartels JE: Feline intravenous urography. *JAAHA* 9:349-353, 1973.
6. Borthwick R, Robbie B: Large volume urography in the cat. *J Small Anim Pract* 12:579-583, 1971.
7. Borthwick R, Robbie B: Urography in the dog by an intravenous transfusion technique. *J Small Anim Pract* 10:465-470, 1969.
8. Kneller SK: Role of the excretory urogram in the diagnosis of renal and ureteral disease. *Vet Clin North Am* 4:843-861, 1974.
9. Lord PE, Scott RC, Chan KF: Intravenous urography for the evaluation of renal diseases in small animals. *JAAHA* 10:139-152, 1974.

10. Root CR: Contrast radiography of the urinary system, in Ticer JW (ed): *Radiographic Technique in Small Animal Practice.* Philadelphia, WB Saunders Co, 1975, pp 396-414.
11. Walker RG, Douglas SW: The use of contrast media in the diagnosis of urinary tract abnormalities in the dog with particular reference to infusion urography: A report of two cases. *Vet Rec* 87:287-289, 1970.
12. Watters JW: Urinary tract radiography—Kidney and ureters. *Compend Contin Educ Pract Vet* 2:224-231, 1980.
13. Zontine WJ: Radiographic interpretation: Excretory urogram. *Mod Vet Pract* 56:106-111, 1975.
14. Biery DN: The upper urinary tract, in O'Brien TR (ed): *Radiographic Diagnosis of Abdominal Disorders in the Dog and Cat.* Philadelphia, WB Saunders Co, 1978, pp 481-542.
15. Feeney DA, Barber DL, Osborne CA: Advances in canine excretory urography, in *Proceedings 30th Gaines Veterinary Symposium.* White Plains, NY, Gaines Dog Research Center, 1981, pp 8-22.
16. Feeney DA, Thrall DE, Barber DL, et al, Normal canine excretory urogram: Effects of dose, time and individual dog variation. *Am J Vet Res* 40:1596-1604, 1979.
17. Saxton HM: Review article: Urography. *Br J Radiol* 42:321-346, 1969.
18. Barber DL, Finco DR: Radiographic findings in induced bacterial pyelonephritis in dogs. *JAVMA* 175:1183-1190, 1979.
19. Finco DR, Stiles NS, Kneller SK, et al: Radiologic estimation of kidney size of the dog. *JAVMA* 159:995-1002, 1971.
20. Barrett RB, Kneller SK: Feline kidney mensuration. *Acta Radiol Suppl* 319:279-280, 1972.
21. Johnston GR, Feeney DA, Osborne CA: Radiographic findings in urinary tract infection. *Vet Clin North Am* 9:749-774, 1979.
22. Feeney DA, Barber DL, Osborne CA: The functional aspects of excretory nephrography: A review, submitted to *Vet Radiol.*
23. Feeney DA, Osborne CA, Jessen CR: Effects of radiocontrast agents on the urinalysis with emphasis on specific gravity. *JAVMA* 176:1378-1381, 1980.

The Excretory Urogram: Part II Interpretation of Abnormal Findings

D. A. Feeney, DVM, MS
Assistant Professor
Department of Small Animal Clinical Sciences
College of Veterinary Medicine
University of Minnesota
St. Paul, Minnesota

D. L. Barber, DVM, MS
Assistant Professor
Department of Anatomy and Radiology
College of Veterinary Medicine
University of Georgia
Athens, Georgia

G. R. Johnston, DVM, MS
Assistant Professor

C. A. Osborne, DVM, PhD
Professor and Chairman

Department of Small Animal Clinical Sciences
College of Veterinary Medicine
University of Minnesota
St. Paul, Minnesota

The excretory urogram may be used to obtain qualitative information about the functional status of canine and feline kidneys by observation of the sequential trends in nephrographic opacity. Comparisons of the degree of initial nephrographic opacification and subsequent trends in nephrographic opacification during excretory urography may suggest the presence of conditions such as contrast medium–induced renal failure, contrast medium–induced systemic hypotension, acute renal obstruction, polyuric renal disease, and glomerular dysfunction. Observation of the size, shape, and distribution of parenchymal opacification of the kidneys during urography assists in diagnosis of renal neoplasms, renal cysts, renal infarcts, hematomas, hydronephrosis, and chronic generalized renal disease (end-stage kidneys). Comparison of structural alterations with the size and shape of the renal pelvis and its diverticula may permit diagnosis of pyelonephritis, hydronephrosis, renal neoplasia, and/or renal calculi.

Excretory urography is an integral part of the evaluation of most patients with suspected urinary tract disease. It is used to evaluate the size, shape, and position of various components of the urinary tract.[1-7] Specific situations in which excretory urography is indicated include following severe abdominal trauma and cases of hematuria, dysuria, incontinence, polyuria, oliguria, anuria, and palpable abnormalities.[1,3,7,8] Excretory urography may also be used for evaluation of the upper and lower urinary tract in the presence of abdominal masses of undetermined origin. Involvement (or noninvolvement) of urinary tract structures can be assessed, and the relationship of the masses to the urinary structures may assist in identifying the site or sites of their origin.

Excretory urography may be used in patients with or without azotemia to evaluate renal size or to determine if outflow obstruction has occurred. In humans, failure to correct dehydration prior to administration of radiopaque contrast agents has been associated with adverse reactions involving the kidneys.[9] Occurrence of adverse reactions is more frequent in dehydrated patients with diabetes mellitus, myeloma, and combined renal and hepatic failure than in other dehydrated patients.[9] Based on reports in humans, it has been recommended that excretory urography only be performed on adequately hydrated patients.[3,6]

In general, the radiographic quality (opacification and contrast

Originally published in Volume 4, Number 4, April 1982

enhancement) of the excretory urogram decreases as the degree of renal dysfunction becomes more severe.[10] For this reason, increased doses of radiographic contrast medium have been recommended to improve the quality of the urogram during moderate to severe renal dysfunction.[3,11] Some pathophysiologic alterations in renal function may be associated with specific variation in the sequence of opacification of the kidney during urography (Table I). The radiographic appearance and pathophysiology of these functional abnormalities have been described elsewhere in detail.[3,16] The opacity of the collecting system (pelvis, ureters, and bladder) generally decreases in patients with renal failure because of an obligatory increase in urine volume that reduces the concentration of contrast medium in urine. Reduced opacification of the excretory pathway is not pathognomonic for primary renal failure, however, since it may be associated with an inadequate dosage of contrast medium and nonrenal causes of polyuria.

Contrast medium–induced renal failure has been reported in humans,[17-19] dogs,[3] and cats.[20] The pathophysiology of this disease has not been precisely determined, but it appears to be complex. Possible mechanisms include renal vasoconstriction, direct toxicity to renal tubules, renal vascular occlusion secondary to contrast-induced red blood cell aggregation, and obstruction of renal tubules by Tamm-Horsfall mucoprotein.[17,18] In humans, diabetes mellitus, preexisting renal disease, multiple myeloma, dehydration, and advanced age have been associated with increased risk of contrast medium–induced renal failure.[17-19] The clinical course is usually transient (2 to 37 days) in human patients. It is initially characterized by oliguria and progressive azotemia, followed by increased urine flow rates and subsequent return of normal renal function.[17-19] Although this disorder has not been documented in large numbers of dogs and cats, it is presumed to be potentially reversible. Changes in creatinine clearance have been reported in dogs following contrast medium administration, but the wide degree of renal function impairment among dogs was interpreted to suggest variation in individual susceptibility.[21]

The Nephrogram

Opacification of the renal parenchyma following intravenous injection of contrast medium is termed the

TABLE I

Nephrographic Opacification Patterns Associated with Common Renal Disorders*

Pattern	*Associated Disorders*
Sequential decrease in nephrographic opacity	
A. Good initial opacification followed by progressive decrease in opacity	None[12]
B. Poor initial opacification followed by progressive decrease in opacity	Primary polyuric renal failure Inadequate contrast medium dose Others
Sequential persistence in nephrographic opacity	
A. Fair to good initial opacification followed by persistent opacity	Acute renal tubular necrosis[13] Contrast medium–induced renal failure[14] Systemic hypotension due to radiocontrast agents[13] Others
B. Poor initial opacification followed by persistent opacity	Primary glomerular dysfunction[13] Severe generalized renal disease Others
Sequential increase in nephrographic opacity	
A. Fair to good opacification followed by progressive increase in opacity	Systemic hypotension due to radiocontrast agents[13,20] Acute renal obstruction (probably due to precipitated Tamm-Horsfall mucoprotein in renal tubules)[13] Contrast medium–induced renal failure[14] Others
B. Poor initial opacification followed by progressive increase in opacity	Acute extrarenal obstruction[13] Systemic hypotension existing prior to contrast medium administration[15] Renal ischemia (arterial or venous)[13] Others

*Modified from Feeney DA, Barber DL, Osborne CA: The functional aspects of the nephrogram in excretory urography: A review. *Vet Radiol,* in press.

nephrogram. The components (vascular and tubular) that contribute to the nephrogram have been described.[3,22]

An early vascular nephrogram is a reliable index of renal perfusion. A tubular nephrogram is indicative of the presence of functional renal parenchyma. The normal sequence of opacification and appearance of the normal nephrogram have been described.[3,22] The opacity of the nephrogram is proportional to the dose (in milligrams of iodine) of contrast medium administered.[12] However, the degree of opacity and trends of opacity (e.g., increase, decrease, or persistent) following intravenous administration of contrast medium may be influenced by renal perfusion, nephron function, and patency of the renal outflow tract.[3,4]

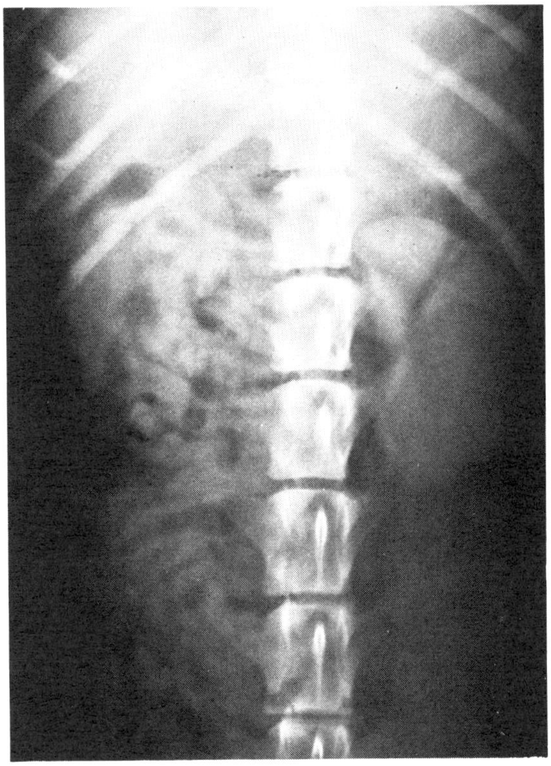

Figure 1A

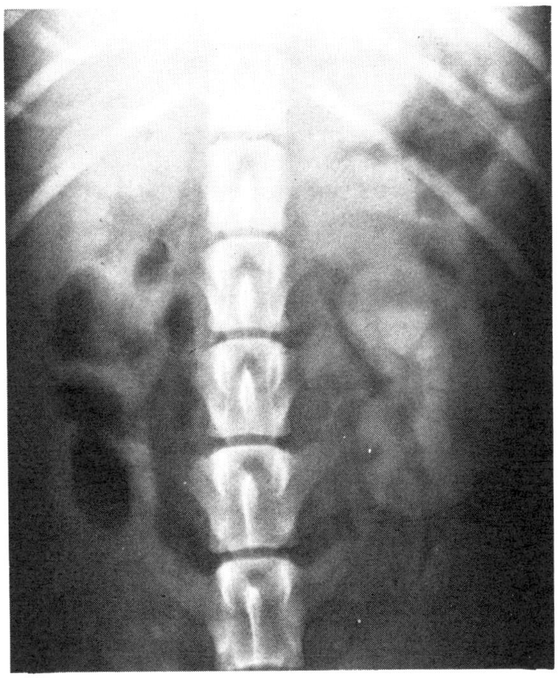

Figure 1B

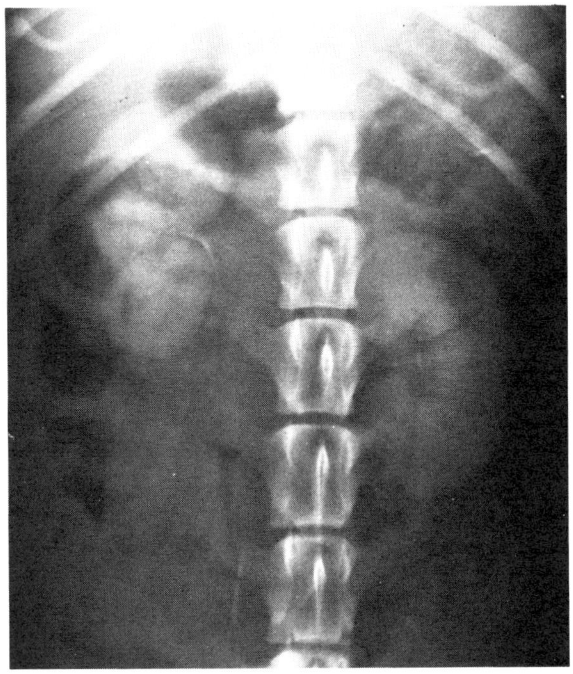

Figure 1C

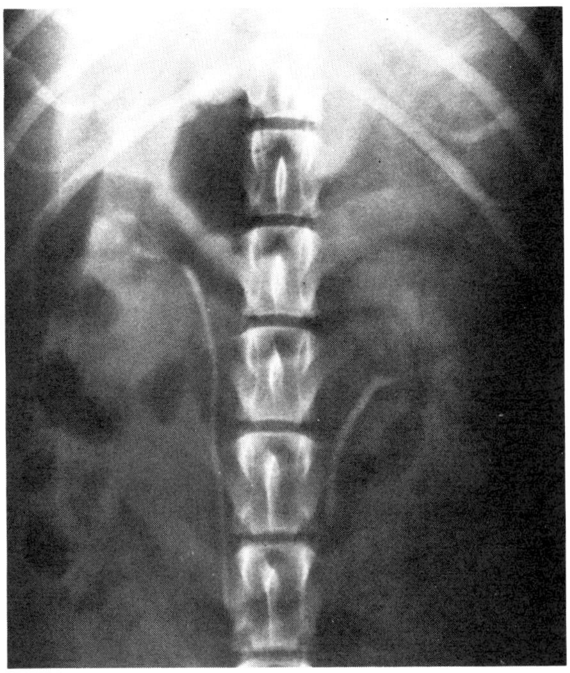

Figure 1D

Figure 1—Excretory urogram of a mature male beagle during systemic hypotension and collapse which occurred following bolus intravenous injection of sodium iothalamate. Ventrodorsal radiographs made at **(A)** 15 seconds, **(B)** 5 minutes, **(C)** 20 minutes, and **(D)** 40 minutes postinjection. Note persistent slightly increasing nephrographic opacity and lack of normal pelvic and ureteral opacification from **A** to **D**. (From Feeney DA, Barber DL, Osborne CA: Advances in canine excretory urography, in *30th Gaines Veterinary Symposium (1981)*. White Plains, NY, Gaines Dog Research Center, 1981, pp 8-22. Reprinted with permission.)

As a general rule, nephrographic appearance should be assessed on each radiograph for variations in opacification, shape, size, and the interface between areas of nonuniform opacification. In addition, after contrast medium injection, the opacity of the nephrograms should be compared in chronologic order to ascertain the sequence of nephrographic opacification. When present, opacification of the collecting system occurs as the nephrogram begins to fade. The maximum degree of opacity of the nephrogram in patients with renal dysfunction is usually observed during the initial vascular phase.[22]

Possible nephrographic patterns found during excretory urography in humans, dogs, and cats are summarized in Table I. In general, the initial opacification refers to findings on 10-second and 5-minute post-contrast medium injection radiographs. *Persistent opacity* and *progressive* changes in opacity (in the table) refer to radiographs obtained 20 minutes or more after injection (including circumstances when radiographs are made 12 to 24 hours after contrast medium injection). Subsequent opacification of the renal pelves, pelvic diverticula, and ureters (pyelogram) is dependent on a number of factors (see discussion in the section about the pyelogram).

An example of an abnormal trend in nephrographic opacity is contrast medium–induced hypotension (Table I). A mature beagle given the routine dose of contrast medium collapsed seconds later. Therapy for hypovolemic shock was immediately initiated and continued throughout the radiographic sequence. Radiographs were obtained during this contrast medium–induced reaction (Figure 1). Note the persistence of, and tendency toward, increased nephrographic opacity through the 20-minute postinjection radiograph. Almost no opacification of pyelographic structures occurred until the animal returned to a nearly normal physiological status 40 minutes following contrast medium injection.

Alterations in renal parenchyma may often be detected by studying nephrographic appearance. An algorithm has been developed in which renal size, renal capsular surface characteristics, and distribution of opacification were used to identify probable causes of specific nephrographio findings (Figure 2). Diseases (such as amyloidosis) that are highly variable in appearance have not been included because they have no predictable trend in architectural alterations.

Localized alterations in nephrographic appearance are usually associated with neoplasms, renal infarcts, solitary renal cysts, hematomas, and/or abscesses.[3] Differentiation of these disorders may be facilitated by examining the interface between normal and abnormal

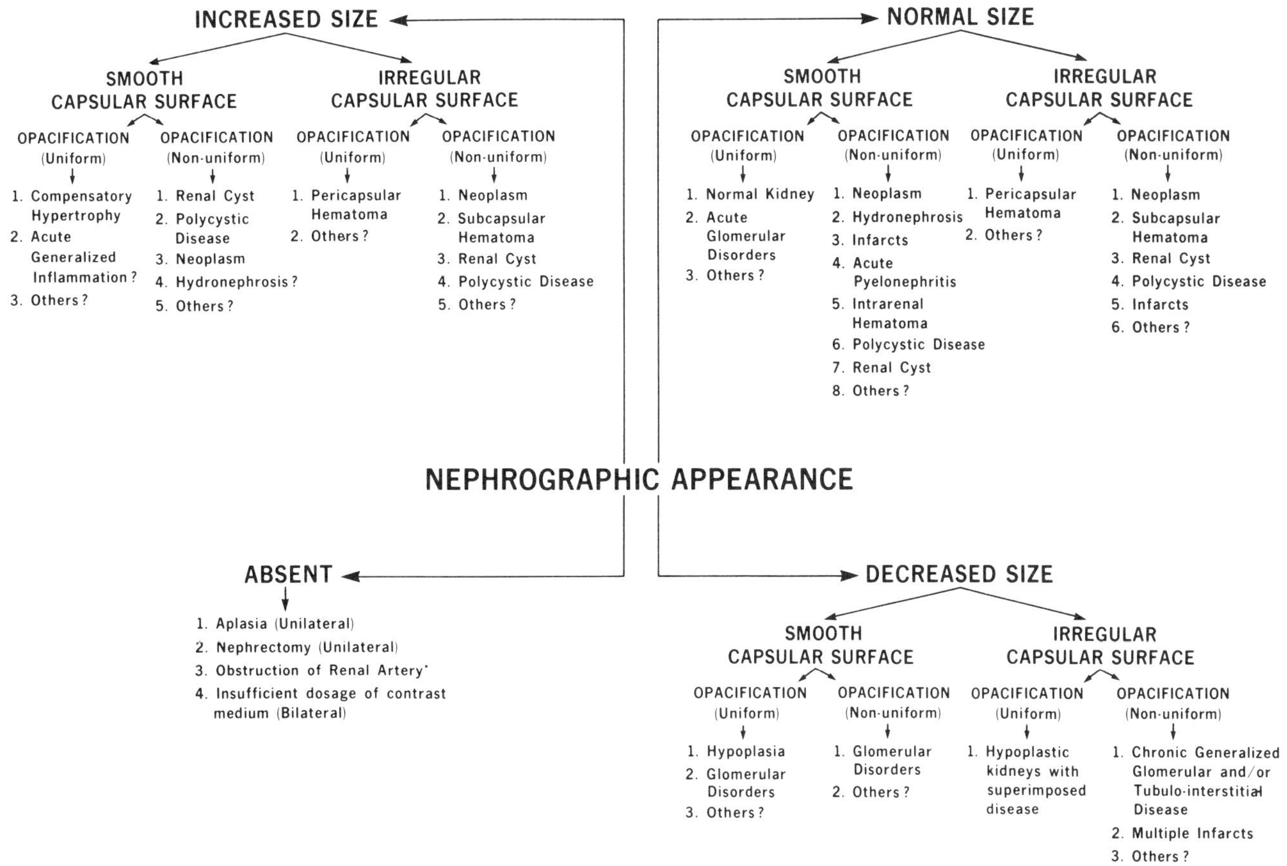

Figure 2—Algorithm for interpretation of nephrographic appearance following intravenous injection of radiographic contrast medium. *Bilateral obstruction of renal arteries would result in death within a few days. (From Feeney DA, Barber DL, Osborne CA: Advances in canine excretory urography, in *30th Gaines Veterinary Symposium (1981)*. White Plains, NY, Gaines Dog Research Center, 1981, pp 8-22. Reprinted with permission.)

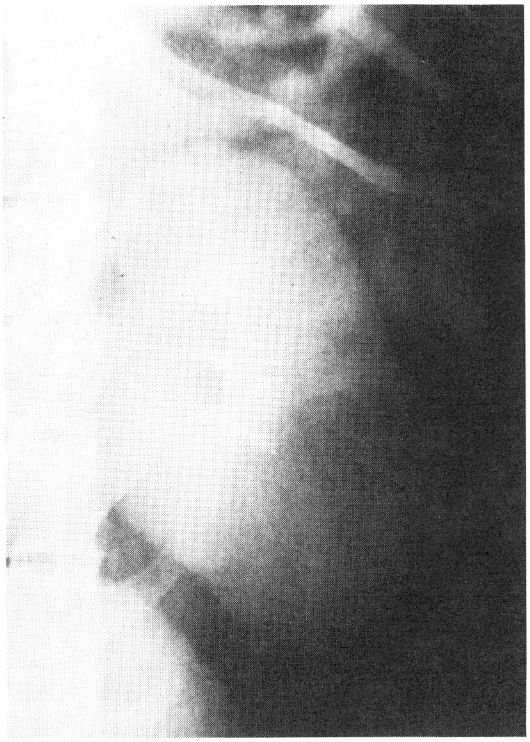

Figure 3—Excretory urogram of a dog with a solitary renal cyst of caudal pole of the kidney. Ventrodorsal view. Note spherical, smoothly marginated area of decreased opacity. (Courtesy of J. Lebel, Colorado State University)

regions. Smooth margins at the interface between lesions and normal kidney are usually associated with renal cysts (Figure 3), whereas an irregular interface is usually associated with neoplasms (Figure 4), infarcts, or hematomas.[3] Moderate hydronephrosis due to ureteral obstruction is an example of a localized parenchymal alteration caused by an abnormality in the collection system (Figure 5).

Generalized alterations in nephrographic appearance are usually associated with advanced hydronephrosis, diffuse infiltrative processes, e.g., lymphosarcoma and feline infectious peritonitis (Figure 6), polycystic disease (Figure 7), congenital renal diseases such as renal dysplasia associated with Lhaso apsos (Figure 8) and Norwegian elkhounds, and chronic generalized renal disorders (Figure 9). Ranking these possible diagnoses in order of probability may be facilitated by knowledge of renal size, capsular surface characteristics (Figure 2), and the history and breed.

The Pyelogram

Opacification of the renal pelves, pelvic diverticula, and ureters is termed the *pyelogram*. Opacification of these structures is due to excretion of contrast medium after it has been filtered and concentrated by nephrons. Detection of concentrated contrast medium in normal renal pelves and ureters three to five minutes after contrast medium administration indicates that renal function is present and that no complete obstruction of the outflow tract exists. Opacity of pyelographic components is related to the dose of contrast medium, state of hydration, degree of renal function, and volume of urine containing contrast medium in the excretory pathway.[9,10,12,23] There is little change in the normal pyelographic appearance following initial opacification except for minor variation in the size of the structures.[12]

Pyelographic alterations caused by common renal diseases are described in Table II. Pyelographic abnormalities in unanesthetized dogs are best assessed on radiographs made 5, 20, and 40 minutes post-contrast

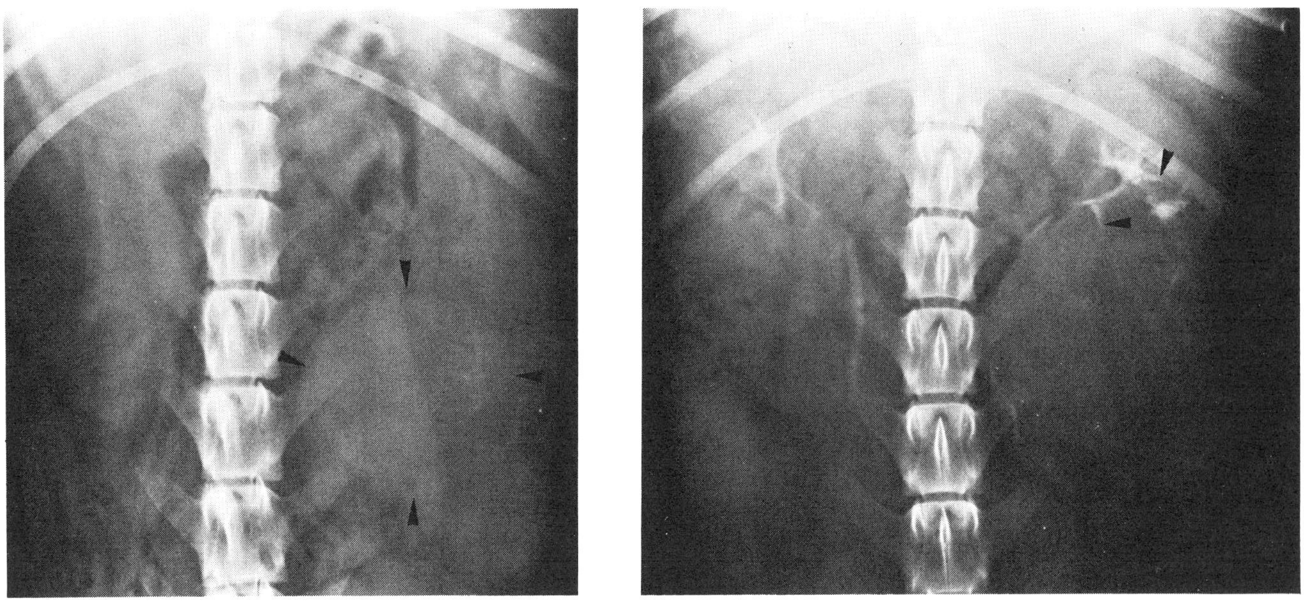

Figure 4—Excretory urogram of a dog with a solitary renal adenocarcinoma of the left kidney. **(A)** Note enlargement of the caudal pole (*arrows*) of the left kidney on survey ventrodorsal radiograph. **(B)** The left renal pelvis is distorted (*arrows*), and the size and shape of the caudal pole of the left kidney are abnormal on this 5-minute postinjection radiograph. Left ureter has been displaced medially by the neoplasm.

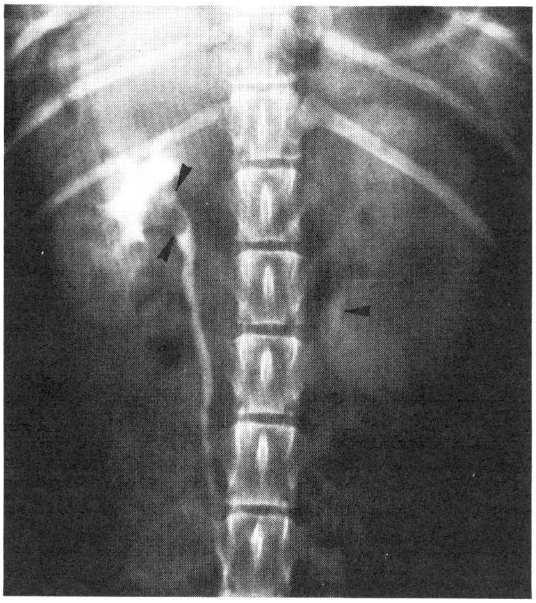

Figure 5—Excretory urogram of a dog with a right renal pelvic calculus and a left ureteral calculus radiographed 20 minute after intravenous injection of contrast medium. Ventrodorsal view. The calculus produces a triangular filling defect (*arrows*) in the dilated pelvis and proximal ureter of the right kidney. The left kidney is enlarged and/or has a perihilar void in nephrographic opacity due to a dilated, nonopacified renal pelvis. A ureteral calculus (*arrow*) located at the medial aspect of the caudal pole of the left kidney caused ureteral obstruction. (From Feeney DA, Barber DL, Osborne CA: Advances in canine excretory urography, in *30th Gaines Veterinary Symposium (1981)*. White Plains, NY, Gaines Dog Research Center, 1981, pp 8-22. Reprinted with permission.)

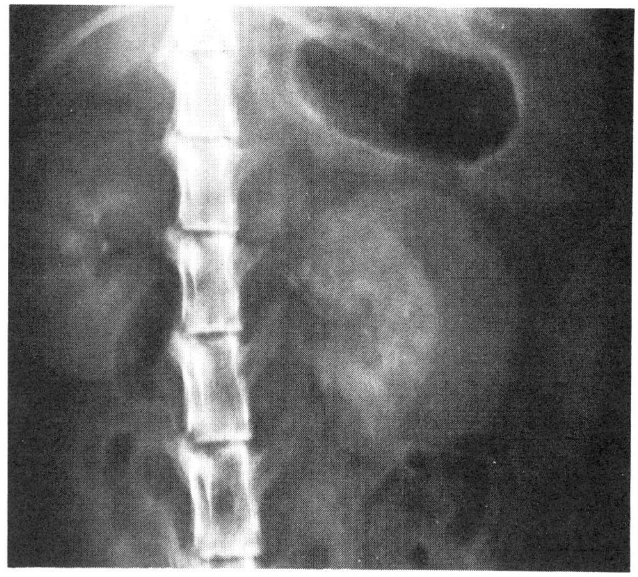

Figure 6—Excretory urogram of a two-year-old cat with mild bilateral renal enlargement due to feline infectious peritonitis. Ventrodorsal view five minutes after contrast medium administration. Uniform nephrographic opacity with poor pyelographic opacity is present. The loss of serosal-surface clarity is due to the presence of peritoneal fluid.

medium injection. Localized distortions of pyelographic structure are usually associated with renal cysts, neoplasms (Figure 4), hematomas, and infarcts.[3] Generalized distortions of pyelographic structure are usually caused by inflammatory disease such as pyelonephritis (Figure 10) and outflow obstruction due to hydronephrosis, or pelvic and/or ureteral uroliths. Uroliths are often associated with obstruction and inflammation (Figure 5).[3] Congenital anomalies such as aperistaltic megaloureter

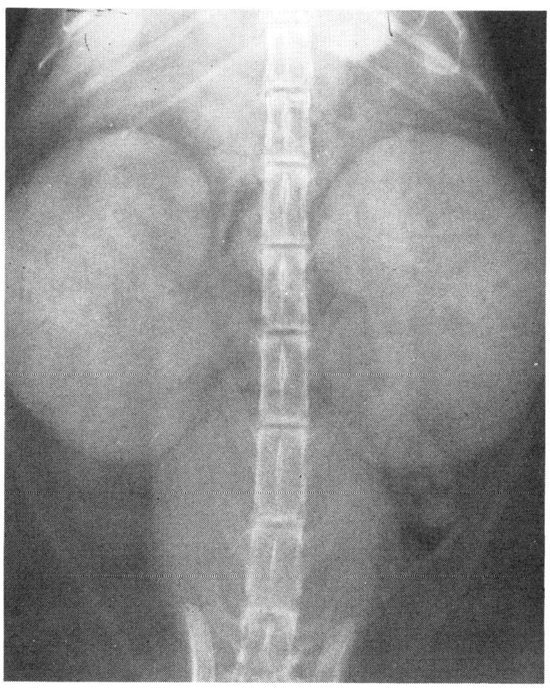

Figure 7A

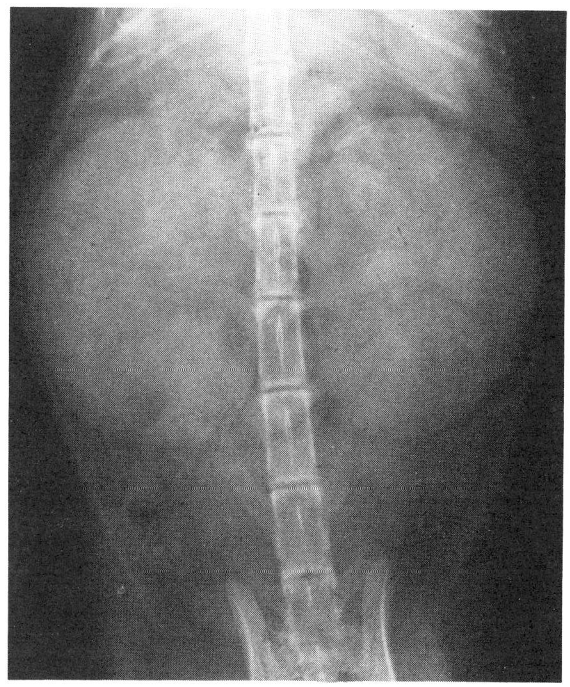

Figure 7B

Figure 7—Excretory urogram of an 11-month-old cat with polycystic kidneys. Ventrodorsal views. **(A)** Note the irregular (patchy) opacification of the enlarged kidneys with no definite renal pelvic opacification, five minutes after contrast medium administration. **(B)** Note the decreased nephrographic opacity and filling of the urinary bladder with poorly concentrated contrast medium 40 minutes after contrast medium administration. Pyelographic opacity is poor as a result of poor renal function, not obstruction.

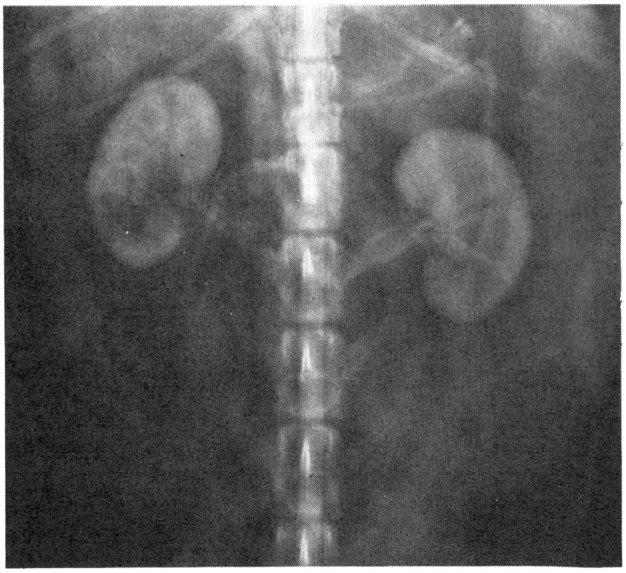

Figure 8—Excretory urogram of a one-year-old male Lhasa apso with chronic progressive generalized renal disease of probable familial origin. Ventrodorsal views. **(A)** Note small kidneys with thin cortices, capsular irregularity, and poor opacification of the right caudal pole on 10-second post-contrast medium injection film.

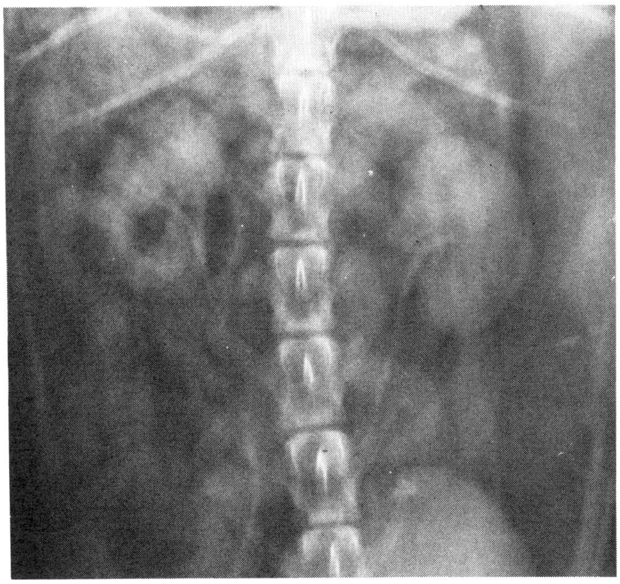

Figure 8—**(B)** Note small kidney with fading nephrogram and poor pyelographic opacification at five minutes after contrast medium administration.

and ectopic ureter may also cause pyelographic changes which resemble or are associated with pyelonephritis (Figure 11). Space-occupying infiltrative diseases such as lymphosarcoma and feline infectious peritonitis may compress the renal pelves and pelvic diverticula (Figure 6),[5] causing distortion and poor opacification. However, alteration of the renal pelves and/or pelvic diverticula with concomitant enlargement of the kidneys is indicative of primary diffuse renal involvement.

Failure of pyelographic opacification following a normal or abnormal nephrogram may be associated with decreased glomerular filtration rate, renal tubular dysfunction, intra- or extrarenal obstruction, premature radiography after contrast medium administration, anuria, oliguria, hypotension, and/or hypovolemia. These factors may cause a delay of minutes to hours from the time of nephrographic opacification to the time of pyelographic opacification. Any delay in pyelographic opacification beyond three to five minutes after contrast medium injection is reason to suspect an abnormality. Such delay should be interpreted in light

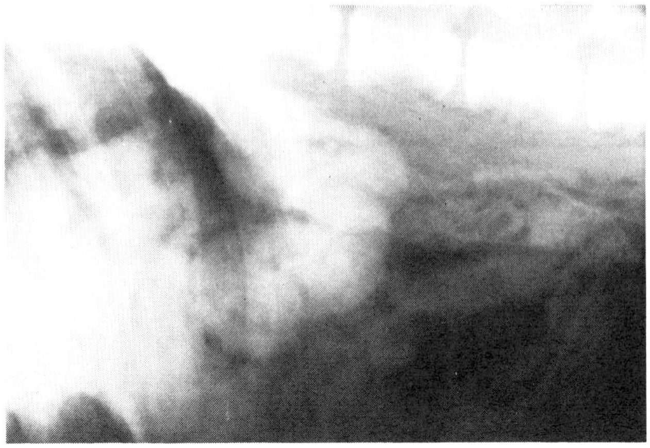

Figure 9—Close-up lateral view of an excretory urogram of end-stage canine kidneys obtained five minutes following contrast medium administration. Note poor opacification, decreased size, and irregular shape of kidneys.

TABLE II

Pyelographic Characteristics of Common Renal Diseases*

- I. Pyelonephritis
  - A. Acute
    - Pelvic dilatation
    - Proximal ureteral dilatation
    - Absent or incomplete filling of diverticula
  - B. Chronic
    - ± pelvic dilatation with irregular borders
    - Proximal ureteral dilatation
    - Short blunt diverticula
- II. Hydronephrosis
  - Pelvic dilatation
  - Dilatation of pelvic diverticula (Note: Diverticula may not be distinguishable if pelvic dilatation is severe)
  - Ureteral dilatation
- III. Neoplasia
  - A. Of renal parenchyma
    - Distortion or deviation of renal pelvis, sometimes with dilatation
    - Distortion or deviation of pelvic diverticula
  - B. Of renal pelvis
    - Distortion or dilatation of renal pelvis
    - Filling defects in renal pelvis
- IV. Uroliths
  - Filling defects in renal pelvis
  - Uroliths usually radiolucent compared to contrast medium
  - May be changes associated with pyelonephritis
  - ±pelvic dilatation

*From Feeney DA, Barber DL, Osborne CA: Advances in canine excretory urography, in *30th Gaines Veterinary Symposium (1981)*. White Plains, NY, Gaines Dog Research Center, 1981, pp 8-22. Reprinted with permission.

of laboratory evaluation of renal function and the status of the patient (e.g., collapsed, depressed, alert).

Evaluation of Excretory Urograms

For optimum consistent results the authors recommend the following sequence of evaluation of excretory urograms. Portions of this sequence may be deleted or modified, depending on the portion of the urinary tract to be specifically examined.

1. Determine that the patient is properly hydrated.
2. Following proper patient preparation confirmed by diagnostic quality survey radiographs, intravenously inject contrast medium at a dosage of 800 mg of iodine per kilogram of body weight.[22]
3. a. Make a ventrodorsal radiograph at 5 to 20 seconds, 5 minutes, 20 minutes, and 40 minutes following bolus intravenous injection of contrast medium.
   b. Make a lateral radiograph 5 minutes following injection.
   c. Make oblique ventrodorsal radiographs 3 to 5 minutes following injection to delineate ureteral termination (bladder, urethra, vagina, or other possible terminating sites).
4. Observe the chronologic sequence and distribution of nephrographic opacity.
   a. Maximum uniform renal opacification should occur immediately after injection, followed by progressive loss of opacity. If this trend is not observed, see Table I.
   b. The renal parenchymal opacity should be uniform with a smooth capsular surface and normal size.[22] If this is not observed see Table II.
5. Observe the chronologic sequence of opacification and size of the pyelographic structures (renal pelves, pelvic diverticula, ureters).[22]

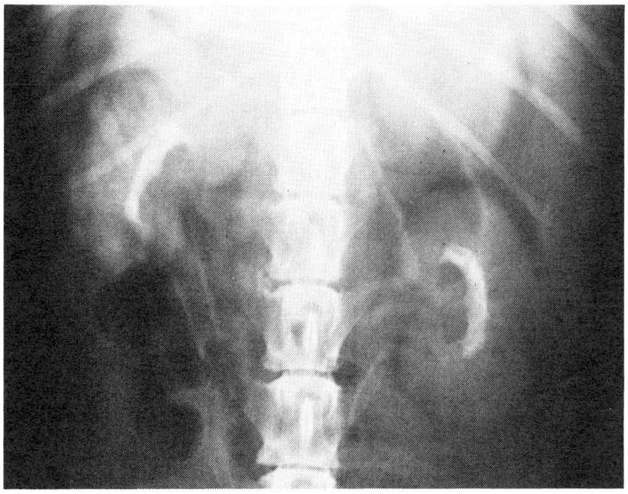

Figure 10—Close-up ventrodorsal view of an excretory urogram of canine kidneys with chronic pyelonephritis obtained 40 minutes after contrast medium administration. Note increased size of renal pelves with short blunted pelvic diverticula. Scalloped renal margins are due to renal scarring.

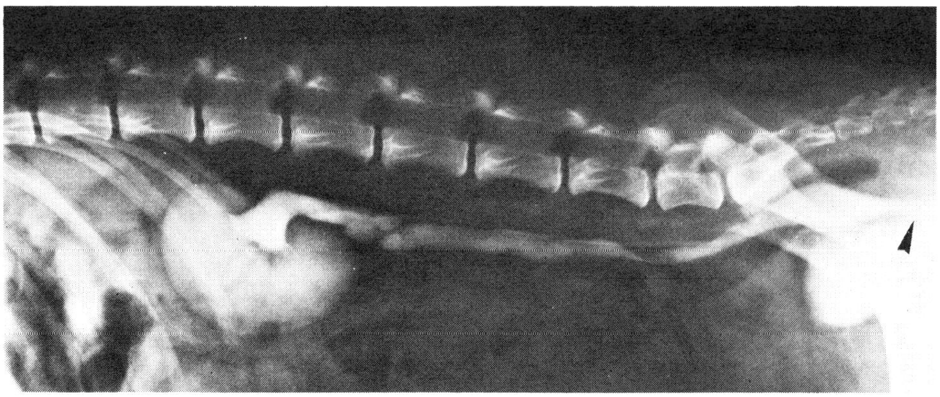

Figure 11A

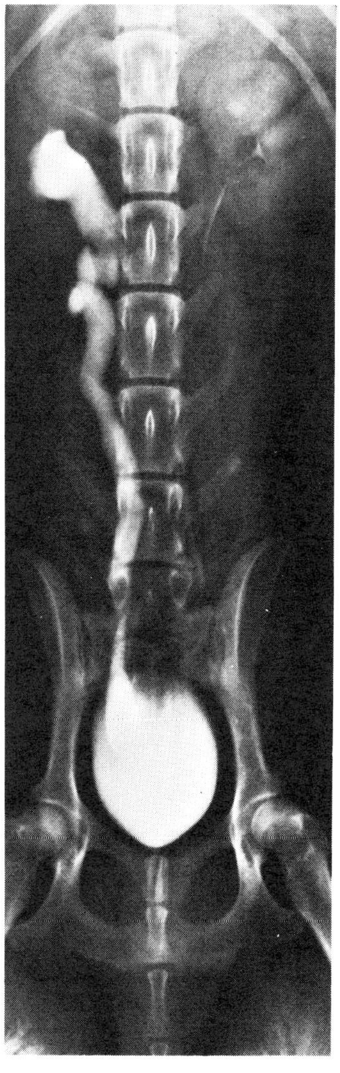

Figure 11B

Figure 11—Excretory urogram of a 1½-year-old Siberian husky with a right ectopic ureter. **(A)** Lateral view obtained five minutes after contrast medium administration. Note dilated renal pelvis and ureter without dilated pelvic diverticula (often associated with pyelonephritis) on the right side. The dilated ureter continues caudally past the trigone (*arrow*). **(B)** Ventrodorsal view obtained 40 minutes after contrast injection. The termination of the abnormal right ureter is not visualized, but contrast medium deposition on the hair of the hindlegs is highly suggestive of incontinence.

a. The pyelogram should be observed 1 to 3 minutes following peak nephrographic opacity and should slowly fade during the following several hours. If not, reexamine the nephrogram (Table I).

b. Measure the width of the renal pelves, pelvic diverticula, and ureters as previously described.[12,22] If abnormal, see Table II.

6. If diseases of the urinary bladder are suspected but retrograde studies are impossible or contraindicated, examine the urinary bladder 30 to 40 minutes postinjection. Lateral, ventrodorsal and, if necessary, oblique views should be obtained at this time to facilitate evaluation of the urinary bladder.

REFERENCES

1. Ackerman N: Intravenous pyelography. *JAAHA* 10:277-284, 1974.
2. Bartels JE: Feline intravenous urography. *JAAHA* 9:349-353, 1973.
3. Feeney DA, Barber DL, Osborne CA: Advances in canine excretory urography, in *Proceedings 30th Gaines Veterinary Symposium.* White Plains, NY, Gaines Dog Research Center, 1981, pp 8-22.
4. Johnston GR, Feeney DA, Osborne CA: Radiographic findings in urinary tract infection. *Vet Clin North Am* 9:749-774, 1979.
5. Kneller SK: Role of the excretory urogram in the diagnosis of renal and ureteral disease. *Vet Clin North Am* 4:843-861, 1974.
6. Root CR: Contrast radiography of the urinary system, in Ticer JW (ed): *Radiographic Technique in Small Animal Practice.* Philadelphia, WB Saunders Co, 1975, pp 396-414.
7. Watters JW: Urinary tract radiography—Kidneys and ureters. *Compend Contin Educ Pract Vet* 2(3):224-231, 1980.
8. Barber DL, Finco DR: Radiographic findings in induced bacterial pyelonephritis in dogs. *JAVMA* 175:1183-1190, 1979.
9. Saxton HM: Review article: Urography. *Br J Radiol* 42:321-346, 1969.
10. Thrall DE, Finco DR: Canine excretory urography: Is quality a function of BUN? *JAAHA* 12:446-450, 1976.
11. Lord PF, Scott RC, Chan KF: Intravenous urography for the evaluation of renal diseases in small animals. *JAAHA* 10:139-152, 1974.
12. Feeney DA, Thrall DE, Barber DL, et al: Normal canine excretory urogram: Effects of dose, time and individual dog variation. *Am J Vet Res* 40:1596-1604, 1979.
13. Fry IK, Cattell WR: The nephrographic pattern during excretory urography. *Br Med Bull* 28:227-232, 1972.
14. Older RA, Kobobkin M, Cleeve DM, et al: Contrast-induced acute renal failure. *Am J Roentgenol* 134:339-342, 1980.
15. Newhouse JH, Pfister RC: The nephrogram. *Radiol Clin North Am* 17:213-226, 1979.
16. Feeney DA, Barber DL, Osborne CA: The functional aspects of the nephrogram in excretory urography: A review. *Vet Radiol,* in press.
17. Ansari Z, Baldwin DS: Acute renal failure due to radiocontrast agents. *Nephron* 17:28-40, 1976.
18. Byrd L, Sherman RL: Radiocontrast-induced acute renal failure. *Medicine* 58:270-278, 1979.
19. Van Zee BE, Hoy WE, Talley TE, Jaenike JR: Renal injury associated with intravenous pyelography in non-diabetic and diabetic patients. *Ann Intern Med* 89:51-54, 1978.
20. Biery DN: The upper urinary tract, in O'Brien TR (ed): *Radiographic Diagnosis of Abdominal Disorders in the Dog and Cat.* Philadelphia, WB Saunders Co, 1978, pp 481-542.
21. Feeney DA, Osborne CA, Jessen CR: Effect of multiple excretory urograms on glomerular filtration of normal dogs. A preliminary report. *Am J Vet Res* 41:960-963, 1980.
22. Feeney DA, Barber DL, Johnston GR, Osborne CA: The excretory urogram: Part I. Techniques, normal radiographic appearance, and misinterpretation. *Compend Contin Educ Pract Vet* 4(3):233-243, 1982.
23. Feeney DA, Barber DL, Culver DH, et al: Canine excretory urogram: Correlation with base-line measurements. *Am J Vet Res* 41:279-283, 1980.

Retrograde Vaginocystography: A Contrast Study for Evaluation of Bitches with Urinary Incontinence

KEY FACTS

- **Retrograde vaginocystography is a relatively simple technique that requires minimal equipment.**
- **The technique is a valuable diagnostic aid, especially in cases of urinary incontinence, vaginal discharge, dysuria, or vaginal abnormalities that prevent digital or instrumental examination.**
- **Room air can be used for the double-contrast cystography but carries the risk of gas embolization; introduction of air should be avoided during vaginocystography because air bubbles inadvertently allowed to enter the vagina may be mistaken for a space-occupying lesion.**
- **Contraction of the constrictor vestibuli muscle under light anesthesia resembles a stricture and should not be interpreted as a pathologic lesion.**

University of Guelph
Renee Leveille, DVM   Matthew A. O. Atilola, DVM, MS, PhD

URINARY problems in bitches are commonly encountered in small animal practice. Clinical examination of the vagina and urethra of bitches, however, is often unsatisfactory.[1] Digital vaginal examination may be restricted by differences in the length or diameter of the vagina and the examiner's digit. Although endoscopy is a valuable diagnostic aid in examining the caudal reproductive tract,[2] lesions of the vaginal and urethral lumina can prevent catheterization or adequate insertion of the endoscope.

Radiographic procedures are often used for localization or verification of diseases originating in or affecting the urogenital tract, investigation of underlying cause of a recurrent urinary tract problem, qualitative assessment of organ function to determine prognosis, and assessment of therapeutic response.[3] A single abnormal presentation on survey radiographs usually is not pathognomonic of a specific disorder but can suggest several different diseases. Radiographic signs on survey film often indicate a need for contrast studies to substantiate findings and to define the disease process more clearly.[4,5]

Retrograde vaginocystography has often been described in the British literature[6-9] but infrequently in North America.[4,7] This article describes the use of retrograde vaginocystography as a contrast study to define abnormalities of the lower urinary tract in bitches.

STUDY POPULATION

Between January 1983 and January 1989, 12,654 dogs were presented to the Small Animal Hospital of the Ontario Veterinary College in Guelph, Ontario, Canada. Of the dogs, 169 (1.3%) bitches were examined for urinary incontinence. The seven bitches in this report were selected on the basis of the diagnostic imaging procedures performed. Four dogs were examined by intravenous urography and retrograde vaginocystography (cases 3 through 6) and three dogs by retrograde vaginocystography only (cases 1, 2, and 7).

From the recorded histories, the age, breed, duration of clinical signs, and the nature of urinary incontinence were determined. Table I summarizes the clinical course of seven cases in which retrograde vaginocystography was performed.

Originally published in Volume 13, Number 6, June 1991

TABLE I
Patients in Which Retrograde Vaginocystography was Performed

Case	*Age (years)*	*Sex*	*Breed*	*Clinical Signs*	*Duration*	*Radiologic Diagnosis*
1	1	Intact female	German shepherd	Urinary incontinence, vaginal discharge, pollakiuria	10 months	*Retrograde vaginocystography*: vaginal structure and possible short urethra, cystitis
2	1	Intact female	Tibetan terrier	Urinary incontinence, recurring urinary infection, pollakiuria, hematuria, dysuria	3 months	*Retrograde vaginocystography*: vaginitis
3	3	Intact female	Golden retriever	Urinary incontinence, perivulvar dermatitis	2 years	*Intravenous urography and retrograde vaginocystography*: left ectopic ureter
4	0.5	Intact female	Labrador retriever	Urinary incontinence	3 months	*Intravenous urography*: dilated left renal pelvis and ureter; *retrograde vaginocystography*: left ureter enters the vagina
5	5	Spayed female	English springer spaniel	Urinary incontinence	5 years (intermittent)	*Intravenous urography and retrograde vaginocystography*: no abnormal findings
6	7.5	Intact female	Husky	Urinary incontinence	5 months	*Intravenous urography*: dilation of right ureter; *retrograde vaginocystography*: right ectopic ureter
7	14	Spayed female	Irish terrier	Urinary incontinence, hematuria, pyuria, behavior change	1 week	*Retrograde vaginocystography*: no ectopic ureter seen

TECHNIQUE

As for any routine contrast radiographic examination of the abdomen, the bitches were prepared by cleansing the colon and rectum with an enema 24 hours and 3 hours before the procedure. The procedure was performed with standard general anesthetic protocol. Preliminary lateral and ventrodorsal abdominal radiographs preceded contrast cystography and provided evidence of gastrointestinal cleaning as well as satisfactory exposure technique. All catheters and equipment were sterilized and the genitalia cleaned before the lower urinary tract was catheterized.

The procedure was completed in two steps: first was double-contrast cystography; second was vaginourethrography. The bitch was positioned in dorsal recumbency (frog-leg position) for the double-contrast cystogram. A small Foley catheter (10 to 12 gauge) with an inflatable cuff was inserted within the bladder neck. The bladder was emptied, and about 10 ml of a 50% solution of an iodinated contrast medium was introduced. The dog was placed in lateral recumbency and then dorsal recumbency in order to spread the contrast material evenly over the mucosa. Nitrous oxide or carbon dioxide was then introduced. Lateral and ventrodorsal radiographic projections were obtained.

The Foley catheter was removed and the distal tip cut to preserve the cuff. The catheter was then filled with contrast medium before insertion into the vagina in order to avoid introducing air bubbles. The catheter was positioned in the vestibule and the cuff reinflated to prevent leakage of the contrast medium from the vulva. Sometimes it was necessary to close the vulvar lips with tissue forceps to prevent the catheter from slipping out. The dose of 1 ml/kg was injected slowly. Excessive pressure was avoided to prevent vaginal rupture.[9]

THE LATERAL radiographic view, which was exposed at the end of the injection, was the most informative. Ventrodorsal and oblique projections made variable contribution to the studies.

RESULTS

Retrograde bladder filling from ectopic ureters can occur.[7,8,10,11] In our series, the duration of the clinical signs ranged from one week to two years and had been reported as an intermittent problem by some owners.

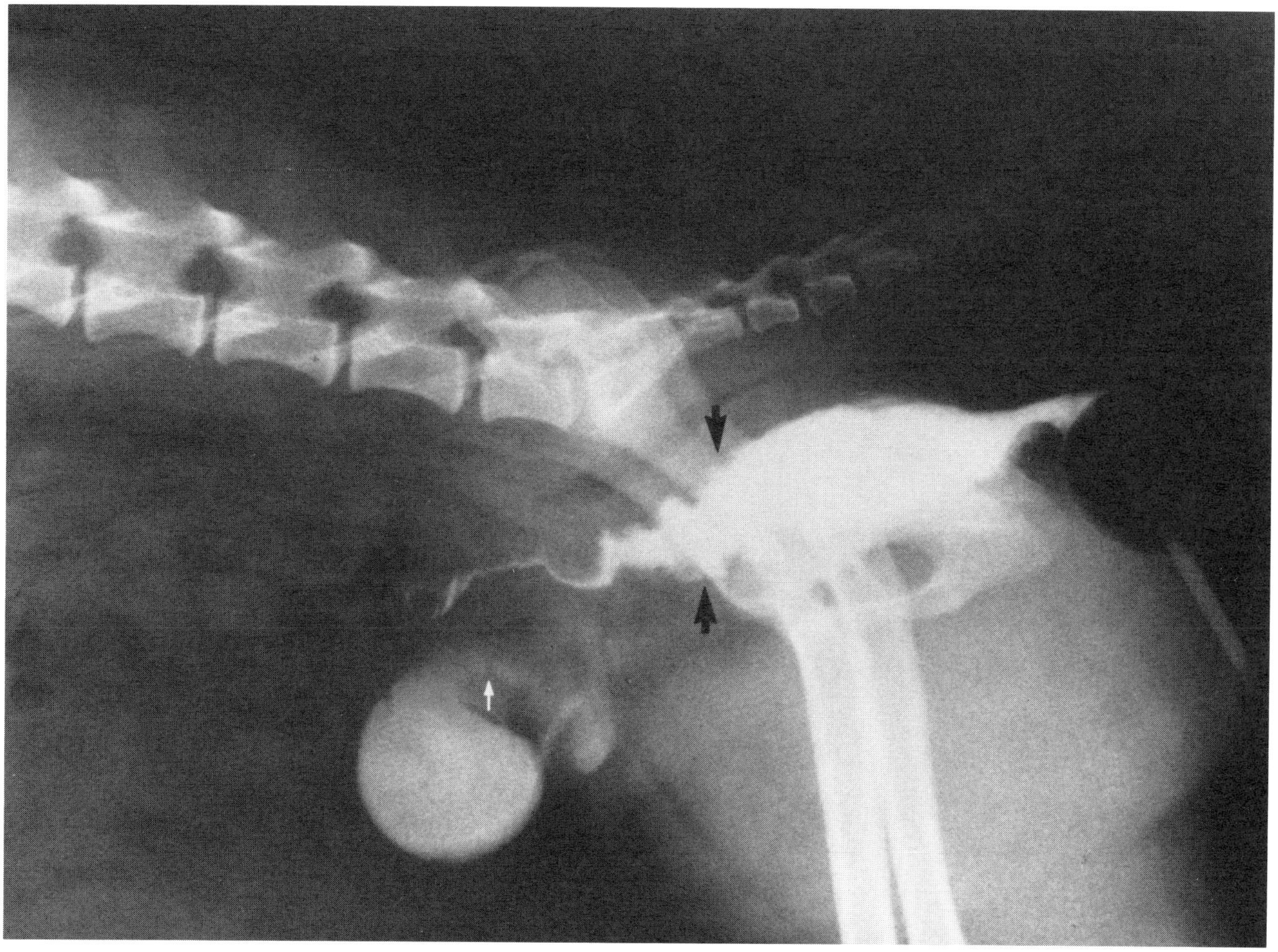

Figure 1—Abnormal retrograde vaginocystography of a one-year-old, intact female Tibetan terrier with vaginitis (case 2). Note the irregular appearance of the vaginal mucosa (*black arrows*). An artifactual luminal defect in the bladder resulting from lack of distention is shown (*small arrow*). A cystography performed afterward eliminated the possibility of mass lesion.

The exact location of the ectopic ureteral orifices was not clearly shown by intravenous urography in cases 3, 4, and 6. Intravenous urography did, however, reveal hydroureter and dilation of the ipsilateral renal pelvis in cases 4 and 6 (Figure 1).

Unlike intravenous urography, retrograde vaginocystography was successful in determining the opening of the ectopic ureter in cases 3, 4, and 6. Each ectopic ureter was confirmed at surgery. In case 7, at necropsy, there was no evidence of ectopic ureter; and the hematuria and pyuria were suspected to originate from an ascending infection.

DISCUSSION

Ectopic ureter is the most frequently diagnosed cause of congenital urinary incontinence.[8] The incidence of unilateral or bilateral ectopia of the ureters in dogs is unknown, and the condition apparently is most common in bitches.[10,12-15] Failure to recognize the condition in male dogs is likely because of lack of incontinence.[10] Confirmation of a tentative diagnosis of ectopic ureter is best made by using positive-contrast radiography of the urinary tract.[12]

Evaluation of the urinary tract by intravenous urography is indicated to confirm the presence of ectopic ureter and to determine whether other abnormalities of the kidneys and ureters are present. Although intravenous urography is an important diagnostic aid, visualization of the urethra and the exact site of termination of the ureters may be difficult.[5]

WHEN an abnormal orifice is detected in the vagina or suspected to be in the urethra, catheterization of the orifice followed by retrograde urethrography can be attempted; but its value is reduced because the catheter in the urethral lumen may obscure or distort a lesion. Voiding urethrography, a commonly used procedure in human patients, has been used in dogs for urethral examinations; but

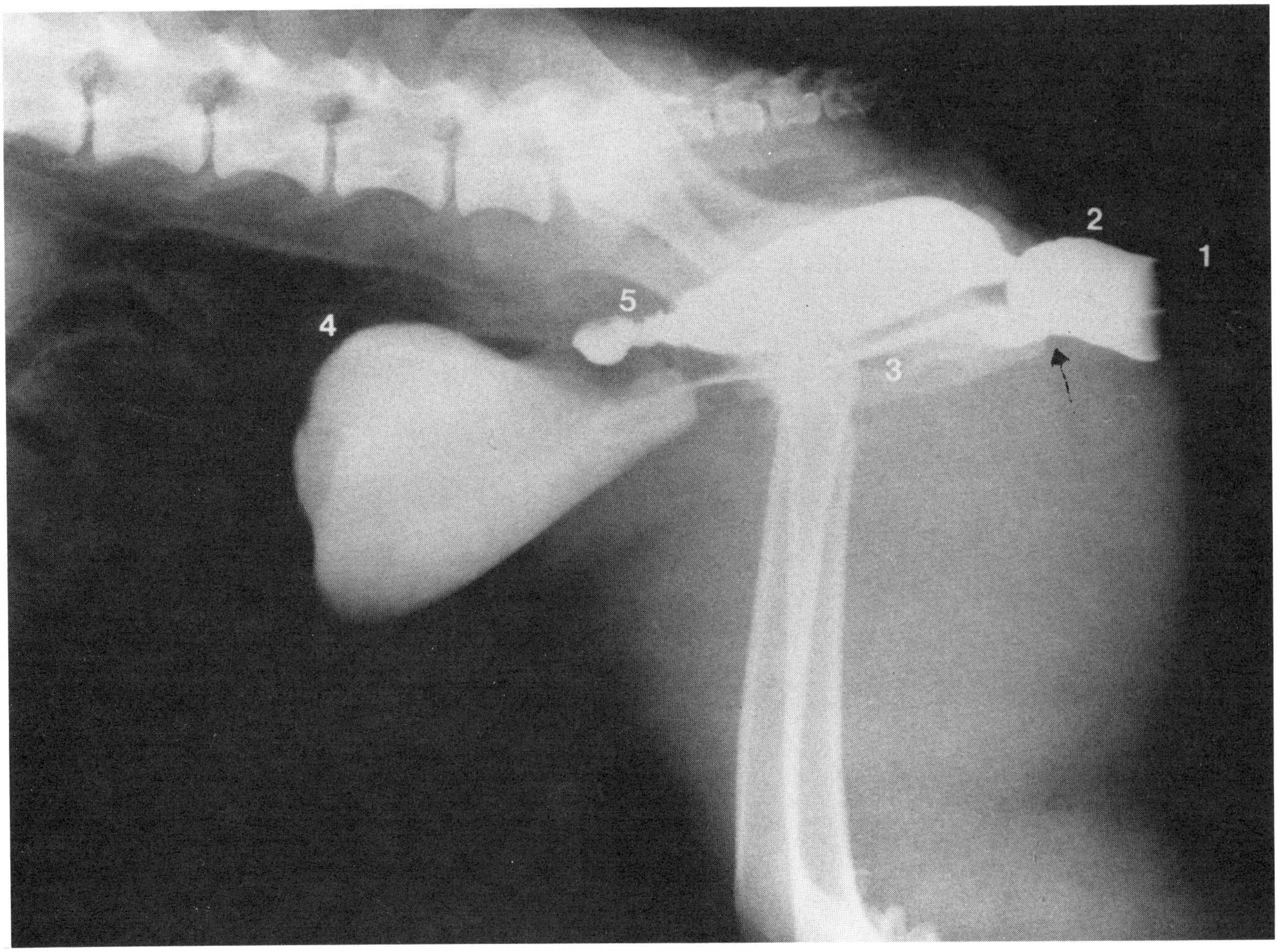

Figure 2—Normal retrograde vaginocystography of a five-year-old, spayed female English springer spaniel (case 5). The *arrow* points to the normal stricture attributable to the contraction of the constrictor vestibuli muscle. *1* = inflated cuff of the Foley catheter, *2* = vagina, *3* = urethra, *4* = bladder (not fully distended), and *5* = cervix.

the difficulty in performing the examination usually results from an inconsistent ability to stimulate urination.[16]

Retrograde vaginocystography has been very helpful in evaluating the terminal orifice of ectopic ureters, the entire length of the urethra, and the vaginal contour (Figure 2). Retrograde vaginocystography is a relatively simple technique that requires minimal equipment. The catheterization of small females may present some difficulties, as in case 7, in which only a vaginogram could be performed.

Room air can be used for the double-contrast cystography; however, it carries the risk of gas embolization.[4] Introduction of air and inadequate anesthesia should be avoided during vaginocystography because air bubbles inadvertently introduced into the vagina may be mistaken for a space-occupying lesion. Contraction of the constrictor vestibuli muscle under light anesthesia does resemble a stricture and should not be interpreted as a pathologic lesion (Figure 2). In estrous bitches, the required dose to fill the vagina is likely to be considerably higher than expected. The effects of endogenous hormones may also explain the larger volume needed in intact bitches.[9]

THE RISK of pyelitis or other urogenital infection is considered minimal with this technique. No side effects were observed in any of the patients. Even when retrograde vaginocystography is diagnostic, intravenous urography is indicated for evaluation of possible additional abnormalities, such as hydroureter and renal hypoplasia.[4]

Although there are many indications for retrograde vaginocystography, investigation of ectopic ureter is the most common[7,8] (Figures 3 and 4). It is also useful in cases of sphincter incompetence and other urethral anomalies because it allows the length and width of the urethra to be assessed, as seen in cases 1 and 5.[17,18] The procedure can be used in patients with other pathologic conditions or malformations, such as ureterovaginal fistula or bilateral dila-

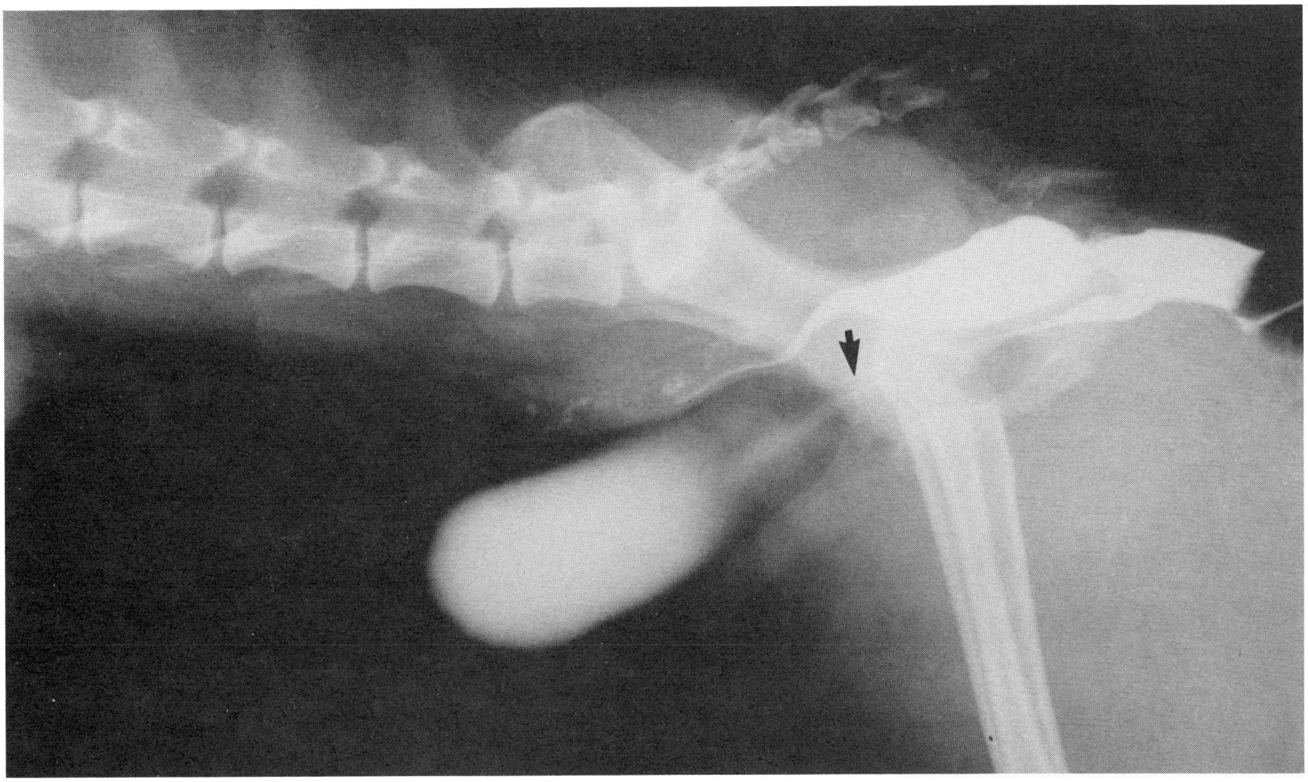

Figure 3—Abnormal retrograde vaginocystography of a two-year-old, intact female golden retriever (case 3). The *arrow* indicates the ectopic ureter.

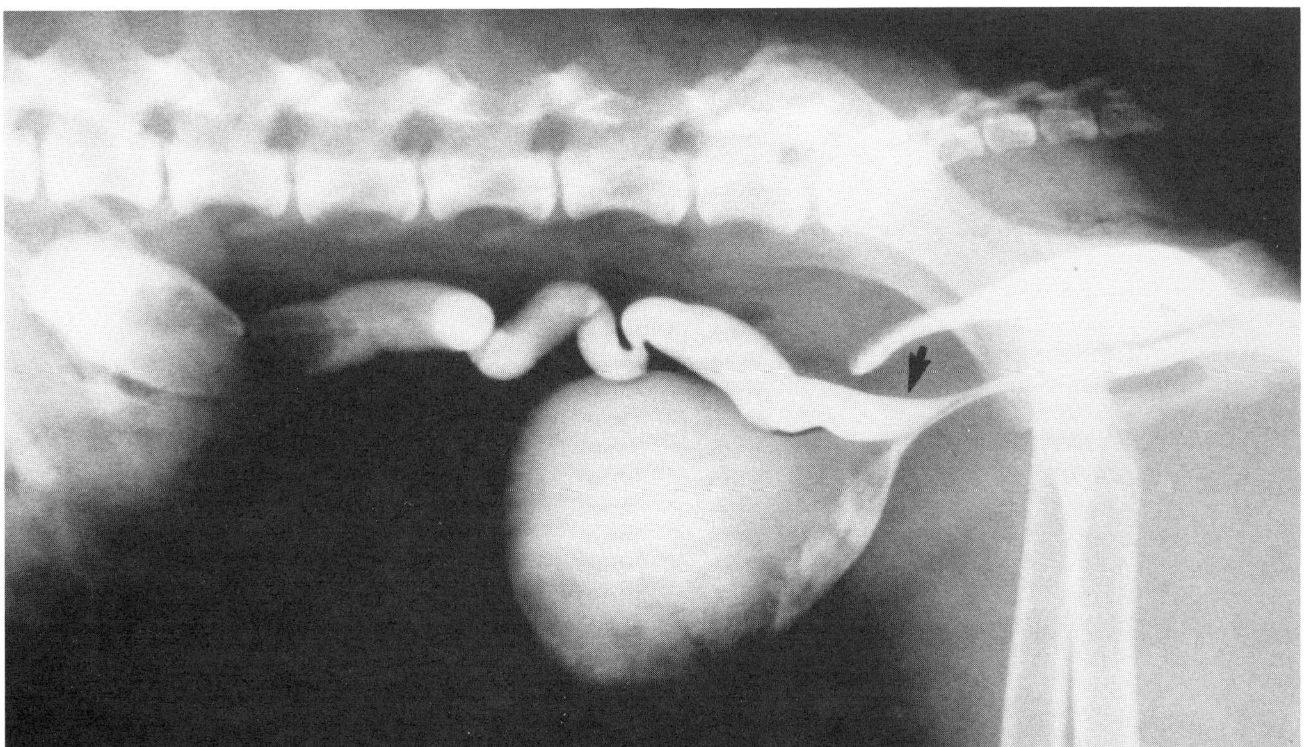

Figure 4—Abnormal retrograde vaginocystography of a six-month-old, intact female Labrador retriever (case 4). The *arrow* indicates the hydroureter and ectopic ureter.

tation of the vagina (intersexuality), and in bitches with vaginal discharge and in which a residual portion of uterus and patency of the cervix can be demonstrated. In addition, retrograde vaginocystography may demonstrate urethral filling defects, rectovaginal fistulae, and vaginal tumors[9] as well as other causes of incontinence (cases 1, 2, 5, and 7).

CONCLUSION

We have found that satisfactory results can be obtained with retrograde vaginocystography; this finding supports a previous report.[7] When adequately performed, vaginocystography can provide essential information about bitches with urinary incontinence. Its accuracy and simplicity make it useful in investigating cases of urinary incontinence, vaginal discharge, dysuria, and physical abnormalities of the canine female lower urinary tract.

About the Authors

When this article was being prepared, Dr. Leveille was affiliated with the Department of Clinical Sciences, Ontario Veterinary College, University of Guelph, Guelph, Ontario, Canada. She is currently affiliated with the Department of Veterinary Clinical Sciences, College of Veterinary Medicine, The Ohio State University, Columbus, Ohio. Dr. Atilola is affiliated with the Department of Clinical Sciences, Ontario Veterinary College, University of Guelph.

REFERENCES

1. Adams WM, Biery DN, Millar HC: Pneumovaginography in the dog: A case report. *J Am Vet Radiol Soc* 19:80, 1978.
2. Lindsay FEF: The normal endoscopic appearance of the caudal reproductive tract of the cyclic and noncyclic bitch: Postuterine endoscopy. *J Small Anim Pract* 24:1, 1983.
3. Feeney DA, Johnston GR: Urogenital imaging: A practical update. *Semin Vet Med Surg [Small Anim]* 1:144–164, 1984.
4. O'Brien TR: Upper urinary tract and radiology of the bladder and urethra, in *Radiographic Diagnosis of Abdominal Disorders in the Dog and Cat*. Philadelphia, WB Saunders Co, 1981, pp 481–694.
5. Adams WM, DiBartola SP: Radiographic and clinical features of pelvic bladder in the dog. *JAVMA* 182:1212–1217, 1983.
6. Douglas SW, Hertage ME, Williamson HD: Contrast media technique, in *Principles of Veterinary Radiography*, ed 4. London, Bailliere Tindall, 1987.
7. Holt PE, Gibbs C, Pearson H: Canine ectopic ureter—A review of twenty-nine cases. *J Small Anim Pract* 23:195–208, 1982.
8. Webbon PM: The radiological investigation of congenital urinary incontinence in the bitch. *Vet Annu* 22:199–206, 1982.
9. Holt PE, Gibbs C, Latham J: An evaluation of positive-contrast vaginourethrography as a diagnostic aid in the bitch. *J Small Anim Pract* 25:531–549, 1984.
10. Smith CW: Bilateral ectopic ureter in a male dog with urinary incontinence. *JAVMA* 177:1022–1024, 1980.
11. Osborne CA, Dieterich HF, Hanlon GF, et al: Urinary incontinence due to ectopic ureter in a male dog. *JAVMA* 166:911–914, 1975.
12. Owen R: Canine ureteral ectopia—A review. Incidence, diagnosis and treatment. *J Small Anim Pract* 14:419–427, 1973.
13. Osborne CA, Perman V: Ectopic ureter in a male dog. *JAVMA* 154:273–278, 1969.
14. Lennox JS, Eger CE, Owen RR: Clinical experiences with the combined technique of ureterovesicular anastomosis for treatment of ectopic ureters. *JAAHA* 12:406–410, 1976.
15. Haynes HM: Ectopic ureter in dogs: Epidemiologic features. *Teratology* 10:129–132, 1974.
16. Ticer JW, Crispin PS, Ackerman N: Positive-contrast retrograde urethrography: A useful procedure for evaluating urethral disorders in the dog. *Vet Radiol* 21:2–11, 1980.
17. Holt PE: Importance of urethral length, bladder neck position and vestibulovaginal stenosis in sphincter mechanism incompetence in the incontinent bitch. *Res Vet Sci* 39:364–372, 1985.
18. Mahaffey MB, Barsanti JA, Barber DI, Crowell WA: Pelvic bladder in dogs without urinary incontinence. *JAVMA* 184:1477–1479, 1984.

Radiographic Aspects of Prostatic Disease in the Dog

Donald E. Thrall, DVM, PhD
Associate Professor
Department of Anatomy and Radiology
College of Veterinary Medicine
University of Georgia
Athens, Georgia

Prostatomegaly is a common malady of aging male dogs. Abdominal radiography and positive contrast, retrograde urethrography play an important role in the assessment of prostatomegaly. Although radiography rarely indicates the exact cause of prostatomegaly, it usually allows the list of differential diagnoses to be narrowed considerably.

Normal Anatomy

The normal prostate gland is a bilobate soft tissue organ that encircles the urethra just caudal to the bladder neck. The prostate is not completely covered with visceral peritoneum (Figure 1). Thus, prostatic disease spreading to periprostatic tissue can involve the intraperitoneal space or the pelvic canal or both.

It has been reported that the relative weight of the prostate, defined as prostatic weight in grams divided by body weight in kilograms, is the same for all dogs except Scottish terriers where it is larger by a factor of four.[1] In the study cited, the author considered benign hyperplasia, present in 63% of the dogs studied, to be normal, and histologic description of the prostates from the Scottish terriers was not given.[1] Thus, the data cannot be considered evidence to support the contention that the prostate of the Scottish terrier is normally larger than that of other breeds, since Scottish terriers in the experimental group may have had prostatic hyperplasia.

Causes of Prostatomegaly

Survey radiographic examination of the caudal abdomen for prostatic disease will be helpful only if the gland is enlarged or has produced detectable alterations in the periprostatic tissues. Glandular enlargement is much more frequently detected than is alteration of the periprostatic tissues without prostatomegaly.

The four major causes of prostatomegaly are *benign hyperplasia, prostatitis,* including abscessation of the prostate, prostatic or paraprostatic *cysts,* and primary or secondary prostatic *tumors.*

Previously published data indicate that the relative size of the prostate is larger with cystic or neoplastic disease than with hyperplastic or inflammatory disease.[2] Also, prostates with cystic or neoplastic disease have a relatively higher degree of periurethral asymmetry than prostates with benign or inflammatory disease have.[2] These facts are important considerations when formulating a list of differential diagnoses for prostatomegaly.

Originally published in Volume 3, Number 8, August 1981

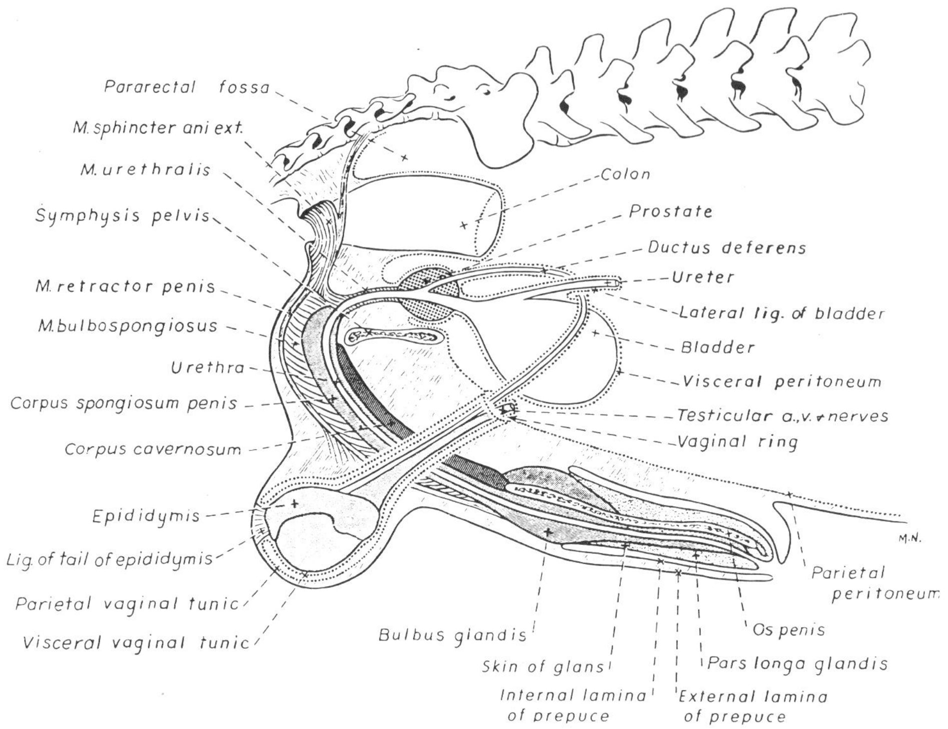

Figure 1—Schematic drawing of the male genital tract in which the relationship of the prostate gland to the peritoneum can be seen. Note that the prostate is not completely covered with peritoneum. (From Evans HE: *Miller's Anatomy of the Dog.* Philadelphia, WB Saunders Co, 1993. Reprinted with permission.)

Radiographic Assessment of Prostatic Disease

Abdominal radiography is an important aid in the diagnosis and management of prostatomegaly. In normal dogs, size and position of the prostate are such that it cannot be identified on survey radiographs of the caudal abdomen. The appearance of prostatomegaly on survey radiographs and the usefulness of special radiographic procedures in evaluating the prostate will be illustrated by the following case studies.

Case 1

A six-year-old male Scottish terrier was presented for intermittent hematuria. The only abnormal physical finding was nonpainful prostatomegaly. In a urinalysis (catheterized sample), occult blood was detected. In lateral abdominal radiographs, two soft tissue masses were present in the caudal abdomen (Figure 2). The location of these two masses was consistent with prostatomegaly that resulted in cranial displacement of the urinary bladder. These masses could not be readily identified on the ventrodorsal projection. It is uncommon to be able to identify a moderately enlarged prostate on the ventrodorsal projection, since it is obscured by the spine, prepuce, and os penis. In an attempt to identify the two soft tissue masses, a positive contrast, retrograde urethrogram was done (Figure 3). In this study, it was

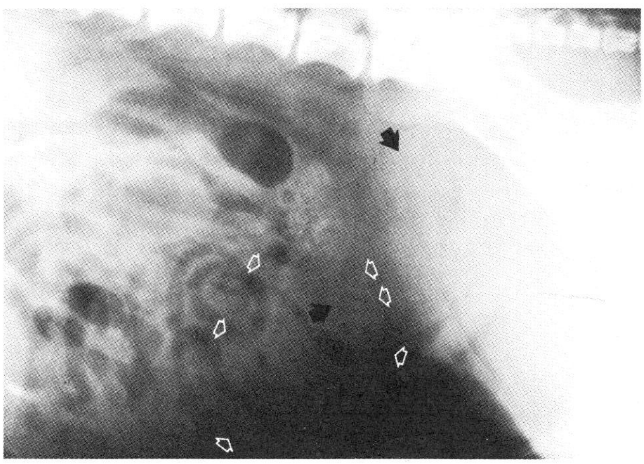

Figure 2—Lateral survey abdominal radiograph in which two soft tissue masses *(arrows)* are present in the caudal abdomen.

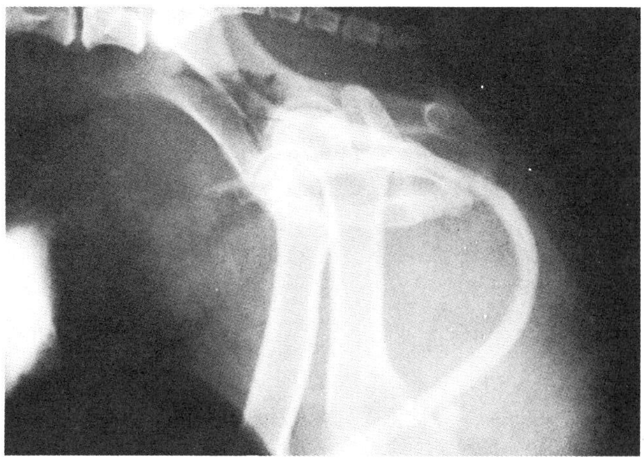

Figure 3—Positive contrast, retrograde urethrogram of the dog in Figure 2. The bladder is displaced cranially by an enlarged prostate. The prostate is symmetric in relation to the urethra. The prostatic urethra appears narrow, but this is not indicative of a stricture (see text).

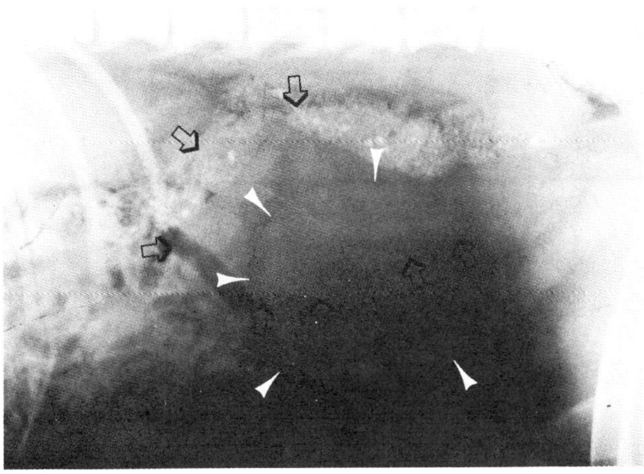

Figure 4A

Figure 4—Lateral (A) and ventrodorsal (B) survey abdominal radiographs in which two masses are present in the caudal abdomen. One mass *(open arrows)* is located dorsally, cranially, and to the right of the other *(white arrows)*.

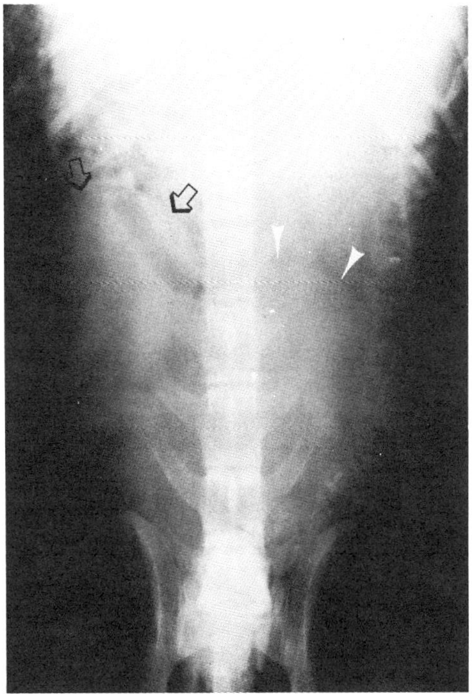

Figure 4B

possible to identify the cranial mass as urinary bladder and the caudal mass as prostate. The prostate had good periurethral symmetry. The diameter of the prostatic urethra in Figure 3 cannot be interpreted as evidence of a stricture. The surrounding enlarged gland may have made the prostatic urethra less distensible than it normally is without disturbing its function. Also, the size of the urethra observed in retrograde urethrography is a function of the rate at which the contrast medium is injected, the resistance exerted by the patient, and the degree of bladder distention.[3]

It is interesting to note that contrast medium did not reflux from the urethra into the prostate. It has been said that urethroprostatic reflux of contrast medium can be used to differentiate between various prostatic diseases.[4] There are, however, data that indicate that such reflux can occur with all four of the previously noted causes of prostatomegaly[2] and can also occur in normal dogs with bladder distention at the time of urethrography.[3] The presence of urethroprostatic reflux of contrast medium is nonspecific and signifies that there are cavitary areas of prostatic parenchyma that openly communicate with the urethra.

To more fully characterize the source of the occult hematuria, a prostatic wash was done. The prostatic wash sample contained only benign epithelial cells. No erythrocytes were found.

Figure 5—Positive contrast, retrograde urethrogram of the dog in Figure 4. The bladder is displaced cranially, dorsally, and to the right by an enlarged prostate gland. The prostate is asymmetric in relation to the urethra.

Figure 5A

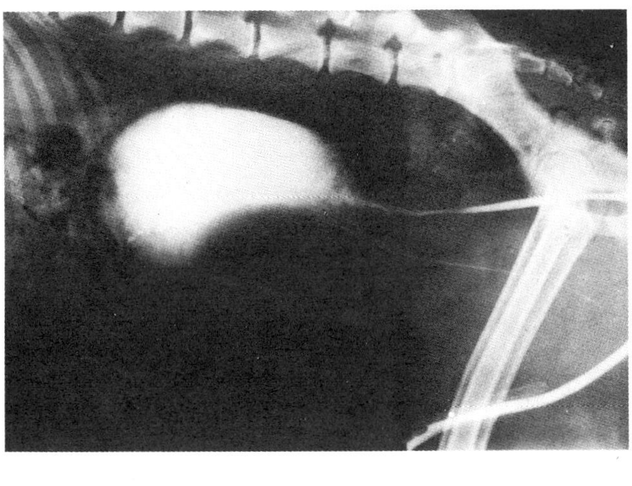

Figure 5B

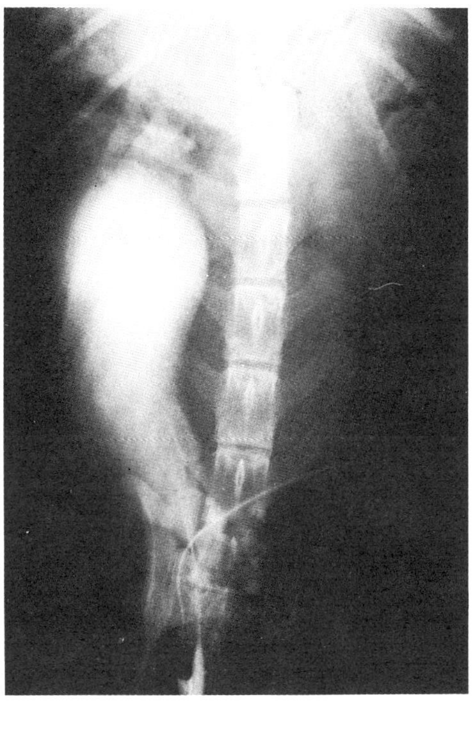

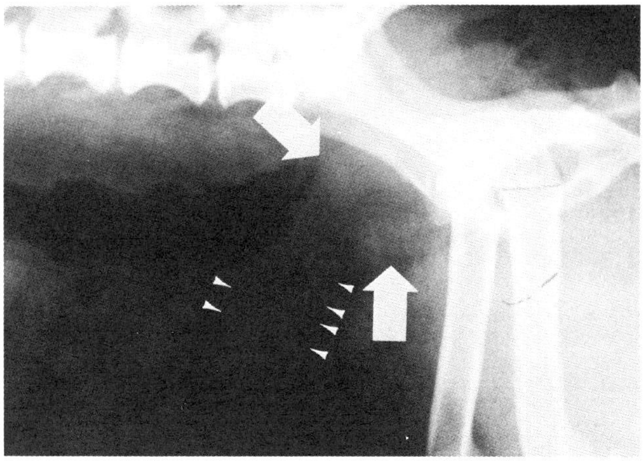

Figure 6A

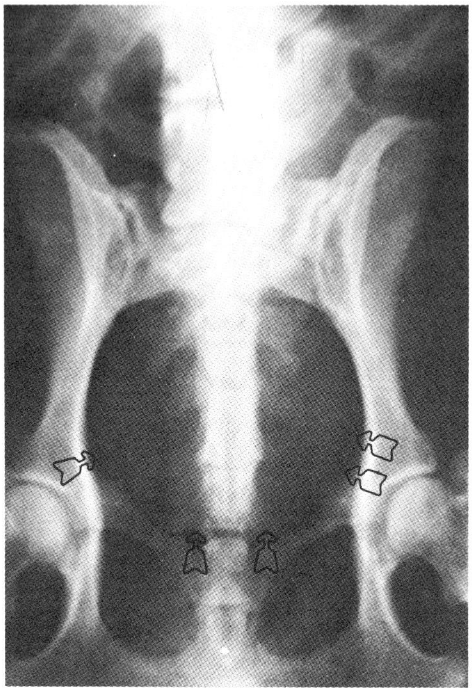

Figure 6B

Figure 6—Lateral (**A**) and ventrodorsal (**B**) survey abdominal radiographs. Two soft tissue masses *(arrows)* are present in **A**. The most caudal mass *(arrows)* is visible in **B**.

The symmetric, nonpainful prostatomegaly, occult hematuria, and normal prostatic wash indicated that benign prostatic hyperplasia was the most likely cause for the prostatomegaly. In patients with prostatic hyperplasia, hematuria may result from stagnation of urine in the bladder or urethra.[4] Benign prostatic hyperplasia is a common cause of symmetric nonpainful prostatomegaly in middle-aged and old male dogs. Prostatitis, the other major cause of symmetric prostatomegaly, could not be substantiated in this patient.

Case 2

A six-year-old male Irish setter was given a routine physical examination. A large mass was palpated in the central abdomen. On survey radiographs of the abdomen, two large soft tissue masses were present in the mid and caudal abdomen (Figure 4). When a positive contrast, retrograde urethrogram was done (Figure 5), the urinary bladder, which was displaced cranially, dorsally, and to the right, was identified as the cranial mass. The caudal mass, which was asymmetric in relation to the urethra, was assumed to be the prostate. Slight urethroprostatic reflux of contrast medium was present. As discussed previously, this was not of assistance in narrowing the list of differential diagnoses. The major possibilities to be ruled out for the asymmetric prostatomegaly in this dog were prostatic cyst, prostatic abscess, and prostatic neoplasia.

The abdomen was explored surgically. A large (20 cm × 20 cm × 20 cm) cystic structure was attached to the left lobe of the prostate by a 2.5 cm stalk. The mass was excised and was subsequently identified histologically as a prostatic cyst.

Case 3

An 11-year-old male Welsh corgi was examined because of chronic hematuria. No physical abnormalities were present. On survey radiographs of the abdomen, two soft tissue masses were present (Figure 6). The caudal mass was thought to be a slightly enlarged prostate. In this case the prostate was visible on the ventrodorsal projection of the abdomen. On a positive contrast retrograde urethrogram, the prostate was slightly enlarged and symmetric in shape, the prostatic urethra was dilated, and urethroprostatic reflux of contrast medium had occurred (Figure 7). The major differential diagnoses for symmetric prostatomegaly are benign hyperplasia and prostatitis. The significance of the prostatic urethral dilatation was unknown, although it has been reported to be associated with prostatitis.[4] The urethroprostatic reflux of contrast medium was not helpful in narrowing the list of differential diagnoses.

In urinalysis of a voided sample, there was mild hematuria, proteinuria and pyuria. A urinalysis of a

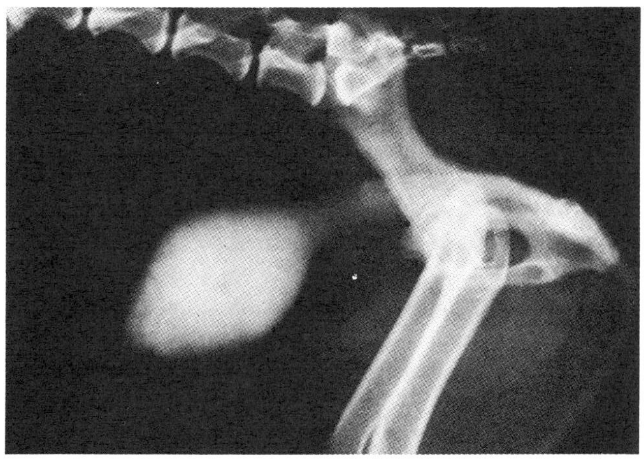

Figure 7—Positive contrast, retrograde urethrogram of the dog in Figure 6. The bladder is displaced cranially by a symmetrically enlarged prostate gland. The prostatic urethra is enlarged and slight urethroprostatic reflux of contrast medium has occurred (see text).

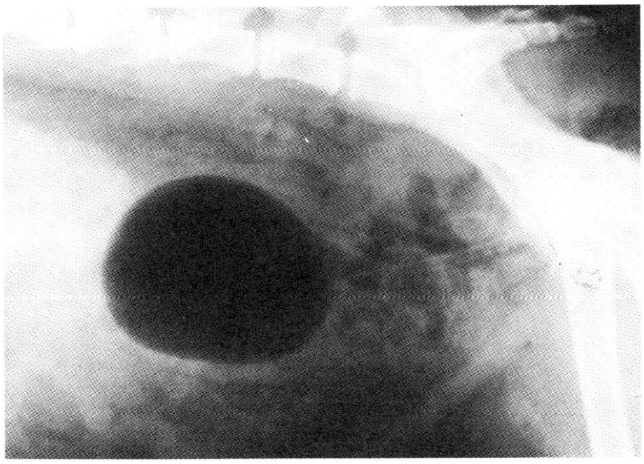

Figure 8—Pneumocystogram from a Boston terrier with prostatic abscessation associated with a Sertoli's cell tumor. Extensive urethroprostatic reflux of air has occurred as a result of parenchymal destruction that communicates with the urethral lumen. Pneumocystography in patients with prostatic disease is hazardous because of possible fatal air embolization.

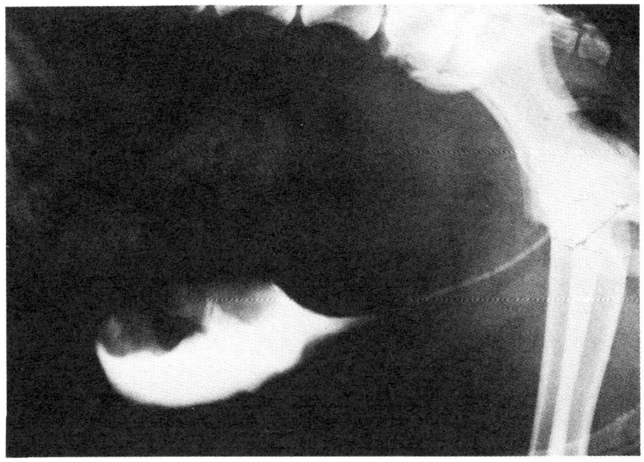

Figure 9—Positive contrast cystogram from a German shepherd with prostatic abscessation associated with a Sertoli's cell tumor. The prostate is asymmetrically enlarged in relation to the urethra. Bladder irregularity is due to exterior compression from bowel. Since the contrast medium was injected into the bladder, urethroprostatic reflux of contrast medium cannot be evaluated.

sample obtained by catheterization was normal. Bacterial culture of the urine was negative. In an ejaculate, degenerate leukocytes were present and a *Streptococcus* was found. The diagnosis was septic prostatitis without abscess formation.

This case represents an excellent example of prostatic infection that has not progressed to abscess formation. In such instances, the prostate is usually symmetric in circumference and in relation to the urethra[2] and parenchymal destruction is not marked. Progression of prostatic infection may result in abscessation of the gland. Also, a preexisting condition may predispose the patient to the development of a prostatic abscess. Two such conditions are prostatic cysts and estrogen-induced squamous metaplasia of the prostate. The radiographic appearance of a prostatic abscess differs from that of prostatitis without abscess formation. Prostatic abscessation commonly results in periurethral prostate asymmetry (Figures 8 through 10). It is difficult to distinguish radiographically between prostatic abscesses, cysts, and tumors.

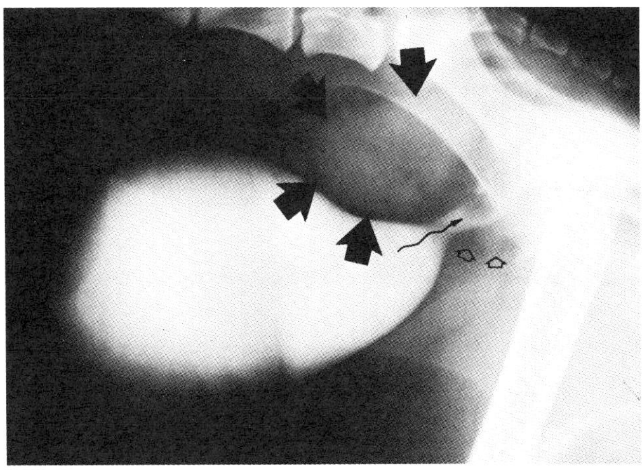

Figure 10—Positive contrast, retrograde urethrogram from an Afghan with a prostatic abscess associated with a Sertoli's cell tumor. The prostate is asymmetrically enlarged in relation to the urethra. Urethroprostatic reflux of contrast medium has occurred in a portion of the gland *(large black arrows)* and no contrast medium is present in the remainder *(open arrows)*. A filling defect, proved to be a blood clot, is present in the prostatic urethra *(curved black arrow)*.

Case 4

A 12-year-old male miniature poodle was examined because of urinary incontinence, tenesmus, and an enlarged prostate. Hemorrhagic urine was observed dripping from the urethral orifice. The prostate was enlarged and irregular. The urinary bladder was distended. The bladder was catheterized and 200 ml of reddish brown urine was removed. The urine was positive for protein (3+) and contained many erythrocytes and leukocytes. Bizarre giant cells with large nuclei were observed in a needle aspirate of the prostate.

On survey radiographs of the abdomen, the urinary bladder contained air and was displaced cranially by a soft tissue mass which was assumed to be the prostate gland (Figure 11). Air in the bladder was probably introduced during the previous catheterization. The presumed prostate gland contained multiple punctate mineralized foci and gas (Figure 11). A positive contrast, retrograde urethrogram confirmed the identity of the mass caudal to the bladder as the prostate (Figure 12). The prostatic urethral mucosa was irregular and the lumen was distended (Figure 12). In addition, the prostate was asymmetrically enlarged in relation to the urethra. From the radiographs, the major differential diagnoses for the prostatomegaly were prostatic abscess and prostatic tumor. Prostatic cyst was considered unlikely because of the extensive irregularity of the prostatic urethral lumen. On chest radiographs, a small (5 mm) interstitial nodule was seen in a cranial lung lobe.

In consideration of the clinical, laboratory, cytologic, and radiographic findings, the tentative diagnosis was

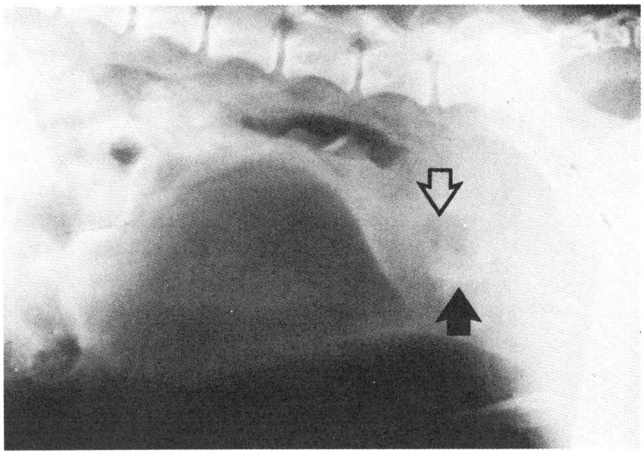

Figure 11—Lateral survey abdominal radiograph in which a gas-distended bladder can be seen. The bladder also contains what appear to be multiple small calculi. A soft tissue mass caudal to the bladder contains gas *(open arrow)* and mineral *(black arrow)* opacities.

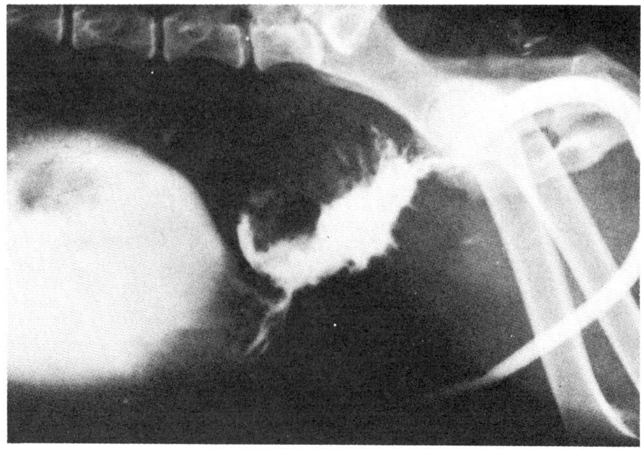

Figure 12—Positive contrast, retrograde urethrogram of the dog in Figure 11. The mass caudal to the bladder is the prostate. The prostatic urethral lumen is enlarged and irregular and there has been some urethroprostatic reflux of contrast medium dorsally.

prostatic tumor with pulmonary metastasis. A poor prognosis was given and the dog was euthanatized. The pathologic diagnosis was prostatic squamous cell carcinoma with pulmonary metastasis.

Prostatic tumors should be included in the list of differential diagnoses for asymmetric prostatomegaly, particularly if prostatic urethral mucosal irregularities can be identified. Sites of spread of prostatic tumors include direct infiltration into the bony pelvis (Figure 13) as well as distant metastasis to the external iliac lymph nodes, lumbar spine (Figure 14), and lungs.

Summary

The radiographic appearance of an enlarged prostate is seldom sufficient to identify the cause of prostatomegaly. Nevertheless, radiographic characteristics of the prostate evaluated by survey radiographs and positive contrast, retrograde urethrography are important in formulating the correct list of differential diagnoses. An important determinant in formulating the list of differential diagnoses is periurethral symmetry. Hyperplastic and inflammatory prostatic diseases (excluding abscessation) tend to result in more symmetric prostatomegaly than do cystic or neoplastic prostatic diseases and prostatic abscesses. Relative size of the prostate is also important since the degree of prostatomegaly seen with cystic and neoplastic diseases is generally larger than that seen with hyperplastic or inflammatory diseases (excluding abscesses).[2] It is important to remember, however, that in the early stages all prostatic diseases may appear radiographically similar.

The main benefit of positive contrast retrograde urethrography is that it allows evaluation of the periure-

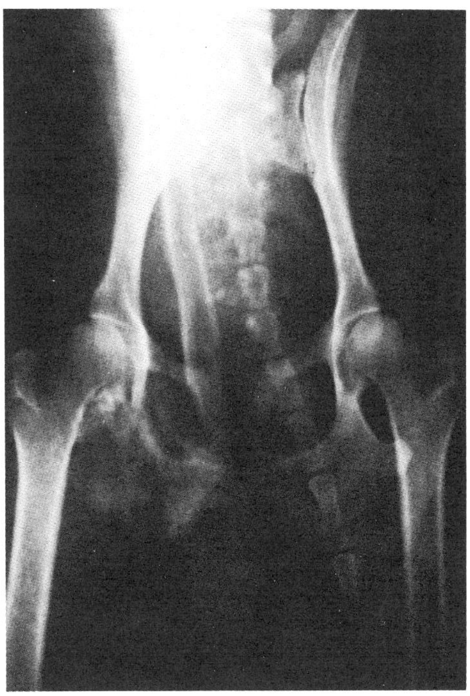

Figure 13—Aggressive osteolytic and osteoblastic lesion of the right ischium due to direct invasion by a prostatic adenocarcinoma.

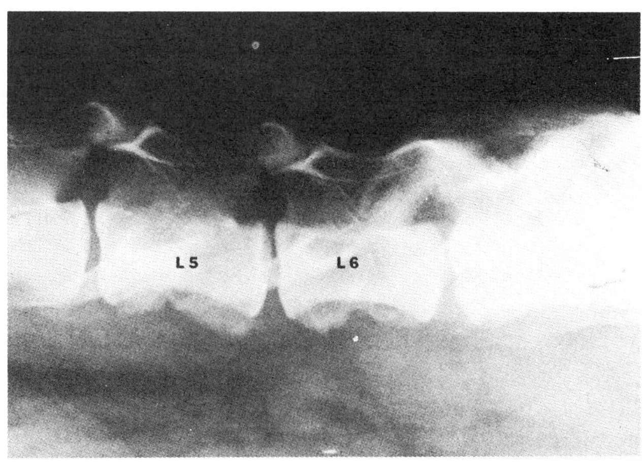

Figure 14—Lateral radiograph of the caudal lumbar spine of a dog in which active periosteal proliferation can be seen ventrally on L_5 and L_6. This periosteal reaction is due to metastasis of a prostatic adenocarcinoma. Lumbar vertebrae are common sites of metastasis for intrapelvic malignancies.

thral symmetry of the prostate. The presence or absence of urethroprostatic reflux of contrast medium during urethrography is of no assistance in formulating the list of differential diagnoses.[2] However, large cavitary prostatic areas identified by urethroprostatic reflux of contrast medium are more suggestive of neoplasia, cysts, and abscesses than of hyperplasia or prostatitis without abscessation. Urethrographic identification of an irregular prostatic mucosal surface is suggestive of a more aggressive prostatic disease such as neoplasia or abscessation. Size of the urethral lumen, evaluated urethrographically, is of little importance in formulating a list of differential diagnoses.

Definitive diagnosis of prostatic disease cannot be made by radiographic means. Radiographic signs must be interpreted in the correct context along with other historical, clinical, and laboratory information before differential diagnoses are listed. Definitive diagnosis of prostatic disease is frequently based upon histopathologic criteria.

REFERENCES

1. O'Shea JD: Studies on the canine prostate gland, I. Factors influencing its size and weight. *J Comp Pathol* 72:321-331, 1962.
2. Stone EA, Thrall DE, Barber DL: Radiographic interpretation of prostatic disease. *JAAHA* 14:115-118, 1978.
3. Losonsky JM, Unpublished data, College of Veterinary Medicine, University of Georgia, Athens, GA, 1981.
4. Greiner TP, Betts CW: Diseases of the prostate gland, in Ettinger S (ed): *Textbook of Veterinary Internal Medicine.* Philadelphia, WB Saunders Co, 1975, pp 1274-1306.

UPDATE

The review of the radiographic aspects of prostatic disease presented in this paper remains correct, although there are two aspects of the topic that deserve comment. First, the difficulty in identifying a slightly or moderately enlarged prostate on a ventrodorsal radiograph of the pelvic region is overstated—a slightly enlarged prostate gland is often clearly seen on the ventrodorsal view. Second, diagnostic ultrasound is a very accurate way to assess prostate size and shape and to detect the presence of mineralization, cysts, or other fluid- or exudate-filled cavities. The availability of ultrasound has decreased the need for cystography/urethrography to evaluate the prostate in many patients. Although special radiographic procedures are still useful for assessment of prostate disease, diagnostic ultrasound can also provide useful information in many cases.

Urethrography and Cystography in Cats Part I. Techniques, Normal Radiographic Anatomy, and Artifacts

Gary R. Johnston, DVM, MS
Daniel A. Feeney, DVM, MS
Carl A. Osborne, DVM, PhD

Department of Small Animal Clinical Sciences
University of Minnesota
College of Veterinary Medicine
St. Paul, Minnesota

The feline urologic syndrome (FUS) (cystitis, urethritis, and urethral obstruction syndrome) is the most common disorder of the urinary tract of cats. Investigations into possible causes have primarily been related to viral, bacterial, or dietery factors that may influence the disease. The radiographic findings in cats with FUS have not been adequately reported. This shortcoming is related to the absence of a standardized technique for cystography and urethrography in cats. The purpose of this article is to (1) describe simple inexpensive techniques of cystography and urethrography in cats, (2) illustrate the normal radiographic appearance of the feline cystogram and urethrogram, and (3) describe and illustrate the technical pitfalls of cystography and urethrography that may simulate the radiographic appearance of inflammatory or neoplastic disease.

The clinical manifestations, incidence, pathogenesis, and medical and/or surgical management of FUS have been described.[1-16] Although a great quantity of information about FUS has been published, the use of different criteria by different investigators in defining this syndrome has resulted in some confusion. The syndrome is primarily encountered in male cats, but females are also affected. The site of urethral obstruction in male cats has been reported to be near the bulbourethral gland,[2] in the membranous (postprostatic) urethra,[2] in the penile urethra,[2] and/or at the tip of the glans penis.[17] Urethral obstruction rarely occurs in female cats. The lumen of the male cat's urethra narrows at the ischiatic arch caudal to the bulbourethral gland and is reported to be a frequent site of obstruction.[2,16,17] However, this report has not been verified in a large series of patients by radiographic techniques. Case reports and textbook reviews of FUS suggest sporadic occurrence of lesions elsewhere, but their frequency of occurrence and significance remain unclear.

Techniques

The paucity of information related to the radiographic appearance of the lower urinary tract (especially the urethra) of cats with FUS is related, at least in part, to technical difficulty in obtaining diagnostic contrast urethrocystograms. To better define the radiographic appearance

Originally published in Volume 4, Number 10, October 1982

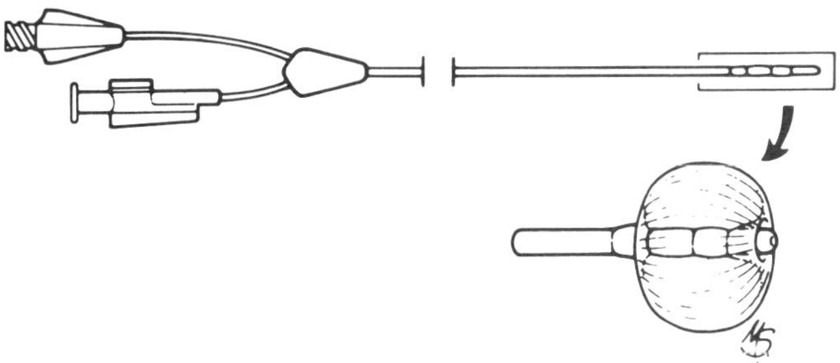

Figure 1—Swan-Ganz flow-directed balloon catheter used for retrograde urethrography in cats.

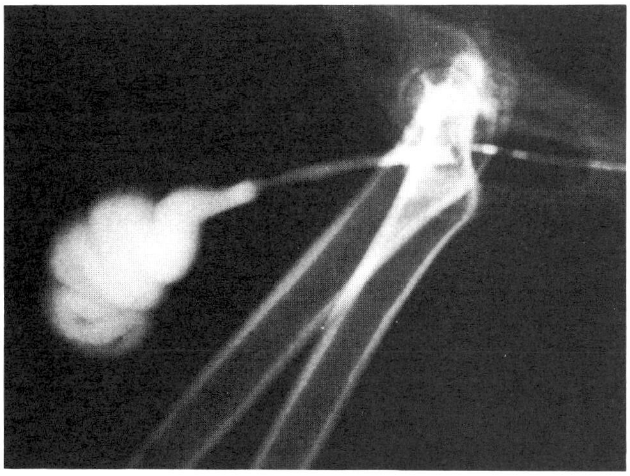

Figure 2—Lateral radiograph of a normal retrograde urethrogram on an adult female domestic shorthair cat. The use of a sterile aqueous lubricant as a diluent increases the viscosity of the contrast medium and facilitates distention of the urethral lumen. The incomplete mixing of the aqueous lubricant and diluted contrast medium with the urinary bladder contents frequently results in a wavy layered radiographic appearance of the positive contrast medium.

of the lower urinary tract of cats with FUS and to localize the site(s) of various abnormalities, a standard protocol for survey and contrast radiographic technique was devised to permit detailed evaluation of the urinary bladder and urethra and to permit comparison of the diagnostic usefulness of different techniques. To obtain radiographs of diagnostic quality within the same time frame, the following sequence was adopted: (1) survey radiography, (2) pneumocystography, (3) double contrast cystography, (4) positive contrast retrograde urethrocystography, and (5) positive contrast antegrade (voiding) urethrography.

Patient Preparation

Proper preparation of the patient is essential to optimal radiographic visualization of urinary tract lesions. Because some radiographic alterations are subtle, it is essential that intestines contain no ingesta and little or no gas. This is especially important if contrast procedures are to be performed. Overnight fasting and a cleansing enema are recommended prior to elective radiography. Water should be available throughout the fasting period.

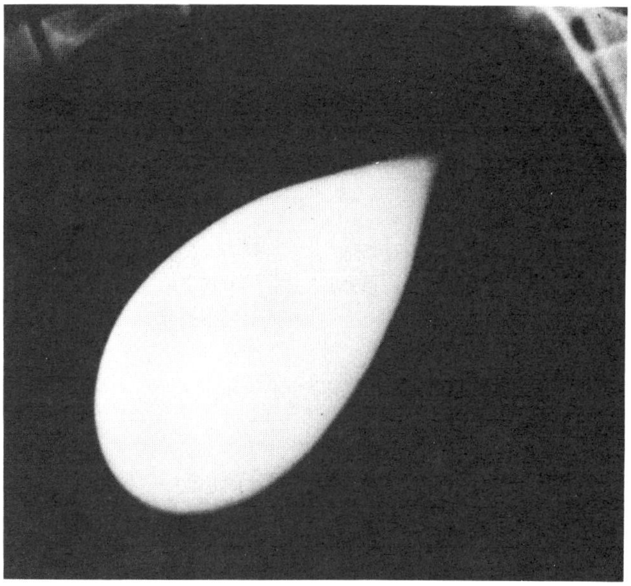

Figure 3—Normal positive contrast cystogram on a two-year-old castrated male domestic shorthair cat. The normal feline urinary bladder varies in configuration depending on the degree of urinary bladder distention. Note smooth mucosal contrast medium margin and tear-shaped configuration.

Pharmacologic restraint is usually necessary to obtain satisfactory films and to minimize the possibility of iatrogenic trauma to the urethra and/or urinary bladder. The authors routinely use ketamine hydrochloride[a] or thiamylal sodium.[b]

Survey lateral and ventrodorsal radiographs should be obtained for evaluation of patient preparation, radiographic technique, and lesions that may be obscured or distorted by contrast radiography.

Prior to contrast radiography the bladder should be emptied by manual compression or with the aid of a 3.5 French catheter.[c] Failure to empty urine from the bladder may simulate bladder-wall thickening during pneumocystography. A "jet stream" encountered during positive contrast retrograde urethrography also may simulate mural thickening because of the incomplete mixing of the positive contrast medium and urine.

Pneumocystography

The authors recommend that the technique of pneumocystography incorporate both partial and complete distention of the urinary bladder with negative contrast media of air, CO_2, or nitrous oxide to aid in detection of small mural lesions. Although embolization may occur following injection of air into the lower urinary tract,[18] in the authors' experience with thousands of cases it has been rare. A lateral radiograph should be obtained after 5 to 8 ml of negative contrast medium have been infused into the urinary bladder via a catheter. Lateral views of a partially distended bladder have been

---

[a]Ketaset®, Bristol Laboratories, Syracuse, NY 13201.
[b]Bio-tal®, Bio-Ceutic Laboratories, Inc., St. Joseph, MO 64502.
[c]Sovereign Sterile Disposable Feeding Tube and Urethral Catheter, Sherwood Medical Industries Inc., St. Louis, MO 63103.

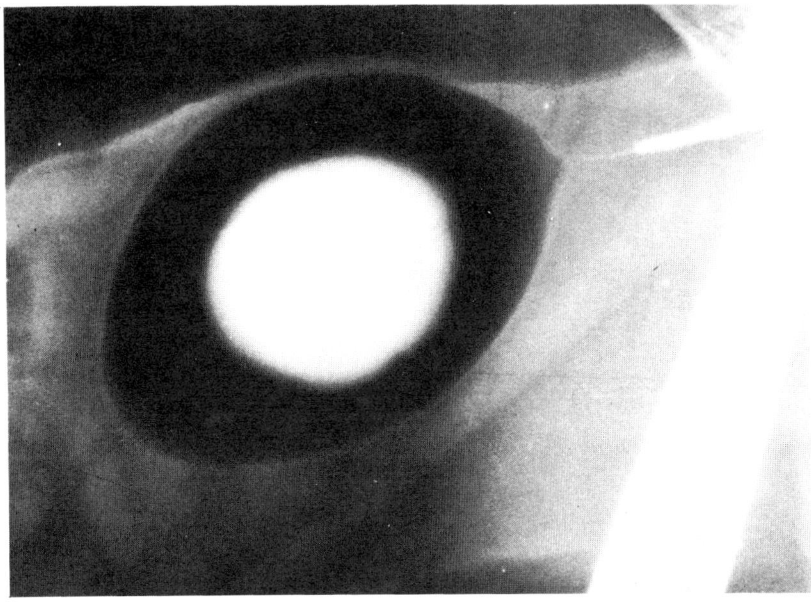

Figure 4—Normal double contrast cystogram of a 14-year-old spayed female domestic shorthair cat. With adequate urinary bladder distention, the urinary bladder wall should have a smooth uniform thickness. The positive contrast medium in the double contrast cystogram should have a smooth interface with the mucosa of the urinary bladder.

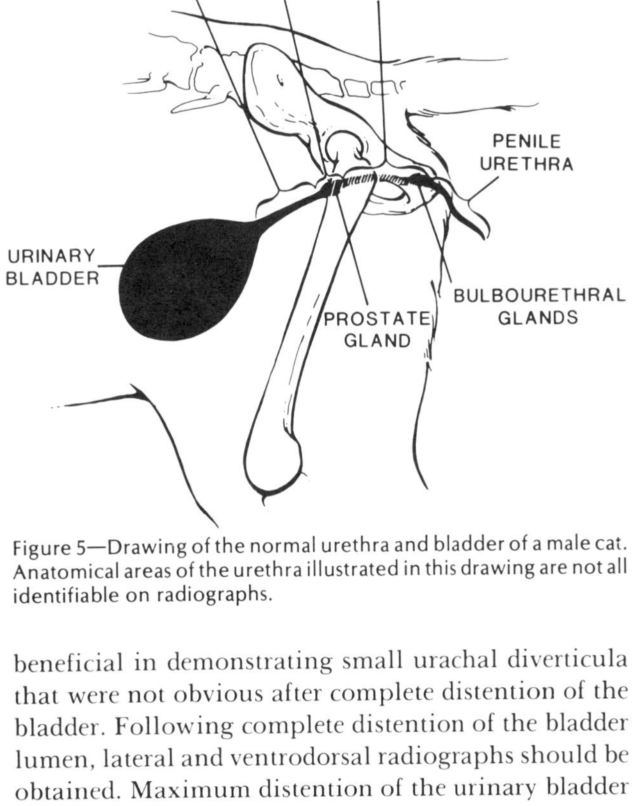

Figure 5—Drawing of the normal urethra and bladder of a male cat. Anatomical areas of the urethra illustrated in this drawing are not all identifiable on radiographs.

beneficial in demonstrating small urachal diverticula that were not obvious after complete distention of the bladder. Following complete distention of the bladder lumen, lateral and ventrodorsal radiographs should be obtained. Maximum distention of the urinary bladder varies in cats with FUS. Volumes of 15 to 45 ml may be obtained without spontaneous voiding in sedated or anesthetized cats. However, absolute values for volume distention should be used with caution because of possible iatrogenic bladder rupture and air embolism. Digital palpation of the bladder, and signs of patient discomfort including abdominal compression and flexion of the rear legs should be used to determine whether the degree of bladder distention is sufficient.

Some cats with inflammatory lower urinary tract disease may be unable to tolerate complete distention of the urinary bladder. If spontaneous voiding occurs following partial distention of the bladder lumen, further attempts to distend the bladder with negative contrast medium are likely to result in spontaneous micturition. Removal of the bladder contents and infusion of 1 to 2 ml of lidocaine hydrochloride[d] may provide sufficient topical anesthesia to permit the desired degree of distention.

Double Contrast Cystography

Following pneumocystography, a double contrast cystogram can be obtained by infusion of 0.25 to 0.75 ml of positive contrast medium into the bladder lumen via a catheter. The authors prefer undiluted meglumine diatrizoate[e] or meglumine iothalamate,[f] although other aqueous organic triiodinated compounds used for intravascular injections may be used. Lateral and ventrodorsal radiographs should be obtained, as described in the section on pneumocystography. This small quantity of contrast material accumulates in the dependent portion of the urinary bladder and facilitates detection of radiolucent free intraluminal filling defects. It also aids in detection of dependent mucosal irregularities that cannot be identified by survey radiography or pneumocystography. Because no effort is made to coat the entire mucosal surface with contrast medium, small mucosal abnormalities may not be observed. If subtle mucosal lesions are suspected, additional views which are intermediate in position to lateral and ventrodorsal views (so-called oblique views) should be obtained. Distention of the bladder lumen with positive contrast

[d]Xylocaine® 2%, Astra Pharmaceutical Products Inc., Worcester, MA 01606.
[e]Hypaque® Meglumine 60%, Winthrop Laboratories, New York, NY 10016.
[f]Conray®, Mallinckrodt Chemical Works, St. Louis, MO 66134.

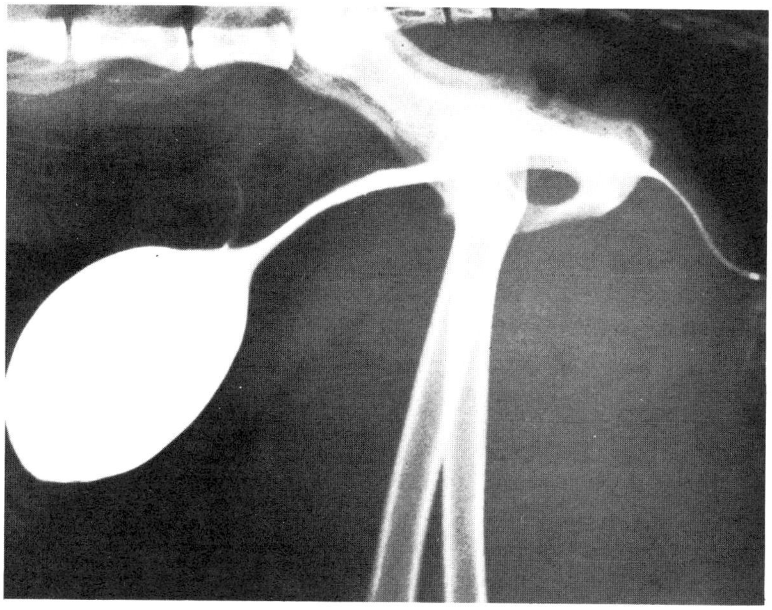

Figure 6A

Figure 6—Normal urethrogram of a four-year-old castrated male domestic shorthair cat. The normal radiographic appearance of the urethra varies depending on the technique of urethrography. Note bilateral vesicourethral reflux. (**A**) Normal retrograde urethrogram.

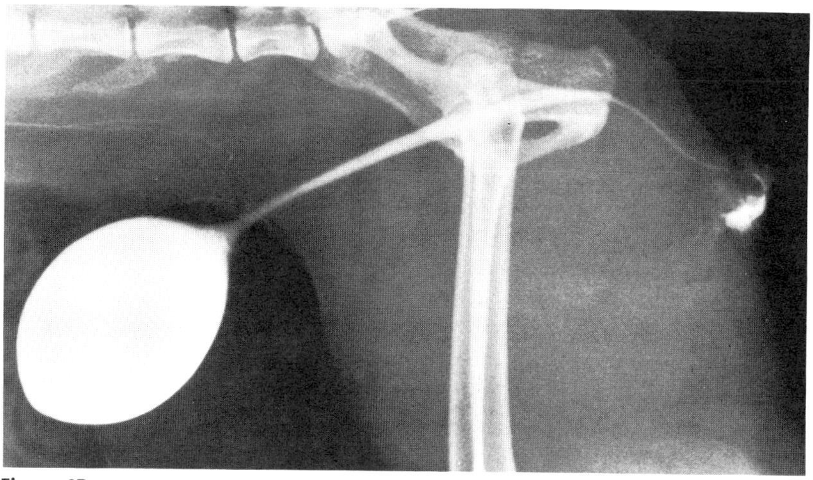

Figure 6B

Figure 6—(**B**) Normal antegrade (voiding) urethrogram performed by external bladder compression using a wooden spoon.

medium (positive contrast cystography) may also be considered.

Positive Contrast Retrograde Urethrocystography

Positive contrast cystography and/or urethrocystography should follow pneumocystography and double contrast cystography for the evaluation of urethral and bladder lesions. Intraluminal, mural, and extraluminal urethral lesions are best defined by positive contrast urethrography. In addition, the positive contrast cystogram or urethrocystogram can detect small urachal diverticula that may not be detectable with negative contrast agents. Mucosal tears and lacerations are better demonstrated by the positive contrast media. Positive contrast media also eliminate the risk of fatal air embolization.

Following double contrast cystography, the bladder contents should be removed. A sufficient quantity of a 5% solution of aqueous positive contrast medium should be infused into the urinary bladder to induce moderate distention of its lumen. The urinary catheter should then be removed. Lateral and ventrodorsal views of the lower urinary tract should be obtained. Alternatively, they may be obtained following distention of the urethra with contrast medium.

Moderate distention of the urinary bladder with positive contrast medium is required to provide sufficient intraluminal pressure to ensure maximum distention of the proximal portion of the urethra during retrograde urethrography. (Complications of this procedure will be discussed in Part II of this article.) The volume of contrast medium required to distend the bladder lumen should be similar to that required to distend it with gas during pneumocystography.

Several techniques for contrast urethrography may be considered. Retrograde or antegrade studies utilizing balloon or nonballoon catheters are recommended for male cats. A 4 French balloon catheter[g] (Figure 1) or a

[g]Swan-Ganz, Flow Directed Balloon Catheter, Edwards Laboratories, Santa Ana, CA 92711.

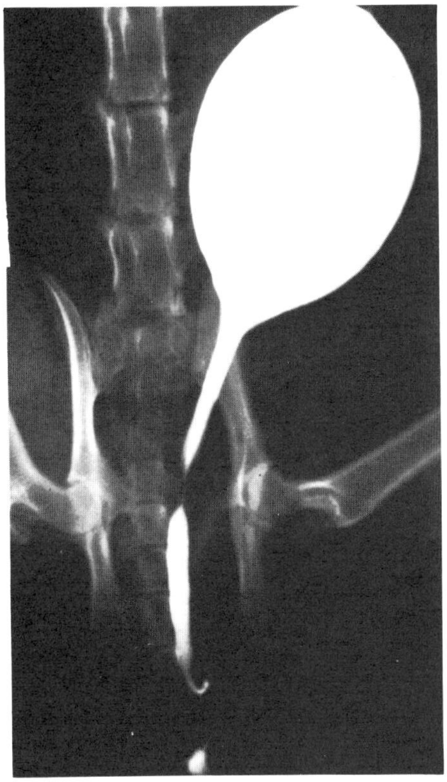

Figure 7A

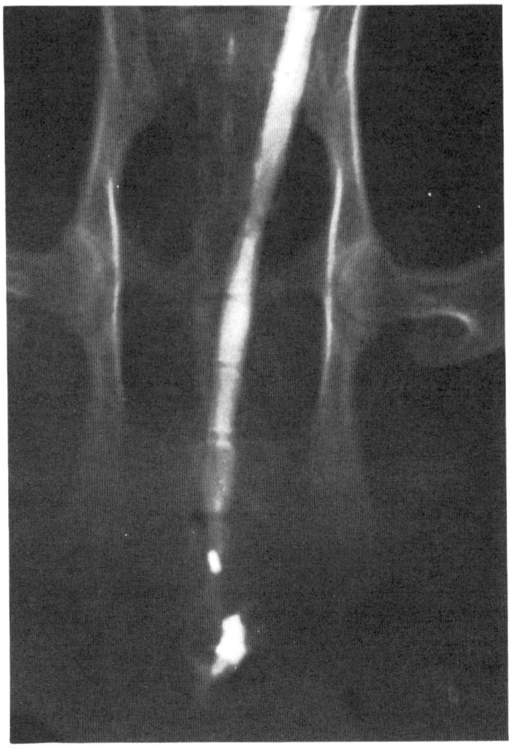

Figure 7B

Figure 7—Ventrodorsal radiographs of positive contrast retrograde urethrograms on a two-year-old male Siamese cat. (**A**) An abrupt narrowing of the prostatic urethra which simulates a partial urethral obstruction is frequently encountered with retrograde urethrography. (**B**) The prostatic urethral luminal narrowing encountered during retrograde urethrography subsequently distended during antegrade urethrography. Suspected urethral strictures should be confirmed and differentiated from spasm by using both retrograde and antegrade urethrography.

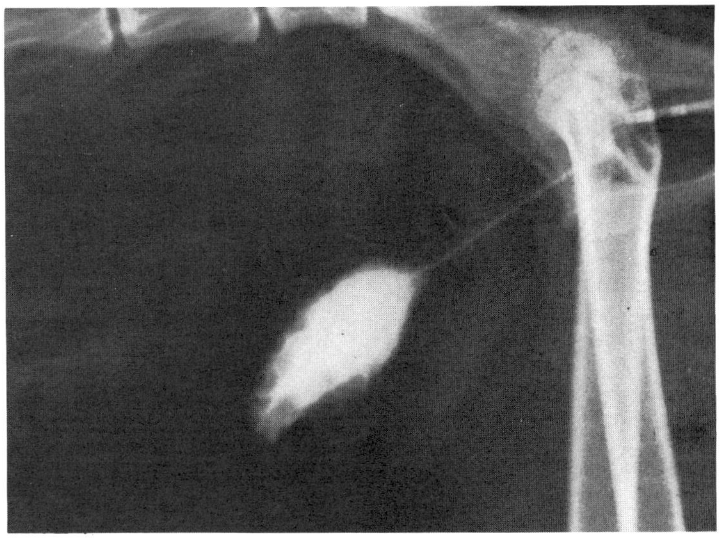

Figure 8A

Figure 8—Lateral radiographs of a retrograde urethrogram on a nine-year-old spayed female domestic shorthair cat. (**A**) Two milliliters of positive contrast medium infused into the urinary bladder resulted in insufficient intravesical pressure to distend the urethral lumen.

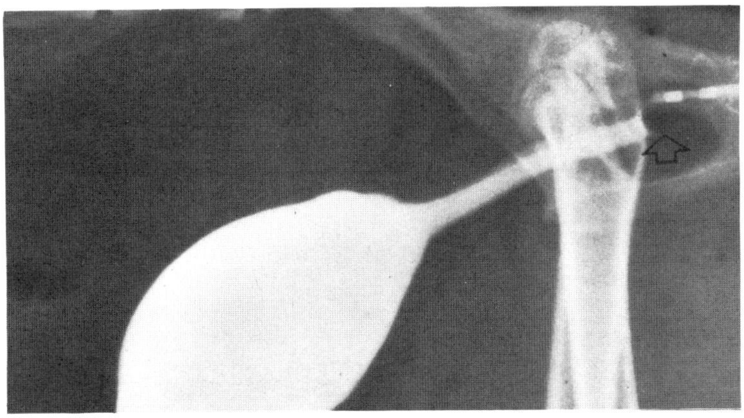

Figure 8B

Figure 8—(**B**) Greater distention of the urinary bladder with positive contrast medium via an inflated balloon catheter (*arrow*) resulted in sufficient intravesical hydrostatic pressure to ensure urethral distention.

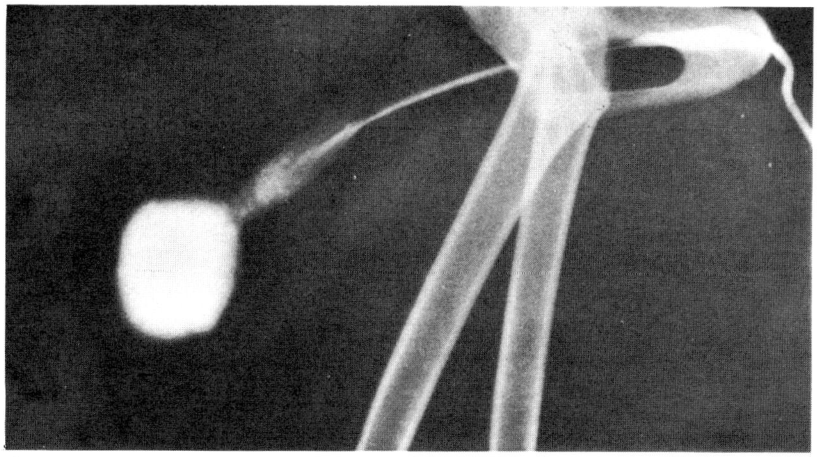

Figure 9A

Figure 9—This series of urethrograms was obtained on a four-year-old male domestic shorthair cat. (**A**) Inadequate urinary bladder distention prior to urethrography has resulted in incomplete luminal distention of the proximal urethra. Failure to remove the contents of the urinary bladder also resulted in a "jet stream" effect of the positive contrast medium, which mimics a mural lesion.

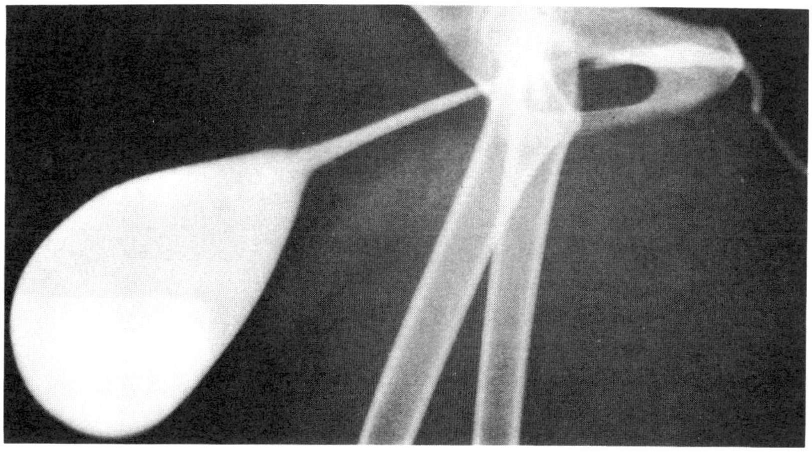

Figure 9B

Figure 9—(**B**) Further infusion of positive contrast media into the urinary bladder provided sufficient intravesical hydrostatic pressure to ensure distention of the proximal urethral lumen. Mixing of the urine with the contrast medium has eliminated the previously encountered pseudomural filling defect.

3.5 French tomcat urethral catheter[h] has been satisfactory. Balloon-tipped catheters have a distinct advantage over other types of urethral catheters in that they prevent reflux of contrast medium through the urethral orifice, thus ensuring proper filling of the urethral lumen proximal to the inflated balloon. Retrograde urethrography in male cats in which a urethral catheter is secured in the penile urethra by external digital compression is not recommended because of potential exposure of personnel to ionizing radiation. Retrograde urethrography of female cats can be performed with the aid of a 4 or 5 French balloon catheter.[g] Satisfactory retrograde urethrograms of the female urethra cannot be obtained with other types of urethral catheters because of reflux of contrast medium around the catheter with subsequent loss through the urethral orifice.

The aqueous organic iodinated contrast media used for contrast cystography are also recommended for contrast urethrography. However, the contrast medium should be diluted 1:3 with sterile distilled water or saline. Reduction of the radiodensity of the contrast medium aids in detection of filling defects that otherwise may be obscured by using undiluted contrast media.

[h]Sovereign Open End Tom Cat Catheter, Sherwood Medical Industries Inc., St. Louis, MO 63103.

Sterile aqueous lubricants[i,j] may be mixed with contrast medium (one part contrast medium to one part sterile saline or distilled water to one part aqueous lubricant) to increase its viscosity and promote distention of the urethral lumen (Figure 2).

The lumen of the balloon catheter should be filled with contrast medium prior to its placement in the urethra to prevent artifacts caused by air bubbles. Care should also be used with balloon catheters to prevent iatrogenic trauma and infection of the urinary tract.

To perform retrograde positive contrast urethrocystography in male cats, the penile urethra is exteriorized and a 4 French balloon catheter is inserted approximately 1.5 cm into the urethral lumen. Lubrication of the catheter tip with an anesthetic lubricant[k] facilitates catheter placement. Inflation of the balloon with 0.5 ml of air helps stabilize the catheter's location. The balloon should not be placed just inside the urethral orifice because the small diameter of the penile urethra at this site will prevent sufficient inflation of the balloon to maintain the catheter's position.

[i]K-Y jelly®, Johnson & Johnson Products, New Brunswick, NJ 08903.
[j]Lubafax®, Burroughs Wellcome Co., Research Triangle Park, NC 27709.
[k]Xylocaine 2% Jelly, Astra Pharmaceutical Products Inc., Worcester, MA 01606.

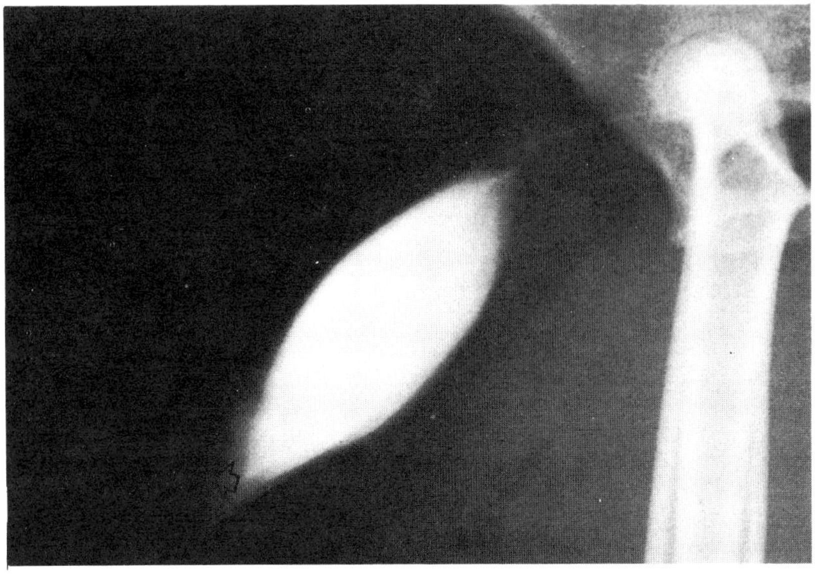

Figure 10A

Figure 10—Lateral positive contrast cystogram on a four-year-old spayed female domestic shorthair cat. (**A**) Improper catheter placement and incomplete distention have resulted in abnormal bladder configuration due to either smooth muscle spasms or catheter pressure. The catheter extends to the cranial tip of the bladder (*arrow*).

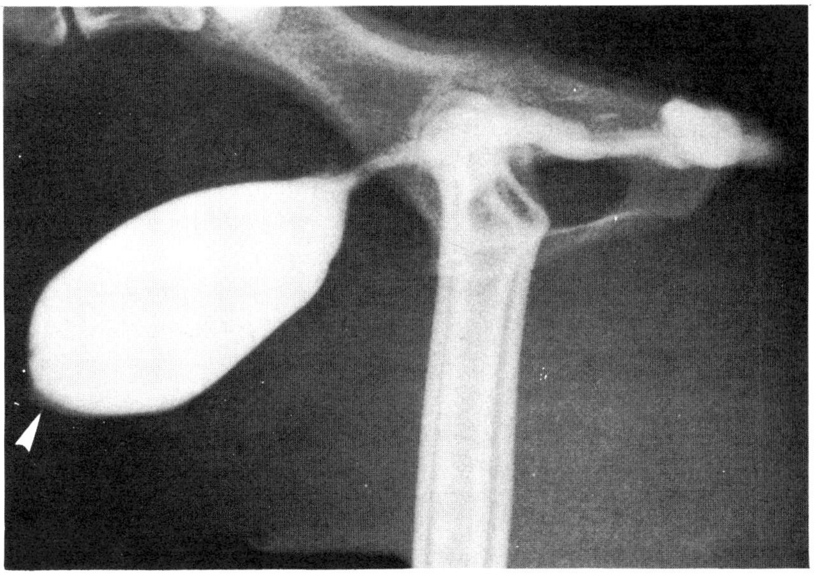

Figure 10B

Figure 10—(**B**) Subsequent catheter withdrawal to the trigone area and further bladder distention resulted in a smooth contour of the urinary bladder wall except for a small remnant of the urachal diverticulum (*arrow*). Pooling of contrast medium in the vagina and vestibule distal to the external urethral orifice is a normal finding with voiding cystourethrography.

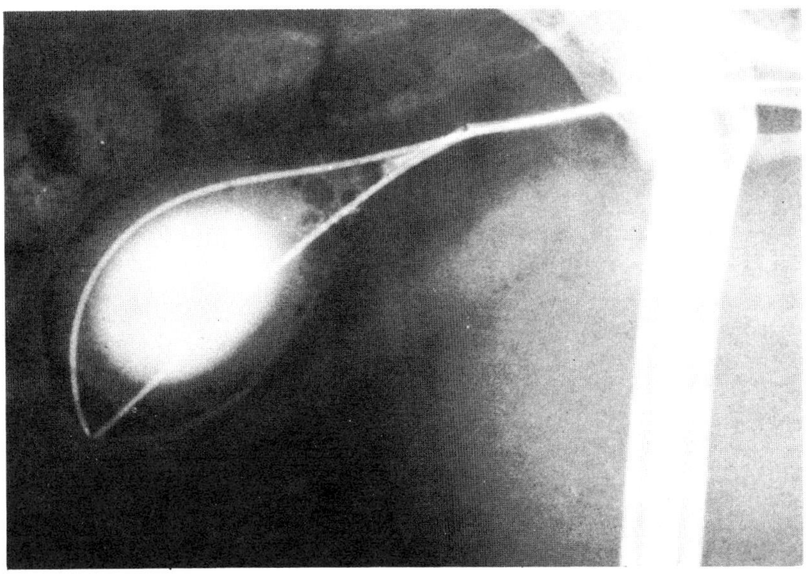

Figure 11—Lateral cystogram on an eight-year-old castrated male domestic longhair cat. Improper placement of nonflexible urethral catheter may cause catheter kinking and may result in bladder and/or urethral trauma. A cystotomy was necessary for removal of the catheter.

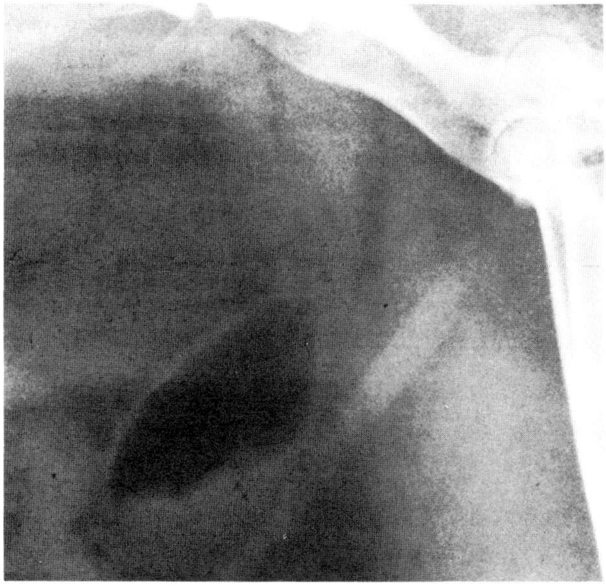

Figure 12A

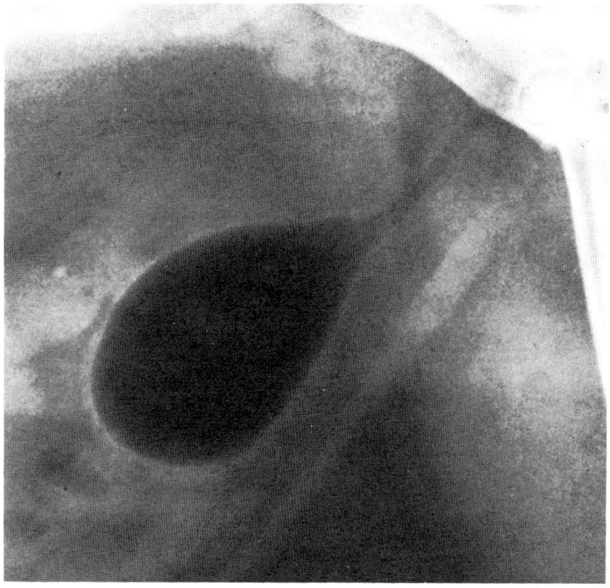

Figure 12B

Figure 12—Inadequate distention of the urinary bladder during cystography or urethrography can result in mural pseudolesions simulating inflammatory or neoplastic disease. This series of pneumocystograms was of an eight-year-old domestic shorthair cat. (**A**) Inadequate urinary bladder distention during pneumocystography resulted in an area of cranioventral thickening suggestive of neoplastic or inflammatory disease. (**B**) Subsequent gas distention of the urinary bladder during pneumocystography has eliminated the previously suspected mural lesion.

Injection of 2 to 3 ml of iodinated contrast medium ensures complete filling of the urethral lumen but may not cause maximal distention. To facilitate maximal distention of the urethral lumen, the radiographs should be obtained slightly before injection of contrast medium through the catheter has been completed.

The procedure for retrograde positive contrast urethrocystography in female cats is similar to that described for male cats. The tip of the balloon catheter should be placed just inside the external urethral orifice. Positioning of the catheter may be verified with the aid of a small otoscope speculum.

Positive Contrast Antegrade (Voiding) Urethrography

Use of balloon catheters for retrograde positive contrast urethrography in nonobstructed cats prevents radiographic evaluation of the portion of the urethra occupied by and distal to the balloon. This portion of the urethra may be visualized by antegrade positive contrast urethrography if necessary. If positive contrast cystography precedes this phase of the study, the bladder will have been filled with contrast medium. If not, the bladder lumen should be distended with an appropriate quantity of aqueous iodinated contrast medium injected via a urinary catheter. Contrast medium can be forced into the urethra with abdominal compression using a wooden spoon placed over the abdomen at a site adjacent to the bladder. Abdominal compression can be induced at the appropriate time by pressing the handle downward. Exposure of the lateral view of the entire lower urinary tract at the time of induced micturition enables evaluation of the distal urethra and the competence of vesicoureteral valves. External abdominal compression with a wooden spoon may produce some distortion of the bladder and proximal urethra.

Antegrade positive contrast urethrocystography may also be considered for evaluation of the urethral lumen of cats that are difficult to catheterize or whose urethral lumina are obstructed. The technique does not require balloon catheters. The urinary bladder is distended with contrast medium either by excretory urography or percutaneous transabdominal bladder infusion via cystocentesis using a 22-gauge, 3-in. spinal needle.[1] Following distention of the bladder, antegrade urethrography can be performed in the manner described for cats without urethral obstruction. Contrast medium may be forced into the urethral lumen by external abdominal bladder compression or by spontaneous initiation of the micturition reflex which can be induced by gradual distention of the urinary bladder during light-plane anesthesia of the cat. Although external abdominal compression of the bladder with a wooden spoon is preferred, some degree of distortion of the bladder and proximal urethra commonly occurs. Appropriate caution should be used to prevent iatrogenic bladder rupture.

Selection of Technique

To compare the diagnostic usefulness of the various radiographic techniques for evaluating the urinary bladder and urethra, each of the described procedures was performed. Although the procedures complement each other and together permit extensive and complete evaluation of the lower urinary tract, it is impractical and usually unnecessary to perform all of the described studies. The authors' recommendations include a min-

[1]Spinal Needle, Becton-Dickinson, Rutherford, NJ 07070.

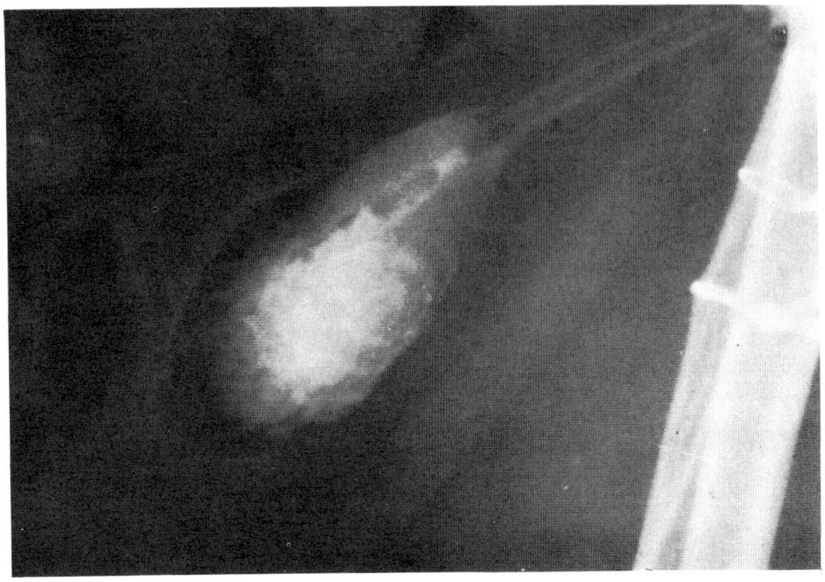

Figure 13—Lateral radiograph of a double contrast cystogram of a six-year-old spayed female domestic shorthair cat. (**A**) Inadequate urinary bladder distention has resulted in an irregular mucosal contrast medium pattern in the dependent portion of the bladder. Diffuse bladder-wall thickening also appears to be present. These findings mimic inflammatory disease of the urinary bladder.

Figure 13A

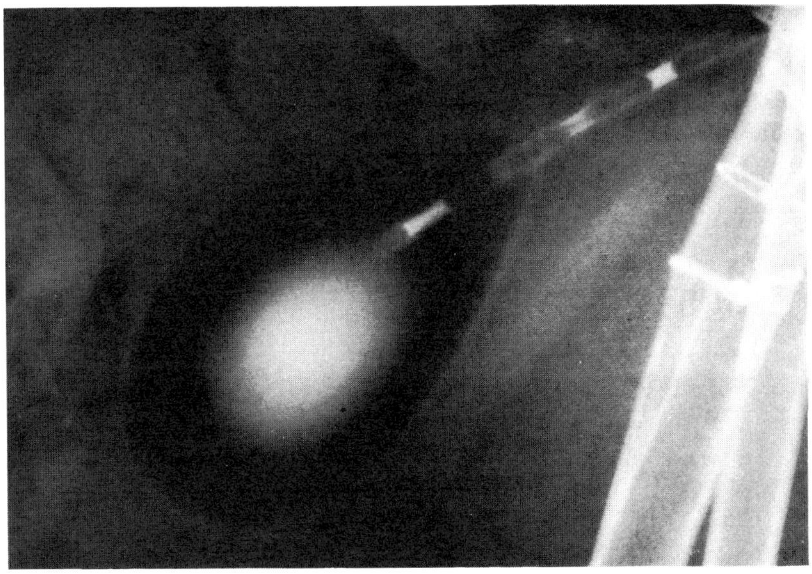

Figure 13—(**B**) Subsequent distention of the urinary bladder has resulted in a normal mucosal pattern and bladder wall thickness.

Figure 13B

imum of eight radiographs: a ventrodorsal and lateral view for two survey radiographs, two for double contrast cystography, two for retrograde urethrography, and two lateral radiographs for antegrade urethrography and partial-distention pneumocystography. They have not evaluated pneumourethrography or double contrast urethrography as diagnostic techniques for urethral disorders because all urethral lesions were considered adequately demonstrated by positive contrast antegrade or retrograde urethrography.

Normal Radiographic Anatomy

Urinary Bladder

The normal feline urinary bladder may be ovoid, ellipsoid, or teardrop-shaped depending on its degree of distention (Figures 3 and 4). The wall of the urinary bladder is normally smooth and has a uniform thickness when distended (Figures 3 and 4). In double contrast cystograms, positive contrast medium in the dependent portion of the bladder lumen has a smooth contour at its interface with the bladder wall (Figure 4).

Urethra

The urethra of male cats may be divided into several anatomical regions on the basis of location and microscopic appearance. They are the (1) preprostatic urethra, (2) prostatic urethra, (3) postprostatic urethra, and (4) penile urethra (Figure 5). Radiographically, the urethra may be divided into (1) the intrapelvic urethra (including preprostatic, prostatic, and postprostatic urethra) and (2) the penile urethra (Figure 6). The normal prostatic urethra is occasionally seen as a narrowed area in the mid-pelvic urethra (Figure 7). Provided adequate pressure is induced in the bladder lumen by distention with contrast medium, the normal urethra of male cats has a continuous and uniformly smooth luminal surface. However, the normal diameter of the urethral lumen is variable. The maximum diameter of the penile urethra

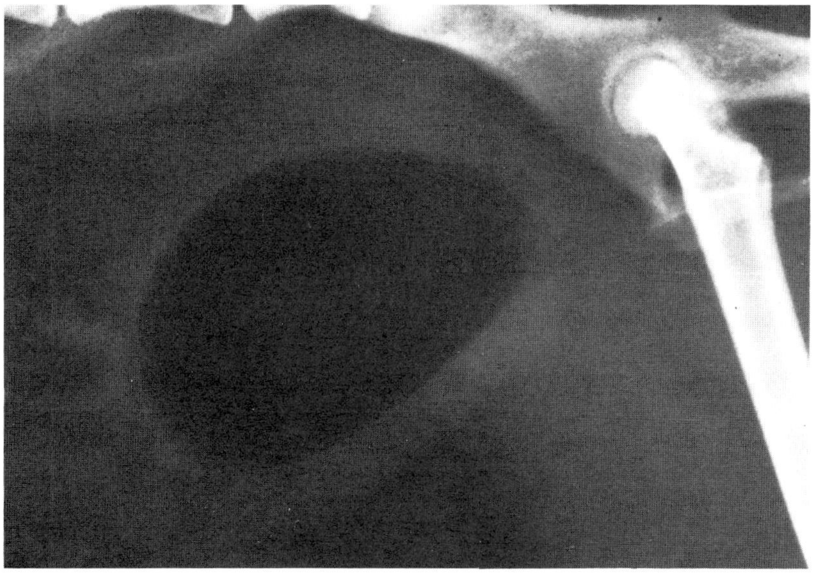

Figure 14—Lateral radiographs of a four-year-old spayed female domestic shorthair cat. (**A**) Intraluminal filling defects with a fluid density may be obscured in the dependent portion of the urinary bladder with a pneumocystogram.

Figure 14A

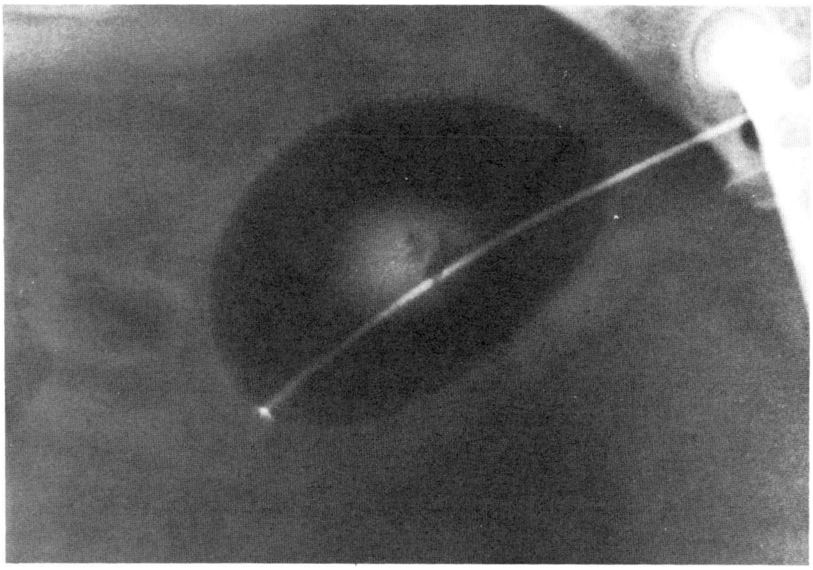

Figure 14—(**B**) Double contrast cystogram demonstrates two filling defects (blood clots) in the dependent portion of the urinary bladder which were not visible by pneumocystography or survey radiography.

Figure 14B

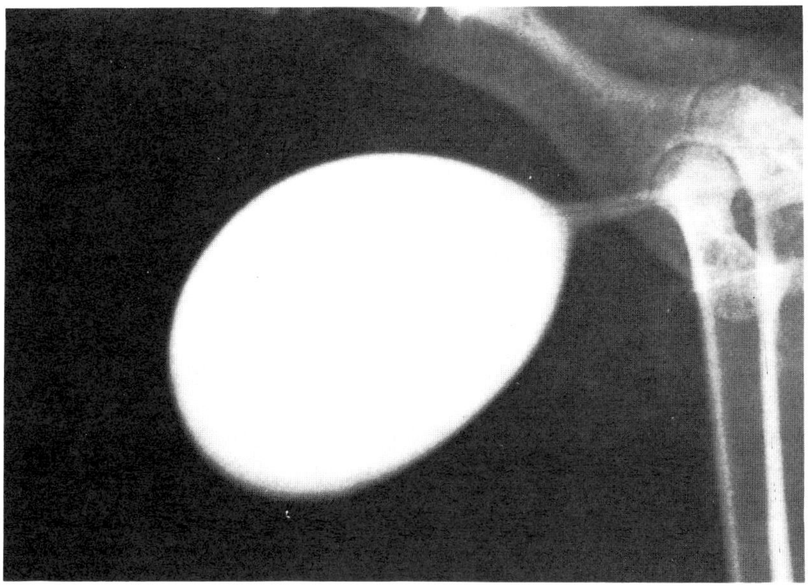

Figure 14—(**C**) Use of undiluted positive contrast medium for urethrocystography also obscures the two filling defects in the dependent bladder previously seen with double contrast cystography.

Figure 14C

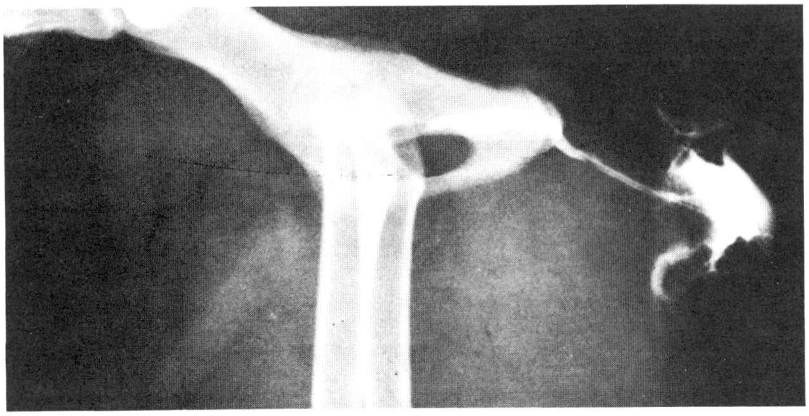

Figure 15—Retrograde urethrograms on the cat in Figure 9. (**A**) The use of a nonballoon catheter for the retrograde injection of positive contrast medium resulted in pericatheter reflux of contrast medium and incomplete luminal distention of the proximal urethra. Incomplete filling of the proximal urethra could be misinterpreted as luminal obstruction.

Figure 15A

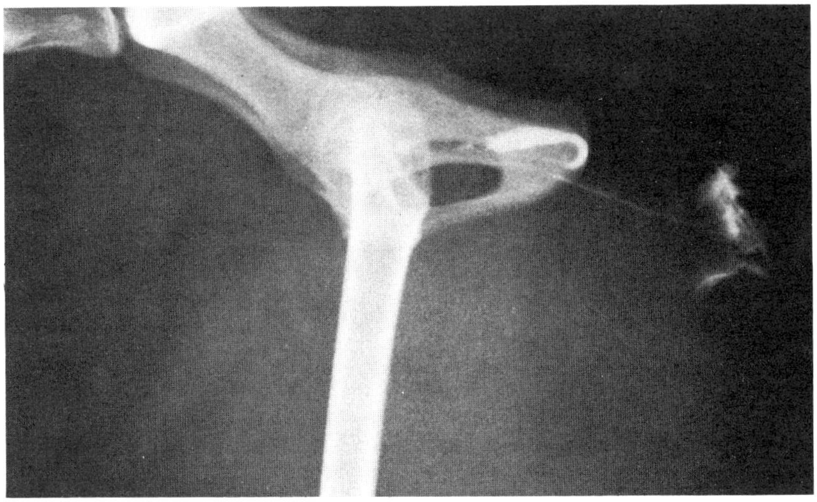

Figure 15—(**B**) Excessive external catheter pressure has caused a flexure in the penile urethra which has resulted in a partial obstruction of the urethral lumen and predisposes to incomplete luminal filling of the proximal urethra and pericatheter reflux.

Figure 15B

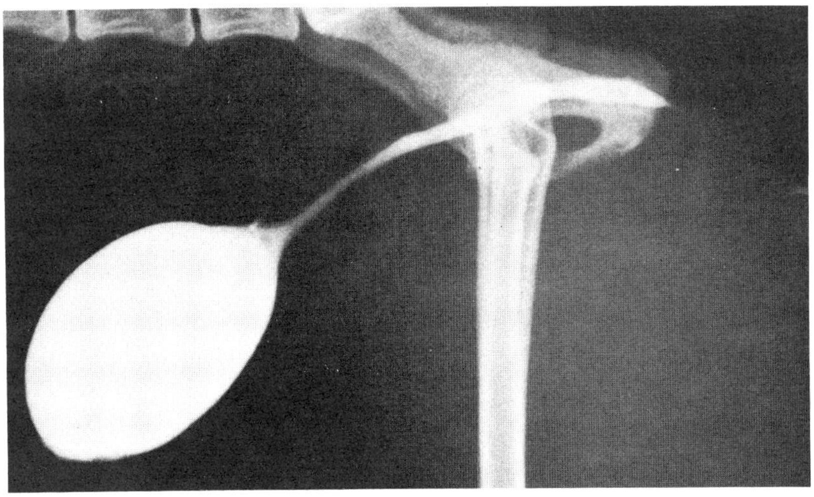

Figure 16—Retrograde urethrogram on the cat in Figure 6. Normal retrograde urethrogram with exposure occurring after the injection of contrast medium was completed. The incomplete filling of the penile urethra was a technical artifact resulting from failure to expose the x-ray film during the contrast medium injection. The filling defect at the bladder neck is an air bubble.

normally occurs at the level of the ischiatic arch. The diameter of the penile urethra becomes progressively smaller toward the external urethral orifice (Figure 6).

The urethra of normal female cats has a uniform diameter throughout its length (Figure 8). As in male cats, the mucosal surface is normally smooth.

Artifacts

Artifacts caused by improper technique during cystography or urethrography may result in radiographic findings that mimic inflammatory or neoplastic conditions. Failure to remove the bladder contents prior to cystography or urethrography may result in pseudointraluminal or mural filling defects following infusion of the positive or negative contrast medium (Figure 9). For cystography, the catheter tip should be placed near the bladder neck, because improper catheter placement can result in an abnormally shaped urinary bladder

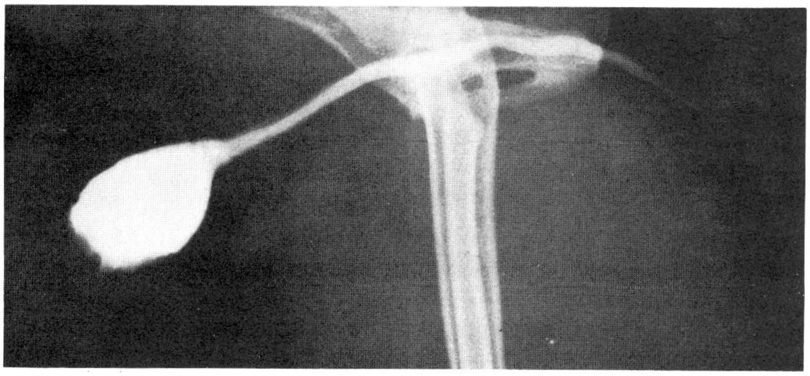

Figure 17A

Figure 17—Antegrade (voiding) contrast urethrocystograms on the cat in Figure 12. (**A**) Variations in urethral diameter are frequently encountered in voiding cystourethrography and may be caused by peristaltic contractions and/or urethral spasms. Note irregular thickening of the bladder wall caused by underdistention of the urinary bladder.

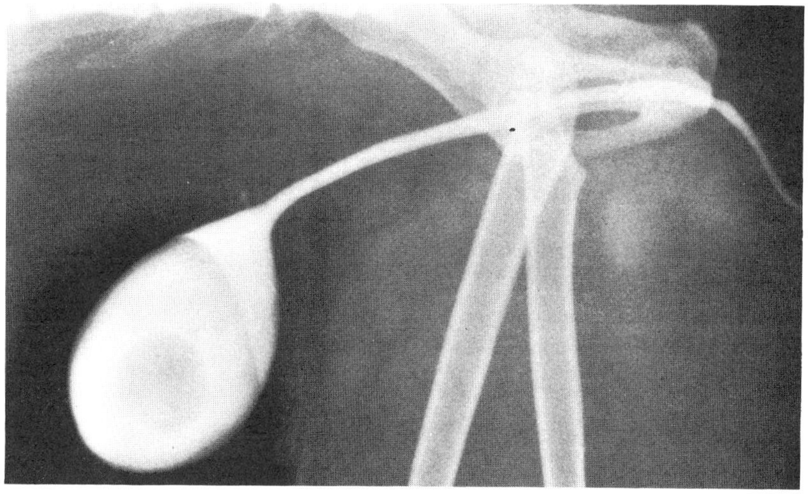

Figure 17B

Figure 17—(**B**) Subsequent voiding cystourethrography performed by external abdominal bladder compression with a wooden spoon eliminated the variations in urethral diameter previously seen. The filling defect in the bladder is an air bubble. A slight amount of vesicoureteral reflux is present.

(Figure 10) or catheter kinking (Figure 11). Inadequate urinary bladder distention, the most common technical pitfall, is associated with normal thickening of the bladder wall that often cannot be distinguished from abnormal bladder-wall thickening. Mural thickening associated with incomplete filling of the bladder may appear diffuse or localized and may simulate inflammation or neoplasia (Figures 12 and 13). Inadequate bladder distention may also result in an abnormally shaped urinary bladder because of extramural compression by contiguous structures. Normal mucosal irregularity suggesting inflammatory and/or neoplastic disease may also be encountered with inadequate bladder distention during double contrast or positive contrast cystography (Figures 8 and 13). A positive contrast cystogram obtained without a preceding pneumocystogram and double contrast cystogram may inhibit visualization of free intraluminal filling defects in the dependent portion of the urinary bladder (Figure 14). Excessive volumes of positive contrast media used in double contrast cystograms may similarly mask free intraluminal filling defects in the dependent portion of the urinary bladder.

Incomplete luminal distention of the urethra commonly occurs during retrograde urethrography of male and female cats. Incomplete urethral distention can be focal, segmental, or generalized and may be caused by technique or urethral disease. Voluntary contractions of the urethralis muscle at the ischiatic arch, smooth-muscle spasms, and peristaltic contractions are the most common causes of focal luminal narrowing and must be differentiated from a urethral stricture. The most common cause of segmental or generalized incomplete urethral distention is inadequate intravesical hydrostatic pressure prior to retrograde urethrography (Figures 8 and 9). Pericatheter reflux of contrast medium around nonballoon catheters is also a common cause of regional or segmental incomplete urethral distention (Figure 15A). Pericatheter reflux of contrast medium with nonballoon catheters used for retrograde urethrography may be influenced by excessive cranial catheter placement, which can result in an iatrogenic flexure of the penile urethra and subsequent partial or complete luminal obstruction (Figure 15B). A slight reduction in prostatic urethral luminal diameter may be encountered with retrograde injection and is considered normal (Figure 7A). Subsequent evaluation of the prostatic urethra with antegrade urethrography by external bladder compression further distends the prostatic urethral lumen (Figure 7B). Incomplete luminal filling in any part of the urethra may occur if the film is exposed after injection of the contrast medium (Figure 16).

Antegrade urethrography associated with spontaneous micturition around the urethral catheter or following gradual overdistention of the urinary bladder may

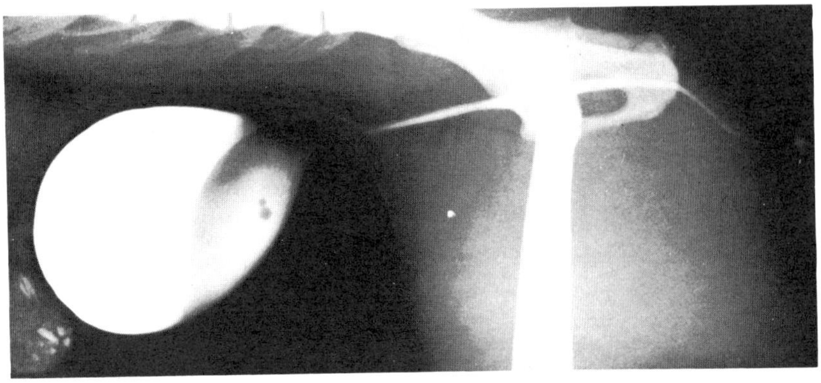

Figure 18—Lateral radiograph of an antegrade urethrogram on a six-year-old male domestic shorthair cat. Improper placement of the wooden spoon for abdominal compression has resulted in compression of the proximal urethra, which simulates urethral disease. Several air bubbles are present in the bladder.

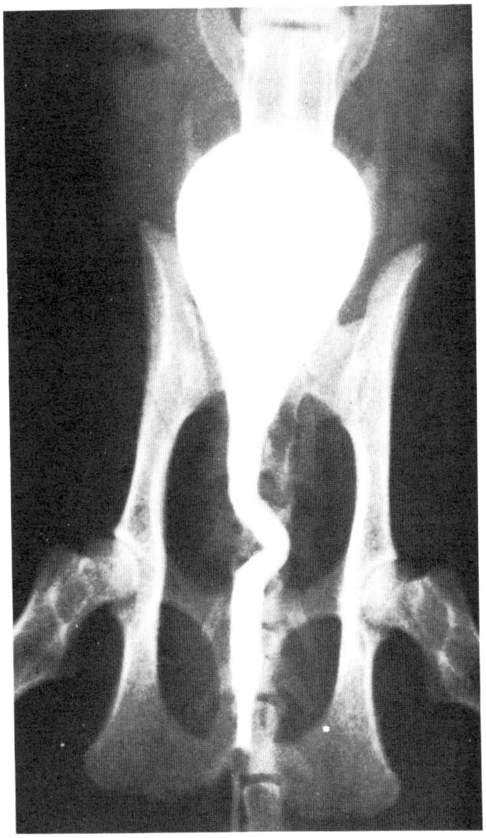

Figure 19—Ventrodorsal radiograph of a retrograde urethrogram on a three-year-old female domestic shorthair cat. The pressure of the abdominal contents on the distended urinary bladder has resulted in caudal displacement of the bladder and a secondary intrapelvic urethral flexure. Flexures, which may mimic extraurethral lesions, can be differentiated by subsequent urethrography with elevation of the caudal abdomen.

result in some areas of incomplete urethral distention because of peristaltic contractions or urethral spasms (Figure 17). Some distortion of the urinary bladder or urethra may occur with external bladder compression (Figure 18). Use of balloon catheters for retrograde injection of contrast media, use of sterile aqueous lubricants as diluents, or use of antegrade urethrography with external bladder compression will distend the urethra and facilitate differentiation of incomplete urethral distention (Figures 7, 9, and 17).

Although adequate distention of the urinary bladder is necessary to ensure urethral distention, iatrogenic urethral flexures may occur because of caudal bladder displacement by cranial abdominal contents. These urethral flexures may mimic urethral displacement by extraurethral lesions and may require further radiographic evaluation (Figure 19).

If a focal urethral stricture is suspected on the initial retrograde urethrogram, a second retrograde study preceded by intraluminal infusion of 0.25 to 0.75 ml of lidocaine hydrochloride may help differentiate a stricture from a urethral spasm. If the focal luminal narrowing persists, antegrade urethrography performed by external bladder compression will distend a nonstrictured urethra.

REFERENCES

1. Foster SJ: "Urolithiasis" syndrome in male cats. A statistical analysis of the problem with clinic observations. *J Small Anim Pract* 8:201-211, 1967.
2. Jackson OF: The treatment and subsequent prevention of struvite urolithiasis in cats. *J Small Anim Pract* 12:555-568, 1981.
3. Osborne CA, Lees G: Feline cystitis, urethritis, urethral obstruction syndrome. *Mod Vet Pract* 59:173-180; 349; 357; 513-520; 669-673, 1978.
4. Feline urolithiasis: Interim report. *Vet Rec* 96:298-299, 1975.
5. Jungreis T: Bladder stones in female cats. *Feline Pract* 5:7, 1975.
6. Pierce D: Feline urolithiasis: A case study. *Feline Pract* 4:30-31, 1974.
7. Lewis LD, Chow FHC, Taton GF, Hamer DW: Effect of various dietary mineral concentrations on the occurrence of feline urolithiasis. *JAVMA* 172:559-563, 1978.
8. Reif JS, Bovee K, Gaskell CJ, Batt RM, Maguire TG: Feline urethral obstruction: A case-control study. *JAVMA* 170:1320-1324, 1974.
9. Rich LJ: Current concepts of feline urethral obstruction. *Vet Clin North Am* 1:245-250, 1971.
10. Rich LJ, Dysart K, Chow FHC,, Hamer DW: Urethral obstruction in male cats: Experimental production by addition of magnesium and phosphate to the diet. *Feline Pract* 4(5):44-47, 1974.
11. Willeberg P: Interaction effects of epidemiologic factors in feline urologic syndrome. *Nord Vet Med* 28:193-200, 1976.
12. Gaskell PJ: Therapy for FUS. *J Small Anim Pract* 19:301, 1978.
13. Robinette JD: Silicone rubber prosthesis for replacement of the urethra of male cats. *JAVMA* 163:285-288, 1973.
14. Whitehead JE: Urolithiasis in the feline. *SAC* 1:307-319, 1961.
15. McCully RM, Lieberman LL: Histopathology in a case of feline urolithiasis. *Can Vet J* 2:52-61, 1961.
16. Richards DA, Hinci PJ, Morse EM: Feline perineal urethrostomy—A new technique for an old problem. *JAAHA* 8:66-73, 1972.
17. Meier FW: Urethral obstruction and stenosis in the male cat. *JAVMA* 137:67-70, 1960.
18. Zontine WJ, Andrews LK: Fatal air embolization as a complication of pneumocystography. *J Am Vet Radiol Soc* 19:8, 1978.

Urethrography and Cystography in Cats Part II. Abnormal Radiographic Anatomy and Complications

Gary R. Johnston, DVM, MS
Daniel A. Feeney, DVM, MS
Carl A. Osborne, DVM, PhD

Department of Small Animal Clinical Sciences
University of Minnesota
College of Veterinary Medicine
St. Paul, Minnesota

The feline urologic syndrome (FUS) is a common urinary tract disorder which affects male and female cats. Many of these cats have a variety of radiographic abnormalities in the urinary tract that may play a role in the cause or may contribute to the recurrent nature of the disease. These anatomical abnormalities can be visualized by uroradiographic contrast procedures. In Part I of this two-part article, the techniques of cystography and urethrography and the normal radiographic appearance of each technique were described. The technical and interpretative pitfalls of these procedures were also discussed. In Part II, the radiographic abnormalities encountered during survey and contrast uroradiography are discussed and illustrated. The complications associated with cystography and urethrography in cats are also described.

Radiographic Abnormalities

Detection of radiographic abnormalities necessitates careful systematic evaluation of both survey radiographs and special uroradiographic procedures. Failure to obtain survey radiographs or to adequately interpret these films prior to cystography or urethrography procedures may lead to an incorrect or incomplete diagnosis.

Survey Radiography

Radiographic evaluation of cats with FUS begins with the systematic evaluation of survey radiographs for abnormalities of size, shape, location, and radiographic density. Abnormalities encountered on survey radiographs do not negate the necessity for further evaluation with cystography and urethrography. Abnormal survey radiographic findings may be suggestive of a lesion that can only be adequately demonstrated with a contrast study.

A markedly distended urinary bladder on survey radiographs is compatible with lower urinary tract obstruction or may be normal. An abnormally enlarged proximal urethra may be suggested on a lateral survey radiograph by the presence of an increased fluid density ventral to the descending colon (Figure 1). An abnormally shaped urinary bladder may also be seen in cats with lower urinary tract disease. The presence of

Originally published in Volume 4, Number 11, November 1982

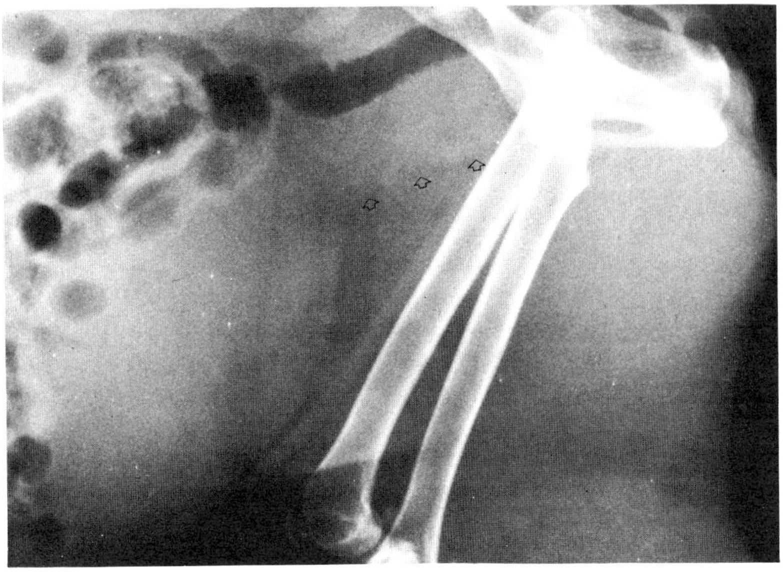

Figure 1—An area of increased fluid density *(arrows)* ventral to the descending colon represented an enlarged proximal urethra in an adult male domestic short-haired cat with urethral obstruction. Compare with Figure 20.

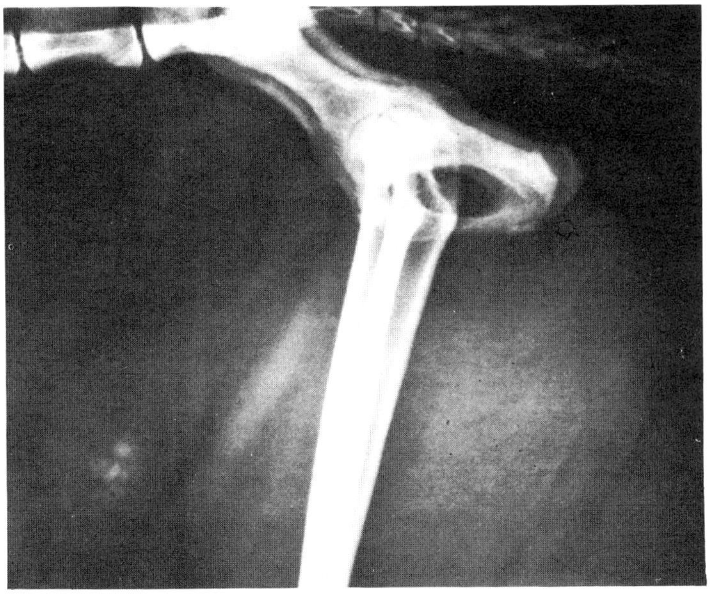

Figure 2—A wedge-shaped protruding fluid density from the cranioventral bladder margin suggestive of a diverticulum, multiple radiopaque cystic uroliths, and a solitary radiopaque urethral calculus *(arrow)* are visible in a five-year-old neutered male domestic short-haired cat with dysuria and stranguria. Compare with cystograms in Figures 10B and 12.

a urachal diverticulum or a persistent urachal ligament of the urinary bladder may be suggested by the radiographic presence of a wedge-shaped protruding fluid density from the cranioventral bladder margin on a lateral recumbent view (Figure 2). However, caution must be used when evaluating abnormalities of urinary bladder shape because superimposed fluid-filled bowel may simulate bladder diverticula. An abnormal location of the urinary bladder may be due to an inguinal or other type of abdominal hernia. Abnormalities such as radiopaque uroliths (Figures 2 and 3), intravesical foreign bodies, and mural calcification of the urinary bladder can have abnormal radiographic densities involving the urinary bladder and/or urethra identified on survey radiographs. Radiopaque uroliths may be single (Figures 3A and 3B) or multiple (Figures 2 and 3C) and may vary in size, shape, and location within the urinary bladder and urethra. Radiolucent densities within the bladder may be visible on survey radiographs. Free intraluminal gas is the most common of these and appears as a smooth round radiolucent density in the bladder silhouette, its location being controlled by positioning (Figure 4). Free intraluminal gas is commonly the result of prior catheterization or transabdominal cystocentesis. Gas located within the bladder wall, emphysematous cystitis, may be more difficult to identify radiographically but usually appears within any or all layers of the bladder wall. Emphysematous cystitis may be secondary to diabetes mellitus or bacterial cystitis. Intraluminal and intramural gas must be differentiated from superimposed gas-filled bowel.

Contrast Uroradiography

Evaluation of cystograms and urethrograms should be systematic and should follow the careful evaluation of survey radiographs. Diagnostic impressions gained from the survey radiographs should be verified with cystography or urethrography. Abnormal radiographic

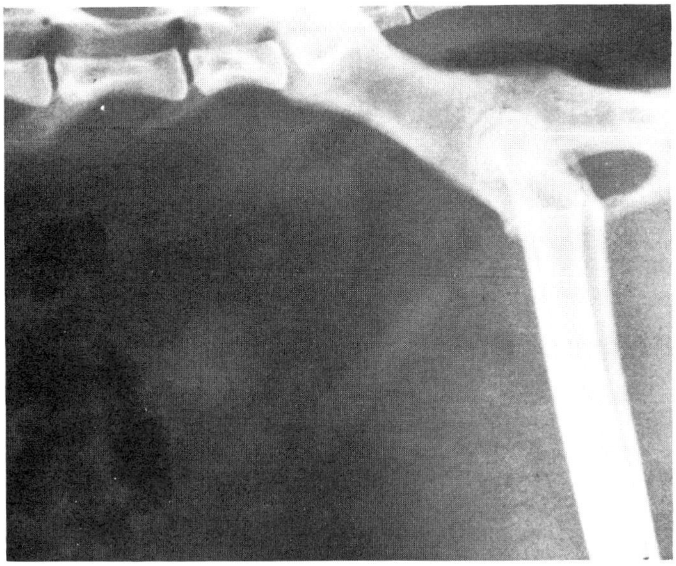

Figure 3A

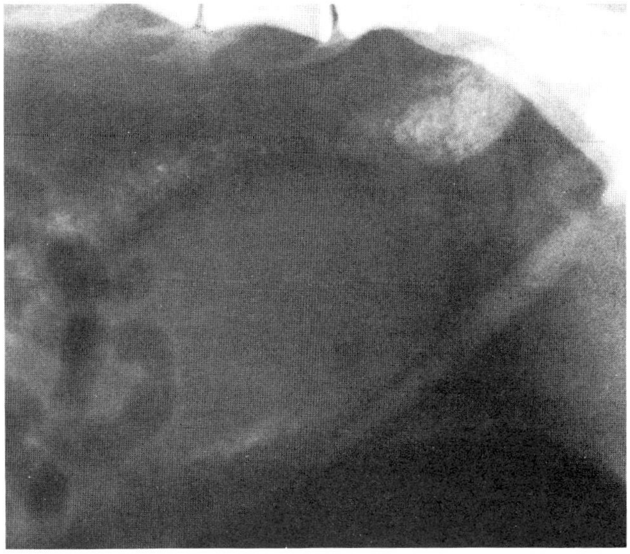

Figure 3C

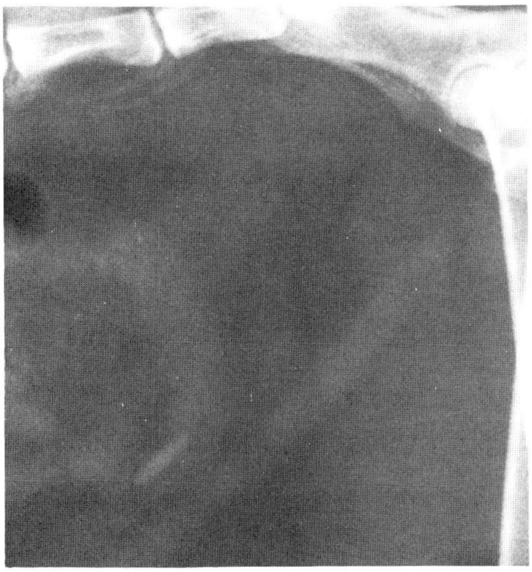

Figure 3B

Figure 3—Uroliths vary in size, number, shape, and location within the urinary bladder and urethra. **(A)** A large spheroidal solitary cystic urolith in a three-year-old male domestic short-haired cat with renal failure. **(B)** Solitary pumpkin-seed-shaped urolith in a 10-year-old spayed female domestic long-haired cat with lower urinary tract disease. Subsequent cystography localized the calculus within the urinary bladder. **(C)** Multiple sandlike cystic uroliths are visible in a one-year-old male Siamese cat with urethral obstruction of three days duration.

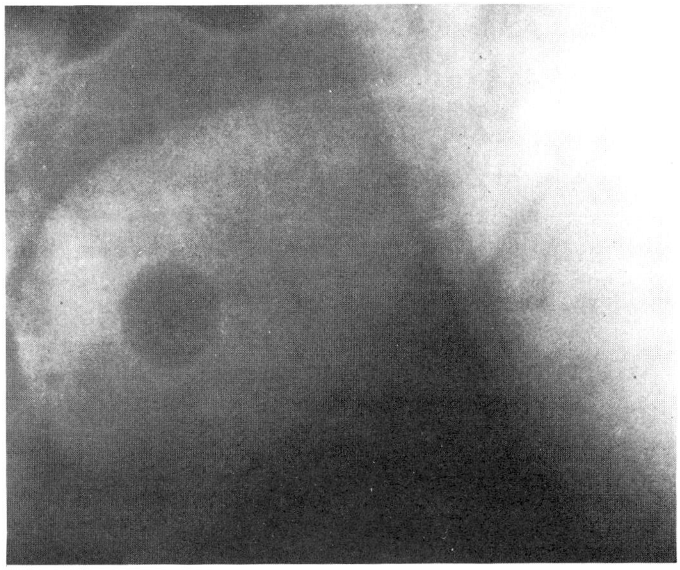

Figure 4—The gas density located in the center of the urinary bladder silhouette on the lateral recumbent survey radiograph represents free intraluminal gas. Prior bladder catheterization, transabdominal cystocentesis, and pneumocystography are common causes of free intraluminal urinary bladder gas.

findings will be described for the following structures: ureters, urinary bladder, and urethra.

Ureters

Vesicoureteral reflux (VUR), although incompletely described, has been reported during cystography and urethrography in cats.[1,2] Information is insufficient to derive meaningful conclusions about the incidence of VUR in normal cats. VUR was encountered in 20 of 53 (37.7%) male and female cats with FUS examined by the authors (Figure 5). Although VUR might theoretically predispose cats with FUS to ascending bacterial infection, this is considered unlikely because of the low incidence of bacterial urinary tract infection present in cats. Focal dilatation of the distal ureter in cats with VUR may be encountered in cats with FUS (Figure 6). Whether this represents a normal variation in anatomy related to overdistention of the urinary bladder or is related to inflammatory ureteral or bladder disease is not known. Other causes of focal or diffuse ureteral dilatation include ureteral ectopia, ureteral calculi, ureteral strictures, and ureteroceles.

Urinary Bladder

The radiographic findings encountered in cats with

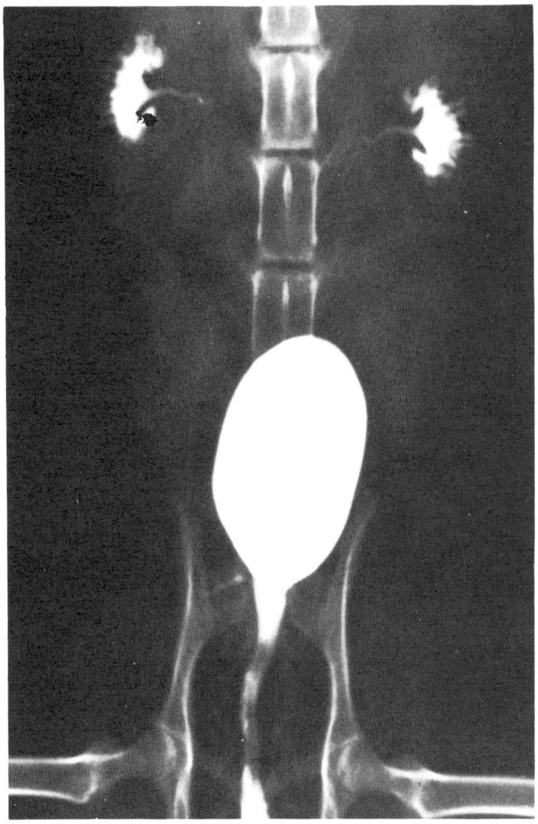

Figure 5—Bilateral vesicoureteral reflux of iodinated contrast medium was encountered during retrograde urethrocystography in a 14-month-old neutered male domestic short-haired cat. The cat had hematuria and dysuria of four months duration and two prior episodes of urethral obstruction. This radiographic finding may or may not be indicative of ascending urinary tract infection.

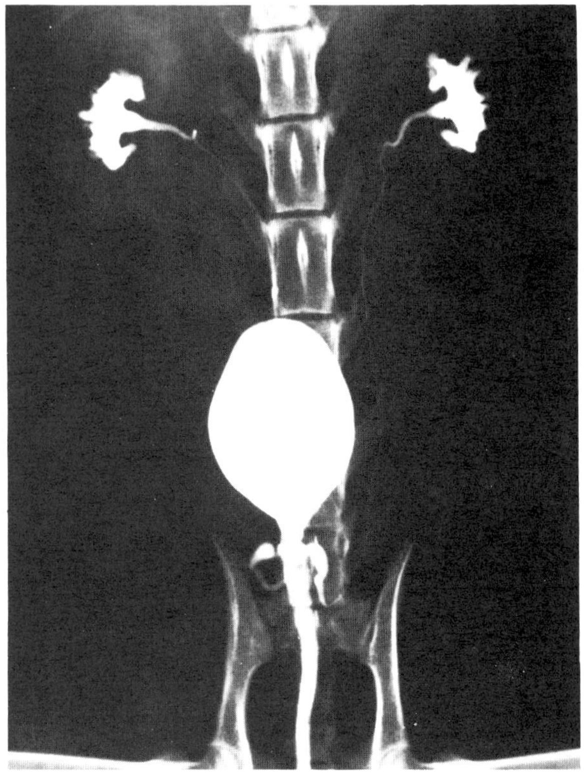

Figure 6—Bilateral focal dilatation of the distal ureters is present with bilateral vesicoureteral reflux during positive contrast cystourethrography in a six-year-old neutered male domestic short-haired cat with intermittent hematuria of several months duration. A perineal urethrostomy had been performed three months previously for episodes of hematuria, dysuria, and stranguria. The cause of localized ureteral dilatation is unknown but may be related to overdistention of a normal urinary bladder or ureteral disease.

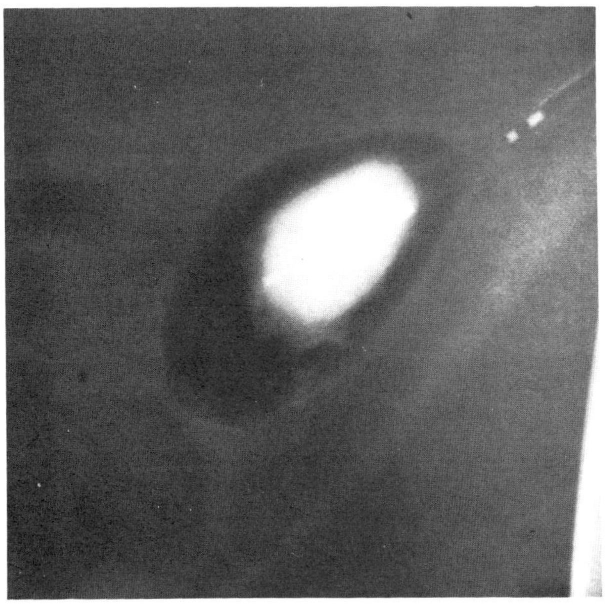

Figure 7A

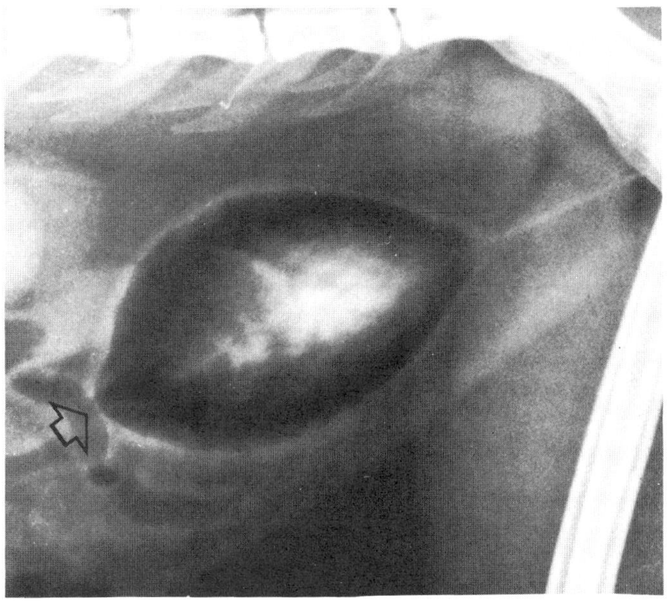

Figure 7B

Figure 7—Mucosal irregularity is frequently present in cats with acute or chronic lower urinary tract disease secondary to neoplastic, infectious, or noninfectious disease. It is best visualized with double contrast cystography and is seen as either a focal or diffuse lesion. **(A)** Focal mucosal irregularity of the cranioventral bladder wall with ulceration was present in an eight-year-old spayed female Siamese cat with hematuria and dysuria of one week duration. **(B)** Diffuse mucosal irregularity and bladder wall thickening are visible in a five-year-old castrated male domestic short-haired cat with hematuria and dysuria of two weeks duration. One episode of urethral obstruction occurred two weeks prior to double contrast cystography. Note the presence of a urachal diverticulum on the cranioventral margin of the urinary bladder *(arrow)*.

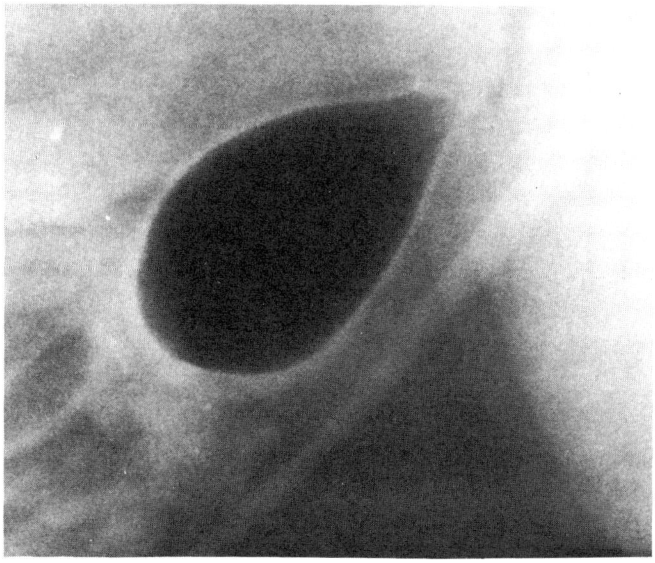

Figure 8A

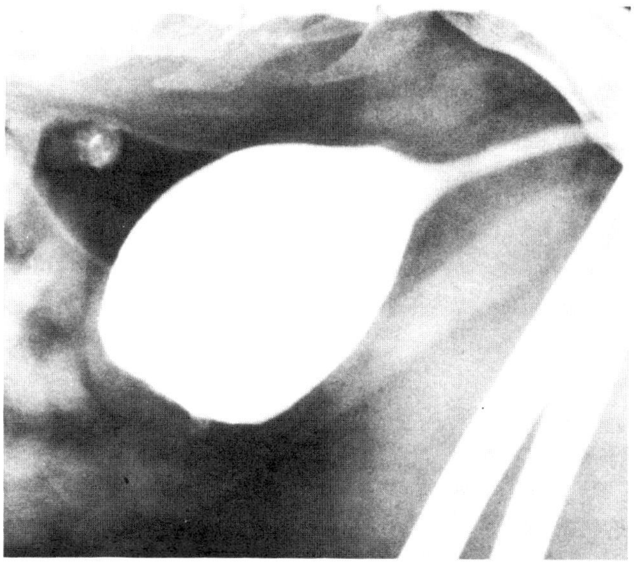

Figure 8B

Figure 8—Mural thickening of the bladder is frequently encountered in cats with lower urinary tract disease and can be due to infectious, noninfectious or neoplastic causes. **(A)** Cranioventral bladder wall thickening is present on pneumocystography in an eight-year-old neutered male cat with hematuria, dysuria, and sterile urine. The cat had a noninfectious, inflammatory cystitis. **(B)** Cranioventral thickening of the bladder wall is visible in an adult male domestic short-haired cat with dysuria and hematuria of two weeks duration. When the clinical signs persisted during medical management of lower urinary disease, the owner requested euthanasia. A transitional cell carcinoma was found.

FUS can vary from no visible radiographic abnormality to severe diffuse involvement of the urinary bladder. For convenience, the radiographic abnormalities encountered in the authors' series of cats with FUS will be described as mucosal or mural lesions or luminal defects.

Mucosal Lesions—Mucosal irregularity may be caused by inflammatory or neoplastic disease. Caution must be exercised in evaluating for mucosal irregularity, because inadequate distention of the urinary bladder can simulate mucosal disease. Although mucosal irregularity can be seen with pneumocystography or positive contrast cystography, subtle lesions are more visible with double contrast cystography. Mucosal lesions are characterized by an irregular interface between the contrast medium and the bladder in the dependent portion of the urinary bladder. Mucosal irregularity may be focal or diffuse (Figure 7). Mucosal ulcerations may be seen in conjunction with mucosal irregularity and are characterized by the ulcerated surface being coated with contrast medium (Figure 7A). Contrast media will also coat the surface of blood clots, and this can simulate ulcerations.

Mural Lesions—If inadequately distended, the normal urinary bladder wall may appear thickened. However, urinary bladder wall thickening may be abnormal and caused by infectious, noninfectious, or neoplastic disease. Therefore, its significance must be evaluated in light of the clinical signs, urine culture, urinalysis, cytology, clinical duration, degree of bladder distention, and prior urethral or bladder instrumentation. Cats with an acute lower urinary tract disease may not have mural or mucosal lesions. The most common location for thickening is the cranioventral bladder wall (Figure 8). Cranioventral bladder thickening is frequently encountered in cats with urachal diverticula. Diffuse mural thickening may be encountered in cats with either acute or chronic lower urinary tract disease. Prolonged bladder distention due to urethral obstruction may result in hemorrhage, edema, and inflammation which can cause diffuse mural thickening (Figure 9). Diffuse cystitis may also be encountered in cats with chronic lower urinary tract disease (Figures 9B and 9C). Diverticula of the urinary bladder may be encountered in male and female cats with lower urinary tract disease and may be congenital or acquired. However, congenital urachal diverticula are considered the most common and may be patent or nonpatent.[4-6] Urachal diverticula have been proposed as significant predisposing factors to lower urinary tract disease.[7] The incidence of urachal anomalies in cats without urinary tract disease is unknown. Pneumocystography or double contrast cystography can demonstrate most urachal diverticula (Figures 7B and 9C), although the smaller diverticula may not be identified unless a positive contrast study is performed (Figure 10). Some urachal diverticula can be difficult to demonstrate by contrast cystography even when a wedge-shaped cranioventral prominence is encountered on survey radiographs. These diverticula may represent stretching of the urachal ligament that attaches the urinary bladder cranioventrally. Urachal diverticula vary markedly in size and shape. They may be wedge-shaped (Figure 7B), pointed (Figure 10A), conical (Figure 10B), or round and cystlike (Figures 9C and 11) and may be associated with attached or free uroliths (Figures 9C and 11A).

Luminal Filling Defects—Luminal filling defects,

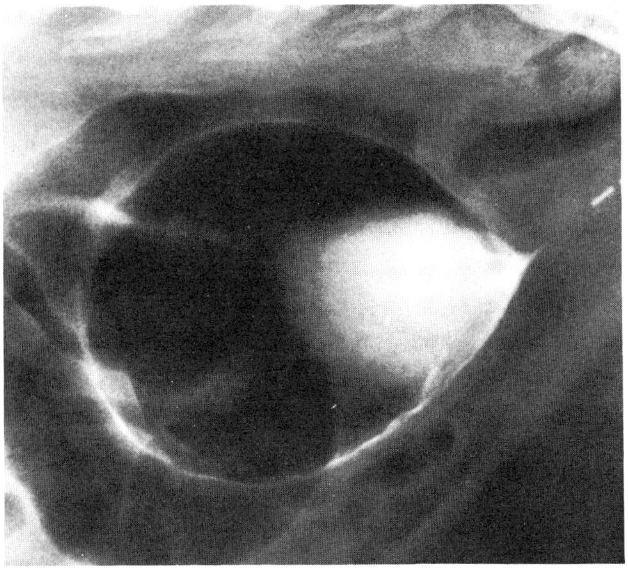

Figure 9A

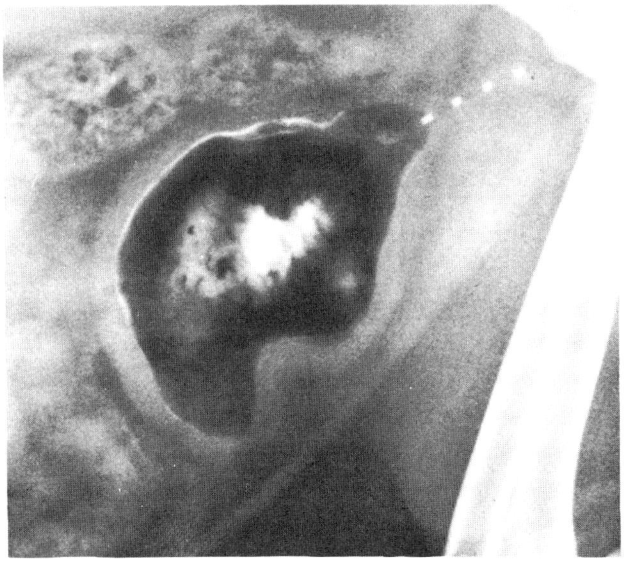

Figure 9B

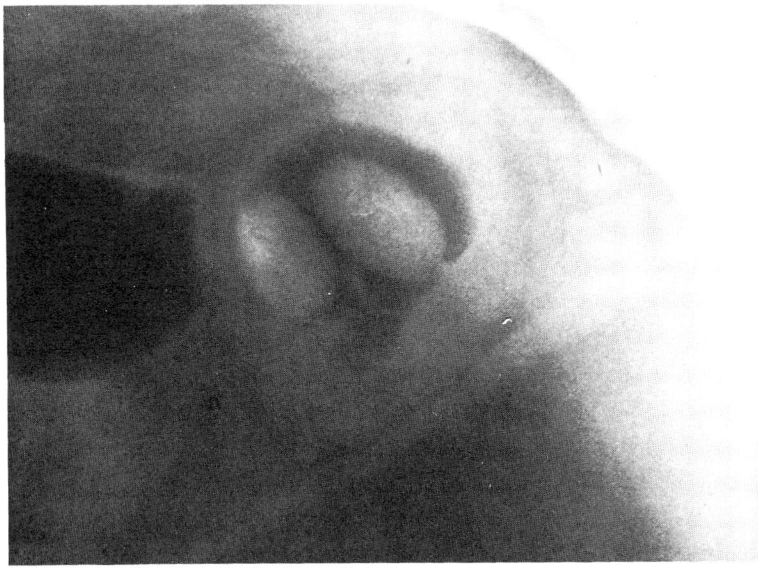

Figure 9C

either free or attached, may be encountered during cystography in cats with lower urinary tract disease. Filling defects are any materials within the bladder that alter normal filling. The differential features of the common filling defects encountered in cats with FUS are listed in Table I.

Free luminal filling defects encountered during cystography in cats with lower urinary tract disease include uroliths (Figures 9C, 11A, and 12), blood clots (Figures 9B and 13), air bubbles (Figure 14), and mucus or matrix plugs (Figures 9B and 15). Uroliths (Figures 11A and 12) and blood clots (Figure 16) may also be attached filling defects. Attached filling defects less frequently encountered during cystography in cats with lower urinary tract disease include neoplasms, submucosal hematomas (Figure 17), polypoid cystitis, ureteroceles and adherent fluid-dense calculi.

Urethra

Urethral abnormalities encountered in the authors' series of cats with FUS include urethral calculi (Figures 10B and 18), urethral strictures (Figure 19), and urethral dilatation (Figures 19 and 20). Female cats are infrequently obstructed by urethral calculi when compared with males. All urethral abnormalities in the authors' prospective evaluation of cats with FUS were confined to males.

Complications

Complications encountered during contrast procedures used for evaluating cats with FUS may be caused

Figure 9—Diffuse thickening of the urinary bladder wall may be encountered in acute or chronic infectious, noninfectious, or neoplastic disease. (**A**) Diffuse mural thickening is seen with double contrast cystography in a six-year-old male domestic short-haired cat five days following relief of urethral obstruction. Overdistention of the urinary bladder of cats may result in urothelial ulcerations, submucosal hemorrhage, edema of the bladder wall, and impaired bladder wall integrity.[3] Radiographically, these lesions are characterized by an increased thickness of the bladder wall. (**B**) Diffuse mural thickening, multiple blood clots, uroliths, and a bladder wall invagination are present in a three-year-old neutered male domestic short-haired cat with hematuria and dysuria of two weeks duration. A perineal urethrostomy for urethral obstruction had been performed five months previously. A second episode of urethral obstruction preceded the survey and uroradiographic contrast studies by four days. A catheterized urine sample was positive for *Proteus mirabilis*. A chronic, necrotic, transmural cystitis was diagnosed histologically. (**C**) Lateral pneumocystogram in a five-year-old male cat with lower urinary tract disease. A perineal urethrostomy had been performed three years previously because of urethral obstruction. Diffuse bladder wall thickening, reduced bladder wall distensibility, two radiopaque cystic uroliths, and a urachal diverticulum are evident. Removal of the penile urethra may alter the normal defense mechanism of the lower urinary tract and predispose the animal to ascending urinary tract infection. Diverticula and other defects may further predispose to urinary tract infection by causing stasis and retention of urine.

TABLE I

Differential Radiographic Characteristics of Intraluminal Filling Defects of the Urinary Bladder

Radiographic Criteria	*Air Bubbles*	*Calculi*	*Sebaceous or Mucous Plugs*	*Blood Clots*
Size	Small to large	Small to large	Small	Small to large
Number	Single, multiple or coalescent	Single or multiple	Single or multiple	Single or multiple
Shape	Commonly round; if coalescing, ovoid or polyhedral	Spheroidal, ovoid, polygonal, pumpkin seed	Spheroidal, ovoid, polygonal, linear	Spheroidal, ovoid, polygonal, linear
Margination	Smooth and distinct	Smooth or irregular, distinct or indistinct	Smooth or irregular, distinct or indistinct	Indistinct and irregular
Location	Commonly at periphery of contrast puddle; if large and coalescing, anywhere	Center of contrast puddle or attached to bladder wall	Center of contrast puddle or attached to bladder wall	Center of contrast puddle or attached to bladder wall
Density				
Survey radiography	Radiolucent	Water-dense (radiolucent) calculi: nondetectable Radiopaque calculi: radiopaque or nondetectable (if small)	Nondetectable	Nondetectable
Pneumocystography	Radiolucent	Water-dense calculi: nondetectable or radiopaque (if attached) Radiopaque calculi: radiopaque	Nondetectable	Nondetectable or radiopaque (attached)
Double contrast cystography	Radiolucent	Water-dense calculi: radiolucent Radiopaque calculi: radiolucent	Radiolucent	Radiolucent
Positive contrast urethrocystography	Radiolucent	Water-dense calculi: radiolucent or nondetectable Radiopaque calculi: radiolucent or nondetectable	Nondetectable	Nondetectable

by the materials or the techniques of cystography and urethrography. These potential complications may compromise the normal defense mechanisms of the urinary system and predispose the patient to urinary tract infection. Fatal complications have not been encountered in the authors' series of cats with FUS.

Materials

Contrast Media

Positive Contrast Media—Meglumine diatrizoate and meglumine iothalamate are triiodinated contrast agents used for cystography and urethrography. Systemic reactions to these radiopaque contrast media are rarely encountered during cystography and urethrography. Local tissue reactions to positive contrast agents have been reported and are related to hyperosmolarity, total volume, method of injection, and duration of contact with the urothelium.[8-12] Concentrations of 5 to 10% of a positive contrast medium are recommended for cystography and are reported to produce minimal inflammatory reaction of the urinary bladder.[8]

Negative Contrast Media—Negative contrast media such as air, carbon dioxide, and nitrous oxide are used in contrast evaluation of lower urinary tract disease. Fatal vascular embolization, an uncommon complication, following pneumocystography with air in dogs and cats, has been reported.[13,14] Carbon dioxide and nitrous oxide are recommended in the presence of urothelial disruption because of their greater solubility in blood compared to that of air. Fatal vascular embolization was not encountered in the authors' series of cats evaluated by pneumocystography or double contrast cystography utilizing air. One case of fatal air embolization following pneumocystography with air was referred to the University of Minnesota Veterinary Hospital for necropsy (Figures 21 and 22).

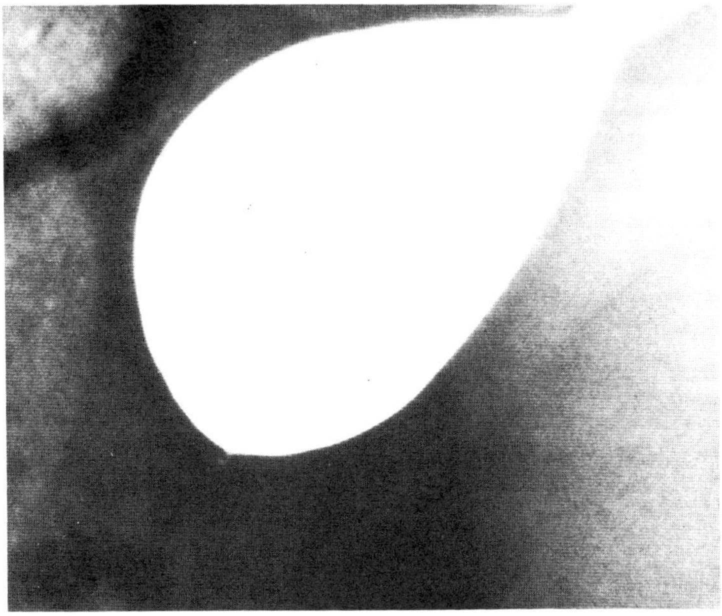

Figure 10A

Figure 10—Some diverticula may be difficult to demonstrate radiographically by pneumocystography or double contrast cystography. (**A**) A small diverticulum was encountered during positive contrast urethrocystography in this one-year-old female Manx cat with intermittent hematuria of one month duration. (**B**) Lateral positive contrast cystogram of the cat in Figure 2. Note cranioventral thickening of the bladder wall in association with a urachal diverticulum and the urethral calculus (*arrow*). Note also that the cystic uroliths visible on the survey radiograph (Figure 2) are obscured by the positive contrast medium.

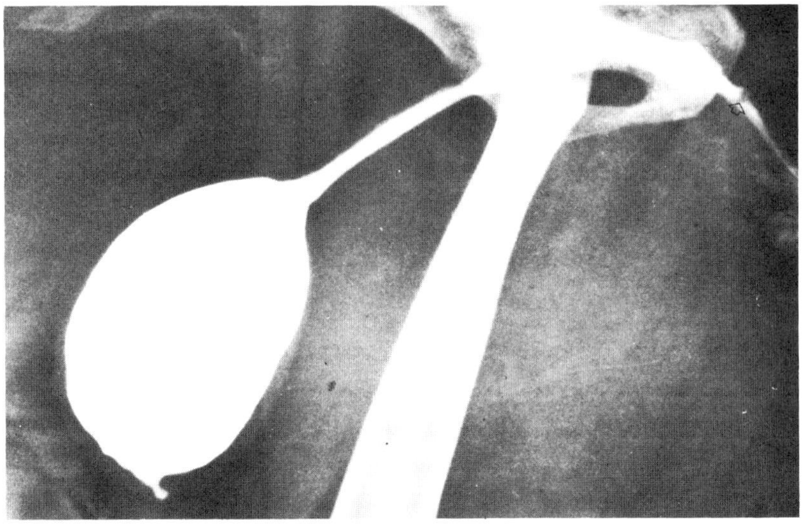

Figure 10B

Figure 11—Urinary bladder diverticula vary in shape, size, and location. (**A**) A cranioventral cystlike diverticulum with cystic uroliths is present in a nine-year-old neutered male domestic long-haired cat. The cat had intermittent lower urinary tract disease of five years duration and no prior history of urethral obstruction. (**B**) A craniolateral cystlike diverticulum is visible in a four-year-old spayed female domestic short-haired cat with hematuria and dysuria of six weeks duration. A surgical biopsy from the resected diverticulum indicated mucosal ulcerations with edema, hyperemia, and hemorrhage. A Gram's stain from the diverticulum revealed no bacteria.

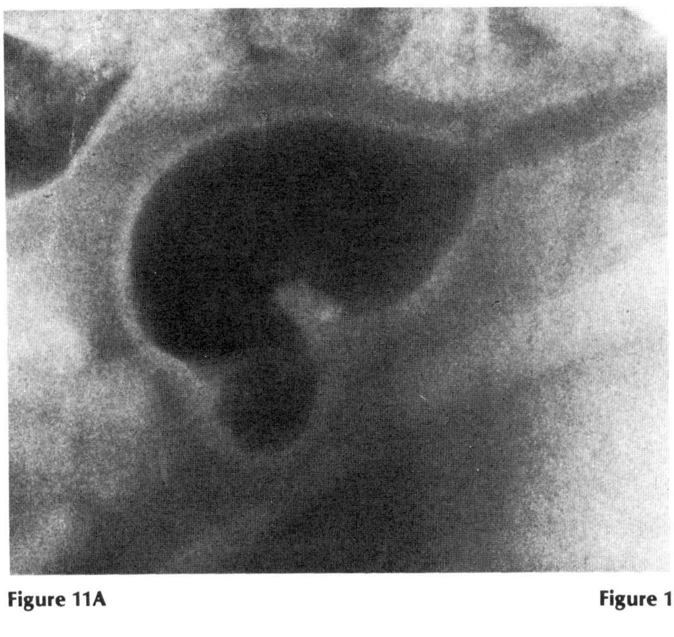

Figure 11A

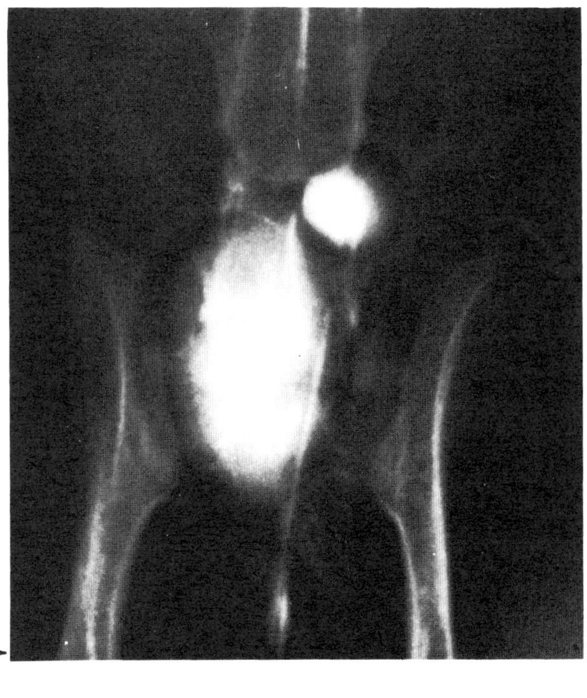

Figure 11B→

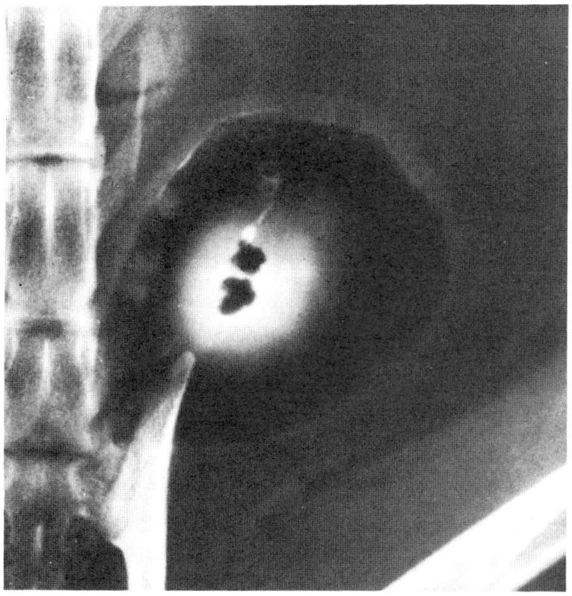

Figure 12—Multiple cystoliths are visible with double contrast cystography in the cat described in Figures 2 and 10B. Variations in radiographic density of calculi are related to their location in relationship to positive or negative contrast media. The urinary bladder wall is also thickened and irregular.

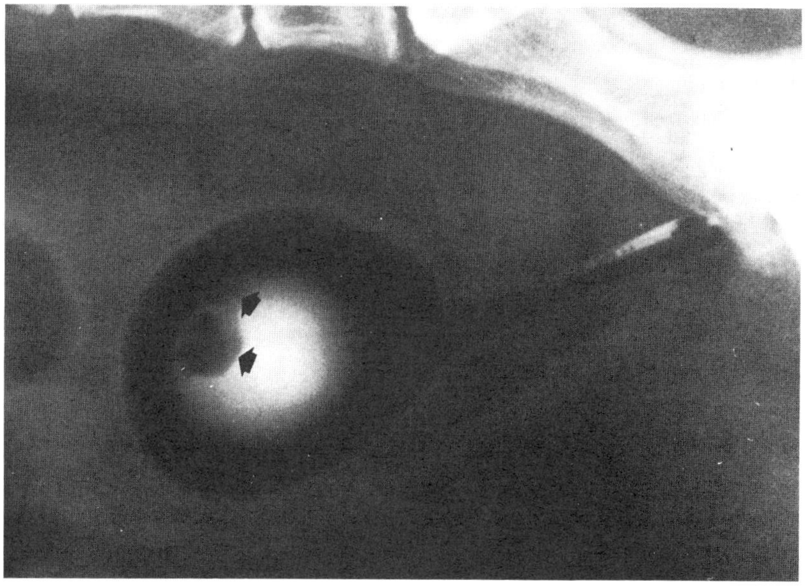

Figure 13—Two free intraluminal filling defects (*arrows*) were visible with double contrast cystography in a six-year-old neutered male Persian cat with intermittent hematuria and dysuria of three years duration. Physical palpation, survey radiography and pneumocystography failed to demonstrate the filling defect. The irregular shape, indistinct borders, and fluid-dense composition of the filling defect are most compatible with blood clots.

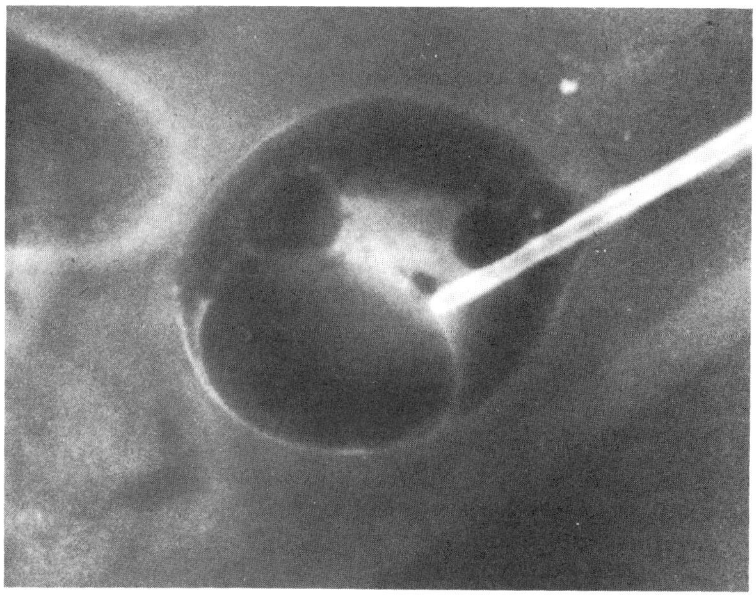

Figure 14—Air bubbles appear as free intraluminal filling defects with positive contrast cystography. Their appearance and location vary depending on the type of contrast medium used and their number and degree of coalescence. Solitary air bubbles are spheroidal and best identified during double contrast cystography at the periphery of the contrast puddle (see Figure 27A). Multiple air bubbles may appear anywhere in the bladder lumen and may be spheroidal, ovoid, or polygonal depending on the degree of coalescence.

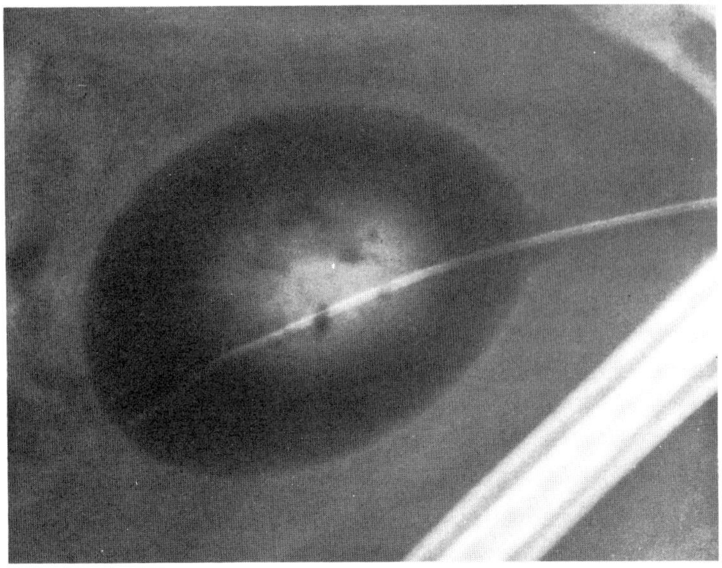

Figure 15—Filling defects are visualized with double contrast cystography in an adult male domestic long-haired cat with hematuria and pollakiuria of six weeks duration. Their variable shapes and irregular, indistinct borders suggest that they are blood clots or mucous plugs. Inability to detect these filling defects during survey radiography and pneumocystography attests to their water density. Mucous and sebaceous plugs, small calculi, and blood clots may be difficult to differentiate radiographically.

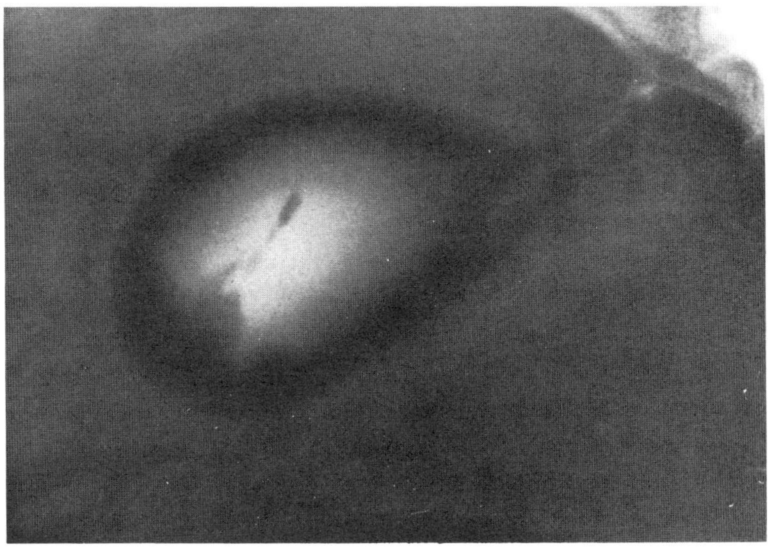

Figure 16—Blood clots visible with cystography may be free intraluminal filling defects (Figure 13) or attached to the bladder wall. Tangential radiographic projections are recommended to optimally demonstrate the site(s) of attachment. Attached filling defects are seen with double contrast cystography in a four-year-old neutered male cat with intermittent hematuria of approximately two years duration. Failure to identify the filling defect by survey radiography or pneumocystography indicates their water composition. Inflammatory polyps or fluid-dense attached calculi must also be considered as radiographic differential diagnoses for the three peripherally located filling defects. The centrally located linear filling defect is a blood clot.

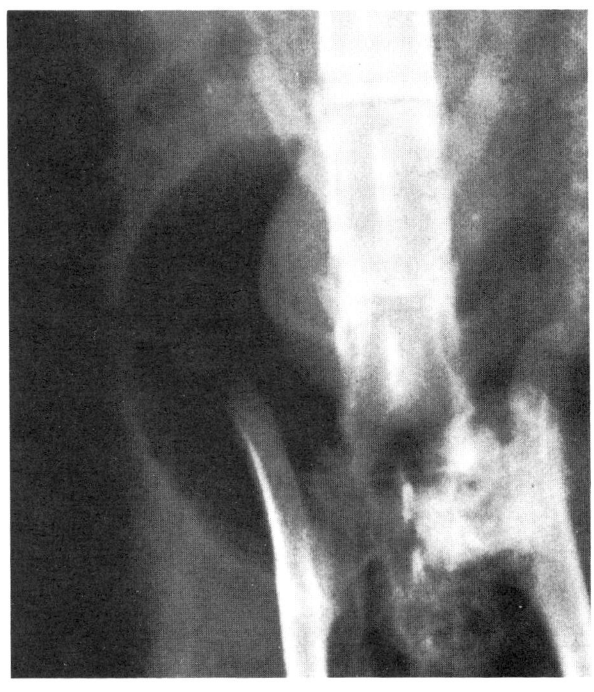

Figure 17—A large soft-tissue-density filling defect is visible with pneumocystography in an 18-month-old neutered male Persian cat with lower urinary tract disease. The histologic diagnosis following surgical resection was an organizing ulcerative submucosal hematoma.

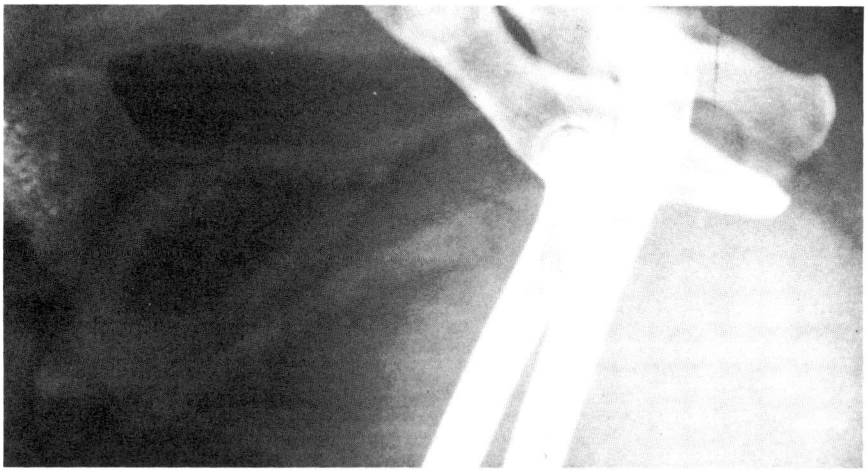

Figure 18—Mutliple cystic calculi and a solitary preprostatic urethral calculus are visible with pneumocystography in a two-year-old male Persian cat with recurrent hematuria following cystotomy for removal of the uroliths. Recurrent urolithiasis must be suspected in cats with clinical recurrence of disease. Although the penile urethra is reported as the most common site of obstruction by calculi, other areas of the urethra may be involved. A perineal urethrostomy may be ineffective if the urethra proximal to the urethrotomy is the site of obstruction.

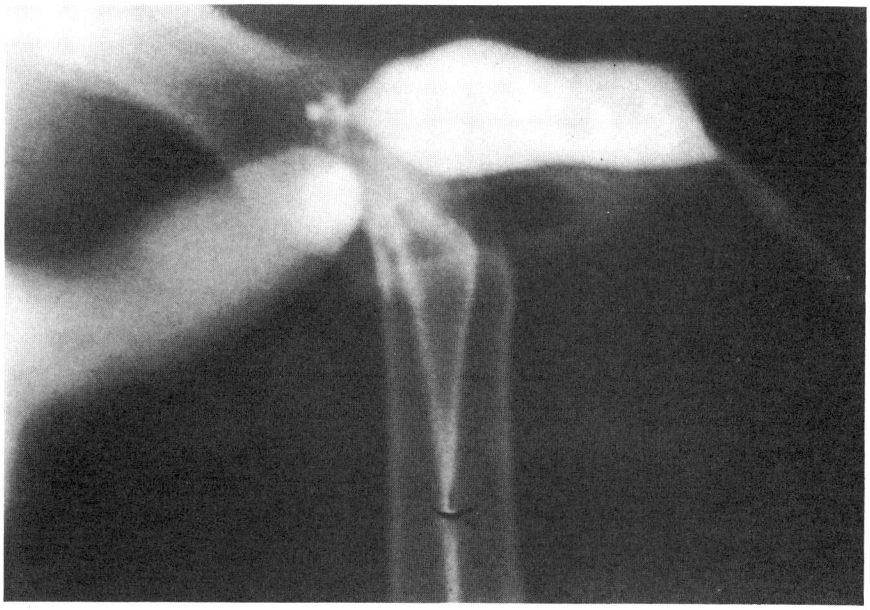

Figure 19—Positive contrast retrograde urethrogram of an eight-month-old male domestic short-haired cat with urinary incontinence and one prior episode of urethral obstruction. Excretory urography excluded ureteral ectopia as the cause of incontinence. Marked urethral dilatation proximal and distal to a stricture in the mid-pelvic urethra is present. On postmortem examination, the stricture was considered congenital.

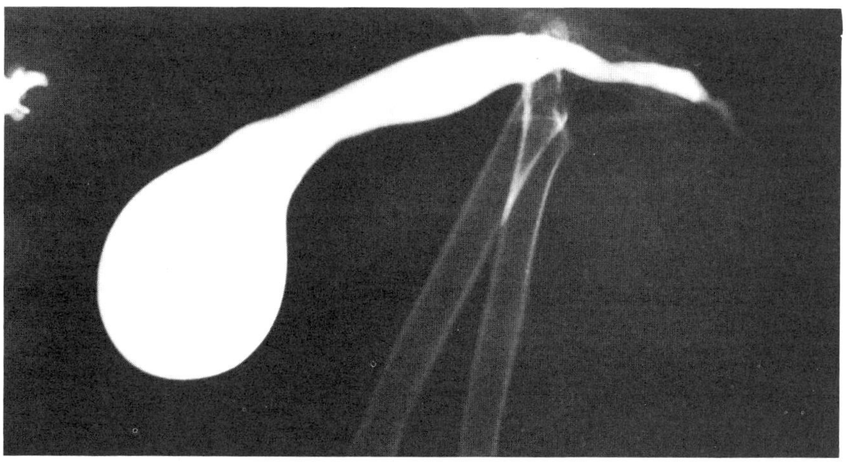

Figure 20—Generalized urethral dilatation is demonstrated with retrograde urethrocystography in the cat described in Figure 1. Histologic diagnosis was a mild inflammatory cystitis. No microscopic urethral lesions were visible. It is not known if the urethral dilatation represented a sequela to chronic partial urethral obstruction or if it was congenital.

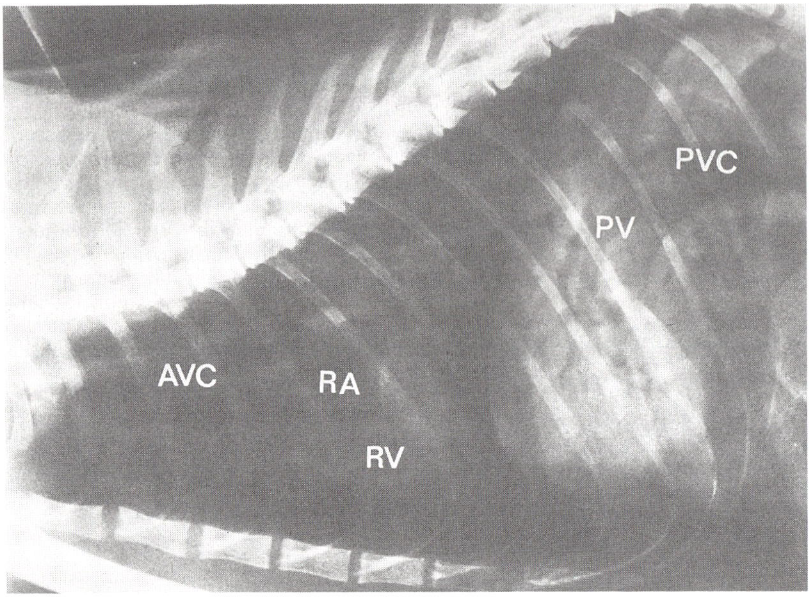

Figure 21—Postmortem radiograph of a four-year-old female domestic short-haired cat that died of vascular air embolism following pneumocystography. Gas is located in the following vascular structures: cranial vena cava (*AVC*), caudal vena cava (*PVC*), hepatic portal veins (*PV*), right atrium (*RA*), and right ventricle (*RV*).

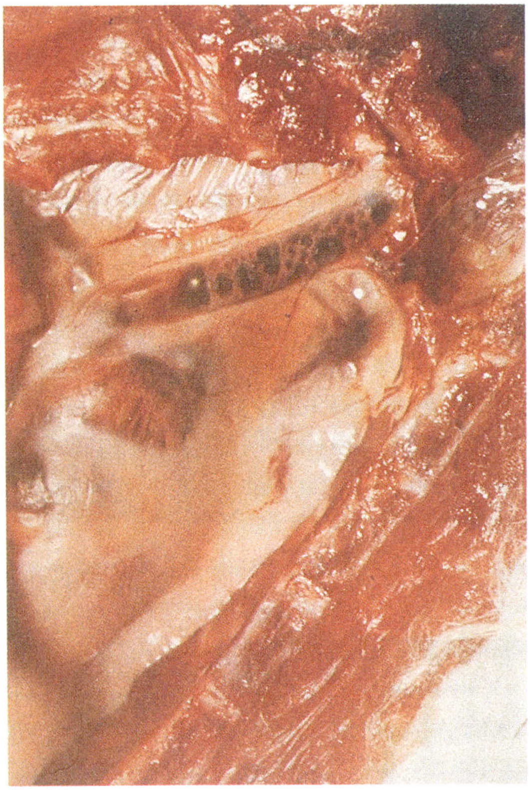

Figure 22A

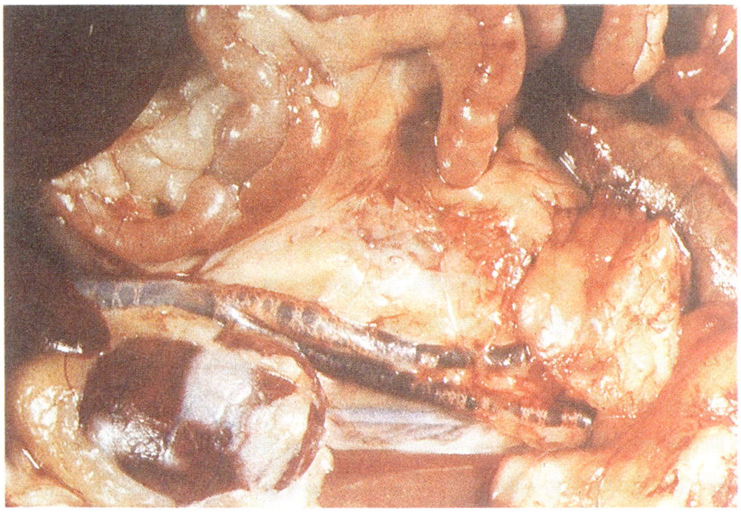

Figure 22B

Figure 22—Necropsy photographs from the cat described in Figure 21. (**A**) Lateral thorax. (**B**) Ventrodorsal abdomen. Note presence of air bubbles in the cranial vena cava (**A**) and portal vein (**B**). The reason for the air in the portal circulation is unknown.

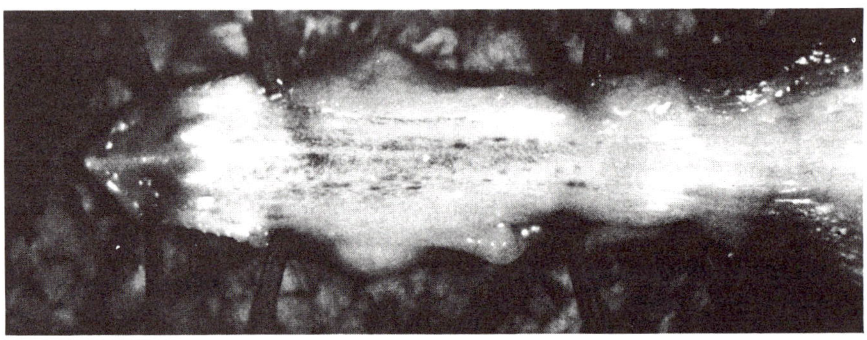

Figure 23—Submucosal urethral hemorrhages are visible in the distal urethra of a normal adult male cat. These lesions were encountered one day following inflation of a balloon catheter for 15 minutes duration in the distal urethra. This is usually considered a reversible complication of balloon catheter urethrography.

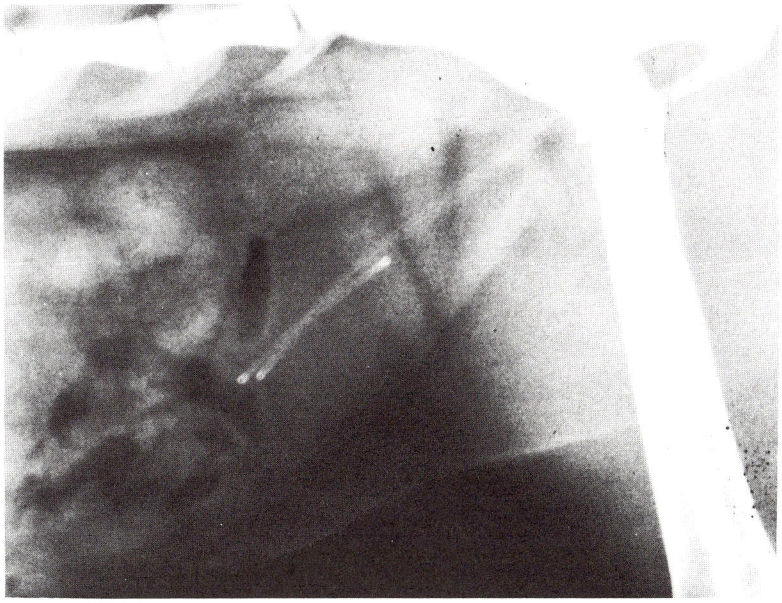

Figure 24—This one-year-old male domestic short-haired cat removed its own stay sutures, which allowed a retrograde migration of the catheter into the bladder. Failure to locate the indwelling catheter by visual examination should alert the clinician that further investigation should be made with survey radiography. Indwelling catheters, particularly in male cats, may allow for ascending bladder infection and a concurrent catheter-induced urethritis.

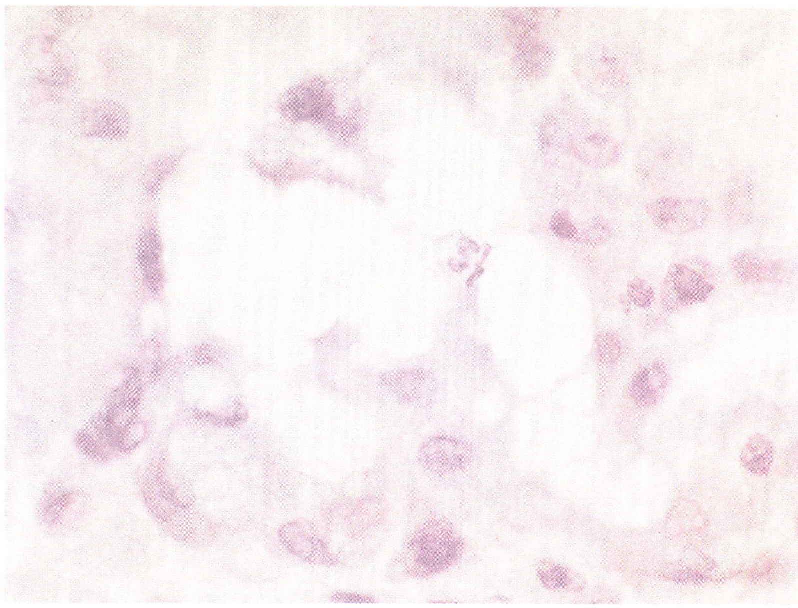

Figure 25—Granulomatous cystitis, characterized histologically by multinucleated giant cells with cytoplasmic inclusions and associated mononuclear inflammatory cell reactions, was encountered in a normal adult female cat following retrograde urethrography where an aqueous lubricant was used as a diluent for the positive contrast medium. Leakage of contrast material into the bladder wall was evident radiographically. (Periodic acid-Schiff stain, original magnification, × 160).

Catheters

Balloon Catheters—Despite the extensive use of balloon-tipped retention catheters for urethrography, there is a paucity of information concerning their potential complications. Submucosal urethral hemorrhages have been reported in the area occupied by an inflated balloon catheter in dogs and cats one day following balloon inflation for 15 minutes (Figure 23).[3] Similar lesions were not encountered in dogs or cats examined 14 days post-balloon inflation[3] for 15 minutes duration, which indicates the reversibility of the urethral lesions resulting from the inflated balloon catheter.

Nonballoon Catheters—Complications resulting from nonballoon catheters may be related to several variables including patient susceptibility, catheter material, catheter size, duration of catheterization, method of urine drainage, and concomitant use of antimicrobial agents.[15]

Catheter kinking or improper placement of a stiff, nonflexible urethral catheter may result in iatrogenic trauma to the urinary bladder or urethra. Mucosal ulcerations and submucosal hemorrhage may reduce the natural defense mechanisms of the lower urinary tract and predispose to infection. Urethral trauma has

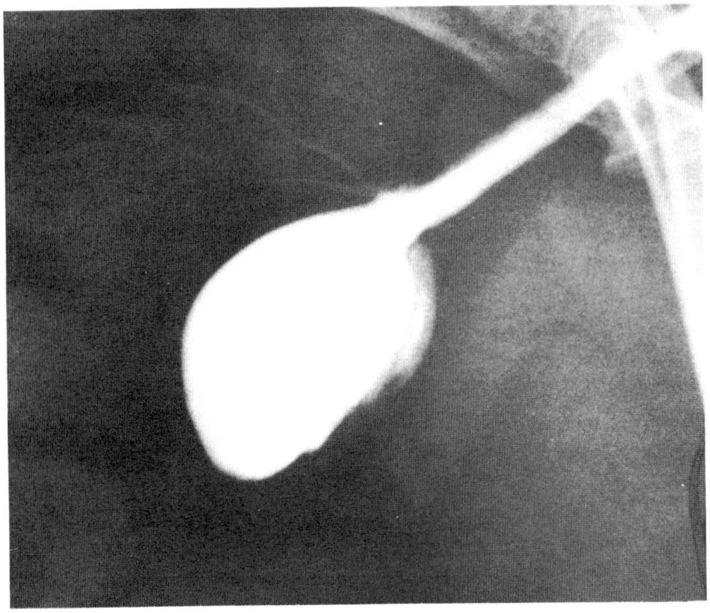

Figure 26A

Figure 26—Acute overdistention of a normal or abnormal urinary bladder during cystography or urethrography in cats can result in (**A**) mural leakage, with confinement of the contrast medium inside the serosal surface, or (**B**) complete disruption of the bladder wall, with escape of the bladder contents into the peritoneal cavity. Cats with lower urinary tract disease may be predisposed to urinary bladder discontinuity because of existing inflammatory disease. Infusion of the urinary bladder in cats with FUS should proceed slowly with external palpation, pericatheter reflux, and retrograde pressure on the syringe plunger as criteria for maximum bladder distention. Note bilateral ureterovesical reflux in **A**.

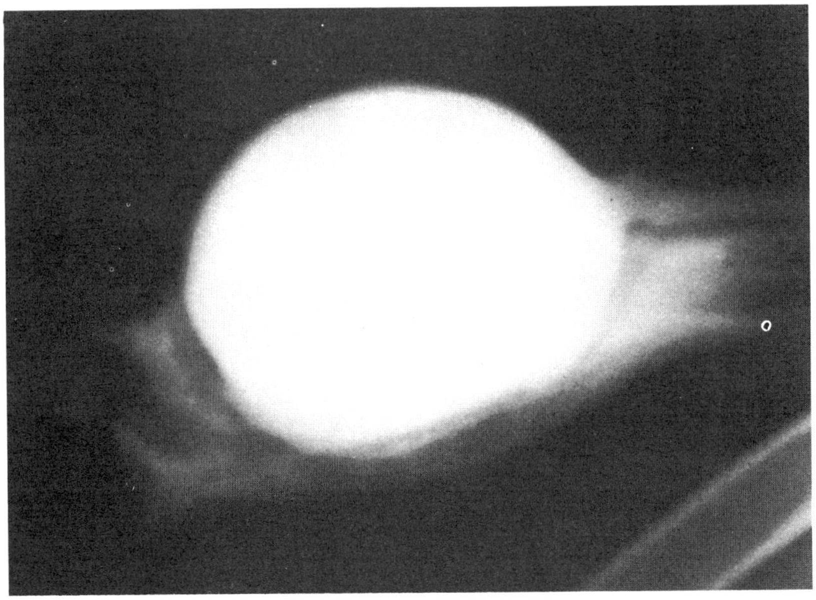

Figure 26B

been infrequently encountered in cats with FUS evaluated by the authors. Coating the catheter with an aqueous lubricant prior to insertion has reduced the occurrence of this complication. The use of soft rubber catheters also minimizes urethral or bladder trauma.

Suture material used to secure an indwelling catheter may be removed by the obstinate patient, and this may result in a retrograde migration of the urethral catheter into the urinary bladder (Figure 24).

Aqueous Lubricants

Surgical lubricating jellies are used to facilitate urethral instrumentation and add viscosity to radiopaque contrast media. Two reports have implicated surgical lubricants in the cause of urethral foreign body granulomas in humans following urethral instrumentation.[16,17] Experimental injection of an aqueous lubricant in laboratory animals has evoked a similar tissue response.[18,19] A similar tissue response in dogs and cats was encountered following retrograde urethrography where an aqueous lubricant was used as a diluent (Figure 25).[3] It is not known whether the granulomatous reaction encountered in these tissues was caused by the aqueous lubricant or other unknown factors. The information, although limited, suggests that these products are not as innocuous as they have been previously suspected to be.

Topical Anesthetics

Topical anesthetics are used to facilitate human and

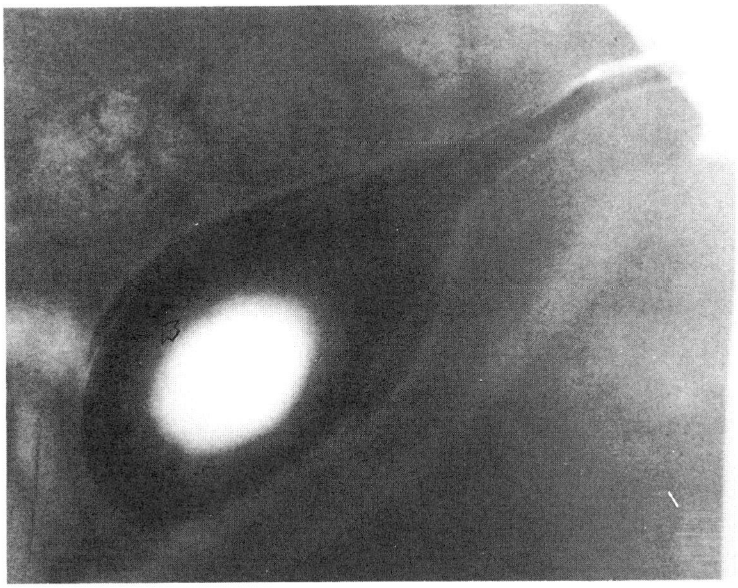

Figure 27A

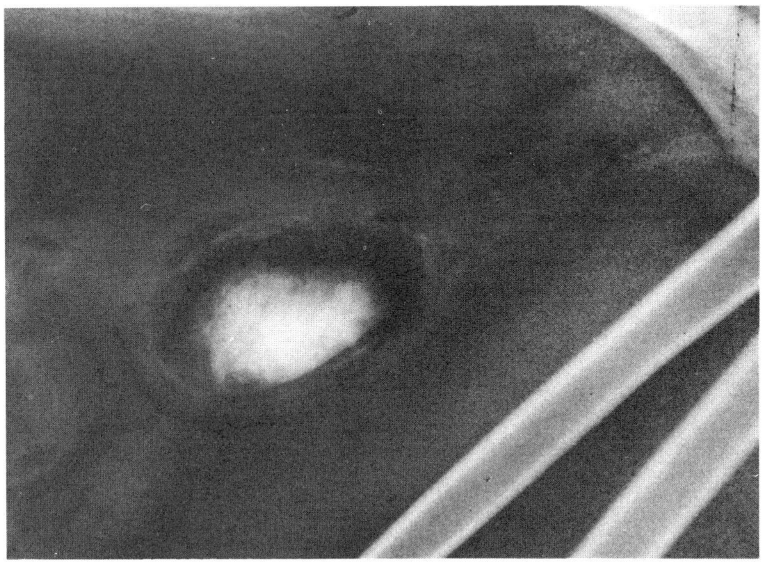

Figure 27B

Figure 27—Emphysematous cystitis may be encountered with bacterial cystitis and other bladder diseases or may be iatrogenic and related to improper use of urinary catheters. Emphysematous cystitis may vary from focal elevations of the urothelium (**A**), to diffuse transmural involvement of the entire wall of the urinary bladder (**B**). Note the presence of air bubbles (*arrows*) at the periphery of the contrast puddle in **A**.

veterinary urologic procedures. Lidocaine hydrochloride is available as a urologic jelly or as an aqueous preparation. Systemic reactions to lidocaine hydrochloride are characterized by central nervous system excitation and cardiovascular depression but are infrequently encountered in humans.[20] Systemic toxicity to lidocaine hydrochloride is variable, depending on the route and speed of administration. Blood levels have not been determined after application of lidocaine to urothelial membranes. To avert potential complication, doses less than 4.5 mg/kg (2 mg/lb) are recommended for cats. Adverse reaction to intravesical infusion of lidocaine hydrochloride has not been encountered by the authors.

Techniques of Urethrocystography

Overdistention

Acute distention of the urinary bladder during cystography or urethrocystography may result in lesions to the urinary bladder and/or urethra. High intravesical pressure and rapid distention of the urinary bladder may impair circulation and can lead to ischemia, venous stasis, and tissue necrosis.[21,22] Overdistention may result in tears in the urothelium, connective tissue, smooth muscle, and blood vessels, thereby predisposing to bladder wall discontinuity.[22] These lesions may compromise the defense mechanisms of the urinary tract and predispose to lower urinary tract infection. Intravesical volumes recommended for cystography and urethrography in dogs and cats vary from 6.6 to 11.1 ml/kg (3 to 5 ml/lb). These volumes may be excessive for cats with lower urinary tract disease and may result in bladder rupture. Radiographically, bladder rupture may vary from mural leakage, with confinement of the contrast medium inside the serosal surface, to complete mural tears, with escape of contrast medium into the peritoneal space (Figure 26).

Macroscopic hematuria is the most frequently encountered complication immediately following cystography and urethrography in male and female cats with FUS. However, the hematuria is temporary and usually subsides in three to five days. Similar findings have been reported in normal dogs and cats following acute bladder distention during retrograde urethrography.[3]

Emphysematous Cystitis

Iatrogenic emphysematous cystitis due to the radiographic procedures has been encountered in cats and may range from focal to diffuse elevation of the urothelium to a transmural involvement of all layers of the urinary bladder (Figure 27). Catheter trauma to the urinary bladder mucosa or concurrent inflammatory bladder disease may predispose to vascular embolization of a negative contrast medium. The patient should be closely monitored for cardiovascular collapse if emphysematous cystitis is identified.

Iatrogenic Urinary Tract Infection

Iatrogenic urinary tract infection (UTI) is a serious potential complication of cystography and urethrography in dogs and cats. Potential pathogenic microbes may enter the urinary bladder by several routes. Transport of microbes by the catheter into the bladder during catheterization is considered the common route of infection.[15] Presence of the normal bacterial flora in the distal urethral mucosa results in the transport of some organisms into the bladder whenever a urinary catheter is used but can be minimized by the use of sterilized catheters and aseptic catheterization techniques. Microbes may also ascend through the catheter lumen when a nonsterile catheter or syringe serves as a source of microbial contamination. Motile bacteria may enter the urinary bladder in the absence of retrograde flow if a continuous column of urine exists in the catheter between the source of contamination and the bladder.[15] Motile bacteria may also ascend the urethral lumen around the outside of the urethral catheter. Compromise of the normal bladder defense mechanisms by catheter trauma or overdistention may further predispose to infection.

Radiographic evaluation of male cats with indwelling urethral catheters for relief of urethral obstruction presents several potential problems to the clinician. Catheter-induced urethritis and bacterial cystitis have been reported in male cats after placement of indwelling urethral catheters.[15,23] These cats may represent a high-risk population predisposed to urinary tract infection because of the presence of the indwelling catheter.

REFERENCES

1. Kipnis RM: Vesicouretheral reflux in a cat. *JAVMA* 167(4):288-292, 1975.
2. Farrow CS: Retrograde urography in the cat. *VM SAC* 69:435-437, 1974.
3. Johnston GR: *Retrograde Contrast Urethrography in the Dog and Cat: Complications and Morphologic Evaluation.* Master thesis, University of Minnesota, 1979.
4. Green RW, Bohning RH, Jr: Patent persistent urachus associated with urolithiasis in a cat. *JAVMA* 158:489, 1971.
5. Hansen JS: Patent urachus in a cat. *VM SAC* 67:379, 1972.
6. Hansen JS: Persistent urachal ligament in a cat. *VM SAC* 67:1090, 1972.
7. Hansen JS: Urachal remnant in the cat: Occurrence and relationship to the feline urological syndrome. *VM SAC* 72:1735-1746, 1977.
8. Breton L, Pennock PW, Valli VE: The effects of Hypaque 25% and sodium iodide 10% in the canine urinary bladder. *J Am Vet Radiol Soc* 19:116, 1978.
9. McAlister WH, Palmer K: The histologic effects of four commonly used media for excretory urography and an attempt to modify the responses. *Radiology* 99:511, 1971.
10. McAlister WH, Shackelford GD, Kissone J: The histologic effects of 30% Cystokon, Hypaque 25%, and Renografin-30 in the bladder. *Radiology* 104:563, 1972.
11. Neustein DH, Herman JR: New urethral anesthetic, clinical evaluation employing new method. *NY State J Med* 67:1401, 1967.
12. Sie CM, Dunbar JS, Wright VJ, Hardwick DF: Contrast media used in cystourethrography. *Invest Urol* 12:434, 1975.
13. Ackerman N, Wingfield WE, Corley EA: Fatal air embolization associated with pneumourethrography. *JAVMA* 160:1616, 1972.
14. Zontine WJ, Andrews LK: Fatal air embolization as a complication of pneumocystography in two cats. *J Am Vet Radiol Soc* 19:8, 1978.
15. Lees GE, Osborne CA: Urinary tract infections associated with the use and misuse of urinary catheters. *Vet Clin North Am* 9(4):713-727, 1979.
16. Climie ARW: Periurethral granuloma due to lubricating jelly. *Harper Hosp Bull* 20:226, 1962.
17. Reed RJ, Smith JL, Sternberg WH: Granulomas induced by surgical lubricating jelly. *Am J Clin Pathol* 36:41, 1961.
18. Blaine G: Experimental observations on absorbable alginate products in surgery. *Ann Surg* 125:102, 1947.
19. Richards CE: Visco-Rayopake in cystourethrography. *J Urol* 58:185, 1947.
20. Covino BG: Systemic toxicity of local anesthetic agents. *Anesth Analg* 57:387, 1978.
21. Finkbeinder A, Lapides J: Effect of distention on blood flow in the dog's urinary bladder. *Invest Urol* 12:210, 1974.
22. Mehrotra RML: An experimental study of the vesical circulation during distention and in cystitis. *J Pathol Bacteriol* 66:79, 1953.
23. Lees GE, Osborne CA, Stevens JB, Ward GE: Adverse effects of open indwelling urethral catheterization in clinically normal male cats. *Am J Vet Res* 42:825, 1981.

Diagnosis and Surgical Management of Osteochondritis Dissecans of the Elbow Joint

J. L. Berzon, DVM
Diplomate, ACVS
Veterinary Specialists of Connecticut
New Britain, Connecticut[a]

Lamenesses that affect the front (pectoral) limbs of actively growing, large dogs are common. Differential diagnoses of metabolic disease processes that affect the elbow joint include the following: osteochondritis dissecans of the medial humeral condyle, fragmented coronoid process, subluxation (elbow dysplasia) caused by asymmetrical growth of the radius and ulna, ununited anconeal process, and ununited medial epicondyle. Several of these conditions result from an abnormal cartilage maturation disturbance called *osteochondrosis*. When a loose or free flap develops over a subchondral osteochondritis defect, the defect is referred to as *osteochondritis dissecans*. Diagnosis of osteochondritis dissecans is based on age, breed, sex, history, and physical and radiographic findings.

The following is a report of osteochondritis dissecans of the distal medial humeral condyle with emphasis on diagnosis and surgical treatment.

A six-month-old, male black Labrador retriever was presented for evaluation of a chronic, weight-bearing, left-forelimb lameness. Physical examination disclosed mild joint effusion of the left elbow joint. Deep pain was elicited by directly palpating the medial joint surfaces and by full extension of the elbow. Analgesics used by other veterinarians that had been consulted only resulted in transient relief of clinical signs.

Radiographs of the affected elbow joint (Figures 1 and 2) revealed a large osteochondritis dissecans lesion and a large, free fragment (joint mouse). Radiographs of the opposite elbow and shoulders were within normal limits. Exploratory surgery of the affected joint was scheduled for the following day.

The patient was preanesthetized with atropine[b] (0.02 mg/kg SQ) and acepromazine[c] (0.02 mg/kg SQ). Induction was completed 30 minutes later with Bio-tal®[d] (10 mg/kg IV); the patient was then intubated and maintained on a semiclosed anesthetic system using a halothane[e]-oxygen mixture. The affected limb was then clipped and scrubbed with Betadine®.[f] Following an orthopedic draping, the medial aspect of the elbow joint was exposed via a 10-cm curved skin incision over the medial humeral epicondyle. An orthopedic stockinette was sewn into place. The median vein, artery, and nerve were located at the cranial margin of the proposed osteotomy site to avoid inadvertent injury. The epicondyle was palpated and predrilled with a 2.0-mm drill. The proximal portion was then overdrilled with a 2.7-mm drill for placement of a lag screw at the time of closure and to ensure exact screw placement prior to osteotomy. The epicondyle was osteotomized with a 10-mm Richards osteotome[g] on its cranial, dorsal, and caudal margins. This allowed the flexor muscles and origin of the medial collateral ligament and joint capsule to be elevated and retracted caudodistally to expose the medial joint surfaces (Figure 3). The large, free fragment was visualized and removed as well as the flap still attached over the osteochondral defect (Figure 4). The osteochondritis dissecans defect was curetted down to a bleeding surface and smoothed with a bone rasp along its edges. The joint was thoroughly irrigated with saline to remove all debris and any additional fragments.

The epicondyle was then reapproximated and held in

[a]Veterinary Specialists of Connecticut is now located in West Hartford, Connecticut.

[b]Professional Veterinary Laboratories, Minneapolis, MN 55437.
[c]Fort Dodge Laboratories, Fort Dodge, IA 50501.
[d]Bio-Ceutic Laboratories, Inc., St. Joseph, MO 64502.
[e]Halocarbon Lab., Hackensack, NJ 08876.
[f]The Purdue Frederick Co., Norwalk, CT 06856.
[g]Richards Manufacturing Co., Inc., Memphis, TN 38116.

Originally published in Volume 5, Number 4, April 1983

place with one large 0.0625 Kirschner wire. The drill hole was tapped with a 2.7-mm ASIF cortical tap, and a 2.7-mm screw and spiked washer were used to secure the fragment in place (Figure 5). (The washer prevents the screw head from sinking into the small epicondylic fragment.)

The screw and washer were covered by closing the fascial layers with 2-0 Vicryl™.[h] The skin was closed routinely with 2-0 Supramid Extra[i] and placed in a modified Robert Jones dressing to control swelling and minimize movement. Postoperative radiographs show accurate screw placement and absence of any fragments (Figure 6).

Suture and bandage removal were performed 10 days postoperatively. Restricted exercise, consisting of leash walking and gentle passive physiotherapy, were advised for four to six weeks until the osteotomy healed. Radiographs at six weeks disclosed good bone healing and no distraction of the osteotomy. Limb usage gradually improved, and at three months the patient was up to a normal exercise level with no clinical signs of lameness.

[h]Ethicon Inc./Pitman-Moore, Washington Crossing, NJ 08560.
[i]S. Jackson, Inc., Alexandria, VA 22303.

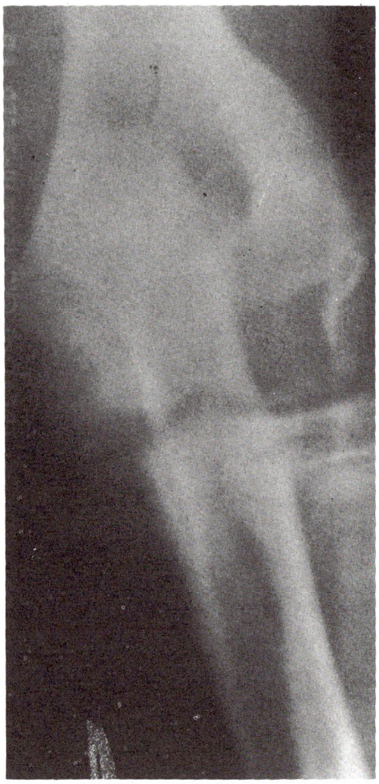

Figure 1—Craniocaudal view of the left elbow joint reveals a large osteochondritis dissecans defect (with large detached fragment) involving the distal medial humeral condyle.

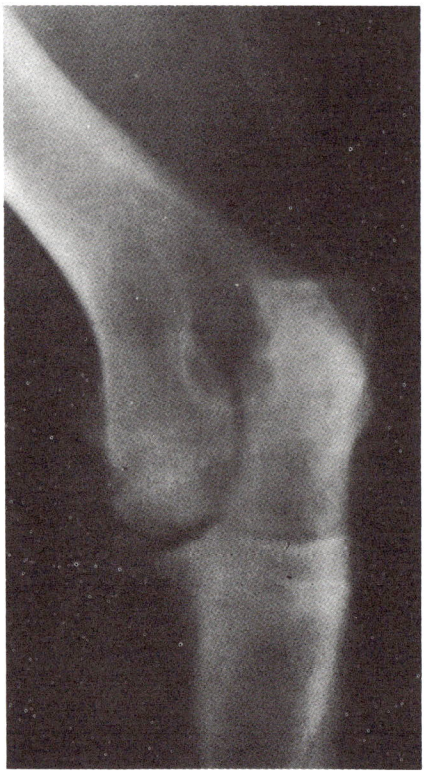

Figure 2—An oblique view of the elbow demonstrates the free fragment and osteochondritis dissecans defect.

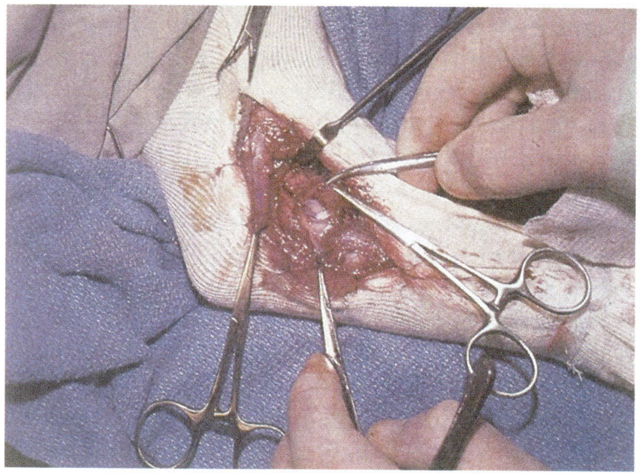

Figure 3—Following completion of the osteotomy, the flexor muscles and origin of the medial collateral ligament are retracted caudodistally to expose the medial articular surfaces.

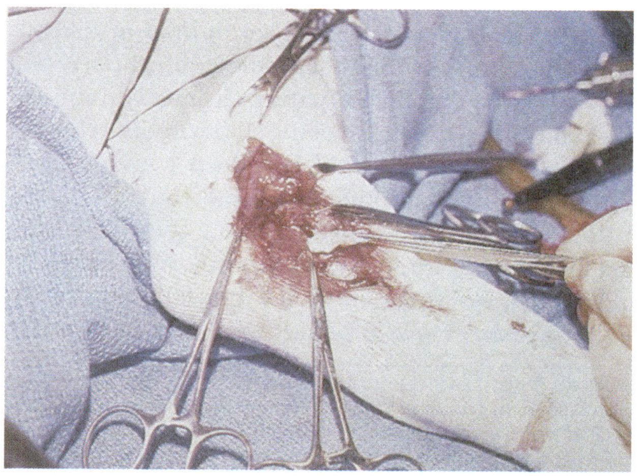

Figure 4—A large free fragment is extracted from the medial compartment of the elbow joint. In this dog, two large osteochondral fragments acting as joint mice (one, 2½ × 2½ cm; the other, ½ × ½ cm) were extracted.

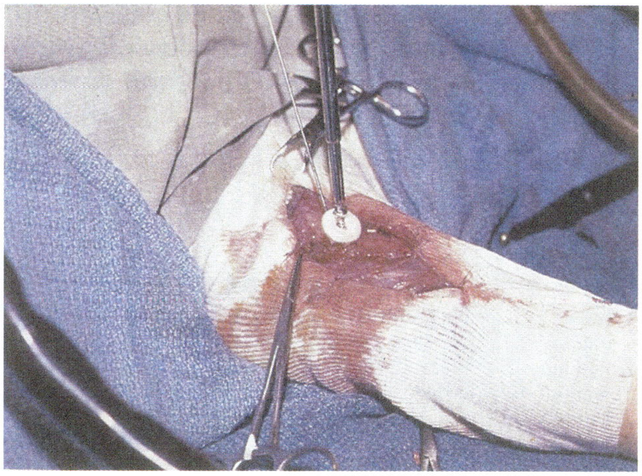

Figure 5—Following a complete joint flush, the predrilled epicondyle is replaced, tapped, and screwed into place using a spiked washer (Kirschner wire is used to hold the epicondyle in place while the screw is placed). The deep and superficial fascial layers are closed to protect the screw head washer from resting directly under the medial skin incision.

Discussion

Osteochondritis dissecans is a well-documented skeletal disorder in growing animals. It has a multitude of potential causes including the following: trauma (microfracture of the articular surfaces), overnutrition, rapid growth and weight gain, environmental factors (e.g., surfaces upon which animals are raised), and interference with the normal ossification of cartilage (endochondral).[1-6]

As they ossify, chondrocytes normally proliferate from the epiphyseal area toward the metaphysis. The growth plate, consisting of layers of chondrocytes, usually maintains a uniform thickness because of the constant state of endochondral ossification occurring on the metaphyseal side of the epiphyseal plate.[7,8] Osteochondrosis is a disturbance of this process in which the articular cartilage displays an irregular arrangement of cells; normal proliferation and differentiation, which allow for ossification, fail to occur. As a direct result, certain areas of articular surface develop abnormally thick zones, and normal bone formation is interrupted. As surrounding areas of normal cartilage ossify, these abnormally thickened areas of cartilage become isolated. These areas are structurally weaker and often develop fissures or cracks within the deep layers. If these fissures reach the articular surface, debris from subchondral clefts and necrotic cartilage are released into the joint space, causing inflammation. This newly opened fissure of cartilage technically represents osteochondrosis. Free flaps of cartilage may form over the defect or may detach and float freely in the joint (joint mice). Environmental influences and repeated microtrauma cause further cleavage and disruption. Healing usually will not take place if a cleaved portion of cartilage remains in place.

Osteochondritis dissecans has been diagnosed in the dog, horse, pig, chicken, cat, and cow.[1-8] It has been reported to affect males more commonly than females (5:3). The age of onset is usually between 3 and 12 months. Breeds of dogs known to be affected include the Bernese Mountain dog, Labrador retriever, dalmatian, golden retriever, Great Dane, boxer, German shorthaired pointer, standard poodle, Old English sheepdog, greyhound, German shepherd, rottweiler, Rhodesian Ridgeback, Great Pyrenees, English setter, Irish setter, cocker spaniel, English springer spaniel, St. Bernard, Newfoundland, Irish wolfhound, whippet, Vizsla, Scottish terrier, border collie, and bull mastiff. Lameness can be uni- or bilateral and is usually seen as a weight-bearing lameness with a gradual onset. Affected animals are markedly lame after extended periods of exercise. Physical examination of involved joints is usually painful on direct palpation and manipulation. Disuse atrophy and joint effusion occur late in the course of disease in association with the development of secondary degenerative osteoarthrosis. Sites of occurrence for osteochondritis dissecans are the following (in order of most common to least): shoulder (caudomedial aspect of the proximal articular surface of the humerus), elbow joint (lateral surface of the medial humeral condyle), stifle joint (medial surface of the lateral femoral condyle), and hock (medial ridge of the medial condyle of the tibial tarsal bone). Osteochondritis dissecans has also been incriminated by some investigators to be the predisposing cause for ununited anconeal process, fragmented coronoid process, aseptic necrosis of the femoral head, retained endochondral cartilage of the distal ulna, hip dysplasia, and other conformational defects (e.g., genu valgum and patellar trochlear hypoplasia).[7-9]

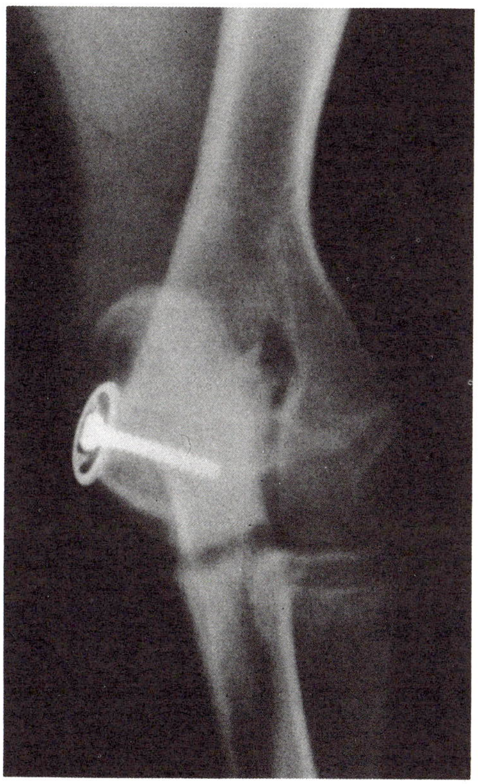

Figure 6—Postoperative craniocaudal view showing screw placement and removal of all fragments.

Conservative management consisting of rest and confinement is used in patients with mild clinical signs and small radiographic lesions with no demonstrable fragments. (Radiographs of both limbs should always be taken for comparison, despite absence of lameness.) Surgical therapy consisting of an exploratory arthrotomy with removal of all free fragments and curettage of the lesion is recommended in all patients with moderate to severe clinical signs, especially those with radiographic evidence of cartilaginous flaps or free fragments.[1]

Summary

Osteochondritis dissecans of the elbow joint is diagnosed by physical and radiographic examination of the affected limb. Surgical therapy is indicated at all times in this joint to restore a more normal articular surface and minimize the potential for secondary degenerative joint disease to develop. Surgical exposure is achieved by osteotomy of the medial humeral epicondyle as described.[10,11] This technique is fast and easy and provides excellent exposure for the complete surveillance of the joint. Replacement of the osteotomy can also be achieved with the use of multiple small Kirschner wires instead of a lag screw technique.

Exercise should be restricted postoperatively for a minimum of four to six weeks to allow the osteotomy site adequate time for healing. Prognosis for soundness is good to excellent if minimal joint disease has occurred at the time of surgical intervention. Patients with moderate to severe degenerative joint disease also appear to benefit. Periodic use of analgesics may still be necessary to control the signs related to degenerative osteoarthritis. Owners must be made aware that a potential genetic basis for the development of osteochondritis dissecans in future progeny may exist.[1]

REFERENCES

1. Berzon JL, Osteochondritis dissecans in the dog: Diagnosis and therapy: *JAVMA* 175(8):796-799, 1979.
2. Belanger LF, Dimond MT, Copp DH: Histological observations on bone and cartilage of growing turtles treated with calcitonin. *Comp Endocrinol* 20:297-304, 1973.
3. Hedhammer A, Wu FM, Krook L, et al: Overnutrition and skeletal disease. An experimental study in growing Great Dane dogs. *Cornell Vet* 64:1-160, 1974.
4. Chineme CH, Krook L, Pond WG: Bone pathology in hypervitaminosis D. An experimental study in young pigs. *Cornell Vet* 66:387-412, 1976.
5. Craig PH, Riser WH: Osteochondritis dissecans in the proximal humerus of the dog. *J Am Vet Radiol Soc* 6:40-49, 1965.
6. Vaughan LC, Jones DGC: Osteochondritis dissecans of the head of the humerus in dogs. *J Small Anim Pract* 9:283-294, 1968.
7. Olsson SE: Osteochondrosis in the dog, in Kirk RW (ed): *Current Veterinary Therapy VI*. Philadelphia, WB Saunders Co, 1977, pp 880-886.
8. Paatsama S, Rokkanen P, Jussila J, et al: A study of osteochondritis dissecans of the canine humeral head using histological, OTC bone, labelling, microradiographic and microangiographic methods. *J Small Anim Pract* 12:603-610, 1971.
9. Berzon JL, Quick CB, Fragmented coronoid process: Anatomical, clinical and radiographic considerations with case analyses. *JAAHA* 16:241-251, 1980.
10. Henry WB Jr, Wadsworth PL, Mehlhoff CJ: Medial approach to elbow joint with osteotomy of medial epicondyle. *Vet Surg*:46-49, April-June 1979.
11. Boudereau RJ, Hohn RB, Bardet JF: Osteochondritis dissecans of the elbow joint in the dog. *JAAHA*, in press.

UPDATE

A more efficient and less traumatic surgical approach to the elbow joint is done without osteotomy of the medial humeral epicondyle. Longitudinal myotomy of the flexor carpi radialis muscle or pronator muscle provides good visualization of the medial joint compartment with minimal trauma. Prognosis for these cases remains fair to guarded, even when surgery is performed soon after diagnosis. Five- to ten-year follow-ups of these cases have found a wide variety of degenerative changes, regardless of the surgical technique performed; the degree of change appears to be related to the severity of the condition at the time of presentation.

Adjunctive therapy such as the postoperative intra-articular administration of hyaluronic acid or Adequan® I.M. (Luitpold Pharmaceuticals, Inc., Shirley, NY) has yielded better clinical results than surgery alone and is worthy of consideration.

Early diagnosis and surgical therapy, combined with a protracted postoperative convalescent period, are critical in the long-term result of this disease.

Diagnosis of Common Developmental Orthopedic Conditions in Canine Pediatric Patients

KEY FACTS

- **Three developmental conditions—ununited anconeal process, osteochondrosis, and fragmented coronoid process—affect the elbow; the conditions cannot be distinguished by signalment, history, and clinical abnormalities.**
- **Avascular necrosis of the femoral head often produces structural failure and collapse of the femoral head resulting in degenerative joint disease.**
- **Palpation of the coxofemoral joint for laxity is the most important procedure for diagnosing hip dysplasia in young dogs.**
- **Panosteitis is often cyclic, and patients may present with a history of shifting-leg lameness.**
- **Hypertrophic osteodystrophy is radiographically characterized by metaphyseal sclerosis and the presence of a coalescing, linear metaphyseal radiolucency situated parallel and subjacent to the physis.**

Louisiana State University
Daniel D. Lewis, DVM   Robert J. McCarthy, DVM   Robert D. Pechman, DVM

DEVELOPMENTAL orthopedic conditions are a common cause of lameness in pediatric canine patients. A consistent, systematic diagnostic approach is critical in establishing an accurate and timely diagnosis.[1–3] A complete history should be obtained before the patient is examined.[1,2,4,5]

Most developmental orthopedic conditions have a latent or insidious onset; many owners are unaware of subtle clinical abnormalities that may have been present for weeks or months.[1] The familial and nutritional history are particularly relevant. Several common developmental orthopedic conditions have an inherited component or have been associated with overnutrition and excessive mineral and vitamin supplementation.[6–11] Most developmental orthopedic conditions have definite breed tendencies, and the clinician must consider the signalment of the patient in light of the history.[1,2,6–17]

A complete physical examination should be performed before specific evaluation of the musculoskeletal system. Special attention should be paid to the respiratory, gastrointestinal, and lymphatic systems in gathering evidence of a systemic disease process.[1–3] Although inappetence, depression, and fever suggest an infectious process, some inflammatory developmental orthopedic conditions can produce a similar clinical presentation.[6,11,12]

In specifically evaluating the musculoskeletal system, the examiner must be attuned to subtle and overt clinical signs and cognizant of the clinical abnormalities typically produced by each developmental orthopedic condition.[1,2,5,6] In addition, several specific examination procedures can aid the veterinarian in detecting clinically silent developmental orthopedic problems that might cause lameness.[1,2,5,7,18,19]

When the history and physical examination have been completed, the clinician should have localized the involved region and derived a differential diagnosis.[4,5] Radiography remains the most important diagnostic modality for substantiating or refuting the clinical diagnosis.[20–22] This article focuses on the clinical and radiographic diagnosis of the most common developmental orthopedic conditions that affect pediatric canine patients.

Originally published in Volume 14, Number 3, March 1992

OSTEOCHONDROSIS

Osteochondrosis is a developmental orthopedic condition in which a disturbance in the normal process of endochondral ossification results in thickening or retention of articular or physeal cartilage. The articular cartilage of the epiphyses of the long bones is most frequently affected. The thickened articular cartilage is prone to fibrillation, fissuring, and separation. If a cartilage flap develops, intra-articular inflammation and degenerative joint disease may result and the condition is more appropriately described as osteochondritis dissecans.[9,17,23–27]

OSTEOCHONDROSIS occurs most frequently in rapidly growing, male, large- and giant-breed dogs.[9,17,24,27] Genetic, nutritional, hormonal, and traumatic factors have been implicated in the pathogenesis.[9,17,24,27–40] Osteochondrosis affects many of the joints of the appendicular and axial skeleton; the most common sites of occurrence are the hock, stifle, elbow, and shoulder joint.[9,17,24,27] The clinical and radiographic aspects of osteochondrosis that involves these four sites are detailed separately.

Hock

Although osteochondrosis of the hock may affect any large-breed dog, rottweilers,[41–46] Labrador retrievers,[42,43,45–47] and Australian cattle dogs[41,45,48] are particularly at risk. Affected animals often develop clinical lameness by four or five months of age.[41–48] Most patients display consistent weight-bearing lameness or intermittent non-weight-bearing lameness.[41–48] The affected hock is often held in hyperextension, and muscle atrophy of the limb may be present.[45,46,49] Palpation of the hock demonstrates synovial effusion, which is detected as a fluctuant swelling most easily palpated immediately caudodistal to the malleoli. In more chronic cases, the joint capsule becomes thickened and range of motion is decreased. Extreme flexion or extension of the hock elicits a pain response.[41–48]

The radiographic appearance of osteochondrosis of the hock is variable and depends on the site and extent of the lesion.[44,46] Most patients have a subchondral bony defect with associated subchondral sclerosis (Figure 1A). Mineralized flaps or osteochondral fragments are found in other patients. Degenerative changes, including subchondral sclerosis of the articulating surfaces of the tibia, are frequently present.[41,43–49] The medial trochlear ridge of the talus is affected most often[41–43,45,47–49]; however, lesions that affect the lateral trochlear ridge are being recognized with increasing frequency.[44,46]

Oblique projection radiographs may be necessary to define some lesions, particularly those that involve the lateral trochlear ridge.[41,43,44,46,50,51] The dorsal 45° lateral-plantaromedial oblique projection reportedly is the most useful view in identifying lesions of the lateral trochlear ridge.[44,46] In our experience, the flexed dorsoplantar projection made with a horizontal beam[46] is useful in defining lesions that involve either trochlear ridge.

Stifle

Osteochondrosis of the stifle occurs infrequently.[23,25,28,30,33,52–58] The signalment of affected dogs is similar to that of dogs affected with osteochondrosis at other locations.[25,30,52–58] Seventy-six percent of reported cases have involved male dogs; in 72% of cases, the condition was bilateral.[52] In reports from Europe, German shepherds and Great Danes were predisposed to develop the condition.[25,58]

The onset of lameness is usually insidious and may occur as early as three months of age.[52–57] The lameness is exacerbated by exercise.[52,53,58] Animals that are bilaterally affected generally exhibit only unilateral lameness.[52] Range of motion (especially extension) is decreased, and manipulation of the stifle elicits a pain response. A click may be heard during joint manipulation.[28,52,53,55]

The most common radiographic abnormality associated with osteochondrosis of the stifle is a flattening or subchondral bony defect that involves the medial aspect of the lateral femoral condyle[28,52–58] (Figure 1B). This abnormality should not be confused with the fossa of the long digital extensor tendon[59] or an aberrant attachment of the cranial cruciate ligament.[60] Lesions that affect the medial condyle have been reported in 4% of affected stifles.[52] Detached mineralized cartilage flaps, osteophytes, and degenerative changes may be observed.[28,52–58]

Elbow

Three developmental conditions—ununited anconeal process, osteochondrosis, and fragmented coronoid process—affect the elbow.[61,62] These conditions cannot be distinguished by signalment, history, or clinical abnormalities.[8,9,15–17,24,26,27,61,62]

LAMENESS or a stiff, stilted forelimb gait may be noted first at four to five months of age in dogs with elbow osteochondrosis. Pain on extension of the elbow and joint effusion may be present.[16,17,24,27,61–65] The lesion (a subchondral bony defect that affects the trochlea of the humeral condyle) is best observed radiographically via a slightly oblique, craniocaudal view of the elbow[16,63,65] (Figure 1C). Degenerative changes in the elbow joint may also exist.[63,65] Osteochondrosis of the humeral condyle can be concurrent with fragmented coronoid process.[8,16,17,24,27,61–67]

Shoulder

Although most dogs with osteochondrosis of the scapulohumeral joint do not display clinical abnormalities before six months of age, some dogs develop clinical lameness as early as four months of age.[9,24,27,68–70] Dogs may initially

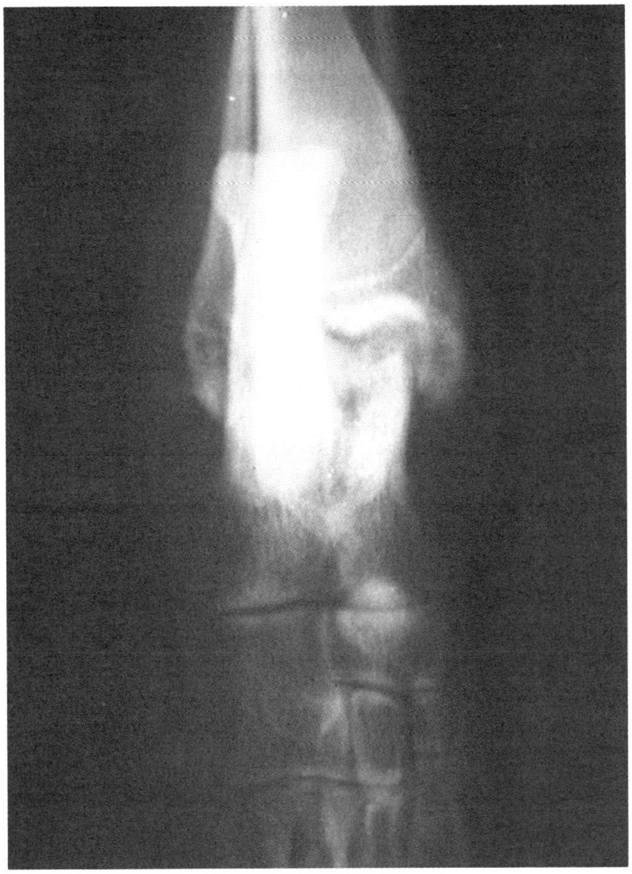

Figure 1A

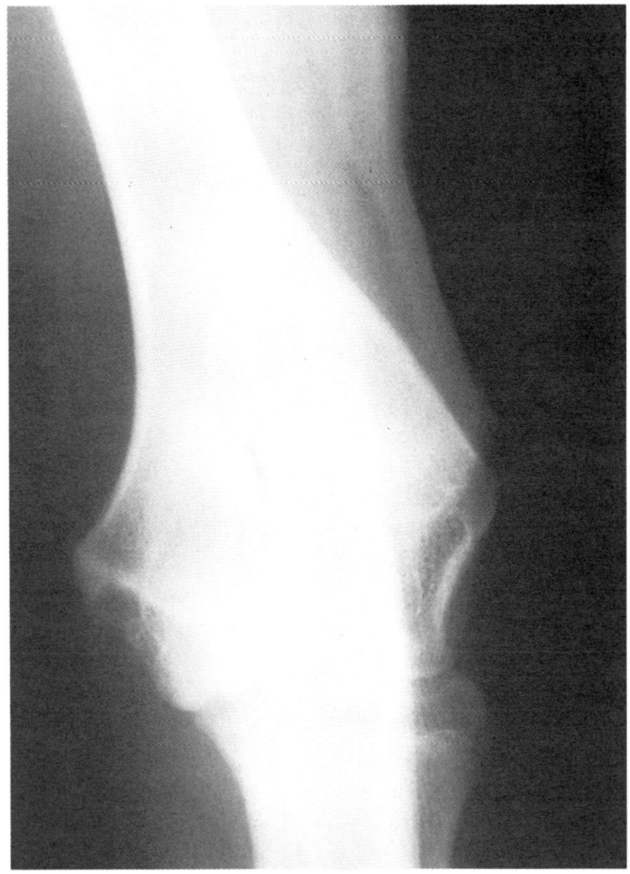

Figure 1C

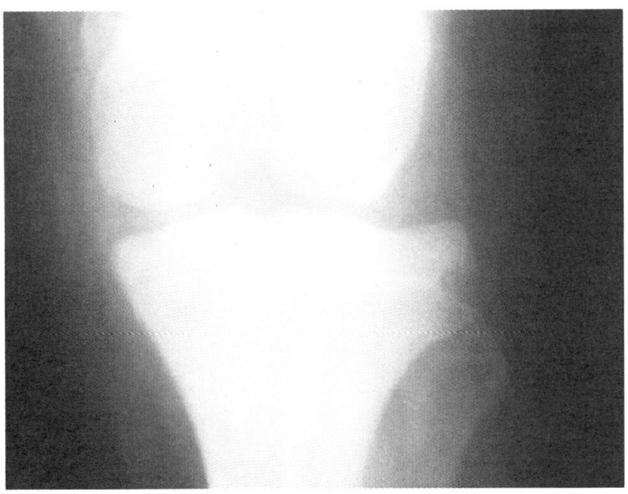

Figure 1B

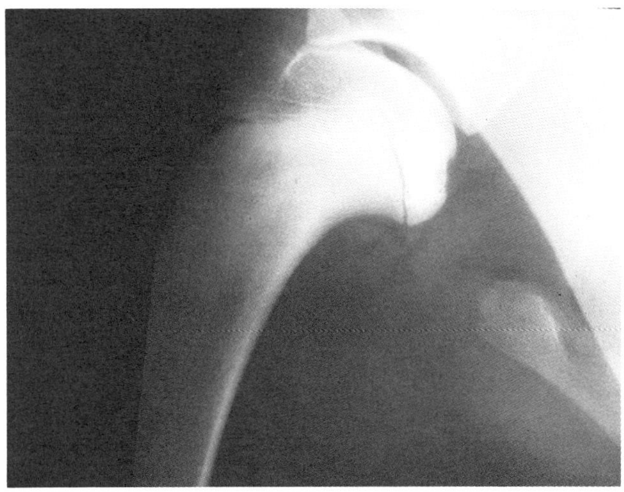

Figure 1D

Figure 1—Radiographic appearance of osteochondrosis at its common sites of occurrence. (**A**) The medial trochlear ridge of the talus. (**B**) The lateral femoral condyle. (**C**) The trochlea of the condyle of the humerus. (**D**) The caudal aspect of the head of the humerus.

have mild, intermittent weight-bearing forelimb lameness; the condition can progress to profound weight-bearing or intermittent non-weight-bearing lameness.[9,17,27,68,69,71] Atrophy of the regional musculature is obvious in severely affected dogs. Flexion and extension of the scapulohumeral joint elicit a marked pain response.[9,17,24,26,27,30,38,39,68–71]

The diagnosis of osteochondrosis is confirmed by the presence of a subchondral bony defect in the caudal aspect of the humeral head, evident on a lateral radiograph of the scapulohumeral joint[68,69,71] (Figure 1D). Radiographic evidence of osteochondrosis of the humeral head is bilateral in 43% to 65% of affected dogs, but only 3% to 5% of patients exhibit bilateral lameness.[72] Positive-contrast arthrography has prognostic value in evaluating the contralateral shoulder in a patient with unilateral lameness and radiographic evidence of bilateral osteochondrosis.[73,74]

BECAUSE cartilage has the same radiographic density as synovial fluid, the only way to distinguish osteochondrosis from osteochondritis dissecans radiographically (unless the cartilage flap has mineralized) is to perform contrast arthrography. The presence of intact thickened cartilage over the subchondral bony defect is a favorable prognostic sign; if contrast medium dissects under the thickened cartilage that overlies a subchondral bony defect (substantiating the presence of a cartilage flap), there is a 50% chance that arthrotomy will be required to remove the flap.[73]

In some patients, the cartilage flap may detach. Contrast arthrography is necessary to identify the flap unless it has mineralized.[72–74] A detached flap that adheres to the synovium of the caudal joint pouch is unlikely to cause lameness. Fifty percent of the dogs with a flap floating loose in the joint space have substantial lameness.[73] Flaps that lodge in the bicipital tendon sheath also are associated with chronic lameness.[72–74]

AVASCULAR NECROSIS OF THE FEMORAL HEAD

Avascular necrosis of the femoral head (Legg-Calvé-Perthes disease) is a developmental condition that occurs almost exclusively in toy and miniature-breed dogs.[13,14,75–77] Males and females are affected with equal frequency. The condition reportedly is unilateral in 84% to 88% of affected dogs.[13,75–78] An incomplete autosomal recessive mode of inheritance has been suggested.[10,75] Aseptic necrosis occurs secondary to vascular compromise of the femoral head. There is subsequent resorption of the necrotic bony trabeculae, which weakens the subchondral bone. This often results in structural failure and collapse of the femoral head with the rapid development of degenerative joint disease.[13,14,75–82]

The process begins at about the time of physeal closure, which may be as early as three or four months of age in toy dogs.[13,14,75–78] Some patients present with subtle weight-bearing lameness during the phase of trabecular resorption before collapse of the femoral head.[13,14,75,78] Pain may be elicited by abduction and extension of the femur.[14,78] As the subchondral bone collapses and degenerative joint disease develops, affected dogs become intermittently or continuously non-weight-bearing on the limb. There is substantial muscle atrophy, and the pain response that is elicited by manipulation of the coxofemoral joint increases in severity.[13,14,75,77,78]

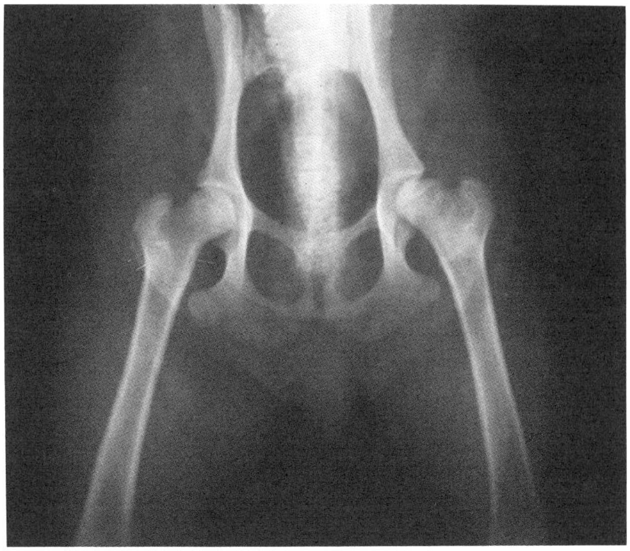

Figure 2—Unilateral avascular necrosis of the femoral head. Structural collapse of the femoral head has resulted in the development of early degenerative changes in the left coxofemoral joint.

THE EARLIEST radiographic abnormality associated with aseptic necrosis of the femoral head is increased radiopacity of the lateral epiphyseal area of the femoral head.[83] This change precedes overt clinical signs and is rarely recognized.[83] Patients with early, subtle clinical signs may have radiographic evidence of focal bony lysis as resorption of the bony trabeculae occurs.[75,77,78,83,84] It is important for clinicians to recognize these early radiographic changes because patients may be managed successfully without surgery if diagnosed at this stage.[85] As revascularization and remodeling progress, structural failure and collapse of the femoral head with the development of degenerative joint disease become evident radiographically[13,14,75–78,83–85] (Figure 2).

HIP DYSPLASIA

Hip dysplasia is the most common developmental orthopedic condition that affects dogs.[7,86,87] The condition is most prevalent in large- and giant-breed dogs.[7,86,87] The development of hip dysplasia is influenced by many genetic, hormonal, and environmental factors.[7,87–97] The coxofemoral joints of affected dogs are normal at birth, but joint laxity develops during the first month of life.[91,96,97–99] Overt clinical abnormalities may be apparent in dogs younger than six months of age, but many dogs lack clinical signs until older. Some dogs have an acute onset of hindlimb

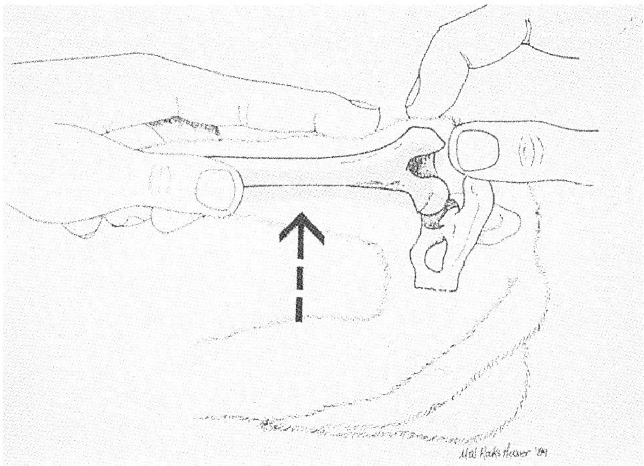

Figure 3—Testing for coxofemoral joint laxity using the technique described by Bardens and Hardwick. The examiner's index finger is positioned over the greater trochanter as a lateral force (*arrow*) is applied to the femur. (From Chalman JA, Butler HC: Coxofemoral joint laxity and the Ortolani sign. *JAAHA* 21(5):671–676, 1985. Reprinted with permission.)

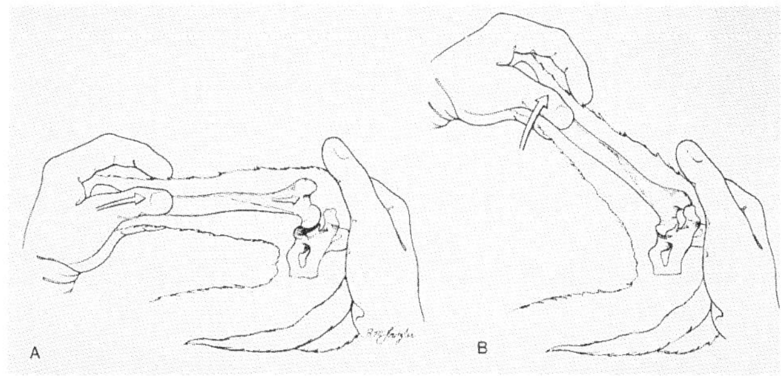

Figure 4—Testing for Ortolani's sign. (*A*) Subluxation of the coxofemoral joint is induced by applying pressure (*arrow*) on the stifle. (*B*) The femur is abducted (*arrow*), and a click is elicited as the femoral head relocates in the acetabulum. (From Brinker WO, Piermattei DL, Flo GL: *Handbook of Small Animal Orthopedics and Fracture Treatment*, ed 2. Philadelphia, WB Saunders Co, 1990, p 277. Reprinted with permission.)

lameness and coxofemoral joint pain; but most dogs have more subtle clinical signs referable to coxofemoral joint laxity and pain, including poor development or atrophy of the pelvic muscle mass, decreased activity, difficulty rising, and so-called bunny-hopping gait.[7,87,100]

Palpation of the coxofemoral joint for laxity is the most important procedure for diagnosing hip dysplasia in young dogs. Coxofemoral joint laxity is assessed in puppies at 7 to 11 weeks of age using the method described by Bardens and Hardwick.[101] In order to be accurate, the examination must be performed with the puppy in a deep plane of anesthesia. Accuracy also depends on the proficiency and experience of the clinician.

THE PUPPY is placed in lateral recumbency. The examiner stands behind the patient, and the proximal diaphysis of the nondependent femur is grasped between the thumb and index finger. The femur is positioned at a 90° angle to the spinal column and parallel to the examination table. The thumb of the opposite hand is placed on the ischiatic tuberosity to provide counter pressure. The index finger of this hand is placed on the greater trochanter and is used to detect joint laxity as the femur is lifted laterally (the examiner's wrist is not flexed). Lateral translation of the head of the femur in the acetabulum, displacing the examiner's thumb positioned over the greater trochanter, indicates laxity (Figure 3). A normal puppy should have less than one millimeter of lateral translation.[101–103]

Many owners do not acquire puppies until they are three or four months of age; by this time, the method of palpation described by Bardens and Hardwick is unreliable.[19,100] The Ortolani and Barlow examinations are used to detect joint laxity in this age group.[19,100,104–106]

For the Ortolani examination, the patient is placed in lateral recumbency and the nondependent limb is grasped at the stifle. The stifle is placed in 90° of flexion; the femur is positioned parallel to the surface of the examination table and perpendicular to the long axis of the pelvis. The examiner's other hand is placed over the sacrum to provide countersupport. Pressure is applied to the stifle. This force is transferred up to the femoral shaft and will result in dorsal subluxation of the femoral head if joint laxity exists (Figure 4*A*). The femur is then slowly abducted as the examiner attempts to elicit a click as the femoral head returns to the acetabulum (Figure 4*B*).

The Barlow examination is accomplished by reversing this procedure. The hindlimb is returned from its abducted position while pressure is applied to the stifle. In a puppy with coxofemoral joint laxity, another click is elicited as the femur is adducted to the point at which the dorsal pressure causes the femoral head to subluxate again.

PATIENTS with hip dysplasia are often in pain and resist palpation of the coxofemoral joints. A patient can only be considered to be negative for Ortolani's sign and Barlow's sign if palpation is performed during heavy sedation or anesthesia.[19,100,105,106]

Radiography is used to confirm the clinical diagnosis of hip dysplasia and to determine whether there are dysplastic or degenerative abnormalities of the coxofemoral joints. The dorsoventral view, adopted by the Orthopedic Foundation for Animals, is unreliable for detecting hip dysplasia in young dogs. Patients in this age group with palpable subluxation of the coxofemoral joint can have normal pelvic radiographs.[100,107,108] As a femur is pulled into

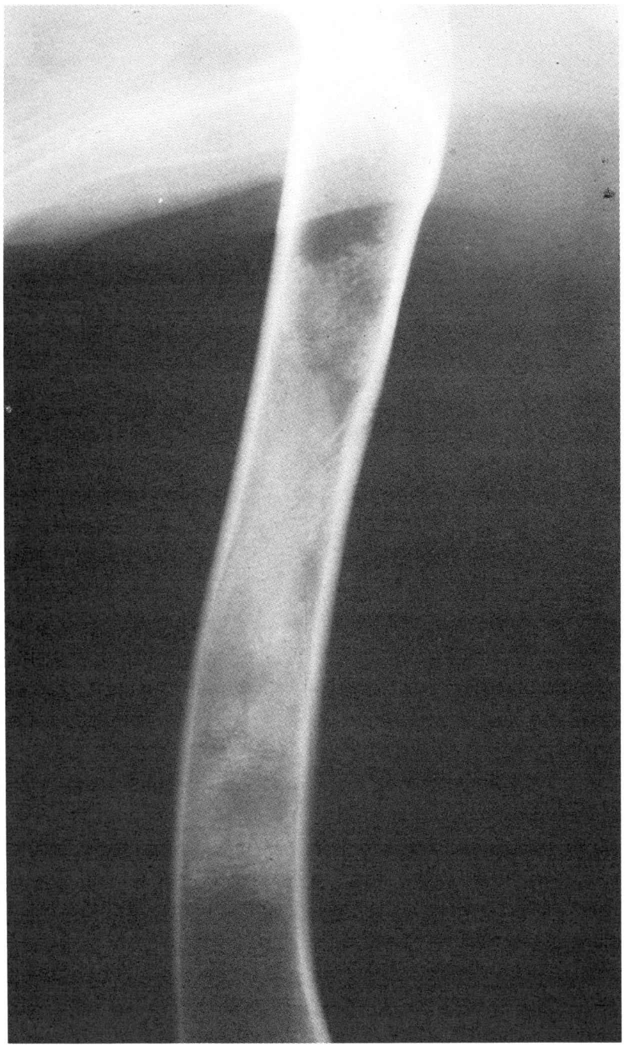

Figure 5—Increased radiopacity of the medullary cavity of the diaphysis of the femur, typical of panosteitis.

full extension and slight internal rotation, lateral displacement of the femoral head from the acetabulum is limited and joint laxity may be masked.[100,107]

The mechanism responsible for attenuating coxofemoral joint laxity is the spiral tension that develops in the fibrous elements of the joint capsule as the femurs are extended.[107] In addition, the synovial fluid (a nondistensible liquid that is incapable of appreciable changes in volume) exerts a hydrostatic vacuum effect that further limits lateral displacement of the femoral head.[107]

Alternative methods for evaluating the coxofemoral joints in dogs with suspected hip dysplasia have been advocated to increase the sensitivity of radiographic detection of hip dysplasia. Smith and coworkers reported a 2.5-fold improvement in sensitivity in detecting joint laxity (compared with the standard extended-femur ventrodorsal projection) by obtaining ventrodorsal radiographs of patients with femurs positioned in a neutral flexion–extension angle while lateral stress was applied to both femurs.[107]

Slocum and Devine developed the dorsal acetabular rim view to define abnormalities of the weight-bearing portion of the coxofemoral joint better.[109] The view is obtained with the patient in ventral recumbency with both femurs positioned in flexion along the body. The x-ray beam is positioned over the dorsal midline and passes through the patient in a cranial-to-caudal direction, longitudinally bisecting both ilia. The dorsal acetabular rim view thus profiles the coxofemoral joint in cross section.[109]

PANOSTEITIS

Panosteitis is an acquired inflammatory condition of unknown cause that affects the diaphyseal and metaphyseal regions of the long bones of large- and giant-breed dogs.[12,110,111] The disease affects males more frequently than females.[110,112,113] The condition is often cyclic or recurrent, and patients typically present with a history of a shifting-leg lameness. Lameness may be accompanied by lethargy, anorexia, and fever. A pain response is elicited when digital pressure is applied to the affected region of the long bones.[12,110–112]

THE EARLIEST radiographic abnormality associated with the condition is an increased radiolucency of the medullary cavity in the region of the nutrient foramen. The phase of increased radiolucency, which corresponds with degeneration of the medullary adipocytes, occurs early in the disease process and is infrequently observed.[110] A hazy or granular increased radiopacity (which may be accompanied by endosteal or periosteal bony proliferation) in the medullary cavity is detected more frequently (Figure 5). This increased radiopacity results from intramembranous ossification of proliferating stromal and adventitial cells of the medullary canal and may not be recognized until 10 to 14 days after the onset of clinical lameness.[110–112]

HYPERTROPHIC OSTEODYSTROPHY

Hypertrophic osteodystrophy (metaphyseal osteopathy, Moeller-Barlow disease, canine scurvy, osteodystrophy I, or osteodystrophy II) is a developmental disease of unknown cause that primarily affects young, rapidly growing, large- and giant-breed dogs.[11,114–116] The condition can affect the metaphysis of any long bone but is most often recognized in the distal radius, ulna, and tibia.[11,114,115] Overnutrition, hypovitaminosis C, excess mineral supplementation, hyperparathyroidism, and hypercalcitoninism have been incriminated in the development of hypertrophic osteodystrophy.[11,114–124] A genetic basis for the disease has not been established, but the condition has been reported to affect an entire litter.[125]

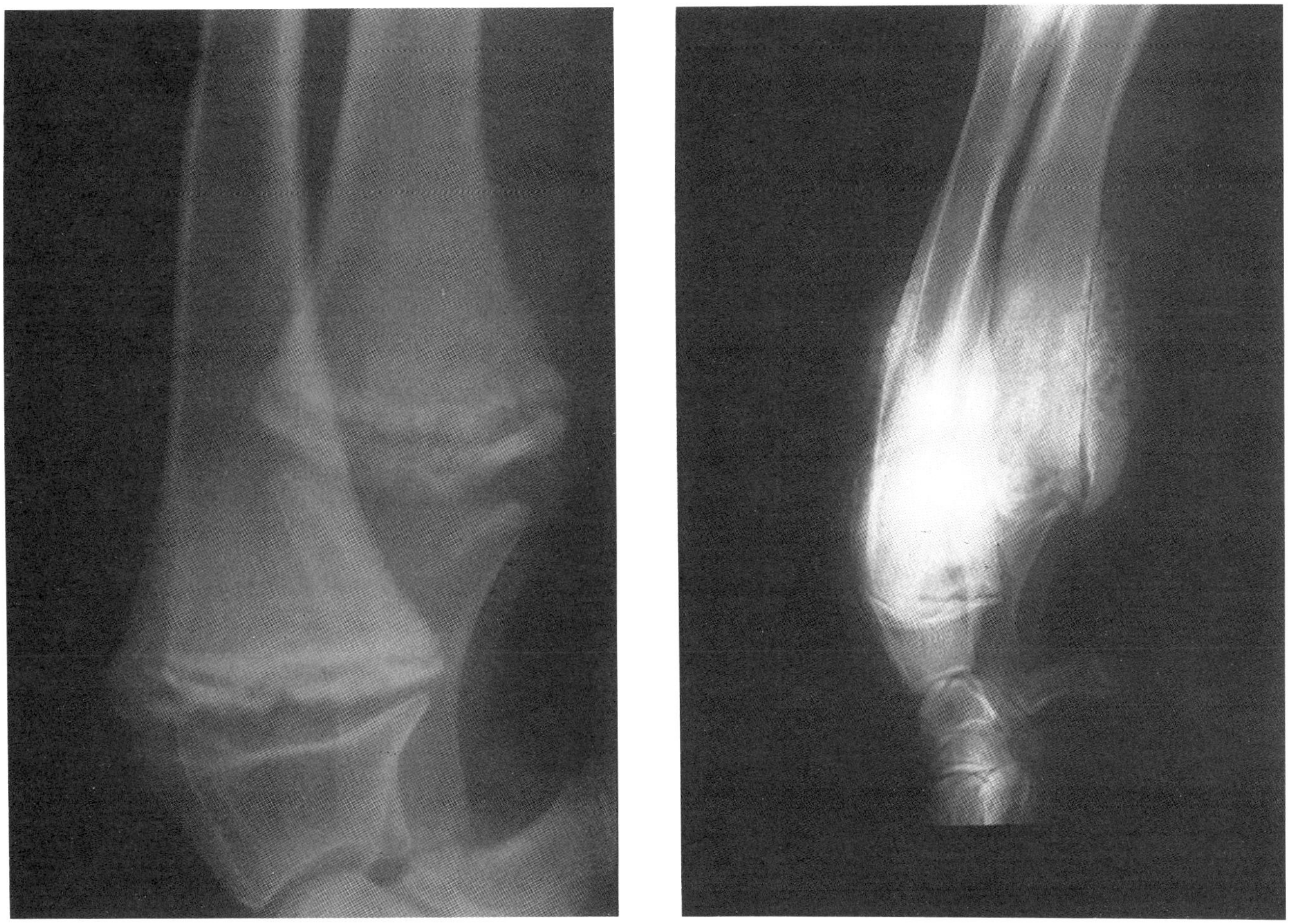

Figure 6A **Figure 6B**

Figure 6—(**A**) The distal antebrachium of a patient with hypertrophic osteodystrophy characterized by metaphyseal sclerosis and a coalescing, linear radiolucency subjacent to the physis. (**B**) As the condition progresses, extensive metaphyseal periosteal new bone can form.

Clinical signs may develop between two months of age and the time of growth plate closure but typically manifest between two and four months of age.[11,114,115] Patients that are minimally affected may present with vague symmetric lameness and a reluctance to ambulate. More severely affected dogs may be recumbent, depressed, anorectic, and febrile. The metaphyseal region of affected long bones may be swollen and warm. A pain response is elicited by applying direct digital pressure to the affected metaphysis.[11,114,115]

Hypertrophic osteodystrophy is radiographically characterized by metaphyseal sclerosis and the presence of a coalescing, linear metaphyseal radiolucency situated parallel and subjacent to the physis. This radiolucent zone, which may resemble a second physeal plate, represents an area of suppurative inflammation and hemorrhage[11,114,115] (Figure 6A). As the condition progresses, metaphyseal subperiosteal or extraperiosteal new bone can form[11,14] (Figure 6B). In severe cases, new bone formation may progress to involve the entire diaphysis.[11]

UNUNITED ANCONEAL PROCESS

Ununited anconeal process occurs primarily in large- and giant-breed dogs, most notably in German shepherds.[126–128] The condition affects males approximately twice as frequently as females[128] and is bilateral in 30% of affected dogs.[127,128]

Clinical abnormalities result from progressive degenerative joint disease of the elbow. Affected animals may exhibit lameness as early as four months of age. The lameness is intermittent and may be exacerbated by exercise or prolonged rest.[62,126] Affected dogs may stand or sit with the carpus held in a valgus position and with the elbow abducted, or they may circumduct the antebrachium during the swing phase of the stride. Full extension and flexion of the elbow may elicit a pain response.[126–129] A pain response also can be elicited by applying direct pressure to the anconeal process through the anconeus muscle as the elbow of the patient is held in flexion.[126] Crepitus, synovial effusion, and joint capsule thickening are present in advanced cases.[126–129]

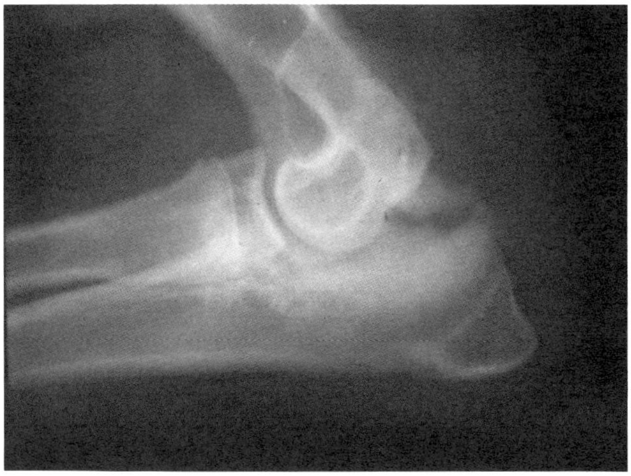

Figure 7—Flexed lateral view of the elbow of a patient with an ununited anconeal process and degenerative joint disease.

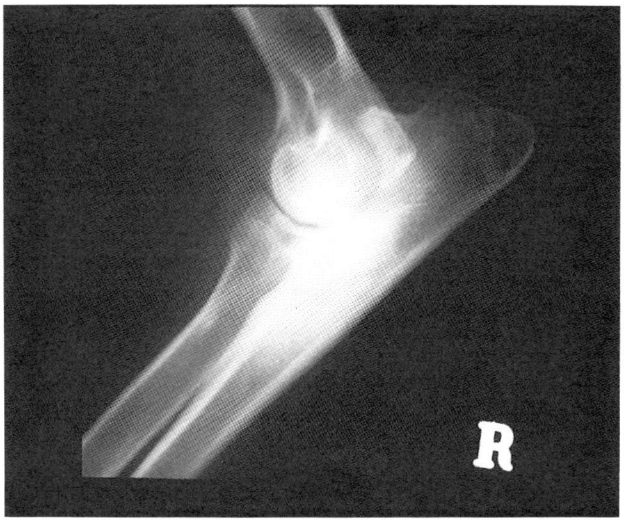

Figure 8—Lateral view of the elbow of a patient with a fragmented coronoid process. There is increased radiopacity of the ulna subjacent to the trochlear notch and coronoid process, osteophyte formation on the anconeal process, and distal subluxation of the humeroradial joint.

The diagnosis is confirmed by a flexed lateral radiograph of the elbow[62,126–129] (Figure 7). In breeds that are predisposed to developing ununited anconeal process, the anconeal process develops as a distinct center of ossification separate from the ulna. In German shepherds, the process begins to mineralize at approximately 12 weeks of age and fuses with the ulna at 16 to 24 weeks of age.[130] A definitive diagnosis of ununited anconeal process thus should not be made before 24 weeks of age.[126] Secondary degenerative changes of the elbow may be present.[62,126–130]

FRAGMENTED CORONOID PROCESS

Fragmented coronoid process is the third developmental condition that affects the elbows of large-breed dogs, particularly retrievers, rottweilers, and German shepherds.[8,16,63,131,132] The cause of the condition is controversial. Originally, fragmented coronoid process was believed to be a manifestation of the osteochondrosis complex[9,63]; pathoanatomic studies have not fully supported this contention.[67] Fissures or fragmentation may result from abnormal stresses placed on the developing coronoid process because of conformational abnormalities of the elbow.[8,67,133–135] The medial coronoid process is most often involved.[8,16,67] The disease is more common in males and is often bilateral.[8] A hereditary basis for the condition has been suggested.[136,137]

CLINICAL signs are rarely noted before five months of age.[8,16,63,131–133,138] Subtle weight-bearing lameness, exacerbated by prolonged rest or exercise, is typical. The onset of the gait abnormality is insidious. As lameness persists, it may increase in severity. Affected dogs often place the carpus in an exaggerated valgus position when sitting or standing and circumduct the antebrachium during the swing phase of the stride.[8,16,62,133] A pain response is usually not elicited unless the elbow is fully extended. Some investigators suggest that the carpus should be placed in a flexed, externally rotated position while the elbow is extended.[126] Joint effusion may be detected as a fluctuant swelling beneath the lateral epicondyle of the humerus.[8]

A fragmented coronoid process is rarely identified radiographically because of superimposition of the medial coronoid process and the head of the radius.[8,62,138–140] The mediolateral (extended and supinated) view made with the elbow maximally extended and supinated 15° reportedly is a superior radiographic projection for demonstrating pathology of the medial coronoid process[140]; however, this view has been of limited diagnostic value in our experience.

A clinical diagnosis of fragmented coronoid process is supported radiographically by the presence of degenerative changes in the elbow in the absence of an ununited anconeal process or osteochondrosis of the humeral condyle.[8,62,138–140] Increased density of the ulna subjacent to the coronoid process and osteophyte development on the anconeal process are early radiographic degenerative changes associated with fragmented coronoid process (Figure 8). Degenerative changes are usually not radiographically evident before patients are seven months of age.[8,62,131,133,138–140] Distal subluxation of the humeroradial joint may be apparent.[8,133,134,136,141] Definitive diagnosis is made at exploratory arthrotomy.

CONCLUSION

The developmental orthopedic conditions discussed in this article are encountered frequently by companion animal practitioners. In order to diagnose these conditions in pediatric canine patients, veterinarians must approach each case in a consistent, systematic manner and be cognizant of the expected clinical and radiographic abnormalities referable to each condition.

About the Authors

Drs. Lewis, McCarthy, and Pechman are affiliated with the Department of Veterinary Clinical Sciences, School of Veterinary Medicine, Louisiana State University, Baton Rouge, Louisiana. Dr. Lewis is a Diplomate of the American College of Veterinary Surgeons, and Dr. Pechman is a Diplomate of the American College of Veterinary Radiology.

REFERENCES

1. Brinker WO, Piermattei DL, Flo GL: *Handbook of Small Animal Orthopedics and Fracture Treatment*, ed 2. Philadelphia, WB Saunders Co, 1990, pp 267–277.
2. Newton CD, Nunamaker DM: *Textbook of Small Animal Orthopedics*. Philadelphia, JB Lippincott Co, 1985, pp 125–128.
3. Alexander JW, Roberts RE: Symposium on orthopedic diseases. *Vet Clin North Am [Small Anim Pract]* 13(1):1, 1983.
4. Lorenz MD, Cornelius LM: *Small Animal Medical Diagnosis*. Philadelphia, JB Lippincott Co, 1987, pp 1–12.
5. McCurnin DM, Poffenbarger EM: *Small Animal Physical Diagnosis and Clinical Procedures*. Philadelphia, WB Saunders Co, 1991, pp 3–15.
6. Shires PK: The musculoskeletal system, in Hoskins JD (ed): *Veterinary Pediatrics: Dogs and Cats From Birth to Six Months*. Philadelphia, WB Saunders Co, 1990, pp 333–357.
7. Rettenmaier JL, Constantinescu GM: Canine hip dysplasia. *Compend Contin Educ Pract Vet* 13(4):643–654, 1991.
8. Lewis DD, Parker RB, Hager DA: Fragmented medial coronoid process of the canine elbow. *Compend Contin Educ Pract Vet* 11(6):703–715, 1989.
9. Olsson SE: Osteochondrosis—A growing problem to dog breeders. *Gaines Prog*:1–11, 1976.
10. Pidduck H, Webbon PM: The genetic control of Perthes' disease in toy poodles—A working hypothesis. *J Small Anim Pract* 19(12):729–733, 1978.
11. Lenehan TM, Fetter AW: Hypertrophic osteodystrophy, in Newton CD, Nunamaker MD (eds): *Textbook of Small Animal Orthopaedics*. Philadelphia, JB Lippincott Co, 1985, pp 597–601.
12. Lenehan TM, Van Sickle DC, Biery DN: Canine panosteitis, in Newton CD, Nunamaker MD (ed): *Textbook of Small Animal Orthopaedics*. Philadelphia, JB Lippincott Co, 1985, pp 591–596.
13. Warren DV, Dingwall JS: Legg-Perthes disease in the dog—A review. *Can Vet J* 13(6):135–137, 1972.
14. Ljunggren G: Legg-Perthes disease in the dog. *Acta Orthop Scand [Supp]* 95:7–79, 1967.
15. Grondalen J: Arthrosis with special reference to the elbow joint of rapidly growing dogs. I. A review of the literature. *Nord Vet Med* 31(1):62–68, 1979.
16. Grondalen J: Arthrosis with special reference to the elbow joint of rapidly growing dogs. II. Occurrence, clinical and radiographic findings. *Nord Vet Med* 31(1):69–75, 1979.
17. Milton JL: Osteochondrosis dissecans in the dog. *Vet Clin North Am [Small Anim Pract]* 13(1):117–134, 1983.
18. Bardens JW, Hardwick H: New observations on the diagnosis and cause of hip dysplasia. *VM SAC* 63(3):238–245, 1968.
19. Chalman JA, Butler HC: Coxofemoral joint laxity and the Ortolani sign. *JAAHA* 21(5):671–676, 1985.
20. Roberts BE: Radiographic examination of the musculoskeletal system. *Vet Clin North Am [Small Anim Pract]* 13(1):19–42, 1983.
21. Morgan JP: *Radiology of Skeletal Disease—Principles of Diagnosis in the Dog*. Davis, CA, Veterinary Radiology Associates, 1981, pp 1–3.
22. Biery DN: Orthopaedic radiography, in Newton CD, Nunamaker MD (eds): *Textbook of Small Animal Orthopaedics*. Philadelphia, JB Lippincott Co, 1985, pp 133–146.
23. Alexander JW, Richardson DC, Selcer BA: Osteochondritis dissecans of the elbow, stifle, and hock—A review. *JAAHA* 17(1):56–66, 1981.
24. Lenehan TM, Van Sickle DC: Canine osteochondrosis, in Newton CD, Nunamaker DM (eds): *Textbook of Small Animal Orthopaedics*. Philadelphia, JB Lippincott Co, 1985, pp 981–997.
25. Punzet G, Walde I, Arbesser E: Zur Osteochondrosis dissecans genu des Hundes. *Kleintier Prax* 20(3):88–98, 1975.
26. Olsson SE: Morphology and physiology of the growth of cartilage under normal and pathologic conditions, in *Bone in Clinical Orthopedics*. Philadelphia, WB Saunders Co, 1982, pp 159–196.
27. Olsson SE: Pathophysiology, morphology, and clinical signs of osteochondrosis (chondrosis) in the dog, in Bojrab MJ (ed): *Pathophysiology in Small Animal Surgery*. Philadelphia, Lea & Febiger, 1981, pp 604–617.
28. Woodard DC: Osteochondritis dissecans in a family of bull terriers. *VM SAC* 74(7):936, 1979.
29. Johnson KA, Dennis KA: Osteochondritis dissecans in a beagle. *Aust Vet J* 54(7):364–365, 1978.
30. Knecht CD, Van Sickle DC, Blevins WE, et al: Osteochondrosis of the shoulder and stifle in 3 of 5 border collie littermates. *JAVMA* 170(1):58–60, 1977.
31. Cordy DR, Wind AP: Transverse fracture of the proximal humeral articular cartilage in dogs. *Pathol Vet* 6(5):424–436, 1969.
32. Mason TA, Lavelle RB: Osteochondritis dissecans of the tibial tarsal bone in dogs. *J Small Anim Pract* 20(7):423–436, 1979.
33. Robins GM: A case of osteochondritis dissecans of the stifle joints in a bitch. *J Small Anim Pract* 11(12):813–817, 1970.
34. Palmer CS: Osteochondritis in Great Danes. *VM SAC* 65(10): 994–1002, 1970.
35. Reiland S: Osteochondrosis in the pig, PhD thesis, Akademisch Auhardling, Stockholm, Sweden, 1975.
36. Hedhammer A, Wu FM, Krook L, et al: Overnutrition and skeletal disease: An experimental study in growing Great Dane dogs. *Cornell Vet* 64(5):1–160, 1974.
37. Van Sickle DC: *Selected Orthopedic Problems in the Growing Dog: An Atlas*. South Bend, IN, American Animal Hospital Association, 1975.
38. Mostosky UV: Osteochondritis dissecans of the canine shoulder: The newer knowledge about dogs. *Proc 13th Gaines Symp*:16–19, 1964.
39. Craig PH, Kiser WH: Osteochondritis dissecans in the proximal humerus of the dog. *J Am Vet Radiol Soc* 6:40–49, 1965.
40. Carrig CB, Morgan JP: Microcirculation of the humeral head in the immature dog. *J Am Vet Radiol Soc* 15(1):28–33, 1974.
41. Rosenblum GP, Robins GM, Carlisle CH: Osteochondritis dissecans of the tibio-tarsal joint in the dog. *J Small Anim Pract* 19(12): 759–767, 1978.
42. Breur GJ, Spaulding KA, Braden TD: Osteochondritis dissecans of the medial trochlear ridge of the talus in the dogs. *Vet Comp Orthop Traum* 2(4):168–176, 1989.
43. Smith MM, Vasseur PB, Morgan JP: Clinical evaluation of dogs after surgical and nonsurgical management of osteochondritis dissecans of the talus. *JAVMA* 187(1):31–35, 1985.
44. Wisner ER, Berry CR, Morgan JP, et al: Osteochondrosis of the lateral trochlear ridge of the talus in seven rottweiler dogs. *Vet Surg* 19(6):435–439, 1990.
45. Beale BS, Goring RL, Herrington J, et al: A prospective evaluation of four surgical approaches to the talus of the dog used in the treatment of osteochondritis dissecans. *JAAHA* 27(2):221–229, 1991.
46. Carlisle CH, Robins GM, Reynolds KM: Radiographic signs of osteochondritis dissecans of the lateral ridge of the trochlea tali in the dog. *J Small Anim Pract* 31(6):280–286, 1990.
47. Olson NC, Mostosky UV, Flo GL, et al: Osteochondritis dissecans of the tarsocrural joint in three canine siblings. *JAVMA* 176(7):635–637, 1980.
48. Johnston KA, Cameron RH, Pettit GD: Osteochondritis in the hock joints of dogs. *JAAHA* 16(1):103–113, 1980.
49. Alexander JW: Osteochondritis dissecans of the hock in the dog. *California Vet* 32(2):9–11, 1980.
50. Aron DN, Mahaffey MB, Rowland GN: Free chondral fragment involving the lateral trochlear ridge of the talus in a dog. *JAVMA* 186(10):1095–1096, 1985.
51. Carlisle CH, Reynolds KM: Radiographic anatomy of the tarsocru-

ral joint of the dog. *J Small Anim Pract* 31(6):273–279, 1990.
52. Montgomery RD, Milton JL, Henderson RA, et al: Osteochondritis dissecans of the canine stifle. *Compend Contin Educ Pract Vet* 11(10):1199–1205, 1989.
53. Robins GM: A case of osteochondritis dissecans of the stifle joints in a bitch. *J Small Anim Pract* 11:813–817, 1970.
54. Lafeber TJ, Beckwith J, Strombeck DR: What is your diagnosis? *JAVMA* 134(6):267–268, 1959.
55. Denny HR, Gibbs C: Osteochondritis dissecans of the canine stifle joint. *J Small Anim Pract* 21(6):317–322, 1980.
56. Knecht CD, Van Sickle DC, Blevins WE, et al: Osteochondrosis of the shoulder and stifle in 3 of 5 border collie littermates. *JAVMA* 170(1):58–60, 1977.
57. Leighton RL: Surgical treatment of osteochondritis dissecans of the canine stifle. *VM SAC* 76(12):1733–1736, 1981.
58. Arbesser E: Osteochondrosis dissecans der Femur-Kondylen beim Hund. *Wien Tierarztl Monatschr* 61(1):303–313, 1974.
59. Losonsky JM, Kneller SK: Misdiagnosis in normal radiographic anatomy: Eight structural configurations simulating disease entities in dogs and cats. *JAVMA* 191(1):109–114, 1987.
60. Dueland R, Sisson D, Evans HE: Aberrant origin of the cranial cruciate ligament mimicking an osteochondral lesion radiographically. *Vet Radiol* 23(4):175–177, 1982.
61. Fox SM, Bloomberg MS, Bright JRM: Developmental anomalies of the canine elbow. *JAAHA* 19(5):605–615, 1983.
62. Goring RL, Bloomberg MS: Selected developmental abnormalities of the canine elbow: Radiographic evaluation and surgical management. *Compend Contin Educ Pract Vet* 5(3):178–188, 1983.
63. Olsson SE: The early diagnosis of fragmented coronoid process and osteochondritis dissecans of the canine elbow joints. *JAAHA* 19(5):616–626, 1983.
64. Denny HR, Gibbs C: The surgical treatment of osteochondritis dissecans and ununited coronoid process in the canine elbow joint. *J Small Anim Pract* 21(6):323–331, 1980.
65. Brinker WO, Piermattei DL, Flo GL: *Handbook of Small Animal Orthopedics and Fracture Treatment*, ed 2. Philadelphia, WB Saunders Co, 1990, pp 505–507.
66. Grondalen J: Arthrosis in the elbow joint of rapidly growing dogs. III. Ununited medial coronoid process of the ulna and osteochondritis dissecans of the humeral condyle. Surgical procedure for correction and postoperative investigation. *Nord Vet Med* 31(12):520–527, 1979.
67. Grondalen J, Grondalen T: Arthrosis in the elbow joint of rapidly growing dogs. V. A pathoanatomical investigation. *Nord Vet Med* 33(1):1–16, 1981.
68. Whitehair JG, Rudd RG: Osteochondritis dissecans of the humeral head in dogs. *Compend Contin Educ Pract Vet* 12(2):195–204, 1990.
69. Vaughan LC, Jones DGC: Osteochondritis dissecans of the head of the humerus in dogs. *J Small Anim Pract* 9(6):283–294, 1968.
70. Rudd RG, Whitehair JG, Margolis JH: Results of management of osteochondritis dissecans of the humeral head in dogs: 44 cases (1982–1987). *JAAHA* 26(2):173–178, 1990.
71. Brinker WO, Piermattei DL, Flo GL: *Handbook of Small Animal Orthopedics and Fracture Treatment*, ed 2. Philadelphia, WB Saunders Co, 1990, pp 486–489.
72. LaHue TR, Brown SG, Roush JC, et al: Entrapment of joint mice in the bicipital tendon sheath as a sequela to osteochondritis dissecans of the proximal humerus in dogs: A report of 6 cases. *JAAHA* 24(1):99–105, 1988.
73. van Bree H: Evaluation of the prognostic value of positive-contrast shoulder arthrography for bilateral osteochondrosis lesions in dogs. *Am J Vet Res* 51(7):1121–1126, 1990.
74. Story EC: Prognostic value of arthrography in canine shoulder osteochondrosis (osteochondritis) dissecans. *Vet Clin North Am* 8(2):301–307, 1978.
75. Nunamaker DM: Legg-Calve-Perthes Disease, in Newton CD, Nunamaker DM (eds): *Textbook of Small Animal Orthopaedics*. Philadelphia, JB Lippincott Co, 1985, pp 949–952.
76. Kemp HBS: Perthes disease: An experimental and clinical study. *Ann R Coll Surg Engl* 52:18–35, 1973.
77. Lee R, Fry PD: Some observations on the occurrence of Legg-Calve-Perthes disease (coxa plana) in the dog, and an evaluation of excision arthroplasty as a method of treatment. *J Small Anim Pract* 10(5):309–317, 1969.
78. Junggren GL: A comparative study of conservative and surgical treatment of Legg Perthes' disease in the dog. *Anim Hosp* 2(1):6–10, 1966.
79. Harrison MHM, Turner MH, Jacobs P: Skeletal immaturity in Perthes' disease. *J Bone Joint Surg* 58B(1):37–40, 1976.
80. Freeman MAR, England JPS: Experimental infarction of the immature canine femoral head. *Proc R Soc Lond* 62:431–433, 1969.
81. Sanchis M, Zahir A, Freeman MAR: The experimental simulation of Perthes' disease by consecutive interruptions of the blood supply to the capital femoral epiphysis in the puppy. *J Bone Joint Surg* 55A(2):335–342, 1973.
82. Zahir A, Freeman MAR: Cartilage changes following a single episode of infarction of the capital femoral epiphysis in the dog. *J Bone Joint Surg* 54A(1):125–136, 1972.
83. Ljunggren G: Legg-Perthes disease in the dog. A case report with special reference to initial radiographic changes. *Clin Orthop* 42(1):32–36, 1969.
84. Hulth A, Norberg UI, Olsson SE: Coxa plana in the dog. A preliminary report of a clinical, roentgenographic, histological, and microangiographic study. *J Bone Joint Surg* 44A(1):918–930, 1962.
85. Gibson KL, Lewis DD, Pechman RD: Use of external coaptation for the treatment of avascular necrosis of the femoral head in a dog. *JAVMA* 197(7):868–870, 1990.
86. Corley EA, Hogan PM: Trends in hip dysplasia control: Analysis of radiographs submitted to the Orthopedic Foundation for Animals, 1974 to 1984. *JAVMA* 187(8):805–809, 1985.
87. Lust G, Rendano VT, Summers BA: Canine hip dysplasia: Concepts and diagnosis. *JAVMA* 187(6):638–640, 1985.
88. Pierce KR, Bridges CH, Banks WC: Hormone induced hip dysplasia in dogs. *J Small Anim Pract* 6(2):121–126, 1965.
89. Pierce KR, Bridges CH: The role of estrogens in the pathogenesis of canine hip dysplasia. Metabolism of exogenous estrogens. *J Small Anim Pract* 8(1):383–389, 1967.
90. Belfield WO: Chronic subclinical scurvy and canine hip dysplasia. *VM SAC* 71(10):1399–1403, 1976.
91. Lust G, Geary JC, Sheffy BE: Development of hip dysplasia in dogs. *Am J Vet Res* 34(1):87–91, 1973.
92. Schales O: Genetic aspects of dysplasia of the hip joint. *North Am Vet* 37(6):476–478, 1956.
93. Jessen CR, Spurrell FA: Heritability of canine hip dysplasia. *Proc Canine Hip Dysplasia Symp Workshop*:53–61, 1972.
94. Riser WH, Larsen JS: Influence of breed somatotypes on prevalence of hip dysplasia in the dog. *JAVMA* 165(1):79–81, 1974.
95. Priester WA, Mulvinill FF: Canine hip dysplasia: Relative risk by sex, size, and breed, and comparative aspects. *JAVMA* 160(5):735–739, 1972.
96. Kasstrom H: Nutrition, weight gain, and development of hip dysplasia: An experimental investigation in growing dogs with reference to the effect of feeding intensity. *Acta Radiol [Suppl]* 344:135–179, 1975.
97. Riser WH, Shirer JF: Correlation between canine hip dysplasia and pelvic muscle mass: A study of 95 dogs. *Am J Vet Res* 28(124):769–777, 1967.
98. Riser WH: The dog as a model for the study of hip dysplasia. Growth form and development of the normal and dysplastic hip joint. *Vet Pathol* 12(4):234–334, 1975.
99. Riser WH: The dysplastic hip joint: Its radiographic and histologic development. *J Am Vet Radiol Soc* 14(2):35–50, 1973.
100. Wallace LJ: Canine hip dysplasia: Past and present. *Semin Vet Med Surg [Small Anim]* 2(2):92–106, 1987.
101. Bardens JW, Hardwick H: New observations on the diagnosis and cause of hip dysplasia. *VM SAC* 63(3):238–245, 1968.
102. Wright PJ, Mason TA: The usefulness of palpation of joint laxity in puppies as a predictor of hip dysplasia in a guide dog programme. *J Small Anim Pract* 18(8):513–522, 1977.
103. Giardina JF, MacCarthy AW: Evaluation of technic for early determination of predysplastic dogs. Hip palpation. *VM SAC* 66(9):878–882, 1971.
104. Ortolani M: The classic: Congenital hip dysplasia in the light of early and very early diagnosis. *Clin Orthop* 119(9):6–10, 1976.
105. Henricson B, Norberg I, Olsson SE: On the etiology and pathogene-

sis of hip dysplasia: A comparative review. *J Small Anim Pract* 7(11):673–688, 1966.
106. Schrader SC: Triple osteotomy of the pelvis and trochanteric osteotomy as a treatment for hip dysplasia in the immature dog: The surgical technique and results of 77 consecutive operations. *JAVMA* 189(6):659–665, 1986.
107. Smith GK, Biery DN, Gregor TP: New concepts of coxofemoral joint stability and development of a clinical stress-radiographic method for quantitating hip joint laxity in the dog. *JAVMA* 196(1):59–70, 1990.
108. Henry JD, Park RD: Wedge technique for demonstration of coxofemoral joint laxity in the canine. *Proc Canine Hip Dysplasia Symp Workshop*:117–126, 1972.
109. Slocum B, Devine TM: Dorsal acetabular rim radiographic view for the evaluation of the canine hip. *JAAHA* 26(3):289–296, 1990.
110. Barrett RB, Schall WD, Lewis RE: Clinical and radiographic features of canine panosteitis. *Anim Hosp* 4(2):94–104, 1968.
111. Bohning R, Suter PF, Hohn RB, et al: Clinical and radiographic survey of canine panosteitis. *JAVMA* 156(7):870–883, 1970.
112. Burt JK, Wilson GP: A study of eosinophilic panosteitis (enostosis) in German shepherd dogs. *Acta Radiol [Suppl]* 319:7–13, 1972.
113. Milton JT: Panosteitis: A review of the literature and 32 cases. *Auburn Vet* 35(3):11–15, 1979.
114. Alexander JW: Selected skeletal dysplasia: Craniomandibular osteopathy, multiple cartilagenous exostosis, and hypertrophic osteodystrophy. *Vet Clin North Am [Small Anim Pract]* 13(1):55–70, 1982.
115. Watson ADJ, Blair RC, Farrow BRH, et al: Hypertrophic osteodystrophy in the dog. *Aust Vet J* 49(9):433–439, 1973.
116. Merillat L: Barlow's disease in a dog. *Vet Med* 31(7):304, 1936.
117. Brinker WO, Piermattei DL, Flo GL: *Handbook of Small Animal Orthopedics and Fracture Treatment*, ed 2. Philadelphia, WB Saunders Co, 1990, pp 554–556.
118. Grondalen J: Metaphyseal osteopathy (hypertrophic osteodystrophy) in growing dogs: A clinical study. *J Small Anim Pract* 17(11): 721–735, 1976.
119. Holmes JR: Suspected skeletal scurvy in the dog. *Vet Rec* 74(29): 801–813, 1962.
120. Meier H, Clark ST, Schnelle GB, et al: Hypertrophic osteodystrophy associated with disturbance of vitamin C synthesis in dogs. *JAVMA* 130(11):483–491, 1957.
121. Bennette D: Nutrition and bone disease in the dog and cat. *Vet Rec* 98(16):313–321, 1976.
122. Riser W, Bingle S: Normal and abnormal growth of the distal foreleg in large and giant breed dogs. *J Am Vet Radiol Soc* 6:50–64, 1965.
123. Watson ADJ: Hypertrophic osteodystrophy: Vitamin C deficiency, overnutrition, or infection. *Aust Vet Pract* 8(2):107–108, 1978.
124. Stogdale L: Foreleg lameness in rapidly growing dogs. *J S Afr Vet Med Assoc* 50(2):61–68, 1979.
125. Woodard JC: Canine hypertrophic osteodystrophy, a study of the spontaneous disease in littermates. *Vet Pathol* 19(4):337–354, 1982.
126. Lenehan TM, Van Sickle DC: Ununited anconeal process, ununited medial coronoid process, ununited medial epicondyle, patella cubiti, and sesamoidal fragments of the elbow, in Newton CD, Nunamaker MD (eds): *Textbook of Small Animal Orthopaedics*. Philadelphia, JB Lippincott Co, 1985, pp 999–1012.
127. Corley EA, Carlson WD: Radiographic, genetic and pathologic aspects of elbow dysplasia. *JAVMA* 147(12):1651, 1965.
128. Sinibaldi KR, Arnoczky SP: Surgical removal of the ununited anconeal process in the dog. *JAAHA* 11(2):192–198, 1975.
129. Brinker WO, Piermattei DL, Flo GL: *Handbook of Small Animal Orthopedics and Fracture Treatment*, ed 2. Philadelphia, WB Saunders Co, 1990, pp 502–505.
130. Van Sickle DC: The relationship of ossification to canine elbow dysplasia. *JAAHA* 2(1):24–31, 1966.
131. Berzon JL, Quick CB: Fragmented coronoid process: Anatomical, clinical and radiographic considerations with case analysis. *JAAHA* 16(2):241–251, 1980.
132. Bennett D, Duff SRI, Kene RO, et al: Osteochondritis dissecans and fragmentation of the coronoid process in the elbow joint of the dog. *Vet Rec* 109(15):329–336, 1981.
133. Wind AP: Incidence and radiographic appearance of fragmented coronoid process. *California Vet* 36(6):19–25, 1982.
134. Wind AP: Elbow incongruity and developmental diseases in the dog: Part I. *JAAHA* 22(6):711–724, 1986.
135. Wind AP, Packard ME: Elbow incongruity and developmental disease in the dog: Part II. *JAAHA* 22(6):725–730, 1986.
136. Bienz HA: Klinische und radiologische untersuchungen uber den fragmentierten processus coronoideus medialis im ellbogengelenk des Berner sennenhundes und der anderen sennenhunde-rassen, Inaugural dissertation, University of Zurich, Zurich, Switzerland, 1985.
137. Guthrie S, Pidduck HG: Heritability of elbow osteochondrosis within a closed population of dogs. *J Small Anim Pract* 31(2):93–96, 1990.
138. Henry WB: Radiographic diagnosis and surgical management of fragmented medial coronoid process in dogs. *JAVMA* 184(7): 799–805, 1984.
139. Robbins GM: Some aspects of the radiographical examination of the canine elbow joint. *J Small Anim Pract* 21(8):417–428, 1980.
140. Voorhout G, Hazewinkel HAW: The radiographic evaluation of the canine elbow joint with special reference to the medial humeral condyle and the medial coronoid process. *Vet Radiol* 28(5): 158–165, 1987.
141. Macpherson GC, Lewis DD, Johnson KA, et al: Fragmented coronoid process associated with premature distal radial physeal closure in four dogs. *Vet Comp Orthop Traum*, submitted for publication.

UPDATE

Since this article was originally published, Daniel D. Lewis, DVM, has moved to the Department of Small Animal Medical Sciences, College of Veterinary Medicine, University of Florida, Gainesville, Florida.

Canine Lumbosacral Diseases: Definitive Diagnosis, Treatment, and Prognosis

KEY FACTS

- **Appropriate therapy and accurate prognosis depend on definitive diagnosis of the specific disease responsible for lumbosacral signs.**
- **Differentiation of diskospondylitis from other lumbosacral diseases is vital because antimicrobial therapy alone is recommended for most cases of diskospondylitis.**
- **Delayed surgical treatment, caused by procrastination or delayed diagnosis, may increase the morbidity associated with degenerative lumbosacral stenosis and its therapy.**
- **Accurate prognosis for neurologic recovery from lumbosacral fracture and luxation is based on neurologic examination and possibly surgical exploration.**

Texas A&M University
Ross H. Palmer, DVM, MS

University of Georgia
Jonathan N. Chambers, DVM

TENTATIVE DIAGNOSIS of lumbosacral disease can be based on a compatible history, signalment, and physical findings. Even though a lumbosacral problem is strongly suspected, appropriate therapy depends on determining a specific cause. The tentative diagnosis can usually be confirmed by a combination of radiography (survey and contrast), electromyography, and high-technology imaging techniques. This article discusses definitive diagnostic steps, proper therapy, and prognosis of lumbosacral diseases.

DEFINITIVE DIAGNOSIS

Radiography

Radiography is the primary method of definitive diagnosis of lumbosacral diseases in dogs. Radiography comprises survey and contrast techniques.

Survey Radiography

Lateral and ventrodorsal survey radiographs are the initial steps in evaluating lumbosacral disease.[1,2] Survey radiography is only diagnostic in conditions that involve bony destruction or displacement, including diskospondylitis, idiopathic lumbosacral stenosis, osseous neoplasia, and traumatic fracture and subluxation.[3-8] Lysis of adjacent end plates, end plate sclerosis, and spondylosis are hallmarks of diskospondylitis.[1,3] Radiographic signs may not be present for four to six weeks after the onset of infection. Radionuclide scanning should be considered in patients suspected of radiographically latent diskospondylitis.[9] Although spondylosis and end plate sclerosis are features of diskospondylitis and spondylosis deformans, vertebral lysis occurs only in the former[9] (Figure 1). Vertebral tumors may also cause osseous lysis but usually do not affect adjacent vertebral end plates.[9] Differentiation of diskospondylitis from other lumbosacral diseases is vital because antimicrobial therapy alone is recommended in most cases of diskospondylitis.

Indirect evidence of degenerative lumbosacral stenosis (e.g., spondylosis deformans, disk space narrowing, end plate sclerosis, and transitional vertebrae) is frequently present on survey radiographs[1] (Figure 2). These findings suggest but do not confirm the diagnosis. Spondylosis may not be as benign a radiographic change as was once

Originally published in Volume 13, Number 2, February 1991

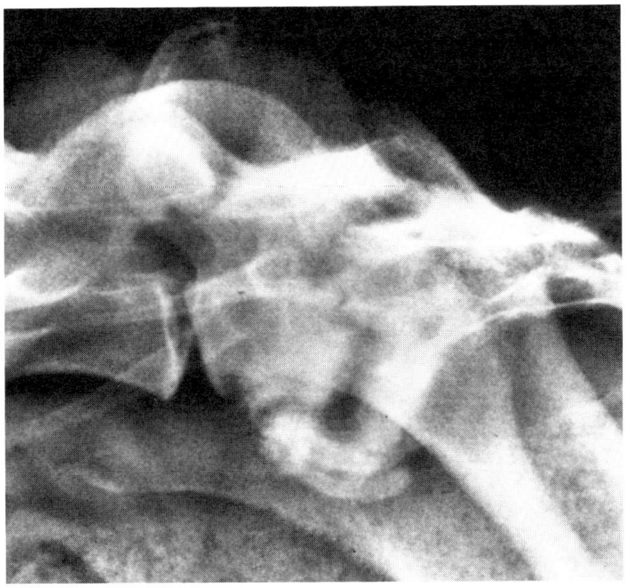

Figure 1—Lateral survey radiograph of an eight-year-old Airedale with pain and difficulty on rising. Lysis of the vertebral end plates distinguishes this case of diskospondylitis from spondylosis deformans. Ventral spondylosis and end plate sclerosis are common features of diskospondylitis and spondylosis deformans.

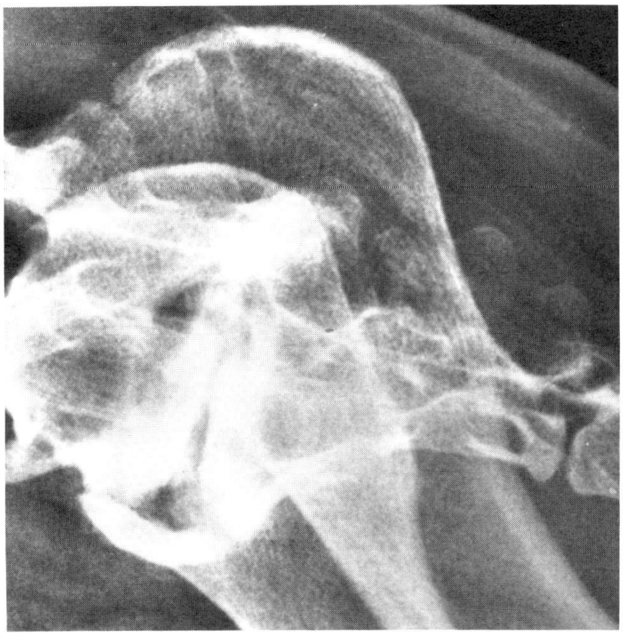

Figure 2—Lateral survey radiograph of a 10-year-old golden retriever with bilateral pelvic limb weakness. Spondylosis deformans, disk space narrowing, and end plate sclerosis suggest degenerative lumbosacral stenosis. Contrast radiography is necessary to confirm the diagnosis. Note the absence of the lytic changes evident in Figure 1.

believed. Although it is often present in asymptomatic dogs, as many as 28% of patients with spondylosis have signs that might be consistent with pelvic limb problems.[10] Spondylosis in the presence of compatible clinical signs is currently considered to be highly suggestive of degenerative lumbosacral stenosis.

In a study of 15 dogs, survey radiography (with supportive historical and clinical findings) was the means of definitive diagnosis of idiopathic lumbosacral stenosis.[4] Subjective observation of vertebral canal stenosis was the radiographic hallmark.[4] Objective means of measuring the vertebral canal failed to differentiate these patients from a normal population.[4] Myelography and intraosseous venography were performed on one patient in this series. Myelography was inconclusive, and venography demonstrated compression at L_7–S_1. Although no other contrast studies were performed in the series, surgical findings did not include disk protrusion. Thickened interarcuate ligament present at surgery suggests that contrast studies may be helpful in definitively diagnosing this ill-defined disease before exploration.

In addition to characterizing osseous changes at the lumbosacral junction, survey radiography can be used to evaluate the contribution of musculoskeletal disease to the clinical signs. Because large-breed dogs (especially German shepherds) are predisposed to hip dysplasia and degenerative lumbosacral stenosis, some weakness or lameness related to hip dysplasia could persist in these patients despite complete resolution of lumbosacral stenosis.

Contrast Radiography

Because clinical signs of lumbosacral disease are usually the result of soft tissue compression of the cauda equina, contrast radiography has become the primary means of definitive diagnosis in dogs.[1] Evaluation of the lumbosacral junction by myelography, vertebral sinus venography, and epidurography have been described and reviewed well.[1,11,12]

Myelography involves the injection of contrast medium into the subarachnoid space. Myelography has been criticized as a method of lumbosacral junction evaluation because the subarachnoid space is tapered or ends cranial to the lumbosacral junction in dogs.[1,13] Stressed views (flexion and extension) may improve the diagnostic sensitivity of myelography.[14]

Several techniques of vertebral sinus venography have been described.[1] Compared with myelography and epidurography, intraosseous venography is technically difficult to perform.[11] If lumbosacral compression is present, three abnormalities may be recognized on the venogram: displacement of the vertebral venous sinuses, narrowing of the sinuses, and obstruction of cranial flow past the compressive mass.[1]

AMONG MANY veterinary radiologists, epidurography is the preferred means of lumbosacral evaluation.[1,11,12] The method combines technical ease and superior sensitivity compared with the other techniques.[11] Epidurography involves the injection of contrast medium into the epidural space. There is a strong correlation between epidurographic and surgical findings.[12] In a recent study, compressive lesions were found at surgery in 96% of dogs with epidurogram findings of 50% elevation of the epidural space or total obstruction to cranial flow of contrast medium[12] (Figure 3). Compressive lesions were found at surgery in 83% dogs with less than 50% elevation of the epidural space. Other suggestive findings included concomitant filling of the epidural space and vertebral venous sinuses as well as extravasation of contrast material into the soft tissue adjacent to the injection site[12]; these suggestive findings can also occur in some normal dogs.

Epidurography is performed in patients under general anesthesia and usually does not require fluoroscopy.[1] After surgical preparation of the injection site, a spinal needle is inserted into the dorsal space at vertebra S_3–Cd_1, Cd_1–Cd_2, or Cd_2–Cd_3.[1] The bevel of the needle is directed cranially and advanced to the floor of the spinal canal. Cerebrospinal fluid cannot be retrieved because the needle is in the epidural space rather than the subarachnoid space. Approximately 0.1 to 0.2 ml/kg of contrast agent is injected.[1]

Although we currently use iohexol, any myelographic agent can be used. Lateral radiographs after injection should include neutral, flexed, and extended (dorsiflexed) positions. Extension often enhances ventral and dorsal compressive lesions. Dorsoventral views should also be taken but are diagnostic in fewer patients.

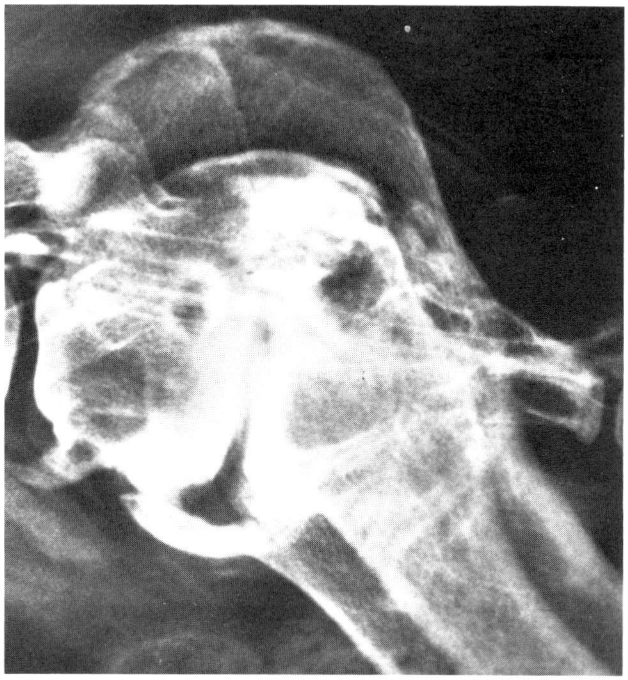

Figure 3—Epidurogram of the patient in Figure 2. There is approximately 50% elevation of the epidural space and subluxation of the lumbosacral space. Disk protrusion, articular facet osteophytosis, and instability were noted at surgery.

High-Technology Imaging

Computerized tomography and magnetic resonance imaging have revolutionized the definitive diagnosis of lumbosacral diseases in humans. In our limited experience, computerized tomography is extremely helpful in characterizing diseases and in preoperative planning in dogs. Contrast studies rely on indirect evidence of compressive soft tissue, but the high-technology techniques allow actual visualization of the compressive soft and bony tissue as well as nervous tissue parenchyma. Until these modalities become practical for veterinary medicine, contrast techniques will be the mainstay of lumbosacral evaluation.

Electromyography

Electromyography can be useful in substantiating a diagnosis of lumbosacral disease and differentiating the disease from musculoskeletal causes of pelvic limb weakness. Although certain electromyographic abnormalities strongly suggest lumbosacral disease, normal electromyographs do not eliminate the possibility of lumbosacral disease.[2,15] Electromyographic changes may indicate neuritis or denervation but cannot distinguish between diseases of the lumbosacrum. Many dogs with pain as the only clinical sign have normal electromyographic results; abnormalities are often found in patients with signs of lower motor neuron disease.[15]

The importance of thorough neurologic examination is apparent. We currently perform electromyography in the major muscle groups of each pelvic limb (the quadriceps group, caudal thigh muscles, and interosseous muscles), the paravertebral muscles, and the muscles of the tail and external anal sphincter to focus surgical therapy to one side of the cauda equina if necessary.

TREATMENT

Definitive diagnosis of the specific disease responsible for the lumbosacral signs is vital to appropriate therapy. Additional considerations are the duration and severity of clinical signs, the intended use of the patient, and the financial constraints and wishes of the client. Treatment can be categorized as nonsurgical (conservative) or surgical.

Nonsurgical Therapy

Diskospondylitis is an infectious disease and thus should be treated with appropriate antibiotics.[9] The selection of antibiotic is based on blood cultures or serologic tests.[9] If the results of the blood culture are negative, *Staphylococcus aureus* is the presumed cause.[9] Oral cephradine (20 mg/kg every eight hours) or cloxacillin (10 mg/kg every six hours) for four to six weeks has been recommended in these instances.[9] Improvement should be evident in five to seven days if the proper antibiotic and dose are being administered.[9] Lack of improvement suggests the need for reassessment, including confirmation of antibiotic dosage and administration, repeated culture, change of antibiotic, and/or surgical curettage and culture of solitary lesions. Cultures from percutaneous aspirates of lumbosacral diskospondylitis lesions can be obtained using fluoroscopy to guide the needle.

In *Brucella canis*-positive dogs, a staged treatment regimen of tetracycline and streptomycin has been recommended together with neutering.[9] Radiographic and clinical evaluation at two-week intervals and blood cultures two weeks after the cessation of antibiotic therapy have been recommended.[9] Treatment duration should vary from 4 to 14 weeks (or more) and should continue at least two weeks after clinical recovery.[3,9] Owners should be informed of the public health significance of *B. canis* infection.

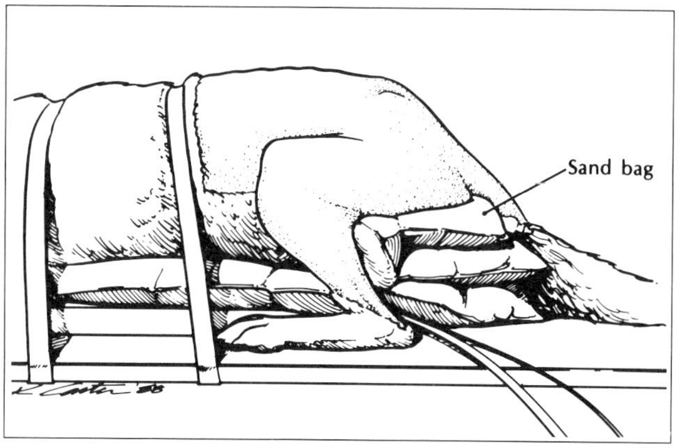

Figure 4—Positioning of a patient for lumbosacral surgery. Sandbags are placed under the tuber ischii to elevate the lumbosacral space, reduce venous congestion, and improve ventilation. (From Chambers JN: Degenerative lumbosacral stenosis in dogs. *Vet Med Report* 1:166–180, 1989. Reprinted with permission.)

IN PATIENTS with degenerative lumbosacral stenosis, nonoperative management is recommended at the first episode of pain only.[2] In obese patients, rest, antiinflammatory and analgesic agents, and weight loss are recommended.[2] The results of conservative therapy are not uniformly successful. Early surgical intervention should be strongly considered in patients with recurrent signs, severe pain, or lower motor neuron signs.[2,15] A delay in surgical treatment because of late diagnosis or procrastination may increase the morbidity associated with the disease and the surgery.[2,15]

Although nonsurgical treatment failed in all 15 reported cases of idiopathic lumbosacral stenosis, resolution of signs followed surgical decompression.[4] Based on this report, conservative treatment apparently is not effective in these patients. Conversely, initial conservative care with rest and antiinflammatory drugs did not alter the surgical prognosis of the disease.

Conservative treatment of lumbar spinal fractures has been reported.[16,17] A successful outcome is possible with conservative care of lumbosacral fractures and luxations in some patients, and such care is an alternative to euthanasia. The difficulty of managing urinary and fecal incontinence must be emphasized to the owner. In general, conservative therapy is considered if there are minimal pelvic limb and urinary bladder neurologic deficits with minimal spinal displacement and instability.[8] Fracture instability is often difficult to judge radiographically, however, and surgical treatment should be considered in most cases.

Lumbosacral neoplasia is uncommon and usually involves a primary bony tumor.[5,7] Because of the poor prognosis associated with most lumbosacral neoplasia, nonoperative treatment is often selected. Definitive diagnosis requires incisional or excisional biopsy via surgical exposure. In our experience, computerized tomography has been helpful in characterizing the tissue of origin before surgical exposure.

Surgical Therapy

Indications for surgical treatment of degenerative lumbosacral stenosis are neurologic deficits, pain that is unresponsive to proper conservative therapy, and frequent recurrences of pain (even if the episodes respond well to conservative treatment). Two surgical techniques have been the recent focus for treatment of these patients. One is directed toward excision of the encroaching tissue[15,18]; the other is aimed at resolution of subluxation via traction and stabilization.[19,20]

FOR BOTH techniques, the patient is positioned in sternal recumbency with the pelvic limbs pulled cranially alongside the trunk to open the interlaminar space.[2] Sandbags or towels are placed to elevate the tuber ischii from the surgical table (Figure 4). This position levels the lumbosacral space, improves ventilation, and prevents vertebral venous sinus congestion secondary to pressure on intraabdominal veins.[2]

Excisional Technique

A routine dorsal midline approach to the lumbosacral space is made.[15,18] The interarcuate ligament is identified and carefully excised from its attachments to the L_7 and sacral lamina (Figure 5, A and B). Epidural fat is visible immediately deep to the ligament. The nerve roots of the cauda equina are often elevated far dorsally in patients with large ventral compressive lesions. The caudal half of the L_7 spinous process and the cranial half of the median sacral crest are removed with a bone rongeur. A dorsal

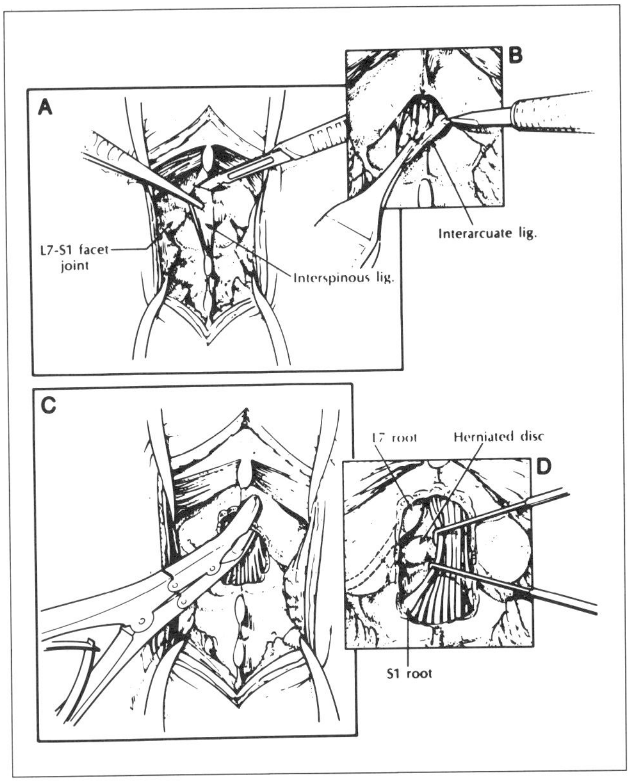

Figure 5—(*A*) Excision of the interspinous ligament. (*B*) Excision of the interarcuate ligament to expose the underlying epidural fat and nerve roots. (C) Laminectomy of L_7 and S_1 to gain wider access to the epidural space. (*D*) Exposure of the L_7 nerve root and intervertebral disk. (From Chambers JN: Degenerative lumbosacral stenosis in dogs. *Vet Med Report* 1:166–180, 1989. Reprinted with permission.)

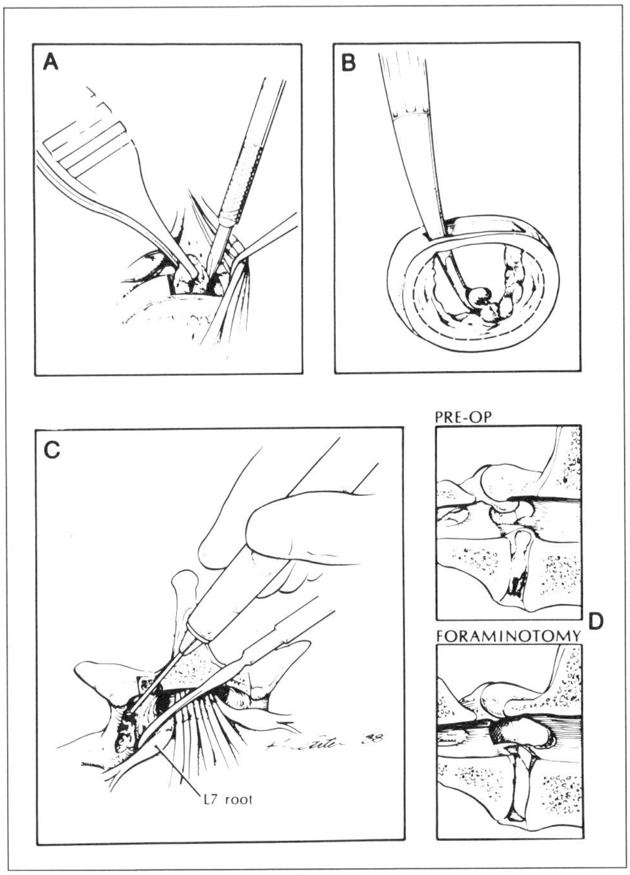

Figure 6—(*A*) Retraction of the cauda equina to allow final excision of disk material after rectangular incisions in the annulus fibrosus have been connected. (*B*) Curettage of the disk space. (C) Technique for removing a compressive osteophyte with a power bur while protecting nerve roots. (*D*) Illustrations before and after foraminotomy and diskectomy demonstrate relief of compressive tissue. (From Chambers JN: Degenerative lumbosacral stenosis in dogs. *Vet Med Report* 1:166–180, 1989. Reprinted with permission.)

laminectomy is performed with bone rongeurs or a pneumatic bur (Figure 5, C and D). Initially, care should be taken to preserve the vertebral pedicles because they support the articular facets.

The nerve roots are inspected with a nerve root retractor. The S_1 nerve roots course parallel the L_7–S_1 facets and run along the lateral aspect of the laminectomy site. It may be necessary to probe beneath the facets gently with the retractor to retrieve the nerve root. The L_7 nerve root is large and lies under the shelf of bone created by the caudal facet of L_7 and the remaining lamina. Extension of the laminectomy further cranially is occasionally necessary to identify and follow this nerve root. Normal nerve roots can be mobilized two or three millimeters without tension. Tension indicates entrapment of the root; the source of entrapment should be identified. Excessive iatrogenic nerve root tension should be avoided.

The cauda equina (excluding the L_7 nerve root) is retracted to one side to view the L_7–S_1 intervertebral disk. Disk protrusion is usually visible as a pearlescent white dome on the floor of the canal. The dome may be a small focal protrusion or may extend the full width of the disk. Wide protrusions can push the more lateral roots dorsally and laterally, making them difficult to see beneath the facets.

The disk is excised by cutting half of a rectangle from the dorsal annulus while the cauda equina is retracted to one side (Figure 6). The cauda equina is then gently retracted to the opposite side, and the rectangular incision is completed. Careful connection of the incisions maximizes the chance of removing the dorsal annulus as a whole rather than in fragments. The disk space is gently evacuated with a curette and rongeurs.

If there is a possibility of entrapment of the L_7 nerve root, the root should be followed to the L_7–S_1 intervertebral foramen. Removal of a hypertrophied joint capsule, interarcuate ligament remnants, remaining dorsal annulus fibrosus, or osteophytes may be necessary to free the course of the nerve root.

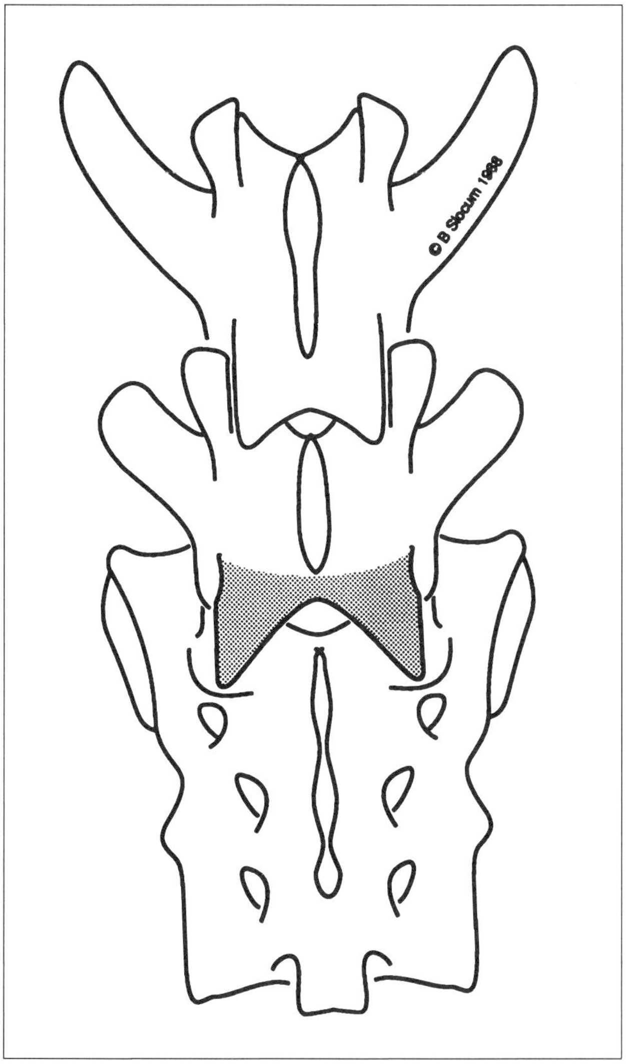

Figure 7A

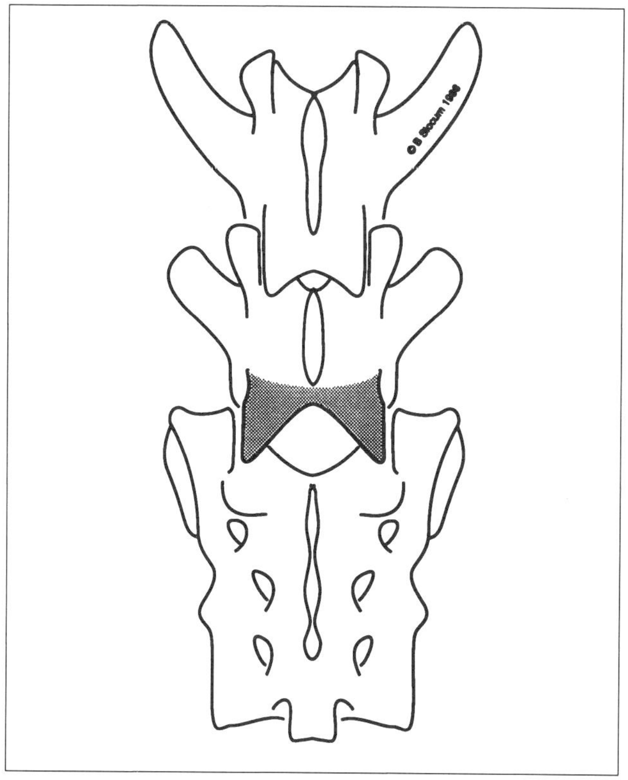

Figure 7B

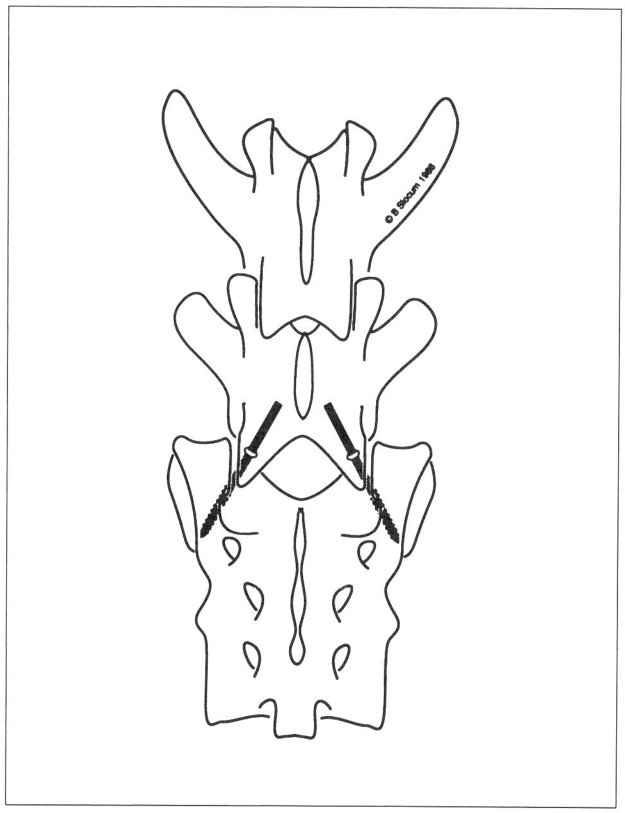

Figure 7C

Figure 7—(**A**) Dorsoventral position of L_7–S_1 subluxation. Note the overlapped position of the articular facets (*shaded*) and the decreased interarcuate space. (**B**) Dorsoventral position of L_7–S_1 after traction. The articular facet joints (*shaded*) have been reduced and the interarcuate space expanded. (**C**) Dorsoventral position of L_7–S_1 after pin fixation. Two partially threaded pins are placed through the L_7 articular facets and into the sacrum to maintain reduction of L_7–S_1. (From Slocum B, Devine T: Optimal treatment for degenerative lumbosacral stenosis: Traction, fixation, and fusion. *Vet Med Report* 1:249–257, 1989. Reprinted with permission.)

To maximize stability, every effort should be made to preserve the pedicle and facets. If necessary, unilateral facetectomy can be performed to eliminate soft tissue or osteophyte entrapment of a nerve root as it exits the intervertebral foramen. Although unilateral facetectomy usually does not jeopardize spinal stability, internal fixation and fusion should be attempted with bilateral facetectomy. Assessment of spinal stability and observation of positional

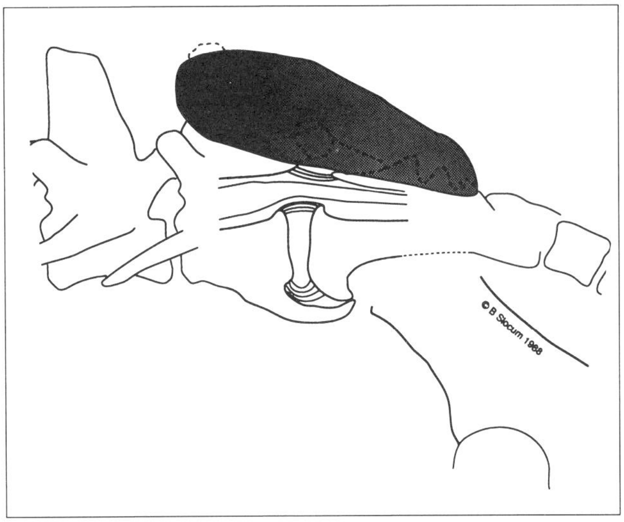

Figure 8A

nerve root impingement in the foramen are accomplished by using towel clamps in the dorsal spinous processes of L_6 and S_2 to mobilize the lumbosacral junction gently.

DEVITALIZED soft tissue is debrided, and the surgical wound is thoroughly lavaged with warm saline solution. A small autogenous fat graft is harvested from the subcutaneous layer and placed over the decompression site. The lumbosacral fascia and superficial layers are closed routinely.

Diskospondylitis patients with moderate to marked neurologic dysfunction may require excision of encroaching tissue and simultaneous culture of the disk space. In our experience, these patients are the exception.

Traction and Stabilization Technique

A standard dorsal midline approach to the lumbosacral spine is performed. The epaxial musculature is retracted from the dorsal spinous processes of L_7 and the sacrum and from the lumbosacral facet articulations. Attachments from the facets and pedicles are not disturbed.[19,20]

A vertebral spreader is positioned with one jaw at the cranial base of the sacral spinous process and the other at the caudal border of the L_7 lamina. The lumbosacral dorsal interarcuate space is expanded until the lumbosacral facets are repositioned in normal alignment (Figures 7A and 7B). To visualize the cauda equina, the interarcuate ligament is incised and reflected. To visualize the L_7–S_1 dorsal annulus, the cauda equina is retracted.

Fixation of the lumbosacral spine under traction is accomplished by directing a 0.062- to 0.125-inch, partially threaded pin through a slightly undersized, predrilled hole in the caudal third of the L_7 articular facet. The pin is seated in the lateral portion of S_1. The free end of the pin is cut at the level of the dorsal spinous process. A similar pin is placed on the opposite side (Figure 7C). A fat graft is placed over the interarcuate space. A corticocancellous bone graft is harvested from the ilial wings and reduced to three-millimeter fragments before placement on the lamina of the sacrum and L_7, over the fat graft and interarcuate ligament (Figure 8). Routine closure is performed.

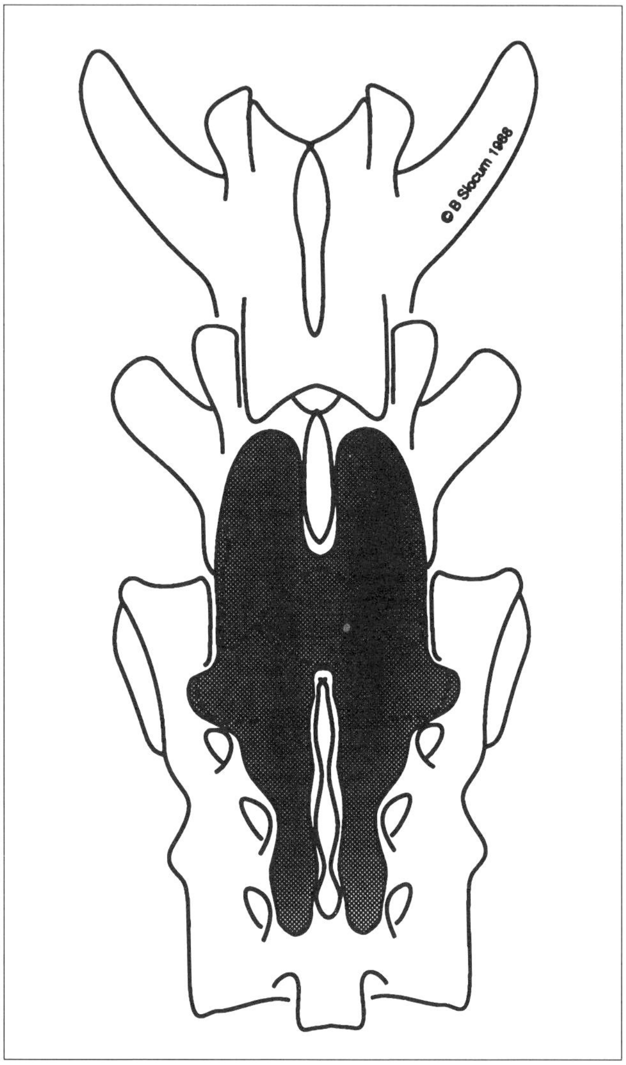

Figure 8B

Figure 8—(A) Lateral view of a cancellous bone graft (*shaded*) contacting L_7 from the dorsal limit of the dorsal spinous process of L_7 and filling the entire region to the sacral spine. **(B)** Dorsoventral view of a cancellous bone graft (*shaded*). (From Slocum B, Devine T: Optimal treatment for degenerative lumbosacral stenosis: Traction, fixation, and fusion. *Vet Med Report* 1:249–257, 1989. Reprinted with permission.)

Surgical Treatment of Fracture and Luxation

The presence of an anal reflex or pain perception in the

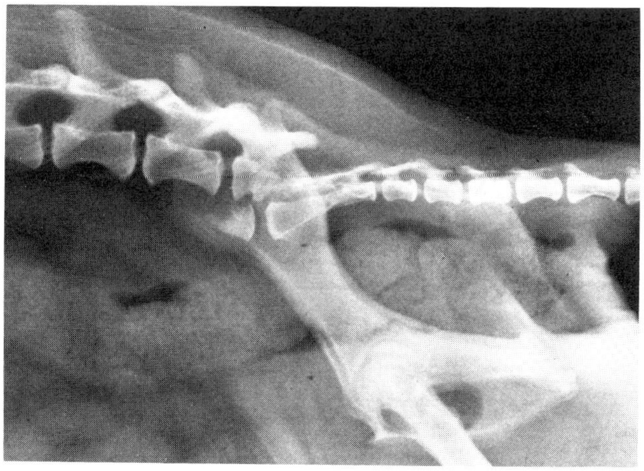

Figure 9A

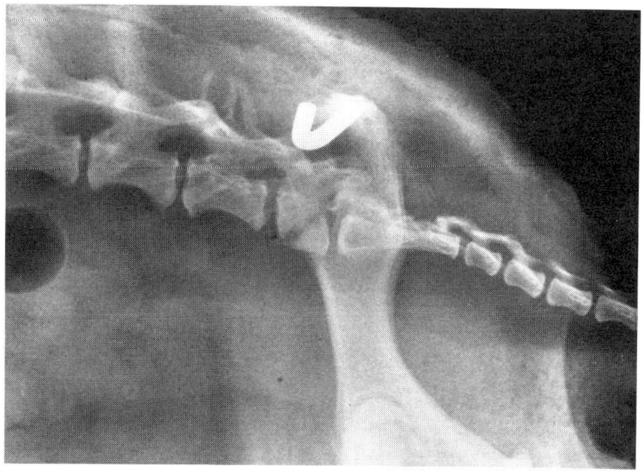

Figure 9B

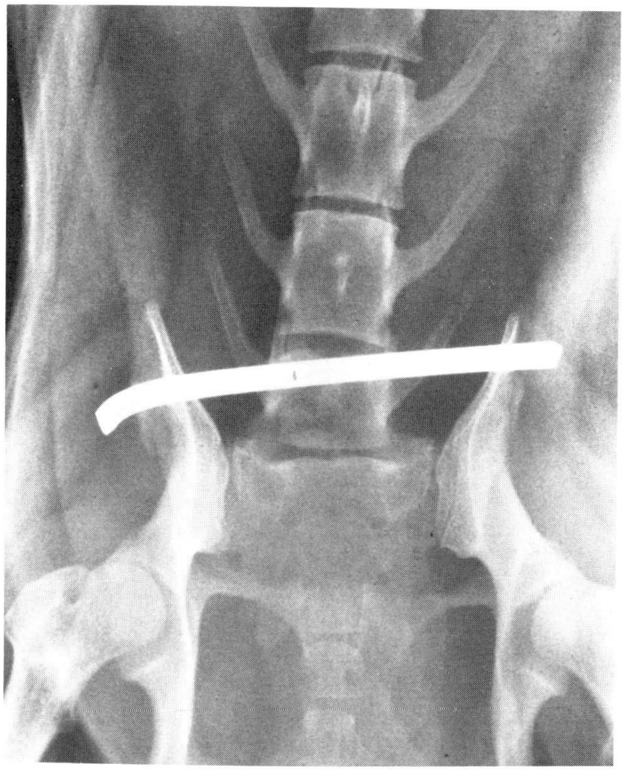

Figure 9C

Figure 9—Radiographs of a four-year-old poodle with an acute onset of pelvic limb paresis and ataxia after being hit by a car. (**A**) Severe displacement of the L_7 body fracture. The patient was weakly ambulatory and demonstrated urinary and fecal incontinence. (**B**) Postoperative reduction of the L_7 fracture with a transilial pin. On surgical exploration, the cauda equina was determined to be anatomically intact. (**C**) Ventrodorsal view of L_7 fracture repair with a transilial pin.

anal or tail region is an indication for surgical reduction and stabilization. If these responses are absent, exploratory surgery can be performed to determine the extent of anatomic nerve root damage.

A standard dorsal midline approach is performed as described. Because most L_7–S_1 fractures and luxations displace ventrally and cranially, reduction is usually achieved by dorsal and caudal retraction of the sacral-pelvic unit (Figure 9A). Reduction is confirmed by proper anatomic alignment of the L_7–S_1 articular facets.

Limited dorsal laminectomy permits visualization of the cauda equina. A transilial pin can be placed while reduction is maintained (Figures 9B and 9C). The pin should pass through one ilial wing, contact the dorsal lamina of L_7, and penetrate the opposite ilial wing.[17] The transilial pin tethers the sacral-pelvic unit to the dorsal lamina of L_7 and thus prevents ventral displacement and luxation. To avoid pin migration and loss of fixation, the ends of the pin should be bent or a threaded pin and washer-nut combination should be used.[17]

Postoperative Care

Exercise restriction is emphasized after surgical treatment of lumbosacral diseases. Restriction for four to eight weeks is recommended after decompressive procedures for stenosis, and restriction for 8 to 12 weeks is suggested after reduction and stabilization of fractures and luxations.[2] Symptomatic treatment for pain relief and appropriate weight reduction are also recommended.[2]

ALTHOUGH there may be improvement within several days of decompression of stenotic vertebral canals, return to normal function and activity level has taken as long as one year with the traction and stabilization technique.[19] Reduction and stabilization of fractures and luxations may result in rapid neurologic improvement, but improvement may be more prolonged or absent. Symptomatic and nursing care of bladder and bowel dysfunction is vital. If the patient is unable to void completely, bladder expression and/or intermittent urinary bladder catheterization is performed at least three times daily.

PROGNOSIS

The prognosis for resolution of signs caused by lumbosacral disease depends on the specific cause, the severity of signs, and the duration of the disease. Patients with degenerative lumbosacral stenosis often improve dramatically after surgery if pain is the only presenting sign.[15,18] In one study, 72% of the dogs were cured by excisional surgery.[15] Patients with chronic lower motor neuron dysfunction had extended and sometimes incomplete recovery after surgery.[15] Only one of eight patients with urinary incontinence at presentation was cured; the other patients had various levels of improvement.[15] Analysis of several reports on surgical management indicates that permanent neurologic injury as a result of surgery is uncommon[15,16,18,19]; a cavalier approach to surgical intervention should nevertheless be avoided.

In the report of idiopathic lumbosacral stenosis, the 15 dogs failed to respond or were refractory to nonsurgical treatments.[4] Surgical decompression of the stenotic canal alleviated clinical signs in all patients.

The most common treatment for lumbosacral diskospondylitis is appropriate antimicrobial therapy. The prognosis for resolution of the disease is good to excellent. In three studies, 84% (32 of 38) of patients with lumbosacral diskospondylitis recovered with antibiotic treatment alone.[3,16,21] In one study, 3 of 21 patients required surgical decompression and antibiotic therapy; all three improved.[3]

After traumatic injury to the lumbosacral spine, thorough neurologic examination is vital for prognostication. The tendency to base prognosis heavily on radiographic displacement must be avoided.[8] Conversely, the ability to stand or walk does not improve the prognosis for recovery of bladder and bowel control.[8] Severe injury is indicated by the absence of motor or sensory function of the tail, an anal reflex and tone, and perineal pain sensation. Despite the apparent severity of the injury, these deficits can resolve.

Reversible neurapraxia cannot be distinguished from irreversible nerve root avulsion on neurologic examination.[8] Surgical exposure of the cauda equina is often the best means for prognosticating in acute lumbosacral trauma patients; the technique permits assessment of anatomic integrity rather than function.[8] Given anatomically intact nerve roots, we usually recommend allowing at least four weeks for signs of improvement. If improvement is evident in this period, continued care and observation are recommended. If there is no improvement, the prognosis is guarded to poor.

Because lumbosacral neoplasia is relatively uncommon, objective prognostication is difficult.[5,8] The prognosis is often poor because most tumors are primary neoplasms of bone origin. Some nerve sheath tumors are benign and potentially resectable with a minimum of neural tissue dissection; resolution or at least control of the disease may be a realistic goal in such cases.[6,7]

About the Authors

Dr. Palmer is affiliated with the Department of Small Animal Medicine and Surgery, College of Veterinary Medicine, Texas A&M University, College Station, Texas. Dr. Chambers is affiliated with the Department of Small Animal Medicine, College of Veterinary Medicine, University of Georgia, Athens, Georgia. Drs. Palmer and Chambers are Diplomates of the American College of Veterinary Surgeons.

REFERENCES

1. Selcer BA: Radiographic imaging of canine lumbosacral diseases. *Vet Med Report* 1:282–290, 1989.
2. Chambers JN: Degenerative lumbosacral stenosis in dogs. *Vet Med Report* 1:166–180, 1989.
3. Gilmore DG: Lumbosacral diskospondylitis in 21 dogs. *JAAHA* 23:57–61, 1987.
4. Tarvin G, Prata RG: Lumbosacral stenosis in dogs. *JAVMA* 177: 154–159, 1980.
5. Lenehan TN: Canine cauda equina syndrome. *Compend Contin Educ Pract Vet* 5(11):941–951, 1983.
6. Luttgen PJ, Braund KG, Brawner WR, et al: A retrospective study of twenty-nine spinal tumors in the dog and cat. *J Small Anim Pract* 21:213–226, 1980.
7. Prata RG: Diagnosis of spinal cord tumors in the dog. *Vet Clin North Am* 7:165–185, 1977.
8. Indrieri RJ: Lumbosacral stenosis and injury of the cauda equina. *Vet Clin North Am [Small Anim Pract]* 18:697–710, 1988.
9. Kornegay JN: Diskospondylitis, in Kirk RW (ed): *Current Veterinary Therapy. VIII.* Philadelphia, WB Saunders Co, 1983, pp 718–721.
10. Morgan JP, Ljunggren G, Read R: Spondylosis deformans (vertebral osteophytosis) in the dog. *J Small Anim Pract* 8:57–66, 1967.
11. Hathcock JT, Pechman RD, Dillon AR, et al: Comparison of three radiographic contrast procedures in the evaluation of the canine lumbosacral spinal canal. *Vet Radiol* 29:4–14, 1988.
12. Selcer BA, Chambers JN, Schwensen K, et al: Epidurography as a diagnostic aid in canine lumbosacral compressive diseases: 47 cases (1981–1986). *Vet Compar Orthop Traum* 2:97–103, 1988.
13. Oliver JE, Selcer RR, Simpson S: Cauda equina compression from lumbosacral malformation and malarticulation. *JAVMA* 173:207–214, 1978.
14. Lang J: Flexion-extension myelography of the canine cauda equina. *Vet Radiol* 29:242–257, 1988.
15. Chambers JN, Selcer BA, Oliver JE: Results of treatment of degenerative lumbosacral stenosis in dogs by exploration and excision. *Vet Compar Orthop Traum* 3:130–133, 1988.
16. Denny HR, Gibbs C, Holt PE: The diagnosis and treatment of cauda equina lesion in the dog. *J Small Anim Pract* 23:425–443, 1982.
17. Slocum B, Rudy RL: Fractures of the seventh lumbar vertebra in the dog. *JAAHA* 11:167–174, 1975.
18. Chambers JN: Optimal treatment for degenerative lumbosacral stenosis: Surgical exploration and excision of tissue. *Vet Med Report* 1:248–252, 1989.
19. Slocum B, Devine T: L_7–S_1 fixation-fusion for treatment of cauda equina compression in the dog. *JAVMA* 188:31–35, 1986.
20. Slocum B, Devine T: Optimal treatment for degenerative lumbosacral stenosis: Traction, internal fixation, and fusion. *Vet Med Report* 1:249–257, 1989.
21. Johnson RG, Prata RG: Intradiskal osteomyelitis: A conservative approach. *JAAHA* 19:743–750, 1983.

UPDATE

High-Technology Imaging

Ross H. Palmer, DVM, MS, Diplomate, ACVS
Larry Y. Kerr, DVM, Diplomate, ACVR
Veterinary Specialty Service of the Santa Cruz Veterinary Hospital
2585 Soquel Drive
Santa Cruz, CA 95065

Since publication of our original manuscript in 1991, we and others have become more experienced and familiar with magnetic resonance imaging (MRI).[1] MRI is emerging as a clinically reliable, noninvasive, high-detail method for diagnostic imaging of the lumbosacral region of dogs. Though exhaustive discussion of the technology behind MRI is beyond the scope of this publication, it must be emphasized that MRI does not use ionizing radiation. Instead, MRI utilizes high-power magnetic fields and radiowave impulses that alter the orientation of protons within a patient's tissue cells, thereby generating a tissue map that can be presented in many planes (most commonly, axial, sagittal, and coronal). Mapping is accomplished by highlighting contrasting responses of tissues to variations in the induced conditions. The conditions can be changed (T1-weighted, T2-weighted, proton-density, and gradient echo images) to intensify the signal emitted from specific tissues.

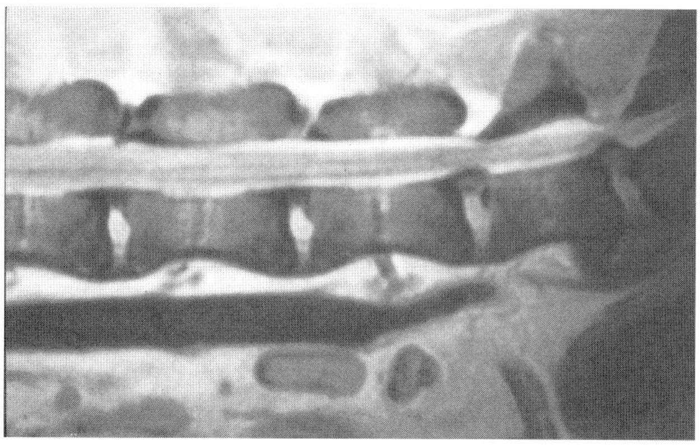

Figure 1—Sagittal proton-density image from the L4 vertebra to the sacrum in a dog with pelvic limb stiffness and lumbosacral pain. Loss of epidural fat is seen at L6–L7 and L7–S1, and displacement of the cauda equina is seen at L7–S1. The nucleus pulposus of L4–L5 and L5–L6 generates a high intensity signal, whereas the lack of intensity of this signal at L6–L7 and L7–S1 is indicative of degeneration.

Our current protocol for MRI scanning is as follows: The attending veterinarian must first have distinctly localized the spinal lesion (in this case, to the lumbosacrum) via neurologic physical examination. In most cases it is not practical to image the entire spine with MRI, as it is with myelography. Before the scan is done, history and radiographs should be used to confirm that there are no ferromagnetic implants (e.g., bone plates, pins, pacemakers, or foreign bodies) in the patient. Depending on the strength of the MRI magnet, it may not be permissible to utilize ferromagnetic monitoring or anesthetic equipment in the room. Our current anesthetic regimen involves slow intravenous infusion of propofol and pulse oximeter monitoring. The patient is anesthetized and carefully placed in dorsal recumbency; the patient must be straight because any tilting or twisting can compromise the diagnostic quality of the image. The MRI unit we presently use has a field strength of 1.5 tesla.

We initially perform T1-weighted sagittal images to evaluate the marrow content of the vertebral bodies to rule out metastatic disease. When disc protrusion is suspected, we perform proton-density sagittal, axial, and coronal images (Figures 1 to 3). It is important to make parasagittal slices from one intervertebral foramen across the central portions of the spinal canal to the contralateral foramen. Close examination of the parasagittal slices is helpful in detecting lateralization of disc protrusions. The foramina should be closely evaluated for nerve root impingement.

(continues on page 286)

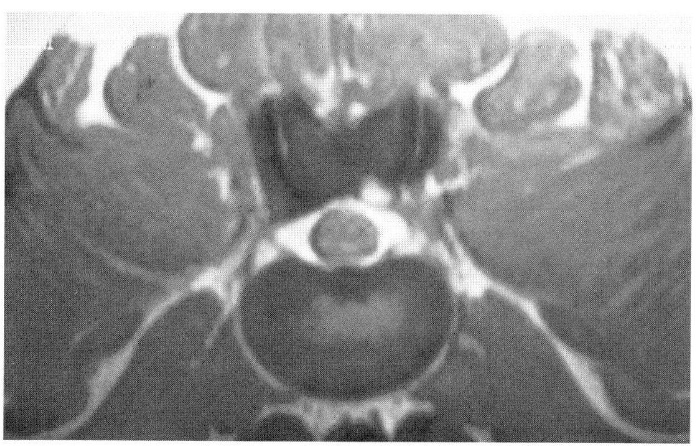

Figure 2—Axial proton-density image through the L5–L6 disc space in the dog in Figure 1 shows the conus medullaris centered in the vertebral canal surrounded by epidural fat. The intervertebral disc has a normal shape.

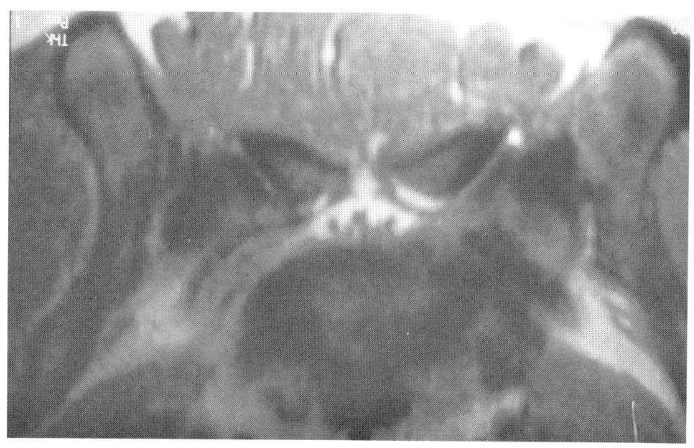

Figure 3—Axial proton-density image through the L7–S1 in the dog in Figure 1 shows loss of epidural fat ventral to the cauda equina and gross distortion of the normal disc architecture. There is apparent lateralized protrusion of the disc obliterating the lateral recess.

Acquired Dysplasias of the Canine Radius and Ulna

Colin B. Carrig, BVSc, PhD
Professor
Virginia-Maryland Regional
College of Veterinary Medicine
Virginia Tech
Blacksburg, Virginia

Jeffrey A. Wortman, VMD, PhD
Assistant Professor
College of Veterinary Medicine
Michigan State University
East Lansing, Michigan

Dogs frequently experience traumas that result in fractures, epiphyseal separations, and soft tissue injuries of varying degrees of severity. Every major fracture of the long bone in an immature animal produces some temporary alteration to the rate of growth of the affected bone, but the changes are usually too insignificant to be recognized clinically. The metaphyseal-epiphyseal junction (i.e., physis) in immature animals is more susceptible to partial or even complete disruption by shearing or compression forces than are the ligamentous structures supporting the joint;[1] thus, it is frequently injured. When injury occurs within the physis of a long bone, there is a possibility of permanent growth alteration. This can lead to angular deformity if there is diminished growth of a portion of the physis of a single bone[2] or if there is retarded growth of one of a pair of parallel bones such as the radius and ulna.[3-5]

The degree of growth alteration will depend on the integrity of the blood supply to the chondrogenic cells[6] and on the growth potential remaining at the time of injury. The type of physeal injury is, therefore, of some predictive value in assessing prognosis following trauma to this part of a bone. Classification of physeal fractures has been proposed in an attempt to relate the type of fracture to the likely degree of growth retardation.[6,7] Crush injuries to the physis have the most profound effect on epiphyseal vessels and are usually associated with greater interruptions to longitudinal growth of the bone.[6,7]

The radius and ulna, a pair of bones closely related to one another, have to grow in a synchronized manner to prevent malalignment of their common articular surfaces and to allow unrestricted growth of the individual bone members. Alterations of normal growth in either the radius or the ulna can result in marked morphologic changes in the adjacent bone, together with abnormalities in the elbow and carpal joints. Dysplasias resulting from abnormal growth of the radius and/or ulna are common orthopedic problems. It will be seen, from consideration of normal growth of the canine radius and ulna, that abnormal development related to asynchronous growth of these bones can result following retarded growth in the proximal radial physis, the distal radial physis, or the distal ulnar physis. Restriction of normal movement between these two bones in relation to one another during growth can also result in abnormal development.

Originally published in Volume 3, Number 6, June 1981

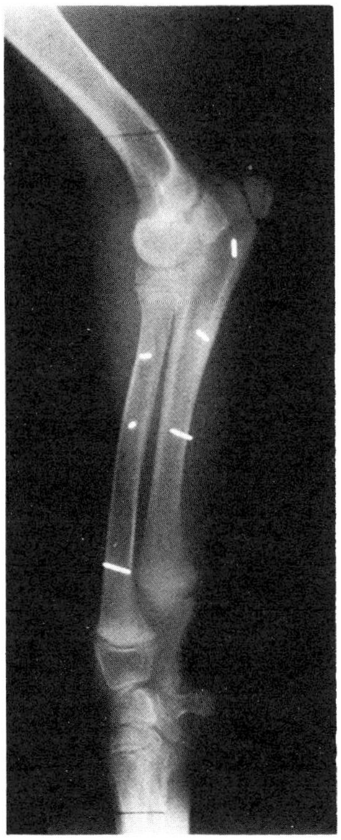

Figure 1A

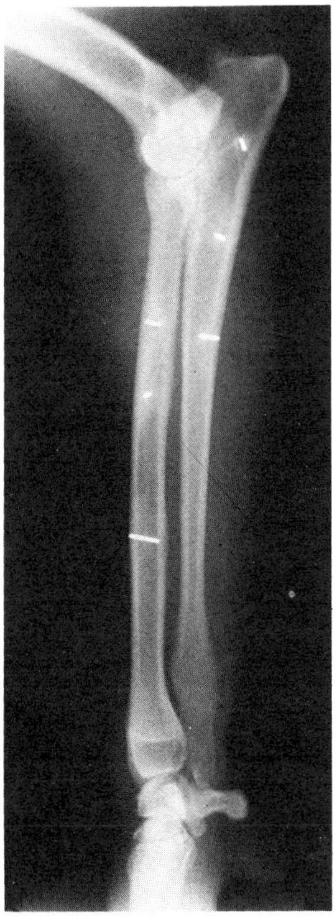

Figure 1B

Figure 1—Lateral radiographs of the radius and ulna of an Australian shepherd dog at 83 days of age (**A**) and 242 days of age (**B**). Marker pins were inserted into the diaphysis of the radius and ulna when the dog was 69 days of age. Note that the distance between the pins in each bone remains unchanged. There is a marked alteration of the relationships between pins in the ulna compared with those in the radius over the period of growth.

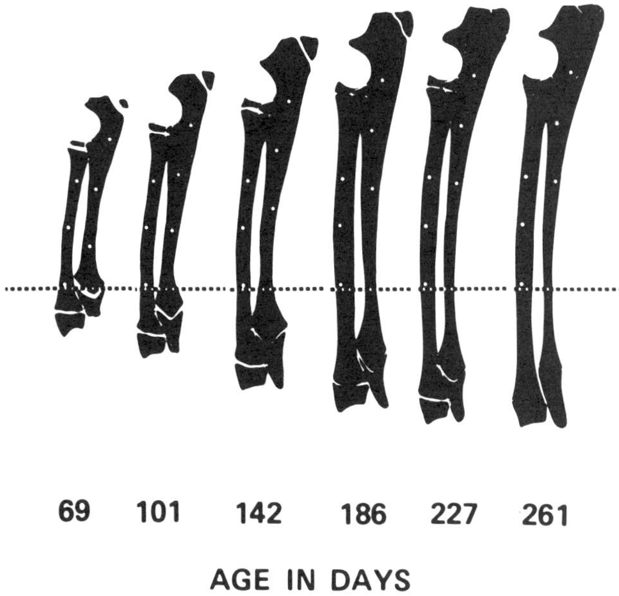

Figure 2—Drawings of lateral radiographs of the radius and ulna of an Australian shepherd dog. Radiographs were taken over the period of growth from 69 days of age. Positions of marker pins in the radius and ulna are indicated. The drawings have been arranged so that the bottom marker pin in the radius lies on the *dotted line*. The relationship of the pins in the radius and ulna changes over the period of growth. Note also that the position of the proximal pin in the ulna maintains a constant relationship with the trochlear notch of the ulna, indicating that longitudinal growth in the ulna distal to the trochlear notch comes exclusively from the distal ulnar physis.

Normal Development of the Canine Radius and Ulna

The radius grows in length from a proximal and distal physis. It articulates proximally with the *capitulum humeri* of the humerus and the radial notch of the ulna. Distally, it articulates with the proximal row of carpal bones and the styloid process of the distal ulna. The radius bears practically all the weight transmitted from the arm to the forearm. The ulna grows from the distal ulnar physis and the ossification center for the olecranon. In some breeds (e.g., the German shepherd and greyhound), an additional ossification center is present in the anconeal process.[8-10] Proximally, the trochlear notch of the ulna articulates with the *trochlear humeri* of the humerus, and the radial notch of the ulna articulates with the articular circumference of the head of the radius. Distally, the ulna articulates with

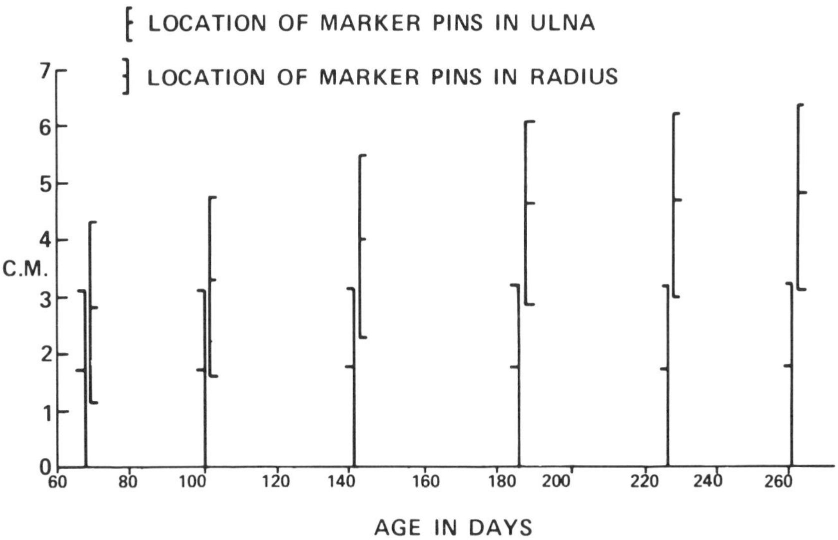

Figure 3—Same dog as in Figure 2. Graphic representation of positions of markers in the radius and ulna over a period of growth. Lack of interstitial growth in either the radius or ulna is indicated by the constant distance between the pins in each bone. Over the period of growth, the pins in the ulna move proximally compared to those in the radius.

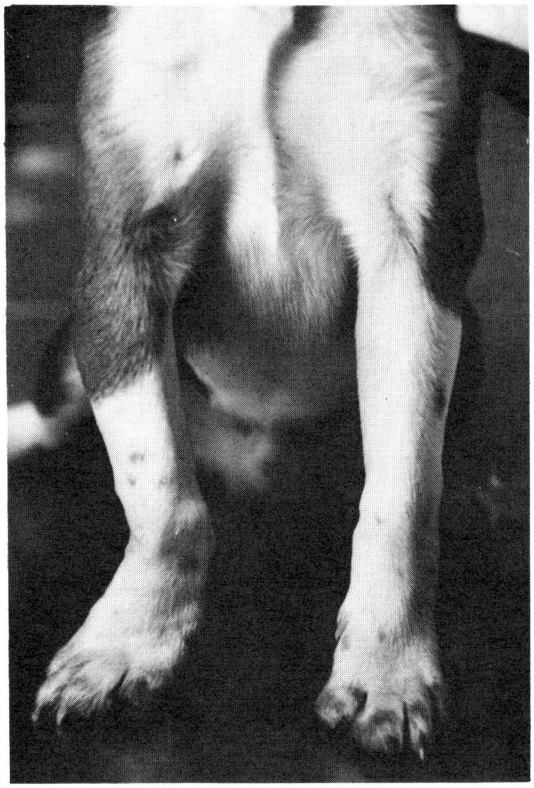

Figure 4—Five-month-old beagle with abnormal development of the right forelimb caused by retardation of longitudinal growth of the ulna. Shortening of the forelimb is seen along with a varus deformity of the elbow, valgus deformity of the carpus, and outward rotation of the paw.

the ulnar notch of the radius, the ulnar carpal bone, and the accessory carpal bone. The radius and ulna are united by the proximal and distal radioulnar synovial joints, the interosseous ligament close to the middle of the radius and ulna, and the radioulnar ligament, which firmly attaches the distal radial epiphysis to the styloid process of the ulna. A much thinner osseous membrane extends proximally and distally from the interosseous ligament.

The age at which radiographic closure of the physes occurs in the radius and ulna varies by breed. Small breeds generally mature at an earlier age than do larger breeds. The age of radiographic closure of the proximal radial physis, the distal radial physis, and the distal ulnar physis has been determined to range between 222 and 250 days in the beagle.[11]

Reports on the contribution of the proximal and distal radial physes to longitudinal growth of the canine radius indicate that variation exists among individual animals. Estimates of the growth contribution of the proximal radial physis differ, with reports of 30%,[12,13] 40%,[14] and 43 to 50%.[15] The distal ulnar physis accounts for 85% of the overall length of the ulna[13,15,16] and 100% of the length of the ulna distal to the elbow joint (Figures 1 and 2). Since the radius grows in length from both the proximal and distal physes and the ulna grows in length below the elbow only from its distal physis, it is apparent that some change in the relationships between the radius and ulna is necessary during growth to maintain alignment between their articular surfaces at the elbow joint. This change can be studied by placing marker pins in the diaphyseal region of the radius and ulna and evaluating their relationships on serial radiographs taken over the period of growth (Figure 2). Movement between the radius and ulna, as well as the absence of interstitial growth in the diaphyseal region of these bones, is demonstrated in Figure 3.

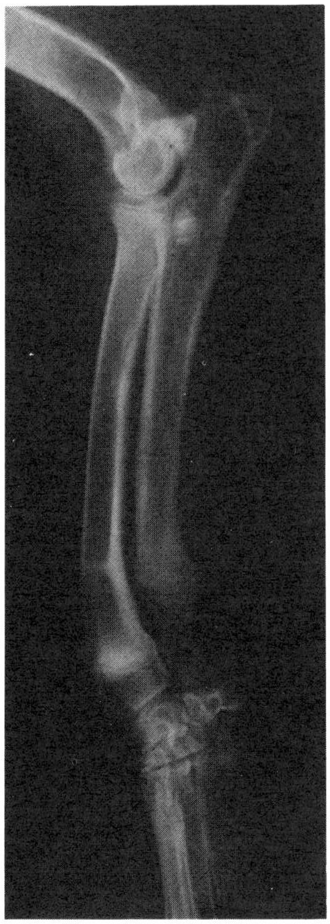

Figure 5A

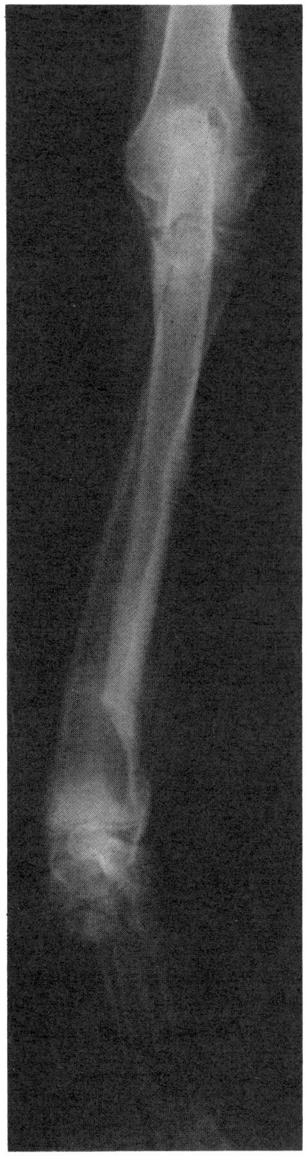

Figure 5B

Figure 5—Lateral (**A**) and anteroposterior (**B**) radiographs of the radius and ulna of a 7-month-old German shepherd with premature closure of the distal ulnar physis. Note that the distal ulnar physis is closed while the proximal and distal radial physes remain open. Reduced longitudinal growth of the ulna has resulted in subluxation of humeroulnar articulation, curvature of the radius, and instability of the carpus. On the anteroposterior radiograph, a varus deformity of the elbow is seen while a valgus deformity is present at the carpus, causing lateral deviation of the paw.

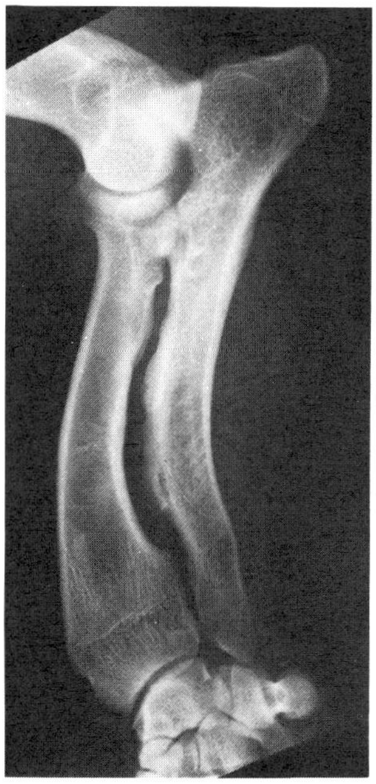

Figure 6—Lateral radiograph of the left radius and ulna of an 18-month-old dachshund with a forelimb lameness. Reduction in longitudinal growth of the ulna has resulted in malalignment of the articular surfaces of the proximal radius and trochlear notch of ulna and subluxation of the elbow joint.

Retardation of Longitudinal Growth

Abnormal growth of the radius and ulna has been described secondary to delayed growth in the proximal and distal radial physes and distal ulnar physis.[17-19]

Retardation of Ulnar Growth

Deformities due to premature closure of the distal ulnar physis are the most common complications of epiphyseal injury in the dog.[4,16,18-20] The conical shape of the distal ulnar physis predisposes the ulnar metaphysis to be forced down toward the epiphysis, regardless of the type of injury sustained.[16] This frequently results in a crush injury to the chondrogenic layer of cells of the physis. Significant retardations of growth of the distal ulnar physis result in a shortened ulna, which restrains growth of the radius, producing cranial bowing of the radius and other deformities. These include shortening of the limb, valgus deformation and external rotation of the carpus and metacarpal bones, elbow subluxation, and subsequent osteoarthrosis of the carpal and elbow joints (Figures 4 and 5).[4,16,19,21-25]

Chondrodystrophic breeds develop forelimb lameness that is due to a relative retardation of the growth of the ulna when compared to the growth of the radius and that results in degenerative changes in the elbow joint (Figure 6).[26,27] These retardations of ulnar growth are apparently developmental and unrelated to epiphyseal injury. Retarded growth of the ulna can also result from retained cartilage cores in the distal ulnar metaphysis (Figure 7). These are most frequently observed in the larger breeds of dog. Often, small retained cartilage cores are not associated with abnormal bone growth;

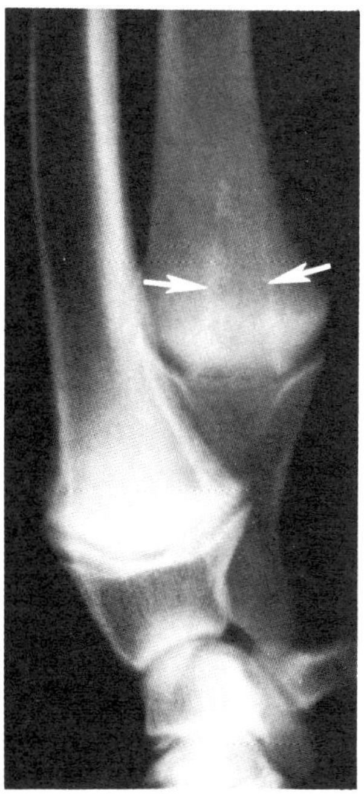

Figure 7—Lateral radiograph of the distal radius and ulna of a 4½-month-old Great Dane. A large, retained cartilage core is present in the distal ulna (*arrows*). Interference with longitudinal growth of the ulna is suggested by a slight degree of curvature in the distal radius. As the animal matured, curvature of the radius became more exaggerated.

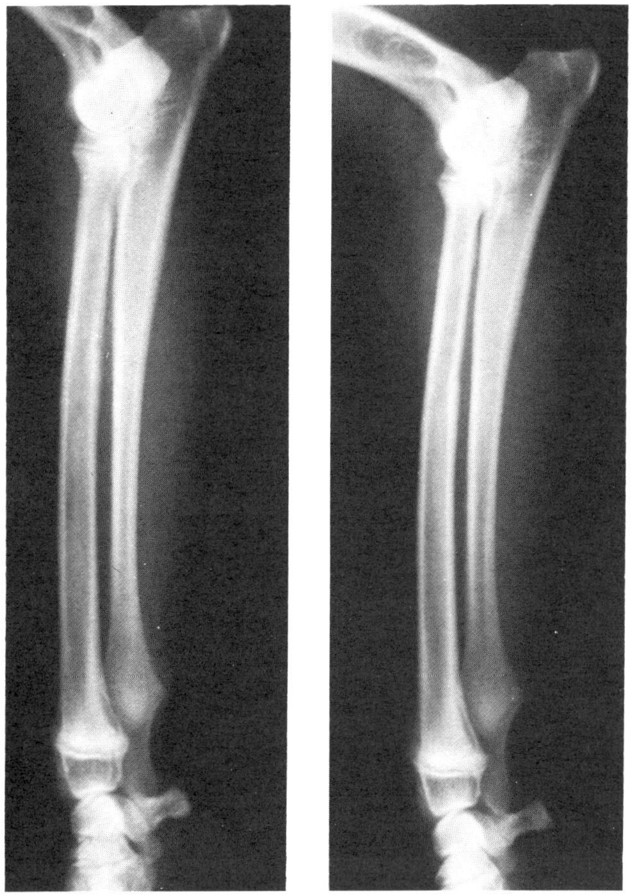

Figure 8A **Figure 8B**

Figure 8—Lateral radiographs of left (**A**) and right (**B**) radius and ulna of a 7½-month-old collie cross. Approximately 10% retardation of longitudinal growth was produced in the right ulna when the dog was 2½ months of age. Apart from reduction in the length of the ulna, only minor morphologic alterations resulted in the right forelimb, as there was an accompanying reduction in longitudinal growth of the radius.

however, when the retained core is large, interference with longitudinal growth of the ulna results and this causes bowing of the radius.

It has been shown that when minor degrees of ulnar growth retardation occur, there is a reduction in growth of the adjacent radius, and while the affected limb is shorter than normal, no gross deformity results (Figure 8).[28] However, when growth retardation of the ulna exceeds the inherent ability of the radius to adjust to this abnormal situation, deformity of both the elbow joint and distal radius results. As the degree of growth retardation in the ulna becomes more severe, the major effect is seen on the distal radius. Marked curvature of the distal radius and disruption of the distal radial physis and carpal joint occur as abnormal stresses are placed on these regions (Figure 9). Major displacements at the elbow joint and disruption of the anconeal process are usually not seen with premature closure of the distal ulnar physis.

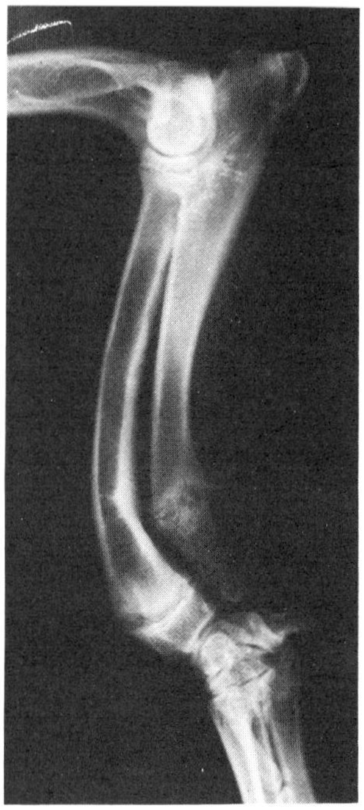

Figure 9A

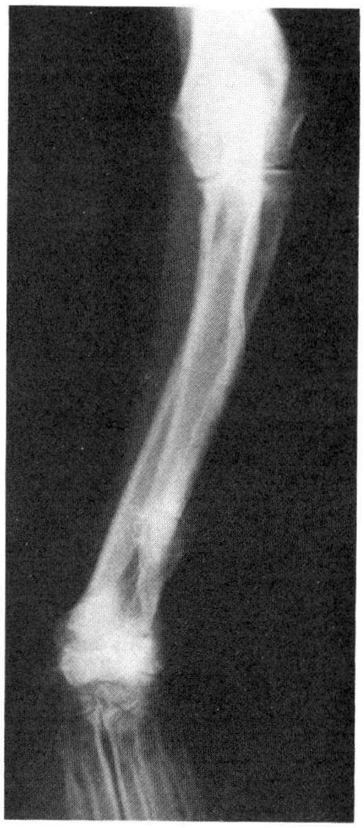

Figure 9B

Figure 9—Lateral (**A**) and anteroposterior (**B**) radiographs of the radius and ulna of a 7½-month-old collie cross following approximately 50% retardation of longitudinal growth of the ulna at 2½ months of age. Changes noted in this case are similar to those shown in Figure 5.

Retardation of Radial Growth

Alteration to longitudinal growth of the radius can originate following trauma to the proximal or distal radial physes. Proximal physeal injuries are apparently uncommon. Premature closure of the proximal radial physis has been described.[19] Radiographic signs include

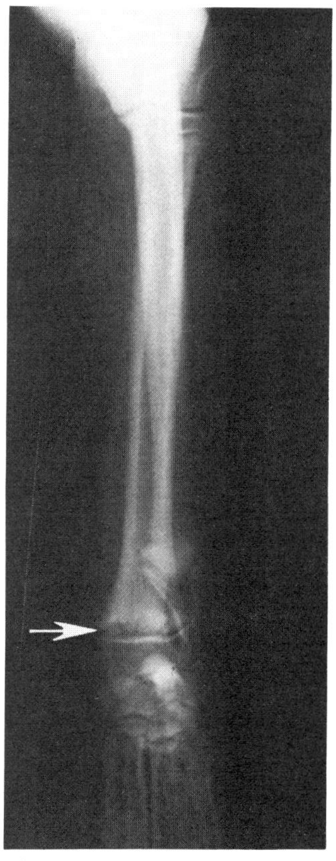

Figure 10A

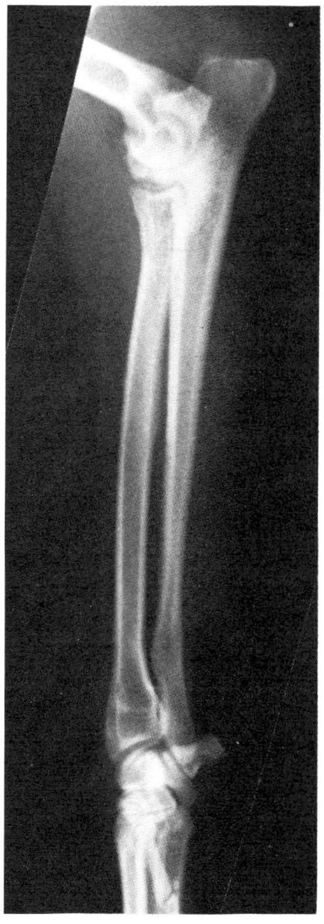

Figure 10B

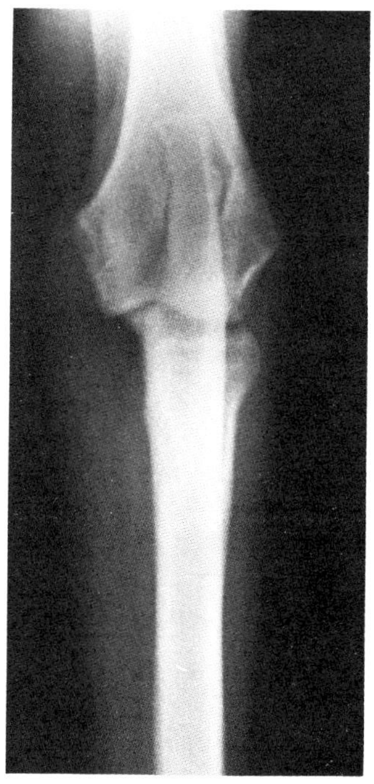

Figure 10C

Figure 10—Anteroposterior radiograph (**A**) of the radius and ulna of a 5-month-old Border collie with trauma to the distal radial physis (*arrow*). The injury resulted in premature closure of the distal radial physis. Laterial (**B**) and anteroposterior (**C**) radiographs of the affected limb at 10 months of age, showing separation between the proximal radius and humerus and malalignment between the articular surfaces of the proximal radius and trochlear notch.

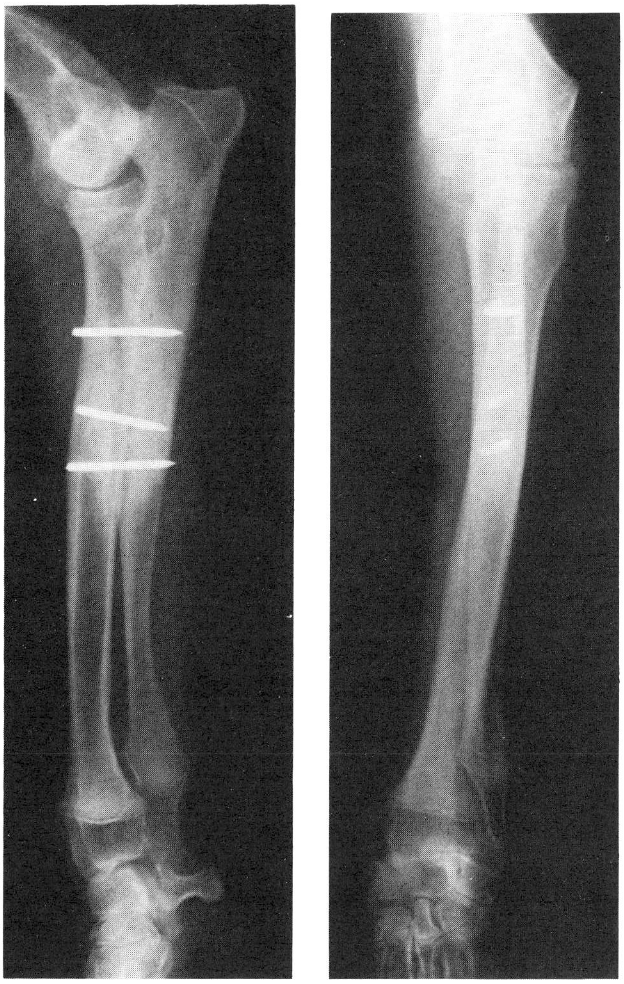

Figure 11A Figure 11B

Figure 11—Lateral (A) and anteroposterior (B) radiographs of the left forlimb of a 5½-month-old Australian shepherd cross, 2½ months after cross-pinning the radius to the ulna. Marked displacement of the humeral condyle from the trochlear notch of the ulna resulted following restriction of the normal shifting that occurs between the radius and ulna during growth.

widening of the humeroradial joint space, with the relationships of the distal radius and ulna remaining normal. The length of the radius is usually reduced only slightly.[19]

When premature closure of the distal radial physis occurs, the resulting retardation of growth can be symmetric or asymmetric depending on the extent and region of the physis that is injured.[29] If the injury affects the lateral part of the physis only, carpal valgus and outward rotation of the paw result. If the entire physis is injured, angular deformity usually does not occur.

Radiographic signs of premature closure of the distal radial physis include reduction in length of both the radius and ulna together with an increase in the humeroradial joint space (Figure 10).[17,19] Instability in the elbow joint results in secondary arthritic changes.[19]

Restriction of Movement Between Radius and Ulna

Considerable movement of the radius in relation to the ulna occurs during normal growth of the canine forelimb (Figures 1, 2, and 3). The morphologic changes occurring after restriction of this movement have been studied by introducing Steinmann pins from the radius to the ulna to effectively prevent changes in the relationship between the diaphyses of the radius and ulna (Figure 11).[14] The changes noted were similar to those occurring following synostosis between the radius and ulna in association with fracture healing in clinical patients (Figures 12 and 13).[30]

Major changes occurred in the relationship between the radius and ulna at the elbow joint. Considerable overgrowth of the proximal radial epiphysis in relation to the trochlear notch of the proximal ulna forced the distal humeral condyle in a proximal direction, and severe damage to the anconeal process of the ulna and

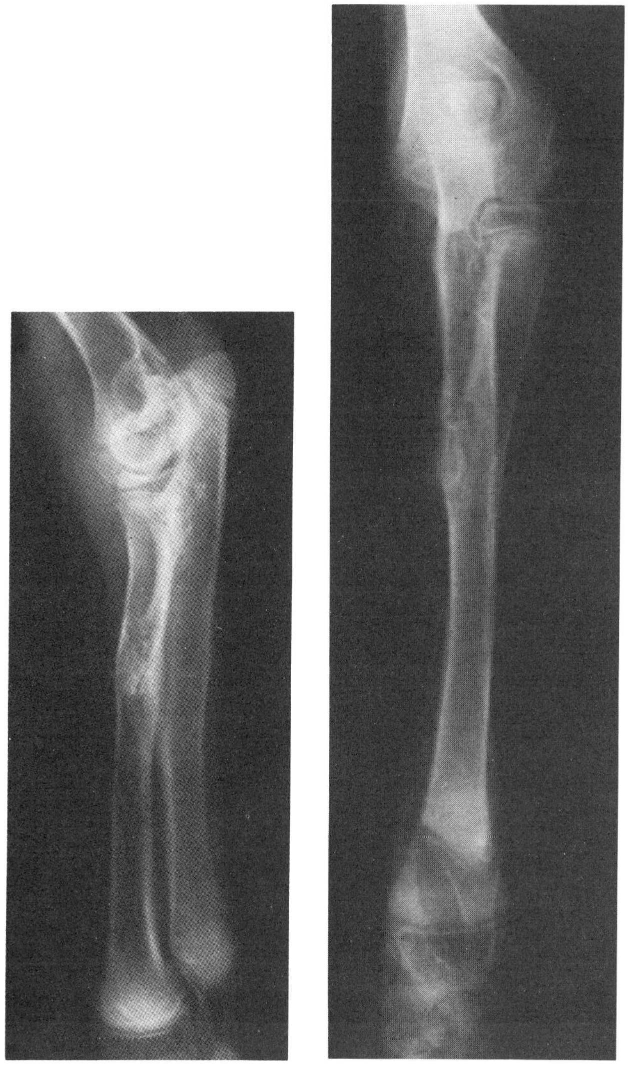

Figure 12A Figure 12B

Figure 12—Lateral (A) and anteroposterior (B) radiographs of the right forelimb of a 5-month-old Doberman pinscher with radioulnar synostosis, which resulted following a fracture 3½ months previously. Marked subluxation of the elbow joint resulted together with disruption of the anconeal process. The similarity in appearance to the experimentally produced radioulnar synostosis can be appreciated by comparing Figures 11 and 12.

the distal humeral condyle resulted. Marked degenerative changes also occurred in the distal half of the trochlear notch (Figure 14). These changes were related to the lack of normal joint contact between the trochlear notch and the humeral condyle which interfered with normal nutrition of the cartilage. The younger the animal at the time of restriction of movement between the radius and ulna, the greater will be the subsequent displacement at the elbow joint and the more severe will be the degenerative changes in the cartilaginous surfaces of the elbow joint. These degenerative changes also occur in clinical cases of radioulnar synostosis.

In experimental dogs with restricted movement between the radius and ulna, it was noted that the overall length of the radius and ulna was not appreciably altered when compared to the normal control limb. Because the relationships between the distal radius and ulna were not appreciably altered, it suggested that stimulation of longitudinal growth from the distal radial physis had occurred. This was possibly caused by traction on the distal radius by the strong radioulnar ligament as the ulna continued to grow distally. Measurements of the percentage contribution of the distal

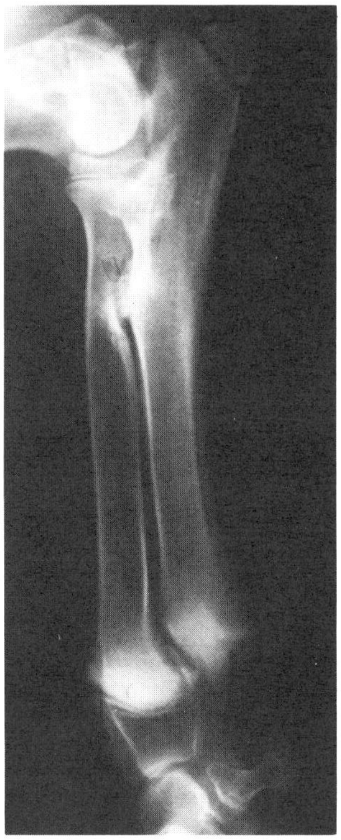

Figure 13A

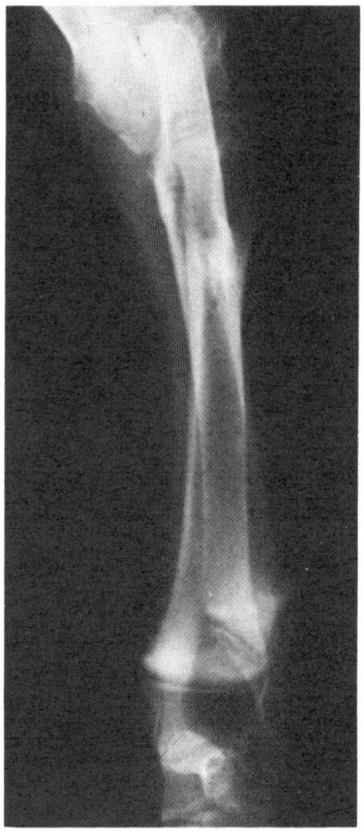

Figure 13B

Figure 13—Lateral (**A**) and anteroposterior (**B**) radiographs of the left forelimb of a 5-month-old German shepherd with radioulnar synostosis following a fracture at 3 months of age. Subluxation of the elbow has resulted, together with separation of the anconeal process.

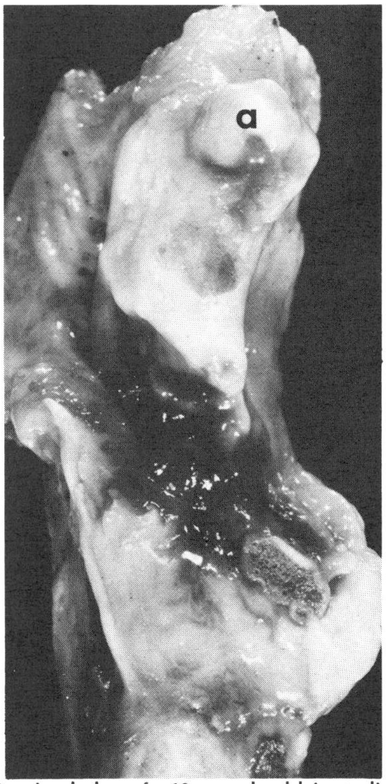

Figure 14—Proximal ulna of a 10-month-old Australian shepherd 7 months after restricting movement between the radius and ulna. The resultant malalignment of the articular surfaces in the elbow joint has lead to severe degenerative changes in the articular cartilage of the trochlear notch. Note that the most severe changes occurred distally in the cartilage that had lost articular contact with the humerus. Degenerative changes also occurred where increased pressure on articular cartilage was present and disruption of the anconeal process (a) is seen.

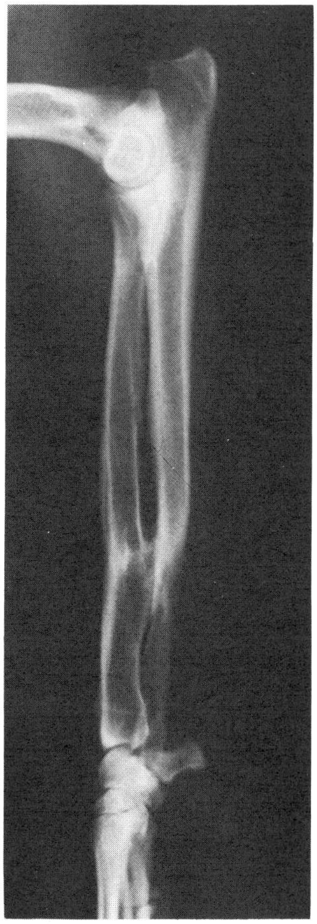

Figure 15A

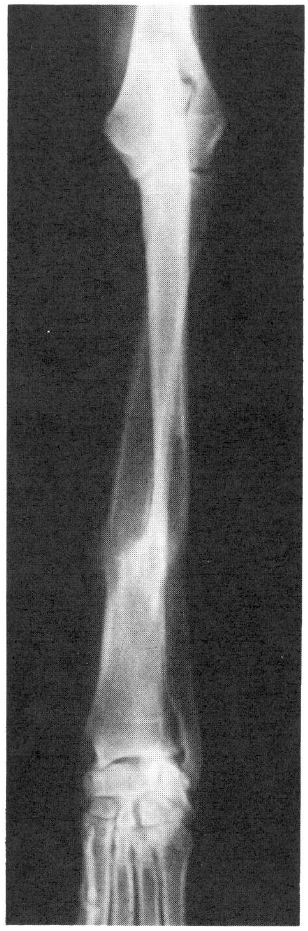

Figure 15B

Figure 15—Lateral (**A**) and anteroposterior (**B**) radiographs of the left forelimb of a 2½-year-old malamute with radioulnar synostosis at 1½ years of age. Because the synostosis between the radius and ulna occurred following skeletal maturity, no major displacement occurred in the elbow joint.

physis to longitudinal growth of the radius indicated an alteration from approximately 60% in the control radius to approximately 80% in the cross-pinned radius.

It is apparent that restriction of movement between the radius and ulna during the period of growth can result in marked alterations to the growth characteristics and morphology of the bones. Surgical procedures on the radius and ulna in the immature patient should minimize factors that could contribute to the limitation of this movement. Optimal realignment and immobilization of fractures involving the radius and ulna should be achieved to minimize synostosis between the bones. Similarly, when metallic fixation devices (e.g., Kirschner apparatus, bone screws) are used on immature patients, care must be taken to insure that they do not cross from the radius into the ulna. Synostosis between the radius and ulna in the mature animal does not result in growth abnormality (Figure 15).

REFERENCES

1. Harsha WN: Effects of trauma upon epiphyses. *Clin Orthop* 10:140-147, 1957.
2. Campbell CJ, Grisolia A, Zanconato G: The effects produced in the cartilaginous epiphyseal plate of immature dogs by experimental surgical traumata. *J Bone Joint Surg* 41A:1221-1242, 1959.
3. Compere EL: Growth arrest on long bones as the result of fractures that include the epiphysis. *JAMA* 105:2140-2146, 1935.
4. Kleine LJ: Radiographic diagnosis of epiphyseal plate trauma. *JAAHA* 7:290-295, 1971.
5. Phemister DB: Operative arrestment of longitudinal growth of bones in the treatment of deformities. *J Bone Joint Surg* 15:1-15, 1933.
6. Salter RB, Harris WR: Injuries involving the epiphyseal plate. *J Bone Joint Surg* 45A:587-622, 1963.
7. Berzon JL: The classification and management of epiphyseal plate fractures. *JAAHA* 16:651-658, 1980.
8. Corley EA: Elbow dysplasia in the German shepherd dog. Doctoral dissertation, Colorado State University, 1966.
9. VanSickle DC: A comparative study of the postnatal elbow development of the greyhound and the German shepherd. Scientific Proc 102nd Annu Meet AVMA. *JAVMA* 147:1650-1651, 1965.
10. VanSickle DC: The relationship of ossification to canine elbow dysplasia. *Anim Hosp* 2:24-31, 1966.
11. Chapman WL, Jr: Appearance of ossification centers and epiphyseal closures as determined by radiographic techniques. *JAVMA* 147:138-141, 1965.
12. Henschel E: Zur Anatomie und Klinik der wachsenden Unterarmknochen. *Arch Exp Veterinaermed* 26:741-787, 1972.
13. Riser WH, Shirer JF: Normal and abnormal growth of the distal foreleg in large and giant dogs. *J Am Vet Radiol Soc* 6:50-64, 1965.
14. Noser G, Carrig CB, Merkley D, Brinker WO: Asynchronous growth of the canine radius and ulna: Effects of cross-pinning the radius to the ulna. *Am J Vet Res* 38:601-610, 1977.
15. Kleine LJ: A radiographic study of experimental premature epiphyseal plate closure of the distal radius and ulna in dogs. Masters thesis, Purdue University, 1967.
16. Skaggs S, DeAngelis MP, Rosen H: Deformities due to premature closure of the distal ulna in fourteen dogs: A radiographic evaluation. *JAAHA* 9:496-500, 1973.
17. Clayton-Jones DG, Vaughan LC: Disturbance in the growth of the radius in dogs. *J Small Anim Pract* 11:453-468, 1970.
18. Morgan JP: Radiology in veterinary orthopedics. Philadelphia, Lea & Febiger, 1972, pp 63-67.
19. O'Brien TR, Morgan JP, Suter PF: Epiphyseal plate injury in the dog: A radiographic study of growth disturbance in the forelimb. *J Small Anim Pract* 12:19-36, 1971.
20. O'Brien TR: Developmental deformities due to arrested epiphyseal growth. *Vet Clin North Am* 1:441-454, 1971.
21. Carrig CB, Morgan JP: Asynchronous growth of the canine radius and ulna—early radiographic changes following experimental retardation of longitudinal growth of the ulna. *J Am Vet Radiol Soc* 16:121-129, 1975.
22. Carrig CB, Morgan JP, Pool RR: The study of degenerative joint disease. *24th Gaines Vet Symp*:12-17, 1974.
23. Carrig CB, Morgan JP, Pool RR: Effects of asynchronous growth of the radius and ulna on the canine elbow joint following experimental retardation of longitudinal growth of the ulna. *JAAHA* 11:560-567, 1975.
24. Kasstrom H, Ljunggren G, Olsson SE: Growth disturbances of the ulna in dogs—A radiographic study. Abstracts of the Third International Conference of Veterinary Radiologists. *J Am Vet Radiol Soc* 14:6, 1973.
25. Newton CD: Surgical management of distal ulnar physeal growth disturbances in dogs. *JAVMA* 164:479-487, 1974.
26. Hitz Von D: Ulnadysplasie biem Bassethound. *Schweiz Arch Tierheilkd* 116:285-294, 1974.
27. Lau R: Inherited premature closure of the distal ulnar physis. *JAAHA* 13:609-612, 1977.
28. Carrig CB, Merkley D, Mostosky UV: Asynchronous growth of the canine radius and ulna: Effects of different amounts of ulnar growth retardation. *J Am Vet Radiol Soc* 19:16-22, 1978.
29. Olson NC, Brinker WO, Carrig CB: Premature closure of the distal radial physis in two dogs. *JAVMA* 176:906-910, 1980.
30. Alexander JW, Walker TL, Roberts RE, Dueland R: Malformation of canine forelimb due to synostosis between the radius and ulna. *JAVMA* 173:1328-1330, 1978.

Radiographic Diagnosis of Long Bone Neoplasms in the Dog

Richard D. Park, DVM, PhD
Professor
Department of Radiology
and Radiation Biology
Colorado State University
Fort Collins, Colorado

Radiographic differentiation of solitary long bone lesions can be difficult. The most frequent differentiation to be made is between long bone neoplasia and acute or chronic osteomyelitis. With a knowledge of the radiographic signs associated with long bone neoplasia, a more accurate differentiation can be made. This article will outline the role of radiology in the diagnosis of long bone neoplasms and establish and review radiographic signs of long bone neoplasia.

Incidence and Distribution

Information regarding incidence and distribution of primary bone neoplasia must be taken into account with the radiographic findings for an accurate diagnosis.

Skeletal neoplasms account for approximately 5% of all neoplasms in the dog.[1] They occur more frequently in large and giant breed dogs than in smaller breeds and have a male-to-female occurrence ratio of 1.2:1.[1,2] The age group having the highest incidence is 8 to 9 years, with high incidence in dogs ranging between 5 and 13 years. A small peak incidence also occurs around 2 years of age.[1,2]

The pectoral limb–pelvic limb occurrence ratio is 1.6:1. The metaphyseal area of the distal radius, proximal humerus, and distal and proximal femur and tibia are sites of highest incidence in long bones.[1-4]

Reported malignant skeletal neoplasms include osteosarcoma, chondrosarcoma, hemangiosarcoma, fibrosarcoma, lymphosarcoma, reticulum cell sarcoma, and plasma cell myeloma. Osteosarcomas are the predominant primary long bone neoplasm in the dog.[1,3]

Radiology

Radiology serves as a diagnostic tool, helps identify the most appropriate biopsy site, and is useful for detecting metastatic lesions throughout the body, e.g., lungs, lymph nodes, or other bones.

All deep, firm extremity swellings should be radiographed on initial presentation. The radiographic examination should not be delayed until the second or third presentation. When a subtle bone lesion present is suggestive of neoplasia, a biopsy should be taken and another radiograph should be made in 7 to 10 days for comparison. Aggressive primary bone neoplasms will usually change considerably and show

Originally published in Volume 3, Number 10, October 1981

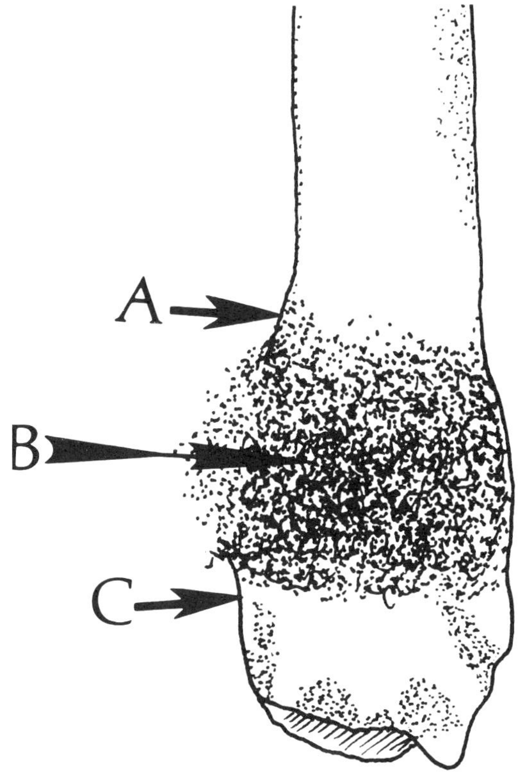

Figure 1A

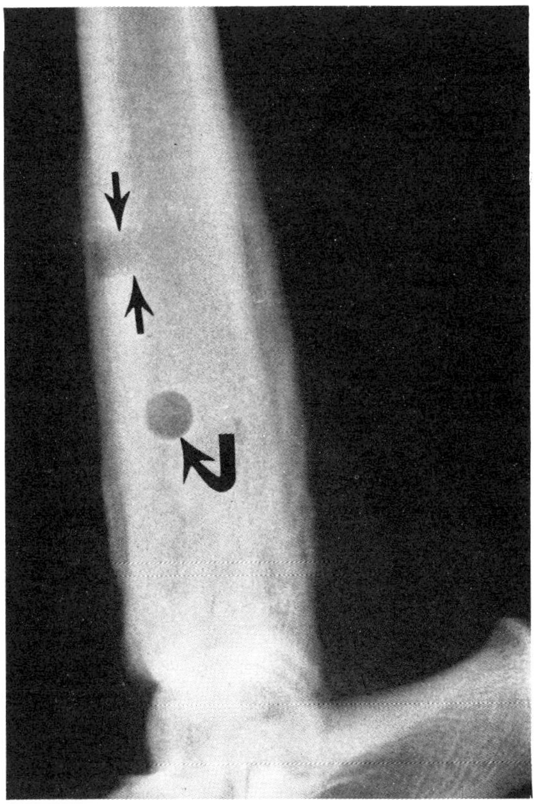

Figure 1B

Figure 1—**(A)** Diagram of biopsy sites for solitary bone lesions. *A* and C represent peripheral biopsy sites. *B* represents the most desirable biopsy site, deep within the central region of the lesion. **(B)** Postbiopsy radiograph of the distal tibia. Two biopsy sites can be identified. One through the center of the lesion directed from lateral to medial *(curved arrow)* and one through the lesion periphery directed from cranial to caudal *(straight arrows)*.

more apparent radiographic signs of primary bone neoplasia on the second examination. More advanced neoplastic lesions are more easily differentiated from other solitary bone lesions. With both subtle and advanced bone lesions suggestive of neoplasia, a biopsy and histopathological examination are recommended for confirmation of the radiographic diagnosis.

Radiographs should be used to determine a biopsy site. The biopsy should be centered over the tumor, and a good sample should be taken from the center of the lesion[3] (Figure 1A). Postbiopsy radiographs can be used to see if the biopsy was properly centered and extended into the central portion of the neoplasm (Figure 1B). A biopsy from the tumor periphery will usually come back inconclusive or will be read histopathologically as reactive bone.[a]

Since metastasis from primary bone neoplasia occurs most frequently to the lungs, a thoracic radiographic examination should be done with all suspect neoplastic bone lesions. Metastasis from primary bone neoplasia to other bones has also been reported.[5-7] A radiographic skeletal survey would be necessary to identify such metastatic lesions.

Radiographic Signs

To help differentiate long bone neoplasia from other solitary bone lesions, a knowledge of the radiographic signs associated with neoplasia is essential.[3] Four areas that should be evaluated on radiographs of solitary bone lesions are the margins, bone cortices, neoplastic matrix (new bone production), and the periosteal reaction (Table I).

[a]*Editor's Note:* Not only can a false result be obtained by sampling the periphery of the lesion, but a diagnosis of necrotic bone can be obtained from samples from the center of a bone tumor. Therefore, many authorities do not agree with this concept of selecting a site for biopsy of a bone tumor. The preferred method is probably to sample both the periphery and the center of the tumor.

TABLE I

RADIOGRAPHIC SIGNS OF LONG BONE NEOPLASIA

Location	*Possible Changes*
Lesion margin	Well-defined Not well-defined (wide transition zone) Does not cross joint space May extend to adjacent bones
Cortex	Erosion Destruction Expansion Punctate lysis
Neoplastic matrix	Intramedullary Extramedullary
Periosteal reactions	Brush border Spiculation Lamination Codman's triangle

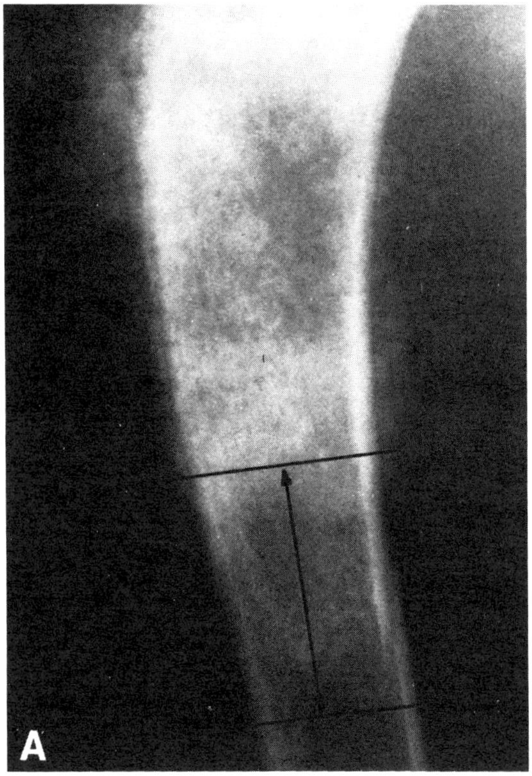

Figure 2A

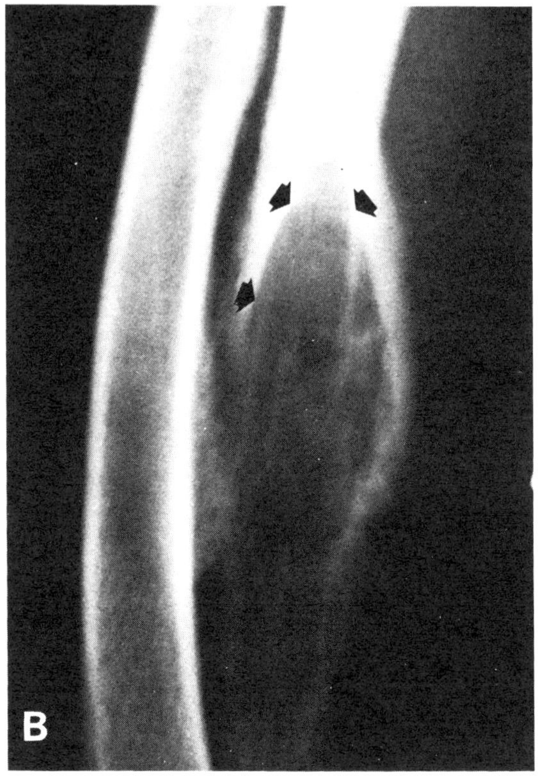

Figure 2B

Figure 2—**(A)** A lateral radiograph of the humerus. A wide transition zone between normal and abnormal bone is present *(arrow* and *lines)*. **(B)** A lateral radiograph of an expansile destructive and productive bone lesion in the distal ulna. The diaphyseal border *(arrows)* is well-defined.

Margination

Since most long bone neoplasms originate in the metaphysis, diaphyseal and epiphyseal margins are present. The diaphyseal margin (Figure 2) may not be well-defined with fast-growing, aggressive neoplasms. These tumors have a long transition zone between normal and abnormal bone. Slow-growing or nonaggressive neoplasms usually have a well-defined diaphyseal margin.[8] Malignant neoplastic margins may or may not be well-defined.

Epiphyseal margins (Figure 3) stop at, or before, the articular cartilage. The primary bone tumor usually does not invade into or across the joint space.

Lateral and medial margins of a primary bone neoplasm may not be confined to one bone in sites where there are paired bones, i.e., radius and ulna, and tibia and fibula (Figure 3). The first response of an adjacent bone is a periosteal reaction. In some cases the response is limited to the periosteum. In other cases the neoplasm may eventually extend into the adjacent bone.

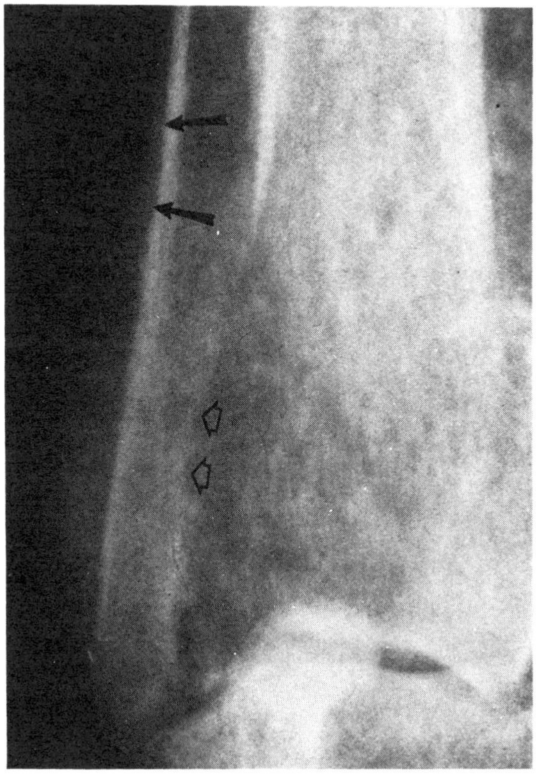

Figure 3—A dorsal palmar radiograph of an osteosarcoma involving the distal radius. The neoplasm extends to the subchondral bone on the lateral distal radius, but does not cross the joint space. Early involvement of the distal ulna is occurring as periosteal reaction on the ulna *(solid arrows)* and mild cortical destruction *(hollow arrows)*.

Cortical Changes

Cortical changes may consist of erosion, destruction, expansion, and punctate lysis. Cortical erosion, large areas of destruction, and expansion are excellent differentiating signs of primary bone neoplasia. Cortical erosive changes seen with primary bone tumors are usually endosteal erosions that produce scalloped or thin cortices (Figure 4). Endosteal erosion may be subtle and is an early sign of primary bone neoplasia.[3]

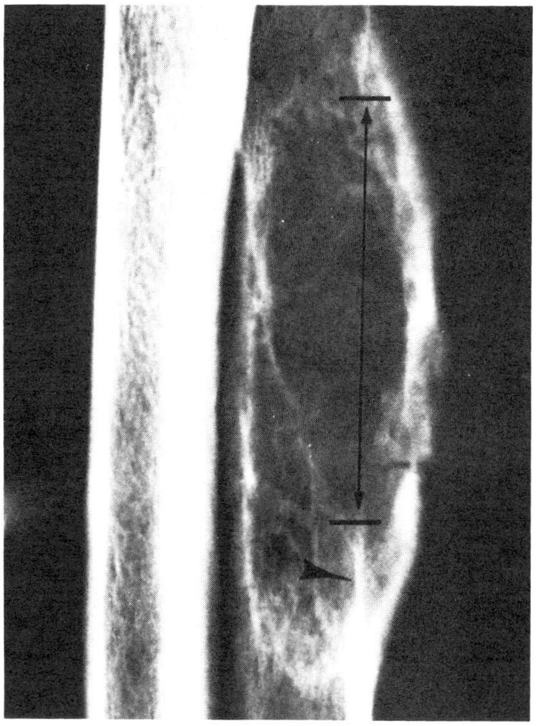

Figure 4—A lateral radiograph of a primary bone neoplasm involving the distal ulna. There is a large area of cortical destruction *(lines* and *arrow)* and an area of endosteal erosion *(arrow)*. Endosteal erosion may occur with or without large areas of cortical destruction.

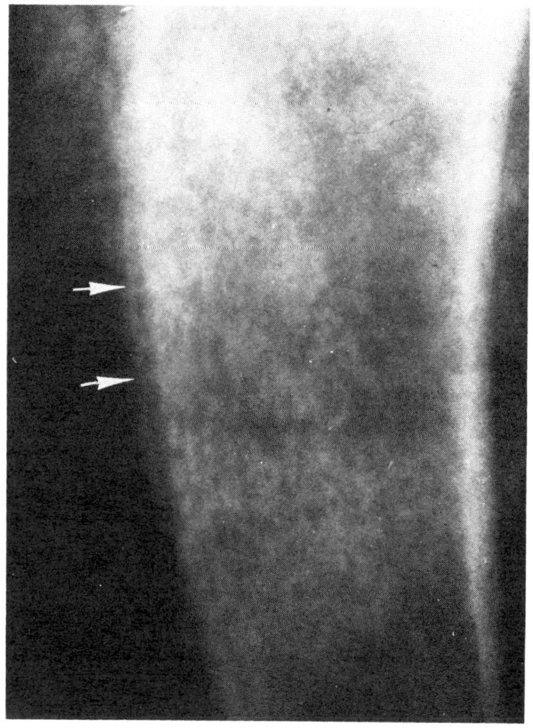

Figure 5—A lateral radiograph of the proximal humeral diaphysis. The primary bone neoplasm is causing punctate areas of cortical lysis most evident throughout the cranial cortex. A laminated periosteal reaction is also present *(white arrows)*.

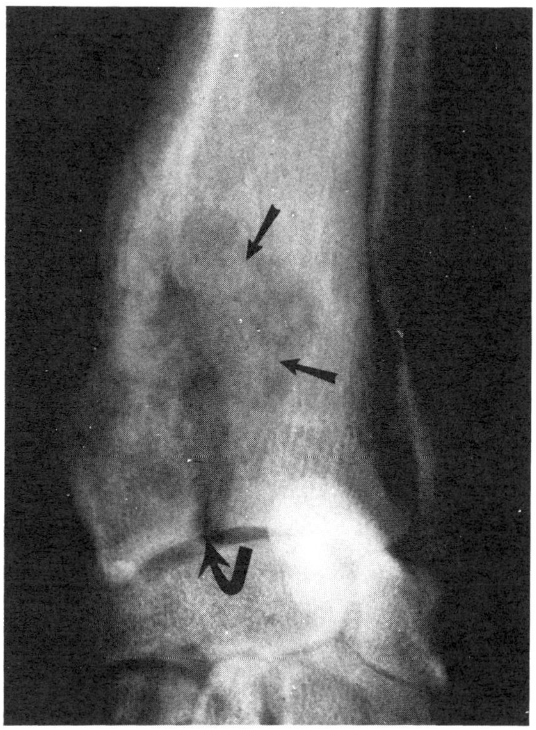

Figure 6—A dorsal palmar radiograph of the distal radius and ulna. Amorphous intramedullary neoplastic matrix is present *(straight arrows)*. This amorphous bone has replaced the normal trabecular bone in one area of the distal radius. The trabecular bone surrounding the lesion is normal. A pathological fracture is also present extending from the medial radial cortex to the radial articular surface *(curved arrow)*.

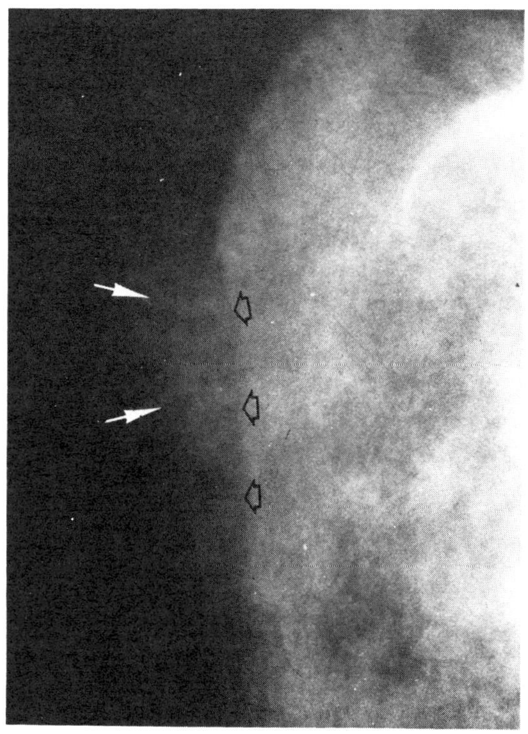

Figure 7—A lateral radiograph of the cranial proximal humerus. Extramedullary neoplastic matrix (new bone production) is extending into soft tissue *(white arrows)* away from the cortex *(hollow arrows)*.

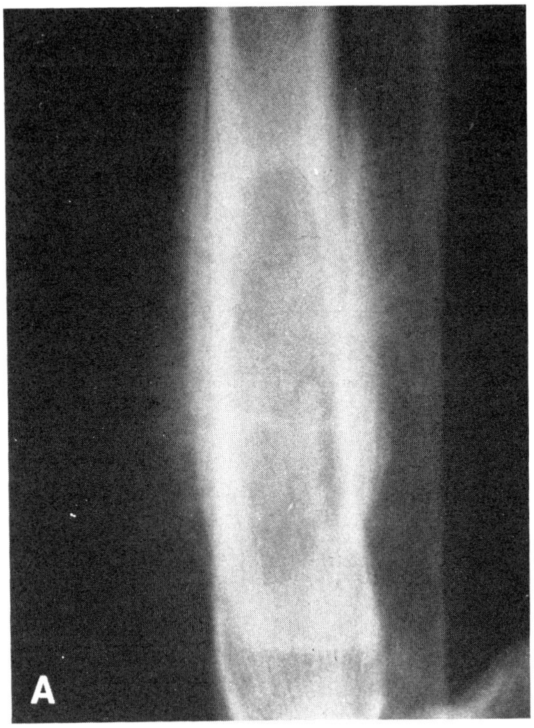

Figure 8A

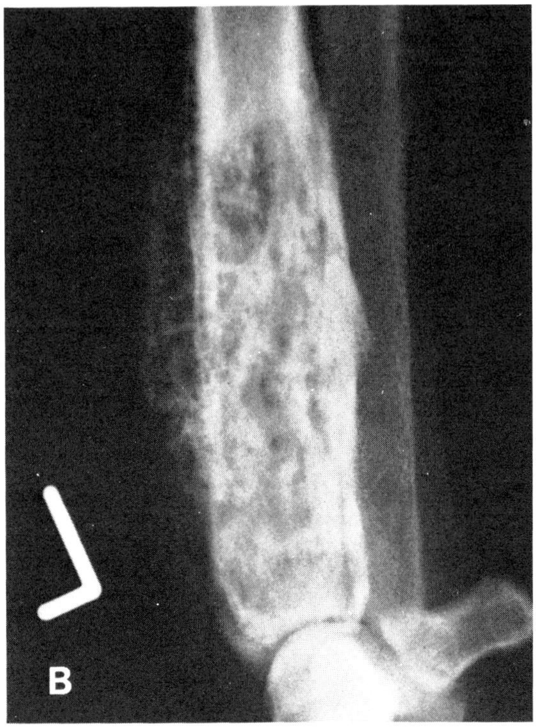

Figure 8B

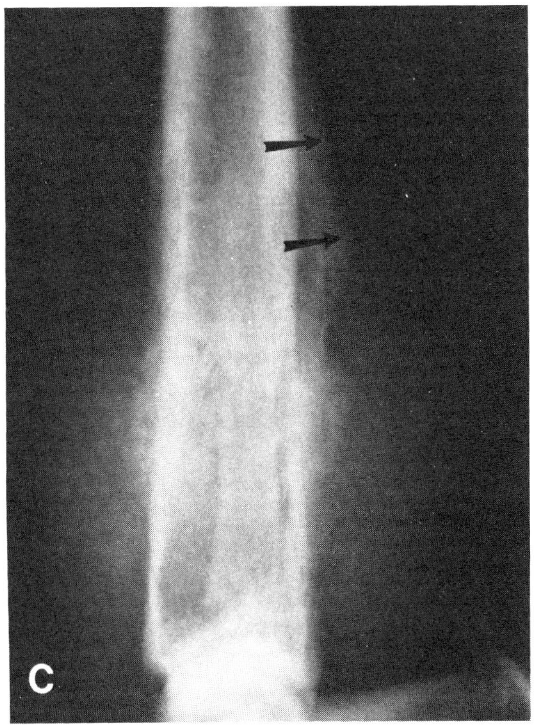

Figure 8C

Figure 8—Examples of periosteal reactions that may occur with primary bone neoplasia: **(A)** brush periosteal reaction; **(B)** spiculated periosteal reaction; and **(C)** Codman's triangle *(arrows)*. See Figure 5 for a laminated periosteal reaction.

Areas of cortical destruction larger than 1 cm may be produced with primary bone neoplasia (Figure 4). Such large areas of destruction occur most frequently with primary bone neoplasia and are seldom seen with other solitary bone lesions.

Cortical expansion may occur with benign neoplasia, cystic bone lesions, and malignant bone neoplasia. The cortex usually remains intact with benign conditions. Malignant primary bone tumors expand and may also cause pathological fractures in the cortex.[9] Large fragments of the cortex may be displaced away from the normal location in such cases.

Punctate cortical lysis is more consistent with acute, active osteomyelitis; however, it may also occur in early cases of neoplastic disease (Figure 5). It is not a good differentiating radiographic sign.

Neoplastic Matrix (New Bone Production)

The production of neoplastic matrix or new bone may be intra- or extramedullary. The pattern may be amorphous, snowflakelike, or sunburst. Neoplastic matrix produced within the medullary cavity replaces normal trabecular bone with bone having one of these patterns (Figure 6). Extramedullary neoplastic matrix production characteristically extends into the soft tissues around the bone (Figure 7). The degree of extension is greater than that of periosteal reactions associated with infectious or inflammatory processes. An early periosteal reaction with a neoplastic lesion may eventually progress to a pattern of extramedullary neoplastic matrix. Intra- and extramedullary neoplastic matrix productions are excellent radiographic signs of bone neoplasia.

Periosteal Reactions

The differentiation of periosteal reactions from extramedullary neoplastic matrix production is not always possible. Periosteal reactions are usually close to the bone surface, whereas extramedullary neoplastic matrix production usually extends into the surrounding soft tissues. Different patterns of periosteal reactions may be seen with malignant bone tumors[3] (Figure 8). Patterns of periosteal response include an irregular brush pattern, spiculation, laminated or onion skin, and a Codman's triangle. An irregular brush pattern is usually seen in early tumor stages. In later stages spiculation and periosteal elevation producing a Codman's triangle may occur. Periosteal spiculation patterns may in some cases represent extramedullary neoplastic matrix production. Codman's triangle is an expansile sign, caused by elevation of periosteum at the tumor margin. It is observed with primary bone neoplasia but also may be seen with traumatic and infectious processes. A laminated or onion skin reaction seldom occurs with primary bone tumors in the dog, but when present it is a good sign of primary bone neoplasia.

By observing and working with the above-mentioned radiographic signs of primary bone neoplasia, a better radiographic differentiation of solitary long bone lesions can be obtained, a proper biopsy site can be identified, and appropriate radiographic examinations to check for metastatic lesions can be initiated.

REFERENCES

1. Brodey RS, Riser WH: Canine osteosarcoma: A clinicopathologic study of 194 cases. *Clin Orthop* 62:54-64, 1969.
2. Brodey RS, Saurer RM, Medway W: Canine bone neoplasms. *JAVMA* 143:471-495, 1963.
3. Ling GV, Morgan JP, Pool RR: Primary bone tumors in the dog: A combined clinical, radiographic, and histologic approach to early diagnosis. *JAVMA* 165:55-66, 1974.
4. Wolke RE, Nielsen SW: Site incidence of canine osteosarcoma. *J Small Anim Pract* 7:489-492, 1966.
5. Brodey RS, Reid CF, Saurer RM: Metastatic bone neoplasms in the dog. *JAVMA* 148:29-43, 1966.
6. Owen LN: An account of multiple osteosarcomata of bone in dogs having multicentric or metastatic origin. *Br J Radiol* 38:520-526, 1965.
7. Weller RE, Pool RR, Hornof WJ: Multiple skeletal metastases of osteogenic sarcoma in a dog. *JAVMA* 175:56-60, 1979.
8. Morgan JP: Systematic radiographic interpretation of skeletal diseases in small animals. *Vet Clin North Am* 4:621-626, 1974.
9. Schneider PR, Stowater JL: Pathologic fractures associated with skeletal metastasis of osteosarcoma in a dog. *JAVMA* 175:61-64, 1979.

UPDATE

Using a core biopsy technique, 83.9% of biopsies from bone neoplasms were positive when taken from the center of the bone lesion as identified on radiographs. Biopsies obtained from the transition zone (periphery) were positive only 54.5% of the time. When biopsies were obtained from both the center and the periphery, 92.3% were diagnosed as bone neoplasia.[1] Therefore, if only one biopsy can be obtained, it should be taken from the central lesion; if two are obtainable, both center and periphery biopsies should be made.

REFERENCE

1. Wykes PM, Withrow SJ, Powers BC, Park RD: Closed biopsy for diagnosis of long bone tumors: Accuracy and results. *JAAHA* 21:489–494, 1985.

Radiographic Diagnosis of Avian Abdominal Disorders

Marjorie C. McMillan, DVM

School of Veterinary Medicine
Tufts University
North Grafton, Massachusetts

Angell Memorial Animal Hospital
Boston, Massachusetts

Windhover Bird Clinic
Walpole, Massachusetts

Many avian diseases create radiographic abnormalities, and failure to recognize them may lead to misdiagnoses and inappropriate treatment. Radiographic examination, however, must complement an accurate history, thorough physical examination, and clinical laboratory data. It is not a substitute for these procedures. The interpretation and significance of certain radiographic abnormalities vary with species, age, sex, and duration in captivity. In addition, the frequency of certain radiographic findings varies with the species of bird under consideration. For example, traumatic injury to the extremities and skull predominates in raptors, whereas infectious diseases and nutritional deficiencies are common in exotic birds.

The radiographic technique used for birds as well as the normal radiographic anatomy of birds are reported in the literature[1,2]; specifically, birds and mammals differ in that birds lack an omentum, well-developed mesenteric attachments, and a falciform ligament. Because of short mesenteric attachments, the abdominal organs of birds remain relatively fixed in position. Fat deposits between organs are minimal, and thus differentiation of specific organ margins is more difficult in birds than it is in dogs and cats. Because only a rudimentary, incomplete diaphragm is present, the cardiac silhouette and bilobed liver blend into a homogeneous soft tissue that has an hourglass appearance on ventrodorsal radiographs. The soft tissue density of abdominal viscera contrasts with the radiolucent surrounding air sacs.

Radiographic findings associated with abdominal disorders are:

1. Changes in the size, shape, position, and density of specific organs
2. Homogeneous abdominal density
3. Loss of abdominal air sac space
4. Visualization of a mass.

Radiographic Abnormalities

Hepatomegaly is a common radiographic finding in psittacines. In a lateral radiograph, the liver normally does not extend beyond the sternum. If the bird is positioned properly for a ventrodorsal view, the liver normally does not extend laterally beyond a line parallel to the sternum connecting the scapula and acetabulum (Figure 1).

Originally published in Volume 8, Number 9, September 1986

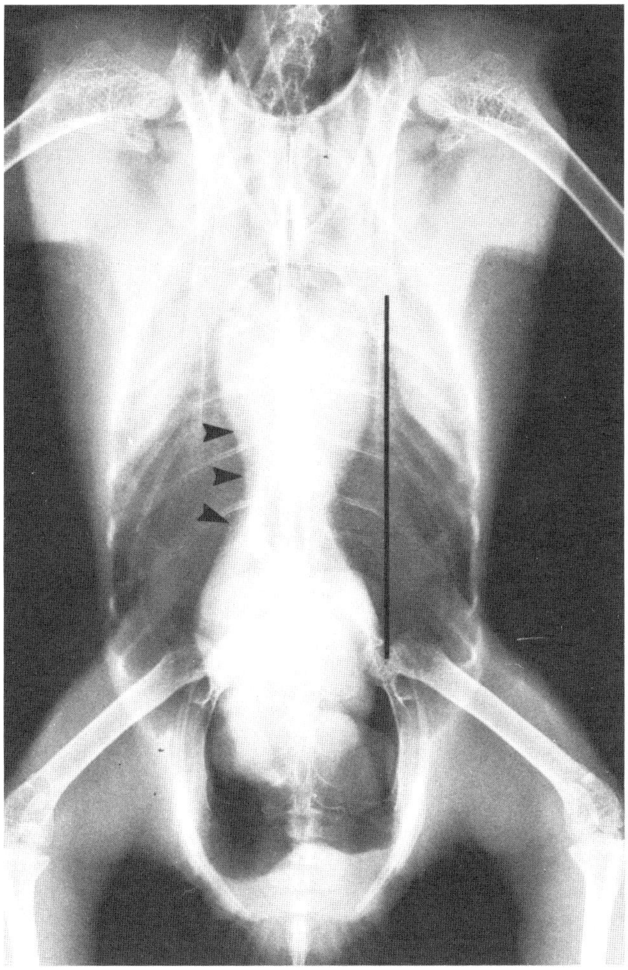

An enlarged liver may cause cranial displacement of the cardiac silhouette, dorsal displacement of the proventriculus, and caudodorsal displacement of the ventriculus. The hourglass configuration of the cardiohepatic silhouette is altered, and the liver is visualized as bulging into the abdominal air sacs. Many viral diseases[3-6] (such as Pacheco's disease, REO [respiratory enteric orphans] disease, Newcastle disease virus, and papovavirus) and bacterial infections (particularly gram-negative organisms, mycobacteria,[7,8] and chlamydia) may result in hepatomegaly (Table I). Often, splenomegaly also is present (Figure 2). Parasites are an uncommon cause of liver disease, although toxoplasmosis in mynahs (*Acridotheres* spp.)[9] and liver flukes in a sulphur-crested cockatoo (*Kakatoe galerita*)[10] have been reported. Such metabolic abnormalities as hemochromatosis in mynahs (*Gracula religiosa*),[11,12] lipidosis in parakeets (*Melopsittacus undulatus*),[13] fatty degeneration, and gout may involve the liver, spleen, kidneys, and heart. Primary and metastatic neoplasia occur most commonly in parakeets; while lymphoma[14,15] (Figure 3), biliary adenocarcinoma, hepatocellular carcinoma,[16] and meta-

Figure 1—Ventrodorsal radiograph of a normal Amazon parrot demonstrates the hourglass appearance of a cardiohepatic silhouette (*arrows*) and the lateral extent of liver (*solid line*). Loss of hourglass configuration or extension of liver lobes beyond the solid line indicates hepatomegaly.

Figure 2—Lateral radiograph of a blue and gold macaw shows splenomegaly (*large arrows*) and kidney enlargement (*curved arrow*) associated with psittacosis.

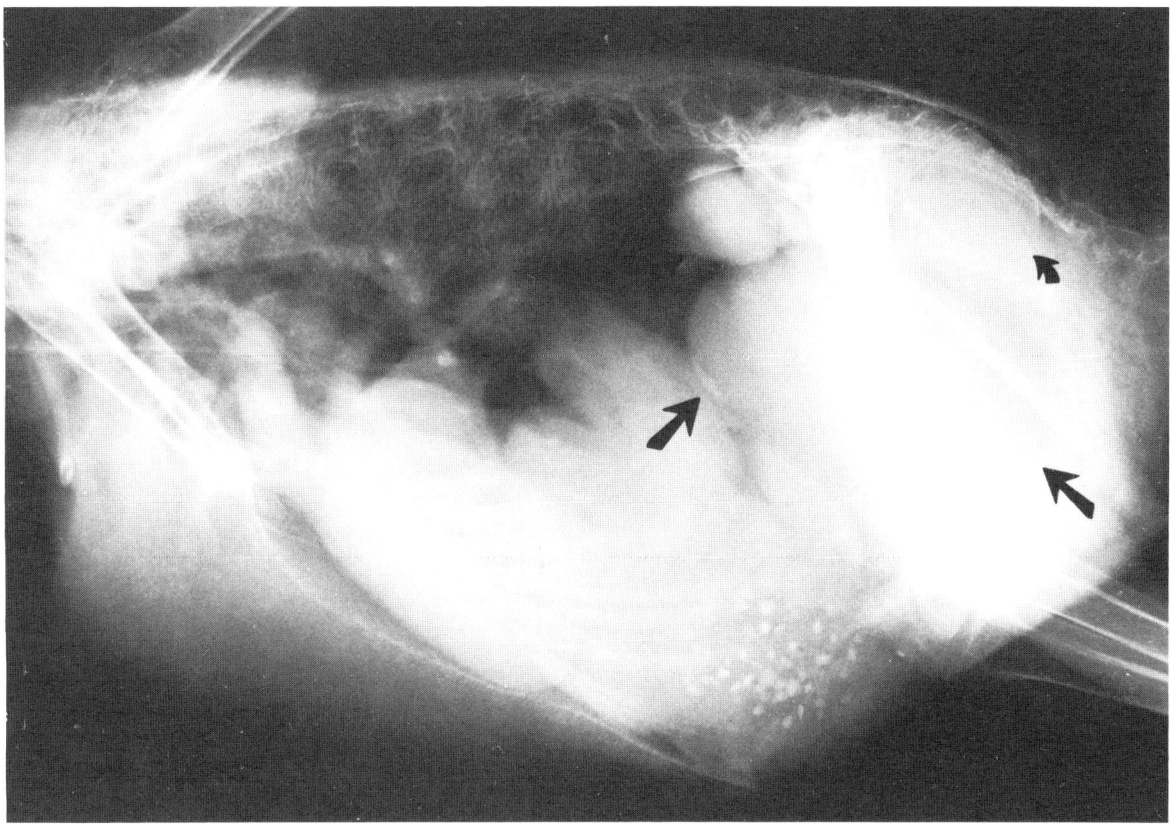

TABLE I
Causes of Hepatomegaly, Splenomegaly, and Nephromegaly

Hepatomegaly	*Splenomegaly*	*Nephromegaly*
Infectious	**Infectious**	**Infectious**
Viral	Viral	Bacterial
Bacterial	Bacterial	Chlamydial
Chlamydial	Chlamydial	
Mycobacterial	Mycobacterial	**Neoplastic**
Fungal		Adenocarcinoma
	Neoplastic	Embryonal nephroma
Neoplastic	Lymphoma	
Primary	Hemangiosarcoma	**Metabolic**
Hepatocellular carcinoma	Fibrosarcoma	Gout
Biliary adenocarcinoma	Leiomyosarcoma	Dehydration
Fibrosarcoma		Lipidosis
Hemangiosarcoma	**Metabolic**	
Hepatoma	Lipidosis	**Cystic**
Lymphoma	Hemochromatosis	
Metastatic		**Toxic**
Adenocarcinoma		Lead
Fibrosarcoma		
Melanoma		
Parasitic		
Toxoplasmosis		
Flukes (cestodes)		
Metabolic		
Hemochromatosis		
Lipidosis		
Fatty degeneration		
Gout		

static adenocarcinoma[16] have been reported in larger psittacines. In mynahs, hepatomas occur in association with hemochromatosis.[17]

The spleen usually is not apparent radiographically (Figure 4). Splenomegaly, often in combination with hepatomegaly, occurs in systemic infections, neoplasia, and such metabolic disorders as lipidosis and hemochromatosis (Table I).

The kidneys are firmly adherent to the synsacrum, have smoothly rounded cranial and caudal poles, are flattened dorsoventrally, and are surrounded by air. The kidneys are best visualized in a lateral radiograph. Obliteration of normal air density surrounding the renal silhouette indicates renal enlargement, dorsal displacement of abdominal viscera, or presence of abdominal fluid (Figure 5). Nephritis from gram-negative bacterial infection and chlamydiosis may cause renal enlargement (Table I).

Dehydration causes increased renal density and, sometimes, renal enlargement. Incomplete clearance and flushing of renal tubules lead to "renal constipation," with an accumulation of uric acid crystals in the kidneys.[18] Theoretically, any condition resulting in impaired renal clearance of uric acid crystals could result in nephromegaly and increased renal density. In addition, changes in kidney size and density are seen in psittacines in association with acute hemolysis caused by lead toxicity.[19] These changes probably are caused by hemoglobin blockage of kidney tubules, with resultant decreased renal tubular function. In contrast to generalized nephromegaly observed in the conditions mentioned, kidney tumors usually cause enlargement of only the cranial or caudal pole with ventral displacement of the ventriculum[2,20] (Figure 6).

Hormonal changes result in cyclic atrophy and recrudescence of the gonads. Hypertrophied testicles are visualized as symmetric enlargements in the ventrodorsal view and as superimposed circular soft tissue masses, cranial and ventral to the kidneys, in the lateral radiograph (Figure 6). An enlarged oviduct results in loss of air sac density below the kidneys and increased soft tissue density in the dorsal abdominal region (Figure 7). Pathologic enlargement of the testicles and ovaries occurs because of neoplasia.[21] In addition, increased medullary bone density occurs in females with ovarian tumors[22] and oviduct abnormalities.

Changes apparent on survey radiographs provide preliminary information for certain disease processes; however, abnormalities of the gastrointestinal tract are best evaluated by barium-contrast examination.[23] As an example, gas in the gastrointestinal tract of birds is abnormal. If an external source of gas (such as tube feeding or aerophagia) is eliminated, a gastrointestinal abnormality is the most likely cause.

Proventricular dilatation,[24] also called *blue and gold ma-*

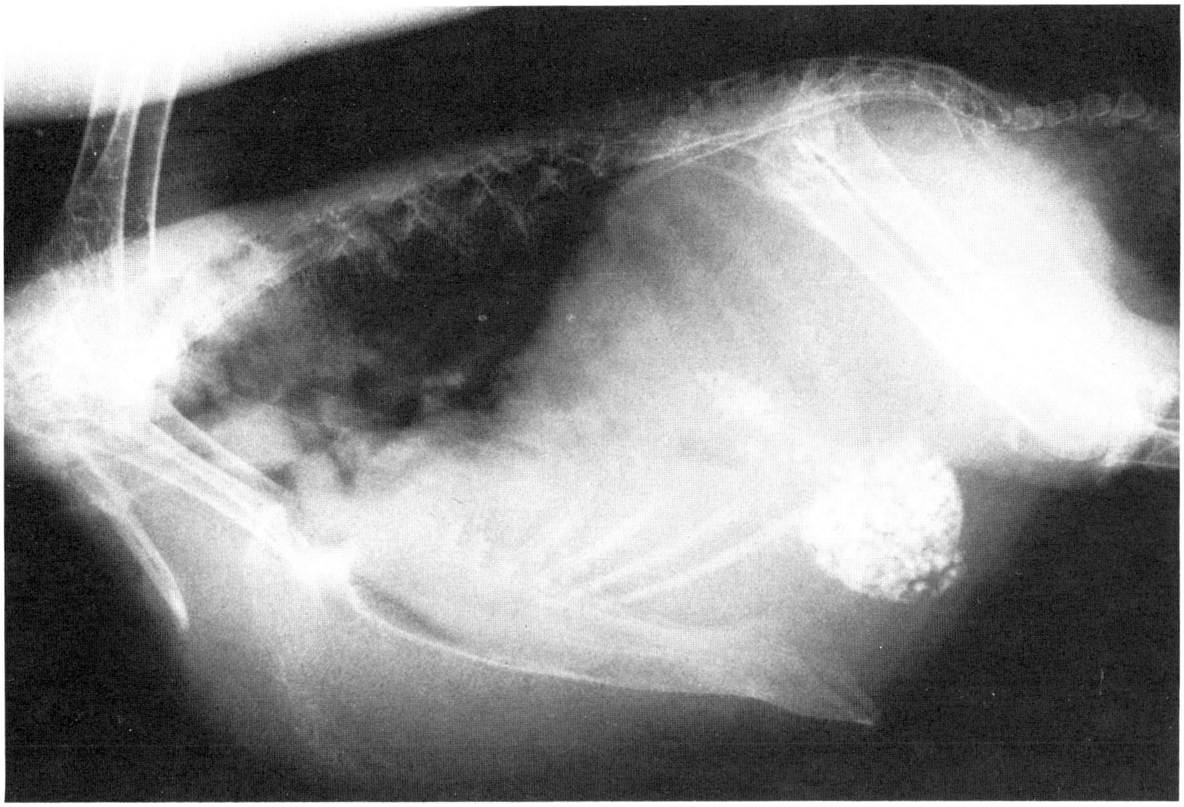

Figure 3A

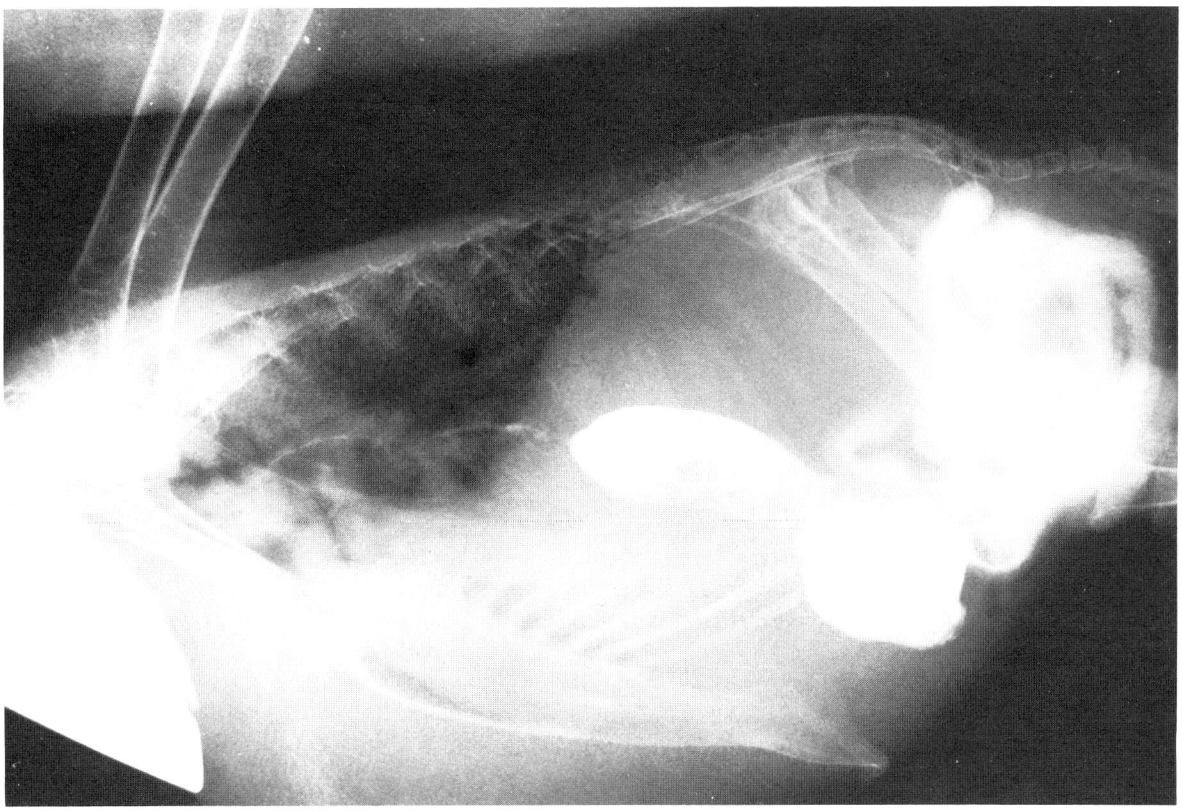

Figure 3B

Figure 3—(**A**) Survey lateral radiograph of an African gray parrot shows dorsal displacement of the proventriculus and caudodorsal displacement of the ventriculus by an enlarged liver. The homogeneous soft tissue mass in the dorsal abdomen obliterates the air sac space below the kidneys and between the lungs and viscera. (**B**) After one hour, the barium-contrast series indicated that the intestines were displaced caudally by a dorsal mass, which was an enlarged spleen. Hepatic and splenic enlargement were caused by lymphosarcoma.

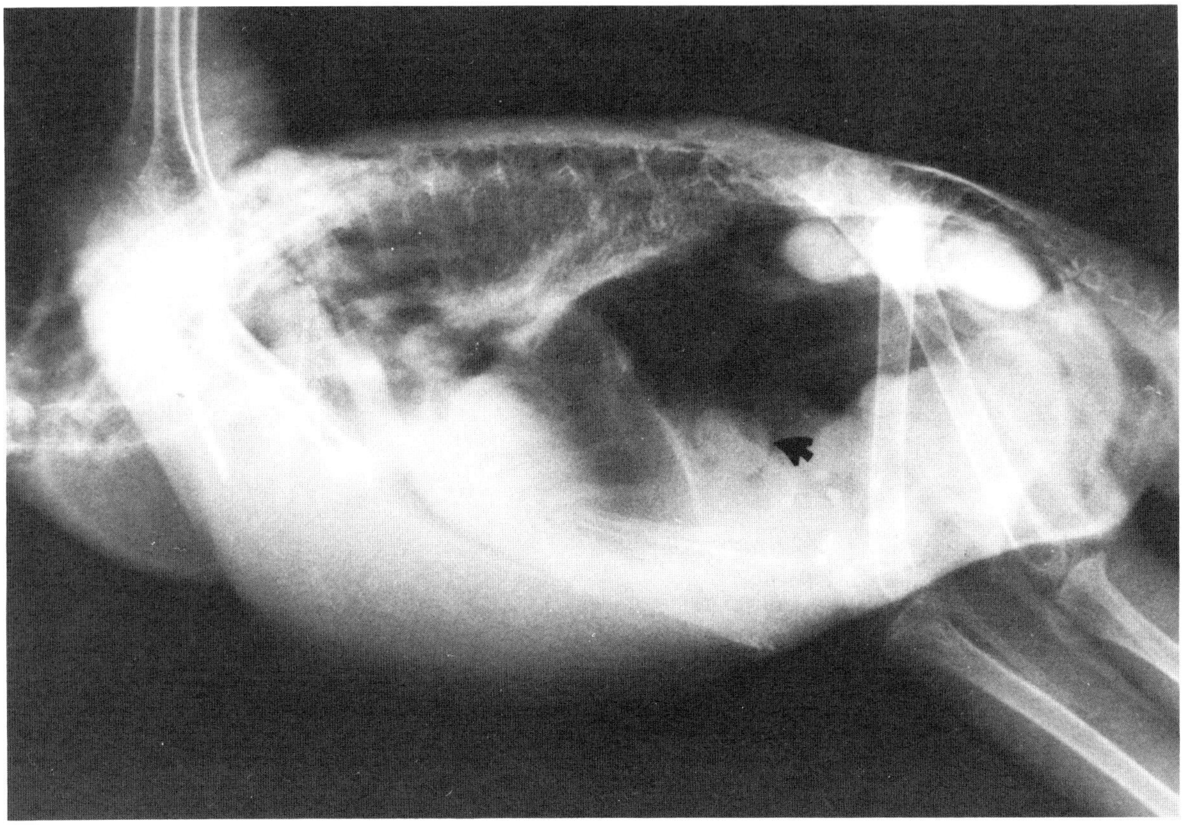

Figure 4—The normal size, shape, and location of the spleen (*arrow*) are apparent in this lateral radiograph of an African gray parrot. Peribronchial infiltrate is present in the hilar and mid region of the caudal lung.

caw syndrome[25] or *infiltrative splanchnic neuropathy*,[3] causes functional ileus resulting in marked gastrointestinal distention. Birds are presented with weight loss, uncontrollable regurgitation, history of passing undigested seeds, and dehydration. In all except a few cases, the disease is fatal. Radiographic changes range from slight distention of the proventriculus with gas to marked distention of the gastrointestinal tract (Figure 8). Barium may persist in the intestinal tract up to 72 hours after administration. The proventriculus is massively distended and may contain food or gas. The ventriculus also is distended and thin walled. The crop is usually distended with fluid. Histologically there is diffuse mononuclear cell infiltration of intrinsic and extrinsic splanchnic nerves supplying the crop, proventriculus, ventriculus, and duodenum. Although most commonly reported in the blue and gold macaw (*Ara ararauna*), the disease occurs in other macaws (e.g., the green-winged macaw [*Ara chloroptera*] and hyacinth macaw [*Hyacinthinus anodorhynchus*]) as well as in cockatoos, conures, and African gray parrots (*Psittacus erithacus*).

Functional ileus also occurs in association with inflammatory processes involving the abdomen. In birds with egg peritonitis, a generalized increased fluid density obscures abdominal detail and dilated gas-filled bowel loops may be apparent. Intestinal serosal adhesions associated with egg peritonitis also result in decreased intestinal motility (Figure 9). Gas-distended loops of intestine are also visualized in conjunction with the massive ascites commonly seen in mynahs with liver failure from hemochromatosis.

Gas and fluid distention of the intestinal tract caused by mechanical ileus can occur from a foreign body obstruction (Figure 10); stricture; neoplasia; and extrinsic masses involving the thyroid gland, oviduct, and spleen. Impaction of the ventriculus with grit results in upper gastrointestinal obstruction (Figure 11). Often these birds have been fed inappropriately sized grit, allowed to eat freely after being deprived of grit for a long period, or have a deprived appetite because of an underlying illness. Radiographs show an increased amount of grit firmly compressed in the ventriculus. Grit also may be visualized in the proventriculus and crop. Barium-contrast examination shows delayed emptying of the crop. Small amounts of barium may pass from the crop, through the ventriculus, and into the intestinal tract.

Atonic distention of the cloaca occurs with spinal trauma and infiltrative neoplastic processes involving the sacral nerves (Figure 12). Obstruction caused by cloacal polyps, papillomas, or adenocarcinoma also causes distention. Laying hens normally have a more dilated cloaca to facilitate passage of eggs; this should not be considered pathologic.

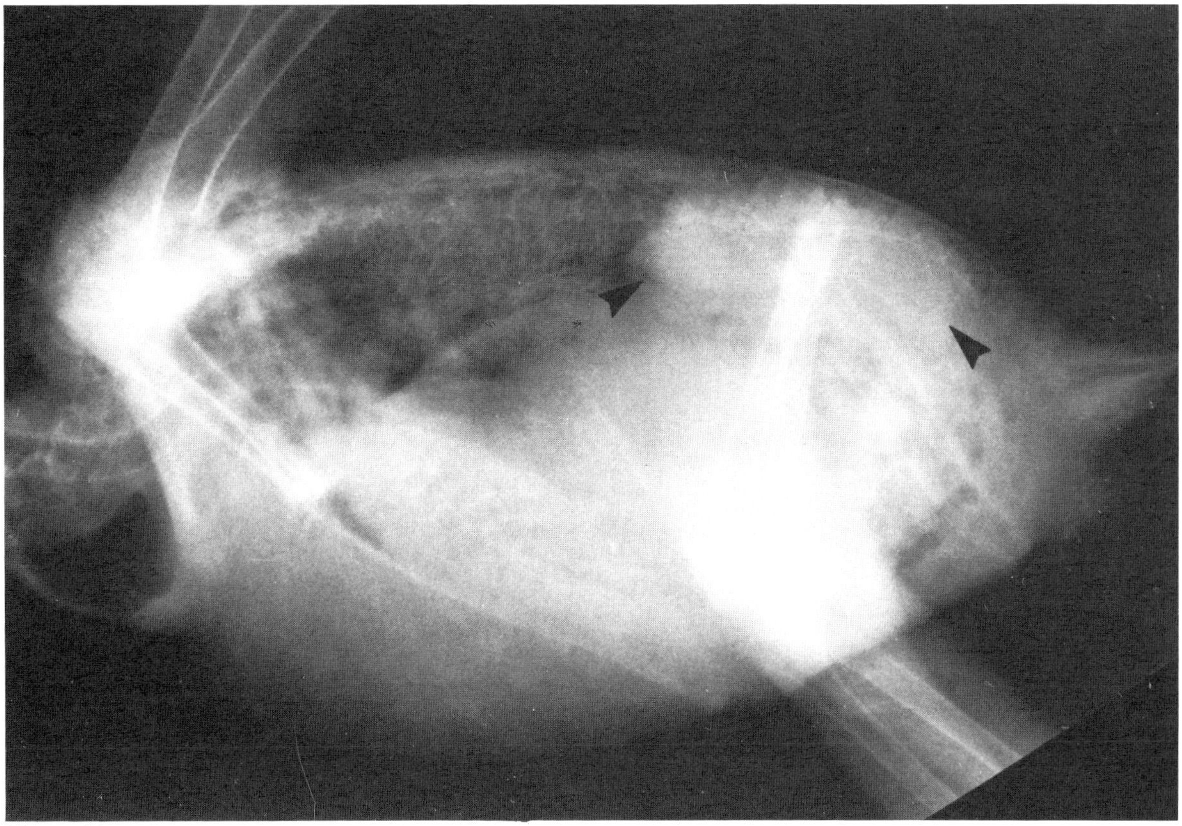

Figure 5A

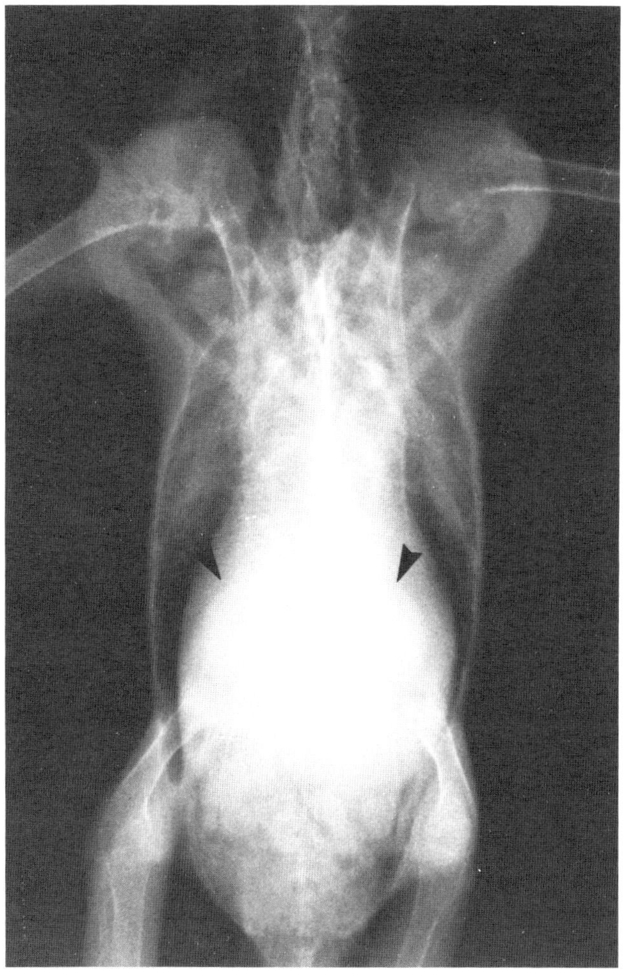

Figure 5B

Figure 5—(**A**) Kidney enlargement (*arrows*) with loss of air sac space ventral and cranial to kidneys is best demonstrated in a lateral radiograph. (**B**) Enlarged cranial kidney pole (*arrows*) is apparent in this ventrodorsal view. Nephromegaly in this Amazon parrot was caused by nephritis from *Escherichia coli* infection.

Additional Imaging Techniques

Urography,[2,26] ultrasonography,[27] and gastrointestinal barium-contrast studies[23] may aid in evaluating abdominal masses.

Urography outlines the kidneys, ureters, and cloaca. Radiographs taken at 10 seconds, 60 seconds, and 2 minutes after administration of contrast material provide the most useful information.[26] Irregularity of kidney size and shape and distention of the cloaca associated with renal neoplasia may be visualized by this means (Figures 6 and 12).

The presence of air sacs makes ultrasound examination difficult in birds. When abdominal fluid obliterates the air sacs, however, abdominal masses may be detected.

A gastrointestinal barium-contrast series helps the veterinarian localize abdominal masses and evaluate mechanical and functional ileus. Displacement of portions of the gastrointestinal tract by extrinsic masses, intraluminal masses, and hypomotility has been reported.

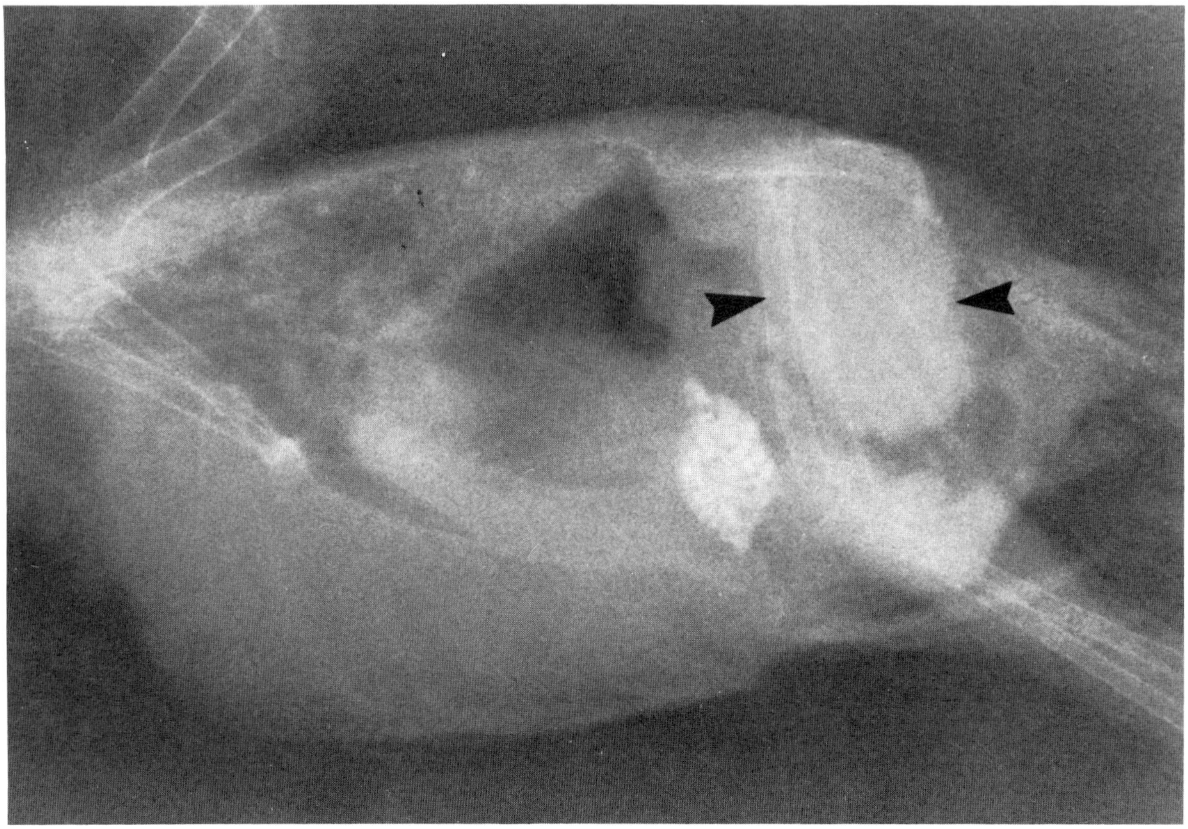

Figure 6A

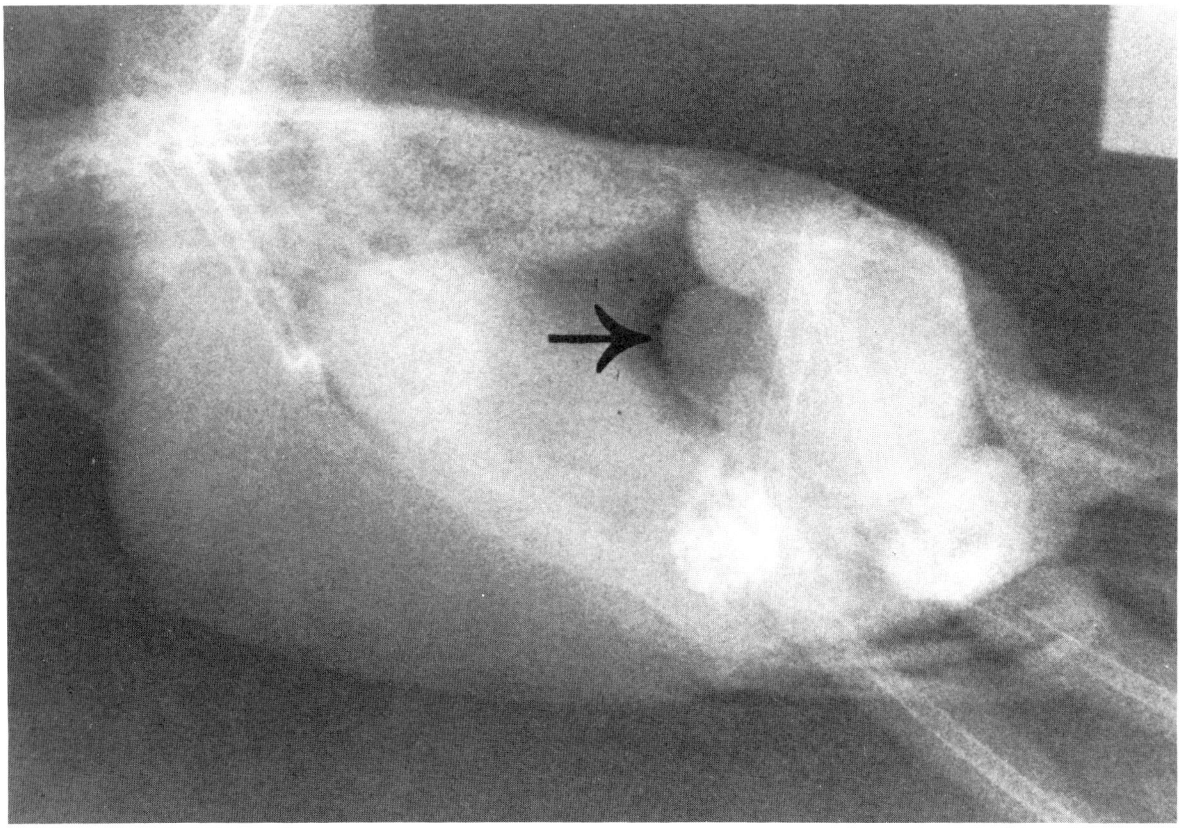

Figure 6B

Figure 6—(**A**) Renal adenocarcinoma (*arrows*) in this budgerigar is producing a large irregular mass from the caudal pole of a kidney. (**B**) The intravenous excretory urogram is enhancing the caudal pole renal adenocarcinoma in another budgerigar. The normal testicle (*arrow*) is ventral to the cranial kidney pole.

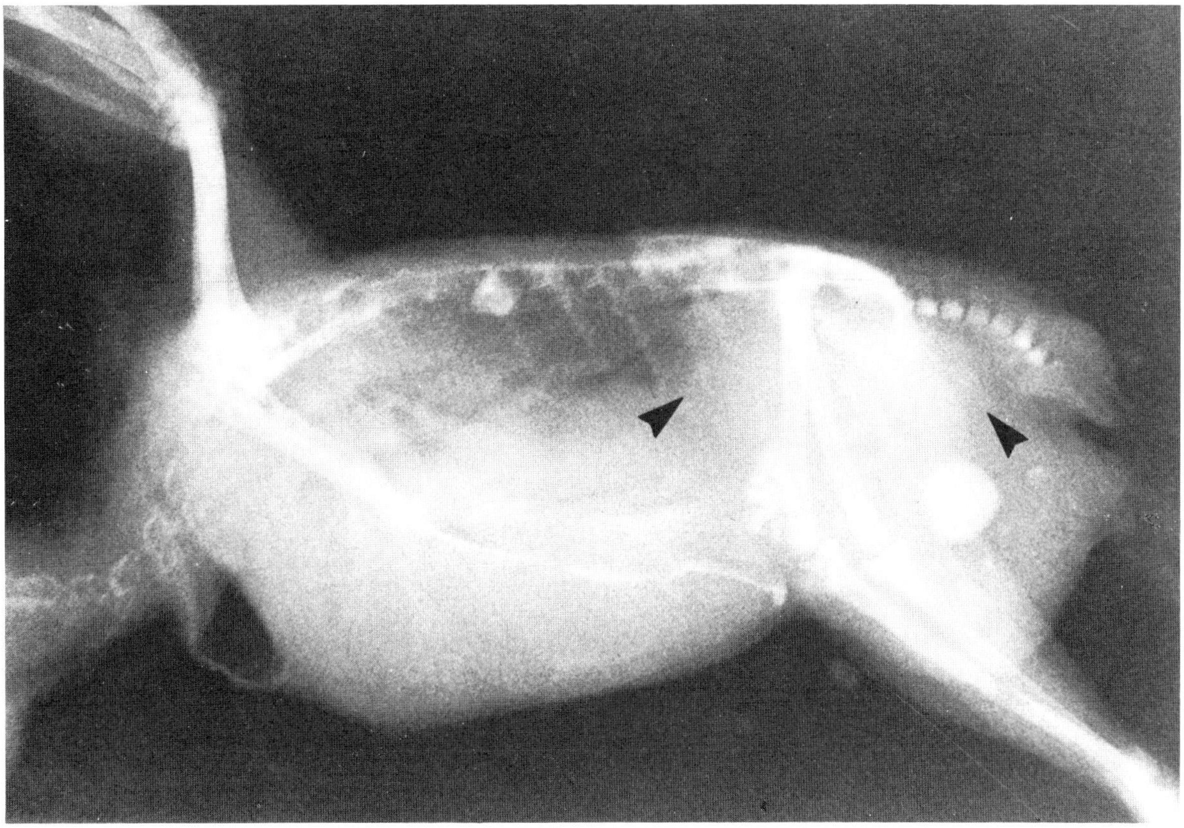

Figure 7A

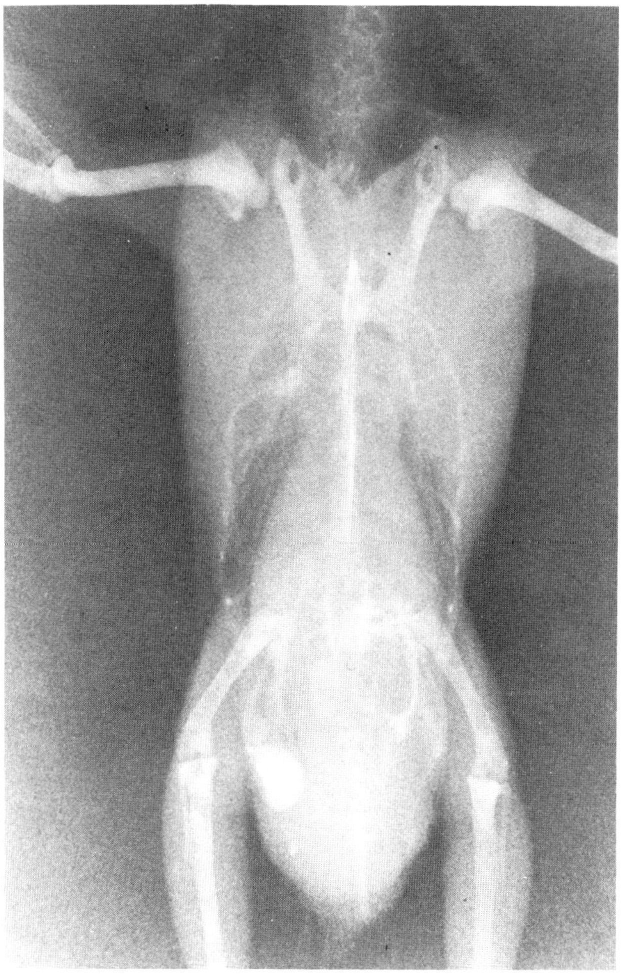

Figure 7B

Figure 7—(**A**) The soft tissue mass (*arrows*) in the dorsal abdomen obscuring visualization of the kidneys is an enlarged oviduct. The ventriculus is displaced cranially, and an abdominal hernia is apparent. (**B**) Mottled increased medullary bone density and well-defined circular regions of increased bone density involve the left pubis and ribs. These changes in budgerigars result from increased estrogen levels.

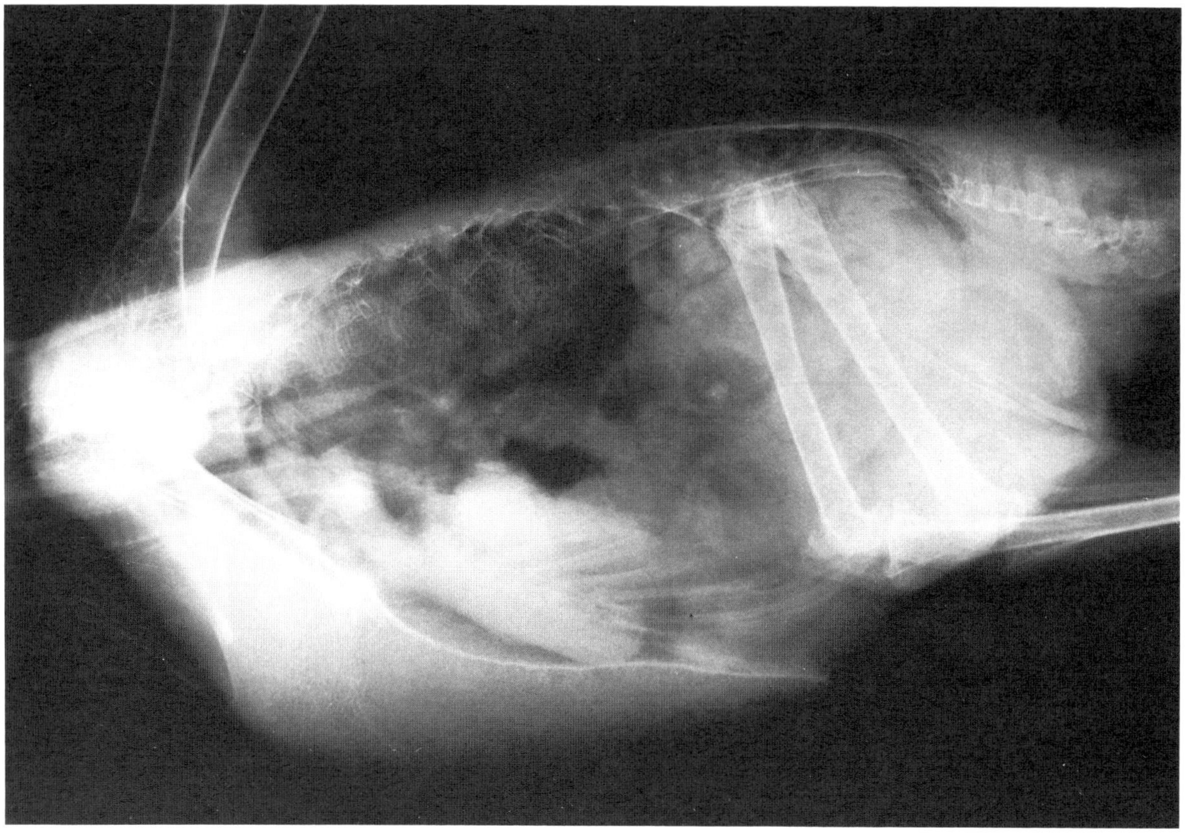

Figure 8A

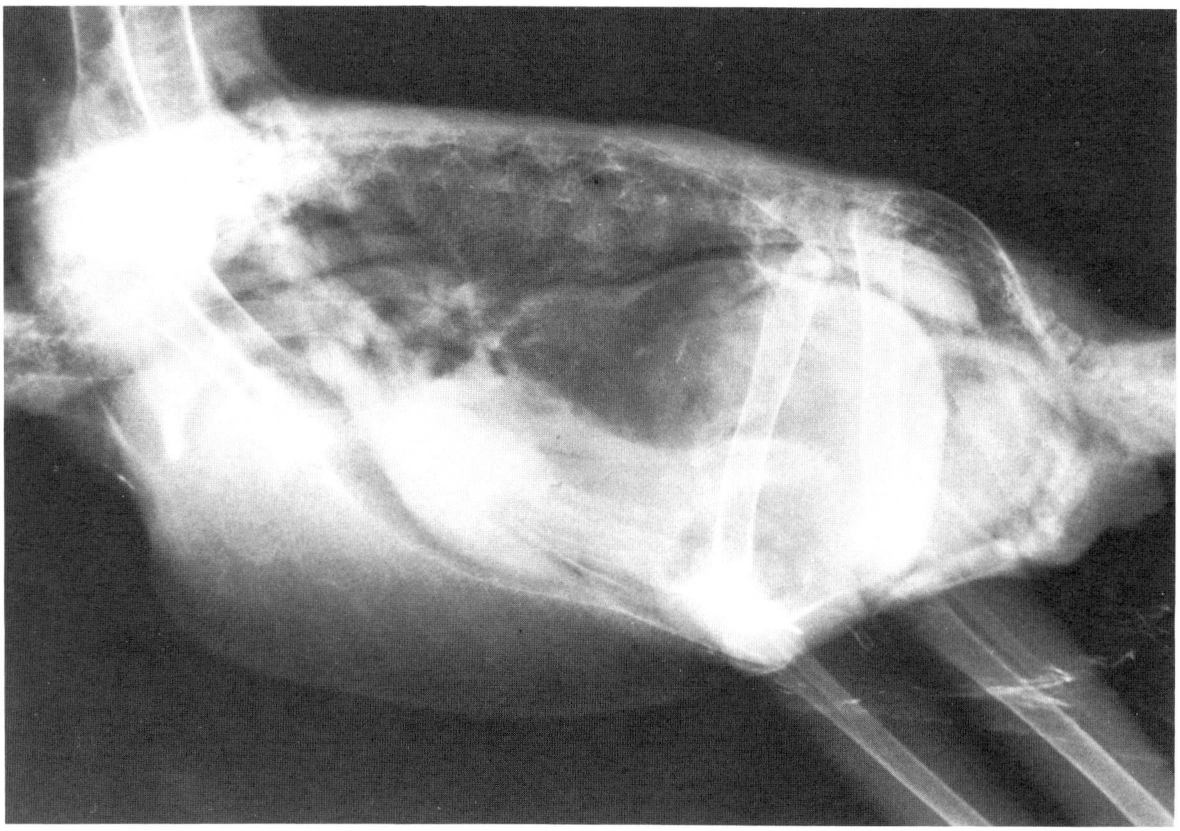

Figure 8B

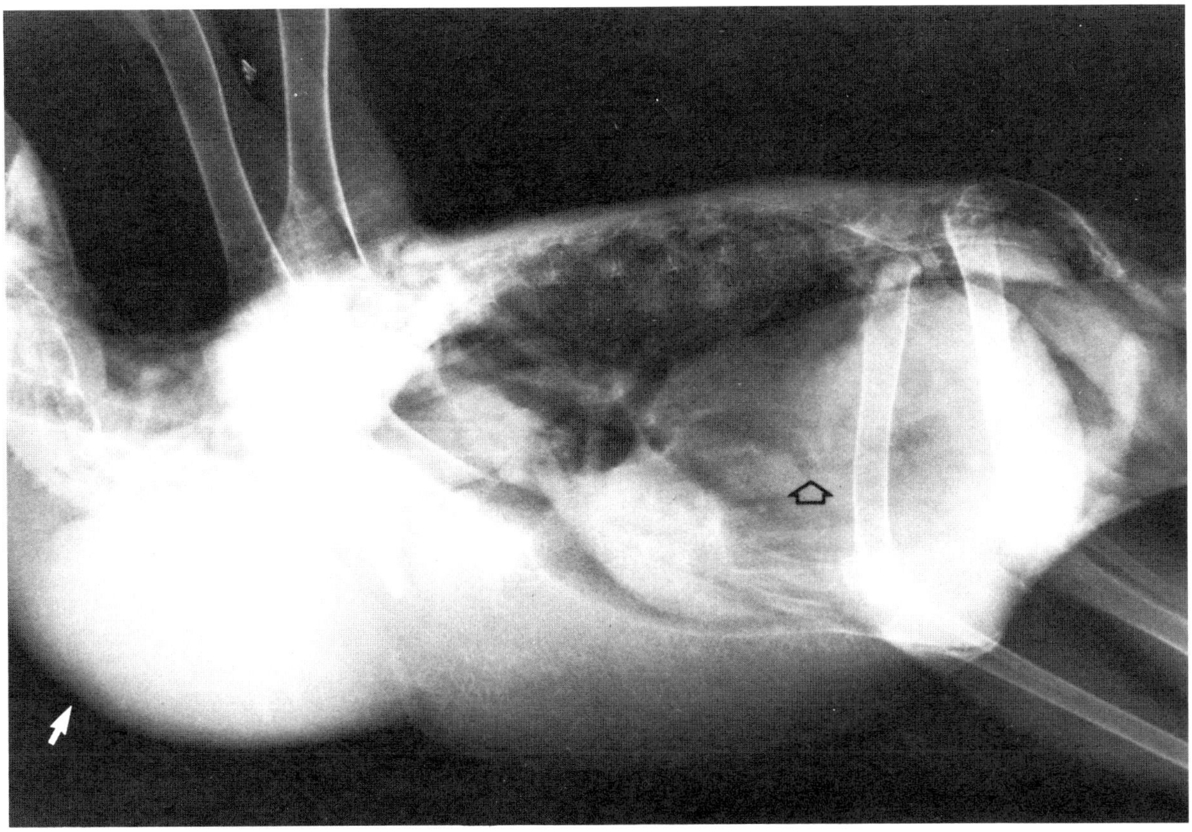

Figure 8C

Figure 8—(**A** through **F**) Radiographic changes associated with infiltrative splanchnic neuropathy. The radiographs are of blue and gold macaws. (**A**) Small amounts of gas and fluid are present in the proventriculus, ventriculus, and intestines. (**B**) Marked distention from the proventriculus and ventriculus being filled with gas and fluid. (**C**) Fluid-filled dilated proventriculus (*open arrow*) and ventriculus. The crop (*closed arrow*) is distended with fluid. (**D**) Ventrodorsal view of the parrot shown in **C**. The distended proventriculus (*open arrow*) could be mistaken for an enlarged liver lobe. (*Figure 8 continues next page*)

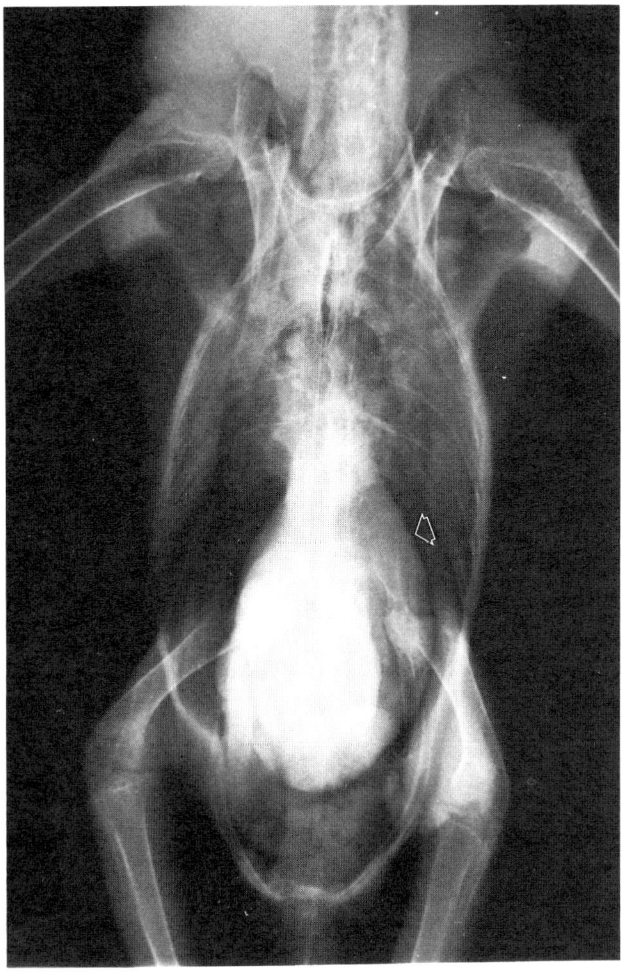

Figure 8D

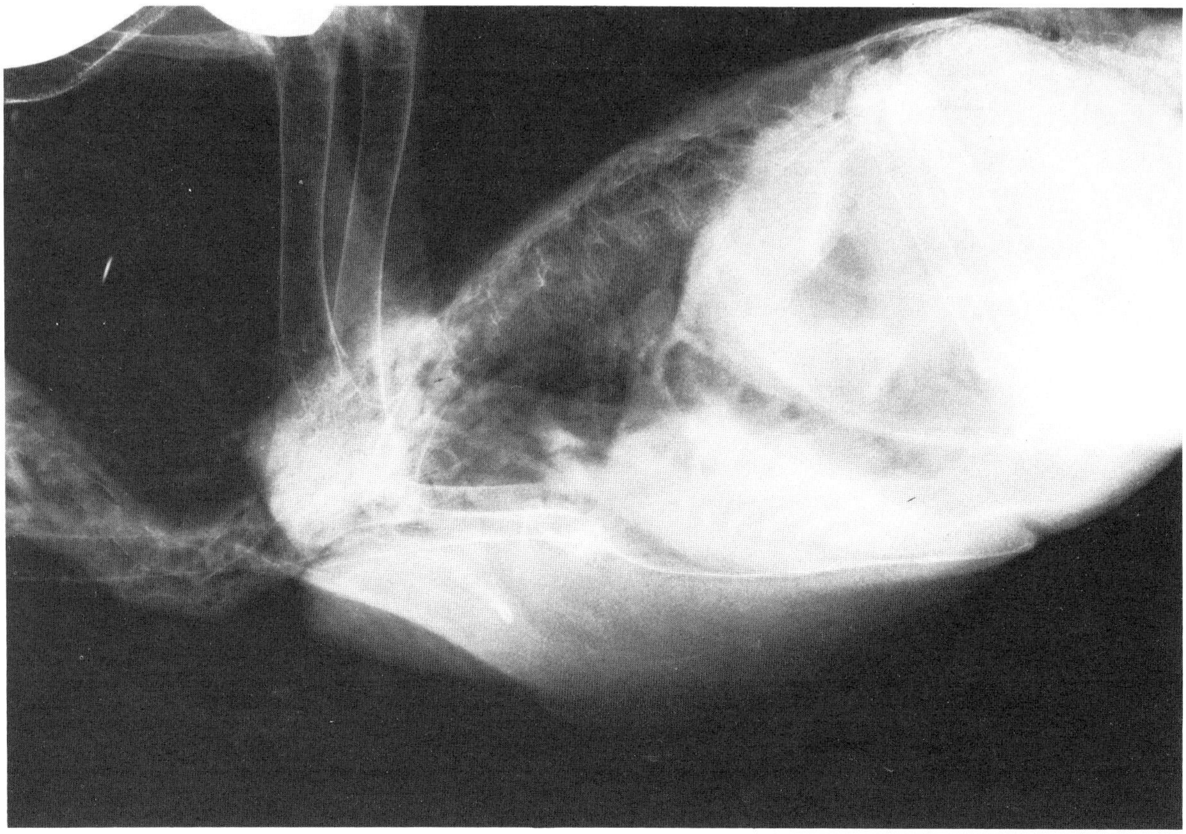

Figure 8E

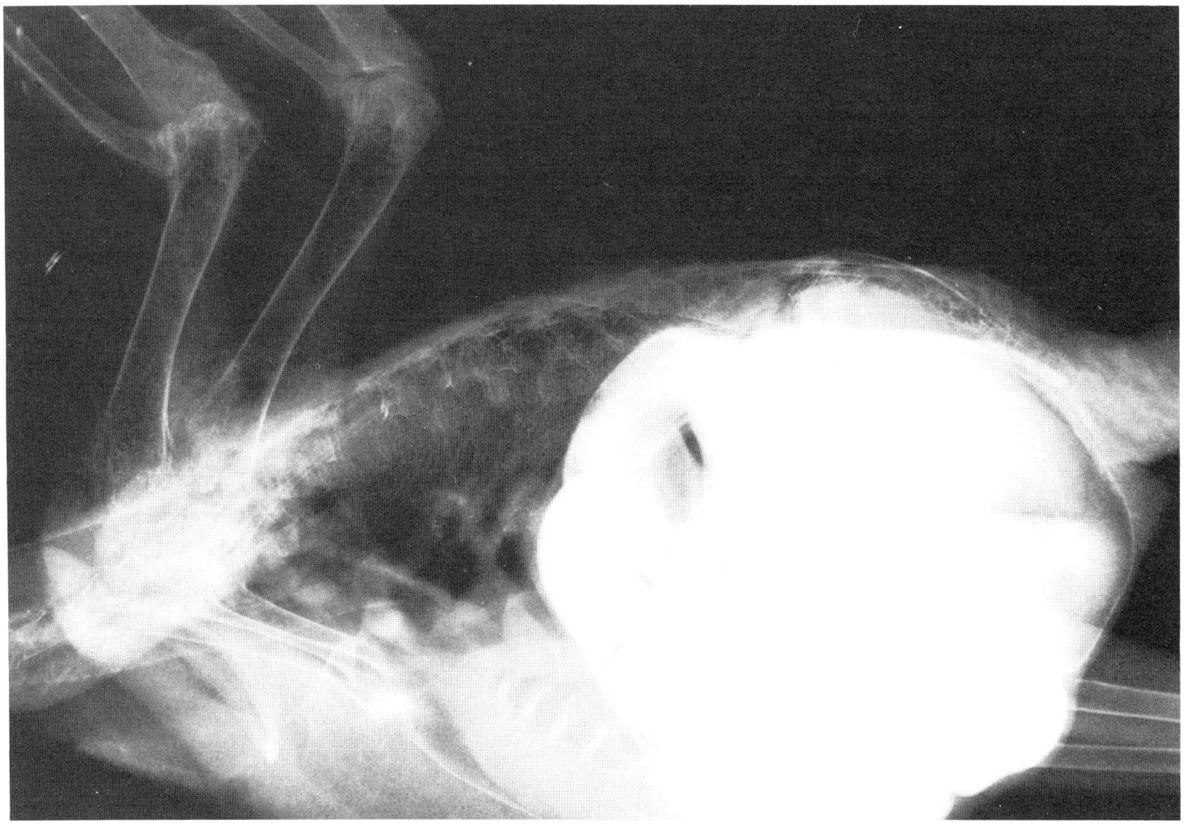

Figure 8F

Figure 8 continued—(**E**) Massive distention from the intestines being filled with gas and fluid because of functional ileus. (**F**) This radiograph shows retention of barium in dilated intestines eight hours after a barium-contrast series.

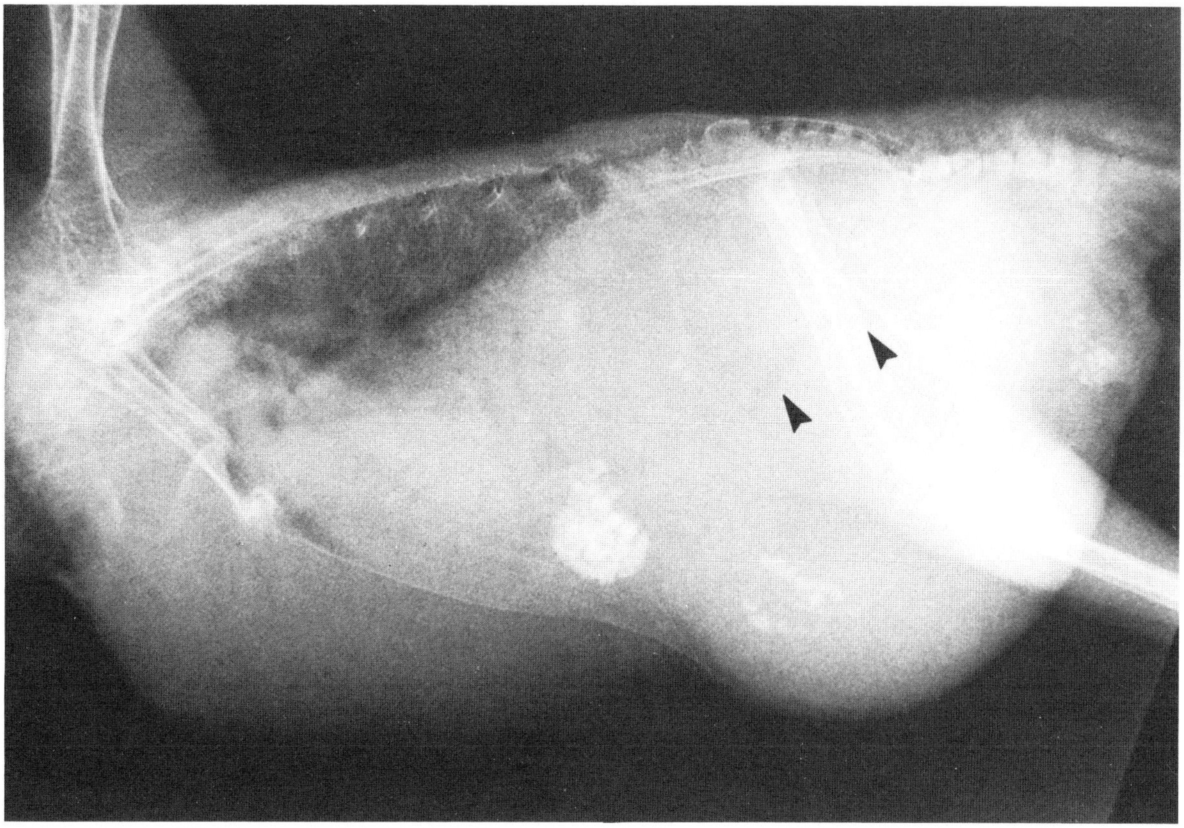

Figure 9A

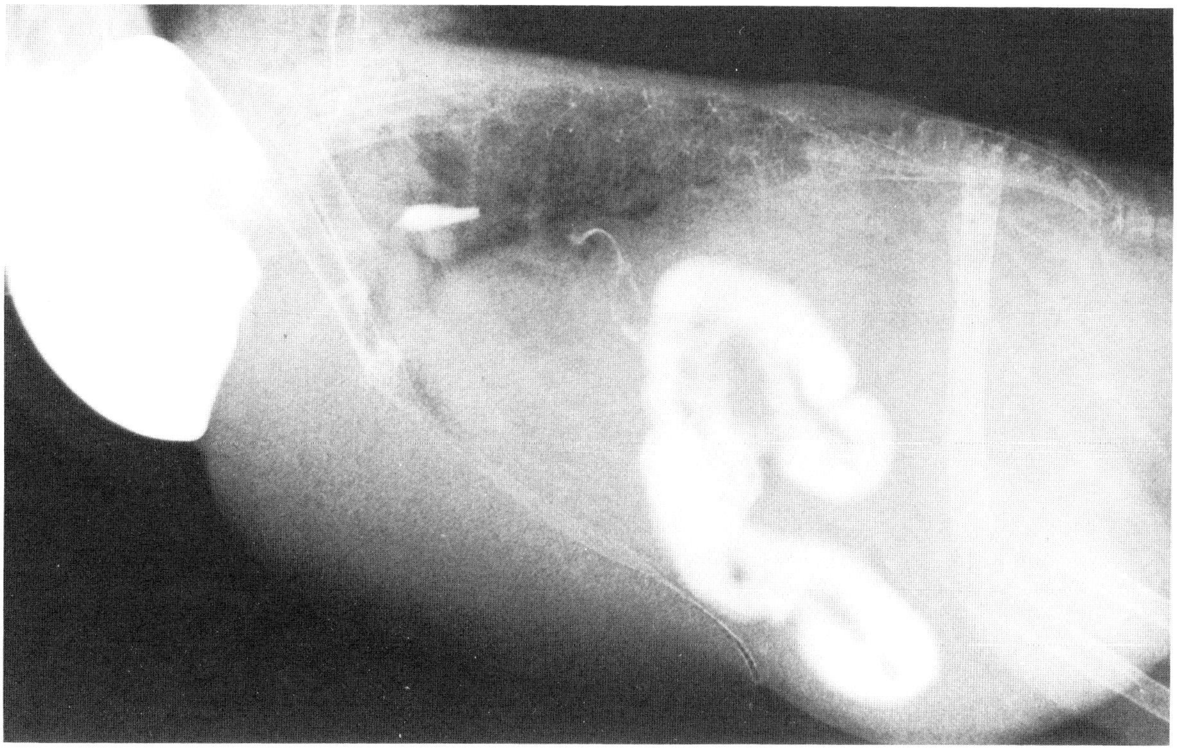

Figure 9B

Figure 9—(**A**) Distention of the abdomen, lack of contrast, and loss of air sac space are caused by abdominal fluid in this female cockatiel. A gas-filled intestinal loop (*arrows*) is present. The ventriculus is displaced cranially. (**B**) This radiograph shows abnormal positioning of the proventriculus, ventriculus, and intestines 30 minutes after a barium-contrast series. The intestines are dilated. Egg peritonitis with abdominal fluid and adhesions is present.

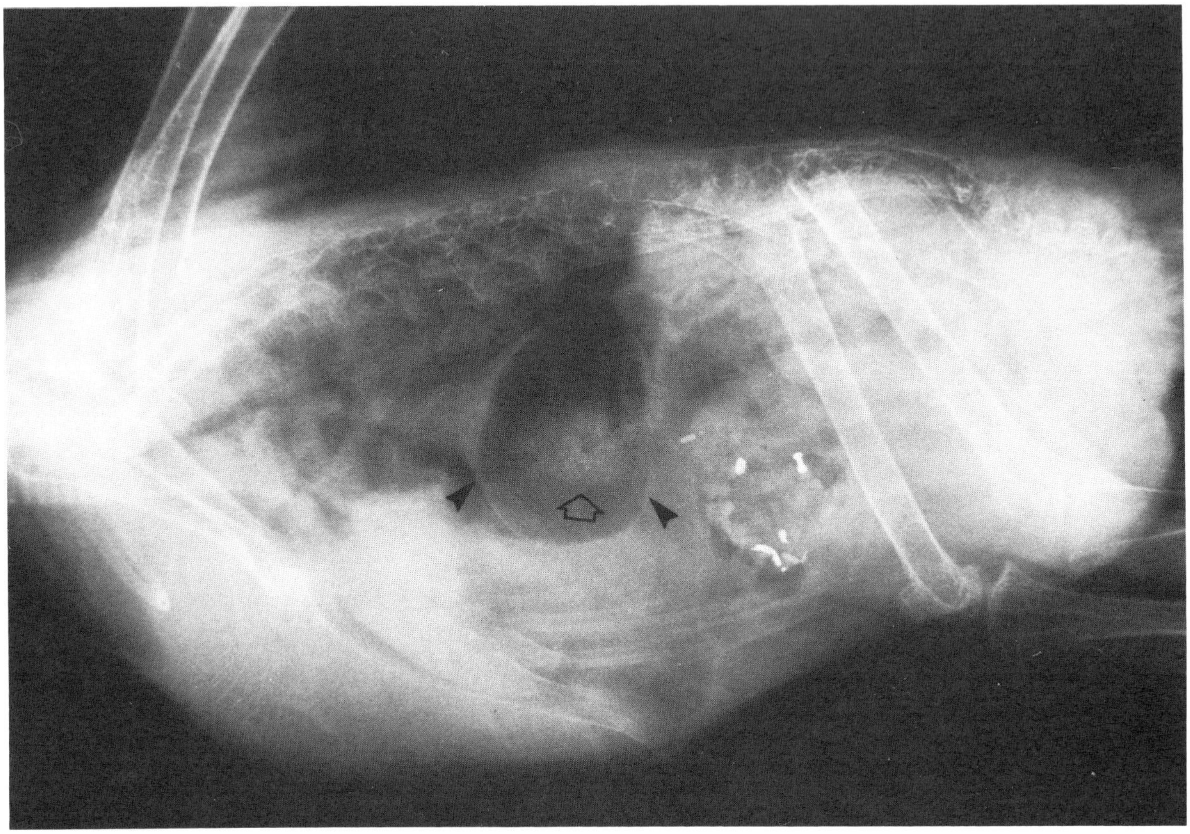

Figure 10A

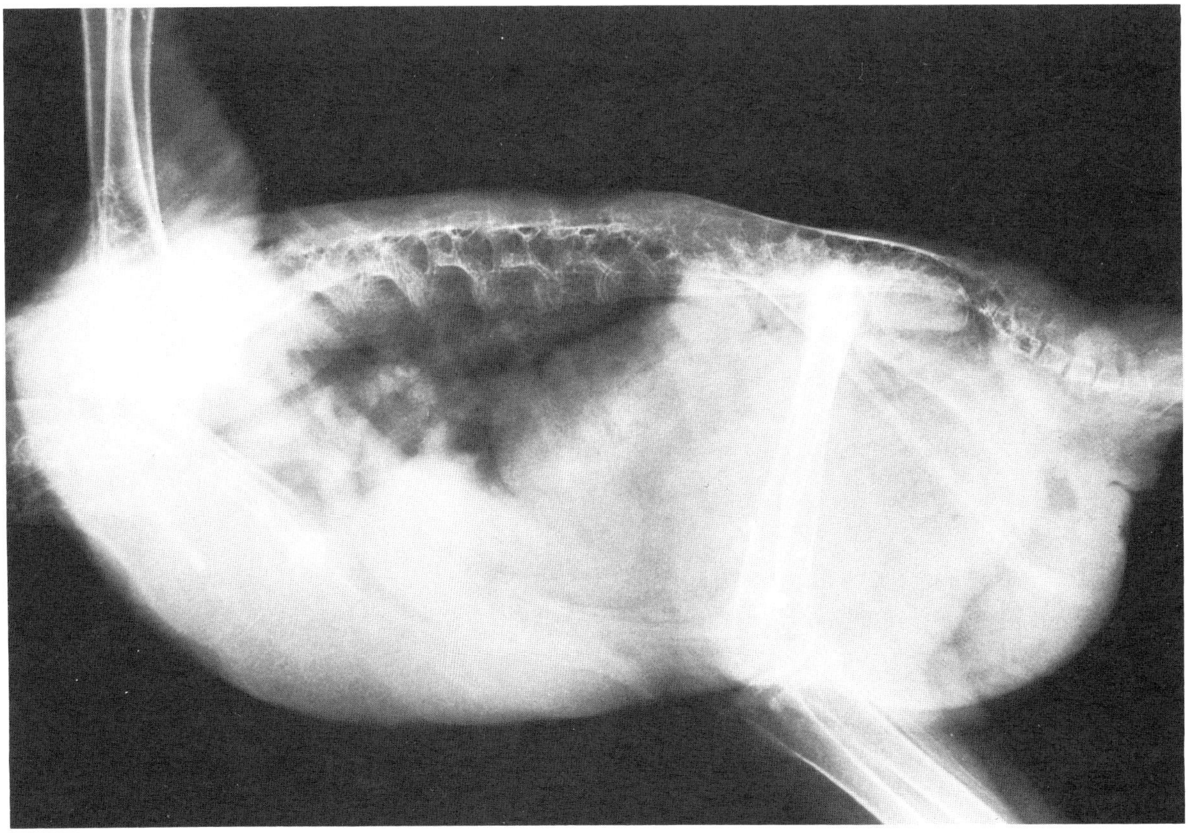

Figure 10B

Figure 10—(**A**) Gaseous distention of the proventriculus (*closed arrows*) and intraluminal foreign material (*open arrow*). Metallic foreign material is present in the ventriculus. (**B**) Radiograph taken 36 hours later shows that the foreign material still persists. Lack of abdominal contrast and mild abdominal distention are attributable to the presence of fluid. This cockatoo ingested a toy that perforated the gastrointestinal tract, causing peritonitis.

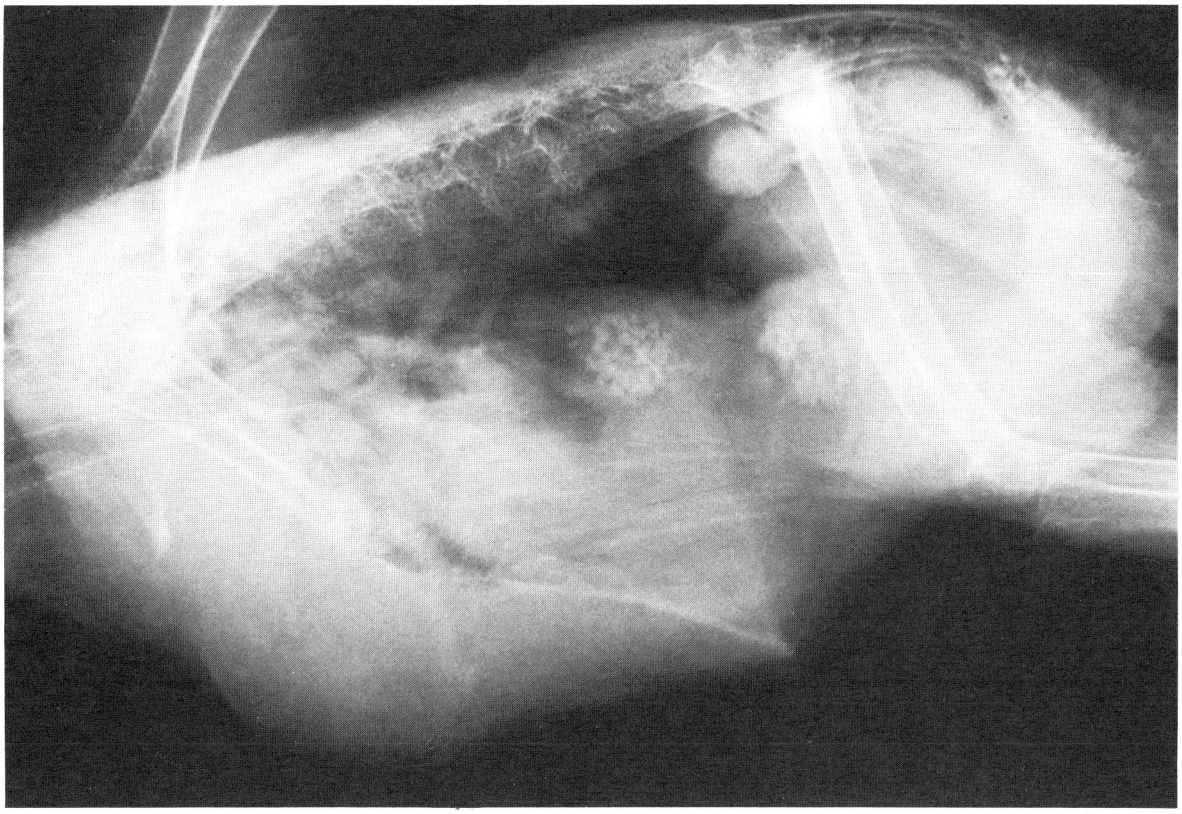

Figure 11A

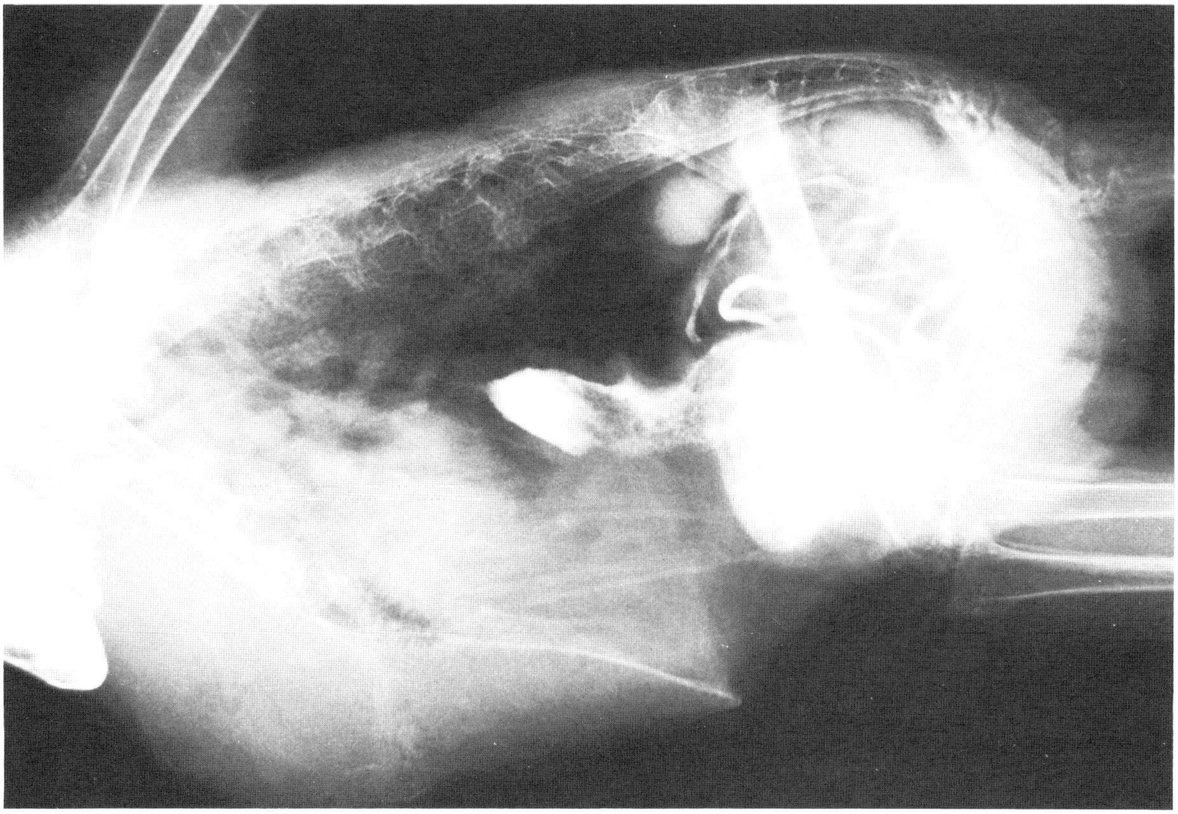

Figure 11B

Figure 11—(**A**) The presence of grit in the proventriculus is unusual. (**B**) A radiograph taken 36 hours after a barium-contrast series shows the barium still present in the crop, proventriculus, and ventriculus. Only small amounts of barium entered the intestines. This Amazon parrot was allowed to consume a large amount of grit after years of no access to grit. The impaction was removed surgically, and the parrot recovered uneventfully.

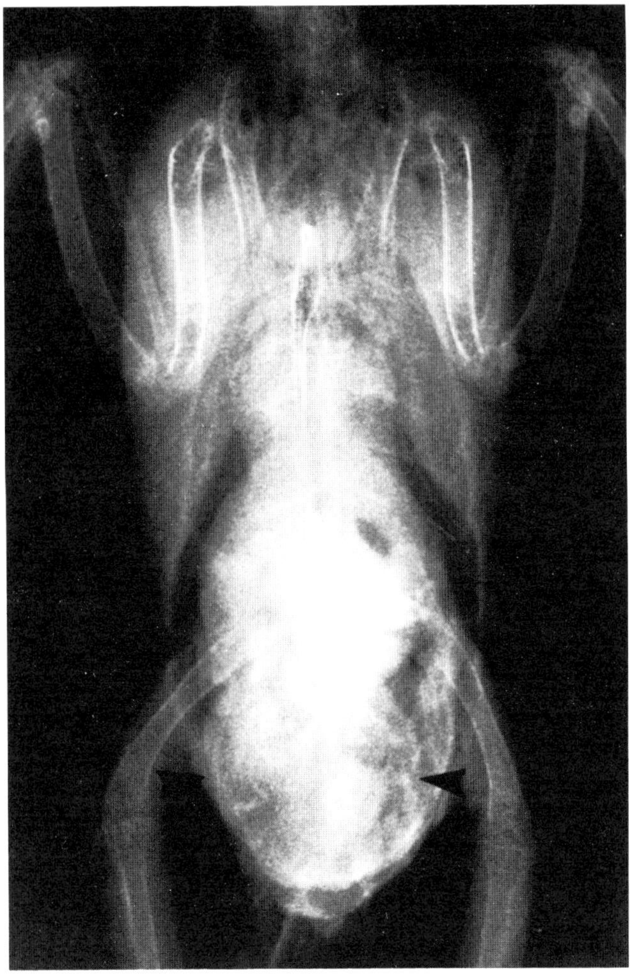

Figure 12—Intravenous excretory urogram shows irregularity in the kidney and distended cloaca (*closed arrows*). On autopsy, this budgerigar had a renal adenocarcinoma with involvement of sacral nerves.

REFERENCES

1. Evans SM: Avian radiographic diagnosis. *Compend Contin Educ Pract Vet* 3(7):660-666, 1981.
2. McMillan MC: Avian radiology, in Petrak ML (ed): *Diseases of Cage and Aviary Birds*. Philadelphia, Lea & Febiger, 1982, pp 329-360.
3. Graham DL: An update on selected pet bird virus infections. *Proc Annu Meet AAV*:267-280, 1984.
4. Gerlach H: Virus diseases in pet birds. *Proc Annu Meet AAV*:87-109, 1983.
5. Clubb SL: Infectious diseases. *Proc Annu Meet AAV*:91-101, 1982.
6. Simpson CF, Hanley JE: Pacheco's parrot disease in psittacine birds. *Avian Dis* 21(2):209-219, 1976.
7. Rosskopf WJ, Woerpel RW, Yanoff SR, et al: Tuberculosis in a parrot. *Mod Vet Pract* 62(10):777-778, 1981.
8. Dolphin RE, Olsen DE, Gallina AM: Tubercular infection in a sulfur-crested cockatoo. *VM SAC* 74(6):833-835, 1979.
9. Dhillon AS, Thacker HL, Winterfield RW: Toxoplasmosis in mynahs. *Avian Dis* 26(2):445-449, 1982.
10. Minsky L, Petrak ML: Diseases of the digestive system, in Petrak ML (ed): *Diseases of Cage and Aviary Birds*. Philadelphia, Lea & Febiger, 1982, pp 432-448.
11. Lowenstine LJ, Petrak ML: Iron pigment in the livers of birds, in Montali R, Migaki G (eds): *The Comparative Pathology of Zoo Animals*. Washington DC, Smithsonian Press, 1978, pp 127-135.
12. Randell MG, Patnaik AK, Gould WJ: Hepatopathy associated with excessive iron storage in mynah birds. *JAVMA* 179(11):1214-1217, 1981.
13. Leav I, Crocker AC, Petrak ML, et al: A naturally occurring lipidosis in shell parakeets, *Melopsittacus undulatus*. *Lab Invest* 18(4):433-437, 1968.
14. Palmer GH, Stauber E: Visceral lymphoblastic leukosis in an African gray parrot. *VM SAC* 26(9):1355-1356, 1981.
15. Petrak ML: Unpublished case material, Angell Memorial Animal Hospital, Boston, MA, 1983.
16. Petrak ML: Case presentations, AFA, Las Vegas, NV, 1980.
17. McMillan MC: Unpublished case material, Angell Memorial Animal Hospital, Boston, MA, 1978.
18. Knox DW: Gout in reptiles and birds, with observations on a comparable syndrome in man, in Montali R, Migaki G (eds): *The Comparative Pathology of Zoo Animals*. Washington DC, Smithsonian Press, 1978, pp 137-141.
19. Woerpel RW, Rosskopf WJ: Heavy metal intoxication in caged birds. Part I. *Compend Contin Educ Pract Vet* 4(10):729-738, 1982.
20. McMillan MC, Petrak ML: The clinical significance of abdominal enlargement in the budgerigar (*Melopsittacus undulatus*). *Compend Contin Educ Pract Vet* 3(10):898-904, 1981.
21. Petrak ML, Gilmore CE: Neoplasms, in Petrak ML (ed): *Diseases of Cage and Aviary Birds*. Philadelphia, Lea & Febiger, 1982, pp 606-637.
22. Schlumberger HG: Polyostotic hyperostosis in the female parakeet. *Am J Pathol* 35(1):1-23, 1959.
23. McMillan MC: Avian gastrointestinal radiography. *Compend Contin Educ Pract Vet* 4(5):273-284, 1983.
24. Ridgway RA, Gallerstein GA: Proventricular dilatation in psittacines. *Proc Annu Meet AAV*:228-230, 1983.
25. Woerpel RW, Rosskopf WJ, Hughes E: Proventricular dilatation and wasting syndrome: Mysenteric ganglioneuritis and encephalomyelitis of psittacines: An update. *Proc Annu Meet AAV*:25-28, 1984.
26. McNeel SV, Zenoble RD: Avian urography. *JAVMA* 178(4):366-368, 1981.
27. Peterson ME, Rantanen NW, Stauber E: Ultrasonic imaging in diagnosis of an abdominal mass in a pigeon. *Mod Vet Pract* 64(10):825-826, 1983.

Radiology of Avian Respiratory Diseases

Marjorie C. McMillan, DVM
School of Veterinary Medicine
Tufts University
North Grafton, Massachusetts

Angell Memorial Animal Hospital
Boston, Massachusetts

Windhover Bird Clinic
Walpole, Massachusetts

The anatomy and physiology of the avian respiratory system result in changes in radiographic patterns that are different from the interstitial, alveolar, peribronchial, and vascular patterns described in mammals. Because birds lack a true pleural space, pneumothorax and pleural effusion do not occur. Pleural fluid is usually attributed to extension from abdominal disease. Avian lungs are firmly attached to the thoracic wall, and thus atelectasis is not associated with thoracic problems. Lung volume remains constant during the respiratory cycle. Because the bronchial tree consists of an interconnecting network of tubules, air bronchograms are not a feature of consolidating pulmonary change. The interstitium is poorly developed so that marked interstitial patterns do not occur radiographically.

Indications

Birds with signs of upper respiratory disease (e.g., sneezing, nasal discharge, and/or infraorbital and periorbital swelling) but that otherwise are healthy may not require radiographic examination on initial presentation. If signs persist or recur after proper medical management, radiographs are indicated. Dyspnea, open-mouthed breathing, wheezing, tail bobbing, coughing, oral abscesses, loss of vocalization, exercise intolerance, abdominal distention, weight loss, and auscultatory abnormalities are indications for radiographic examination.

Preradiographic Considerations

Birds with severe respiratory problems may tolerate only a cursory examination. If respiratory distress is severe or the patient is debilitated, supportive treatment with oxygen and fluids is necessary before physical or radiographic examination. Rapid intramuscular injection of fluids and stabilization in an atmosphere of 40% oxygen before beginning diagnostic procedures may be indicated. In stable patients, an oral speculum allows visualization of the choanal slit, pharynx, glottis, and tongue. Auscultation in a quiet area with a pediatric stethoscope placed over the pectoral region, back, and trachea may reveal abnormal clicks, wheezes, and fluid sounds as well as cardiac murmurs and arrhythmia. Differences in air flow, harshness of sounds, or lack of air flow may be detected if the nostrils are auscultated.

Because abdominal masses or fluid can compromise the respiratory system by extending into the lung or air sacs or by cranial displacement of viscera, abdominal palpation may suggest a cause of respiratory distress.

Originally published in Volume 8, Number 8, August 1986

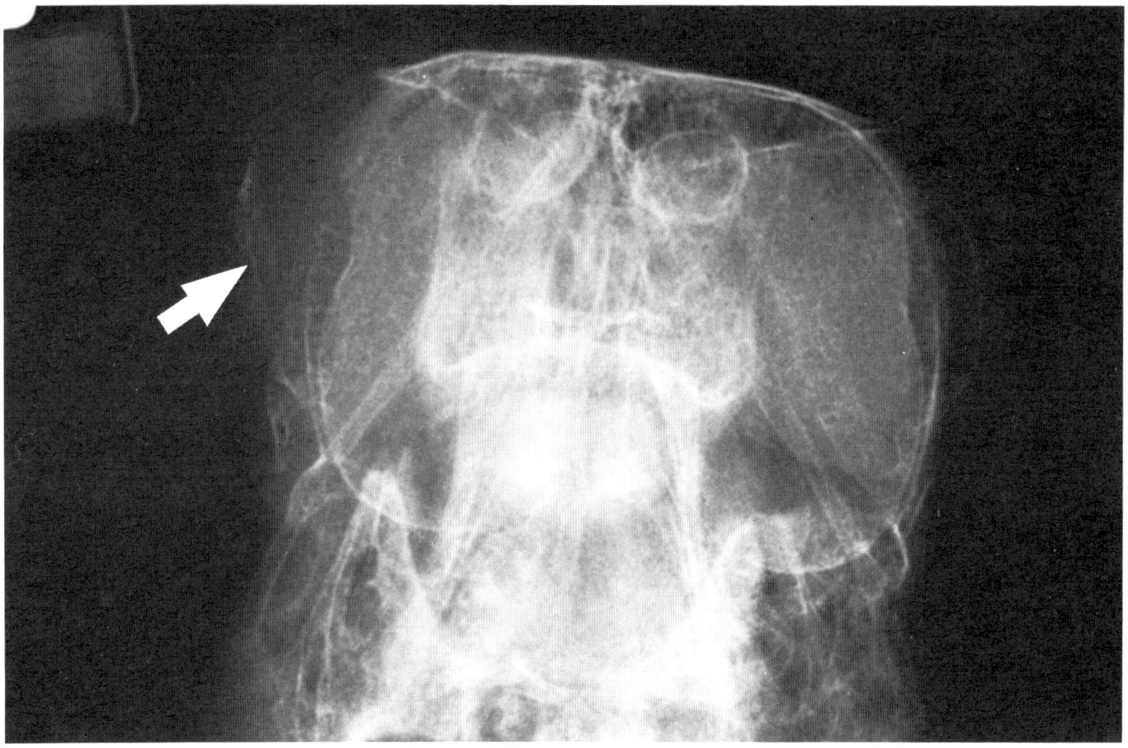

Figure 1—Rostrocaudal view of an Amazon parrot's skull shows a supraorbital abscess displacing scleral ossicle (*arrow*) with no bone erosion.

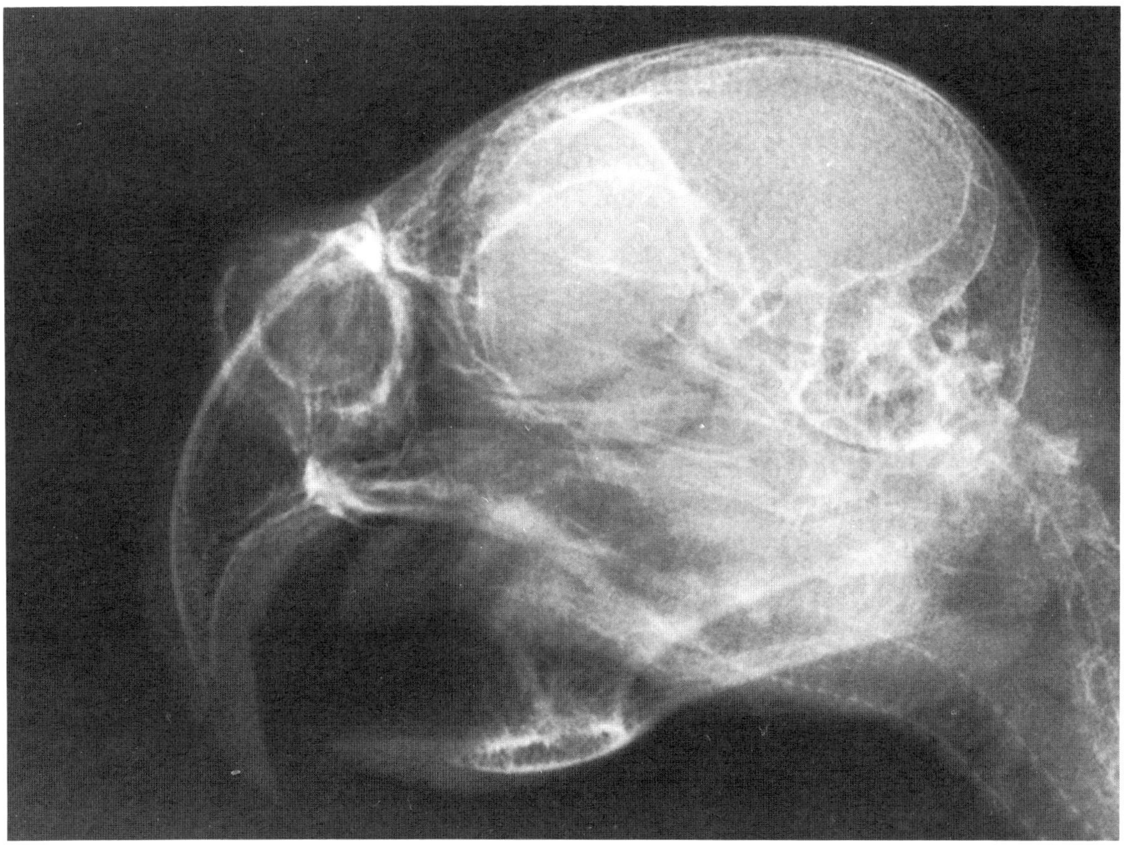

Figure 2—Lateral view of a Senegal parrot's skull demonstrates mineralization within a mass that involved the right nostril. Aspergillosis was diagnosed by biopsy and culture.

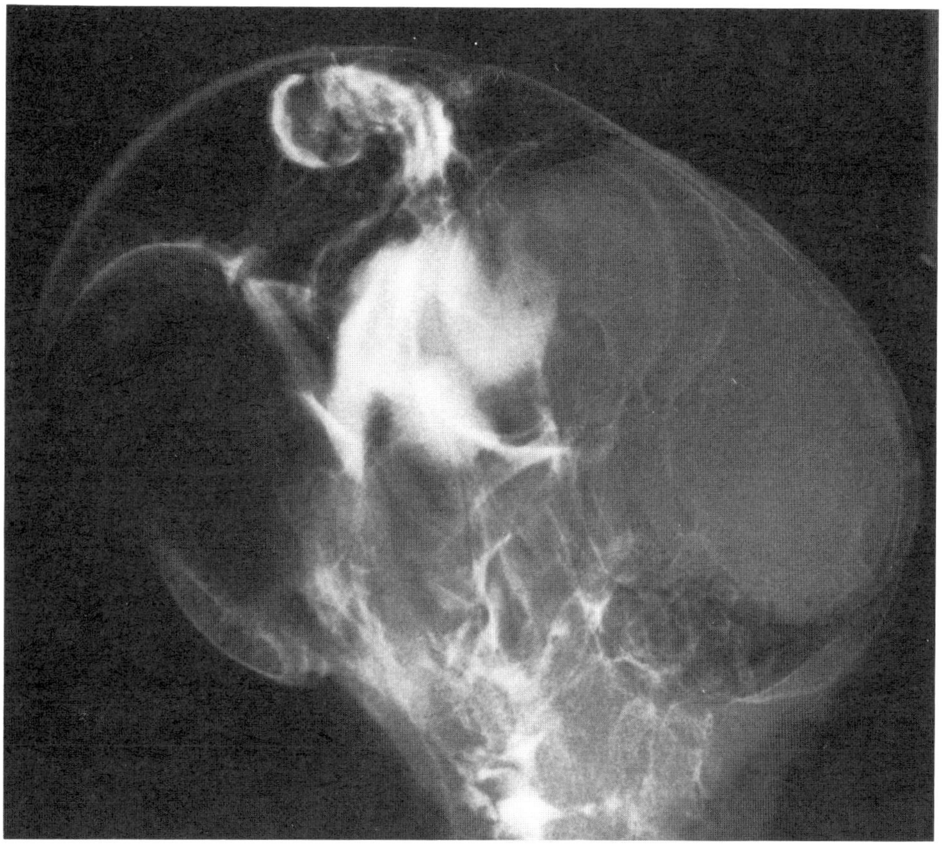

Figure 3A

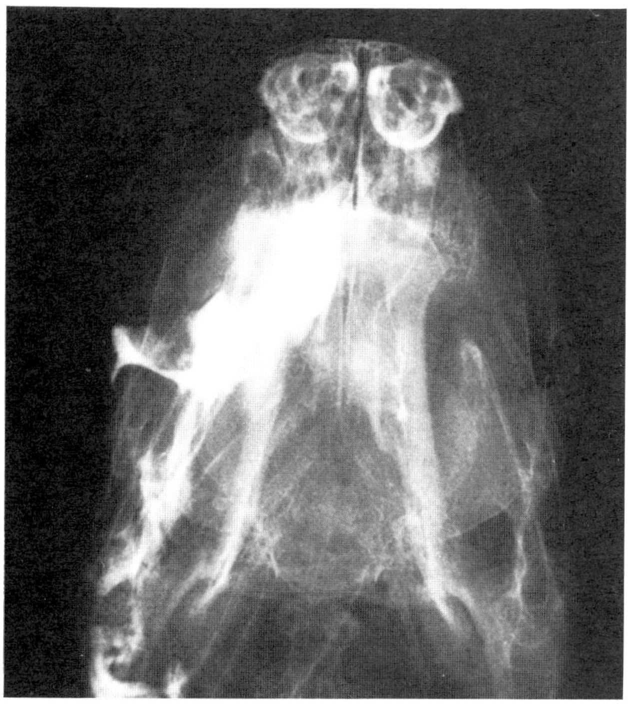

Figure 3B

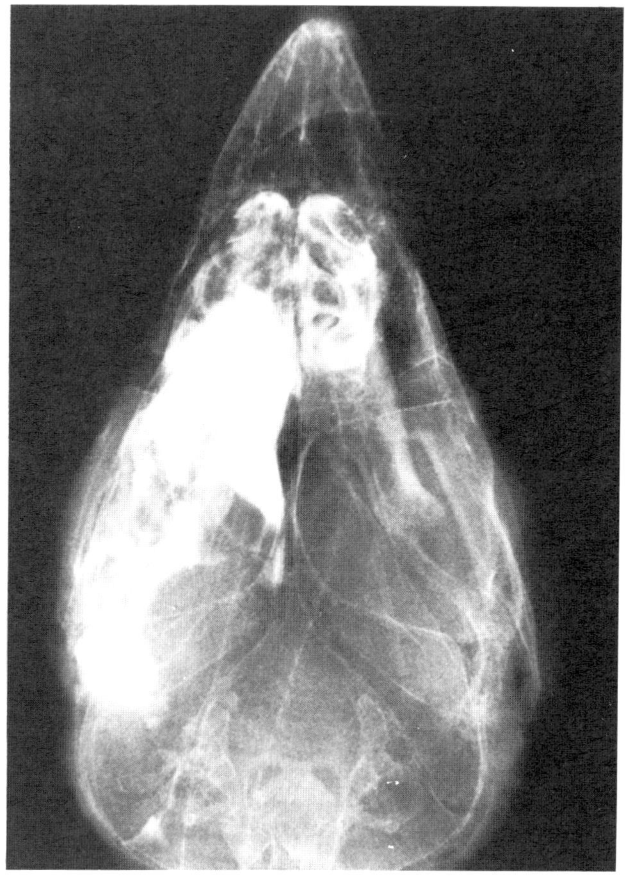

Figure 3C

Figure 3—Positive-contrast sinography of a normal parrot demonstrates the flow of contrast material into the contralateral sinus, nasal cavity, and periorbital and auricular regions. Contrast agent was injected into the right infraorbital sinus. (**A**) Right lateral, (**B**) rostrocaudal, and (**C**) ventrodorsal views.

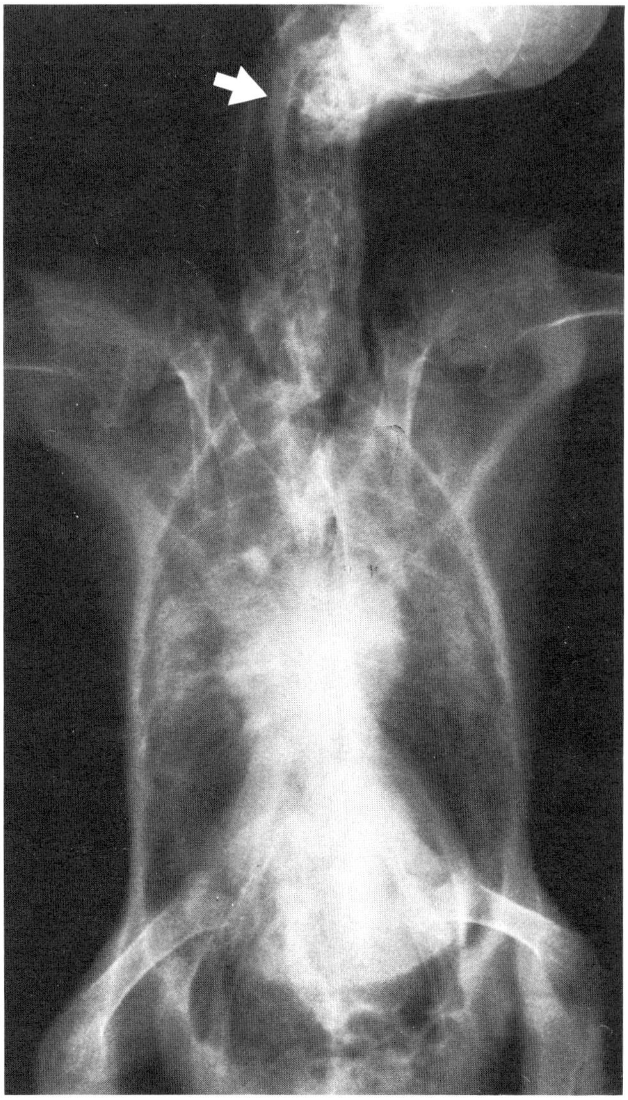

Figure 4—Increased parabronchial pulmonary density is present in the mid portion of both lungs of this parrot. The *arrow* points to a tracheal mass. Aerophagia is apparent. Pneumonia and tracheal abscess were secondary to hypovitaminosis A.

Radiographic Abnormalities

Diseases involving the upper respiratory tract, nasal cavity, infraorbital sinuses, cervicocephalic air sacs, and trachea may show no radiographic abnormalities.

Localized soft tissue densities are often abscesses (Figure 1) and may involve the nasal and oral cavities, periorbital region, or trachea. They are most commonly associated with hypovitaminosis A. Neoplasia is infrequent, but squamous cell carcinoma with bone involvement has been reported.[1] Fibrosarcomas often invade the beak and cause a significant soft tissue mass. Granulomas are the result of chronic rhinitis of bacterial[2] or fungal infection (Figure 2). Parasitic granulomas[3] are infrequent. Localized subcutaneous air pockets and granulomas are reported in association with disease of the cervicocephalic air sac system.[4]

Positive-contrast rhinography and sinography may aid in radiographic evaluation[5] (Figure 3). Studies of normal radiographic patterns in psittacines demonstrate communication between the infraorbital sinus and the nasal cavity, beak, opposite sinus, periorbital region, and tympanic region. This communication helps explain the beak deformities and massive swelling evident around the ocular and aural regions and associated with some of the upper respiratory diseases.

Radiographic changes commonly are caused by lower respiratory tract disorders. These include changes in normal reticular pulmonary pattern, bronchial thickening, abnormal air sac density, subcutaneous emphysema, aerophagia, and discrete masses.

Parabronchial infiltrates cause a blotchy appearance to the usually uniform pulmonary pattern. This change is seen frequently in birds with avian pneumonia along the caudal midlateral aspects of the lungs[6] and is best visualized in ventrodorsal radiographs (Figure 4). Aerodynamics in the

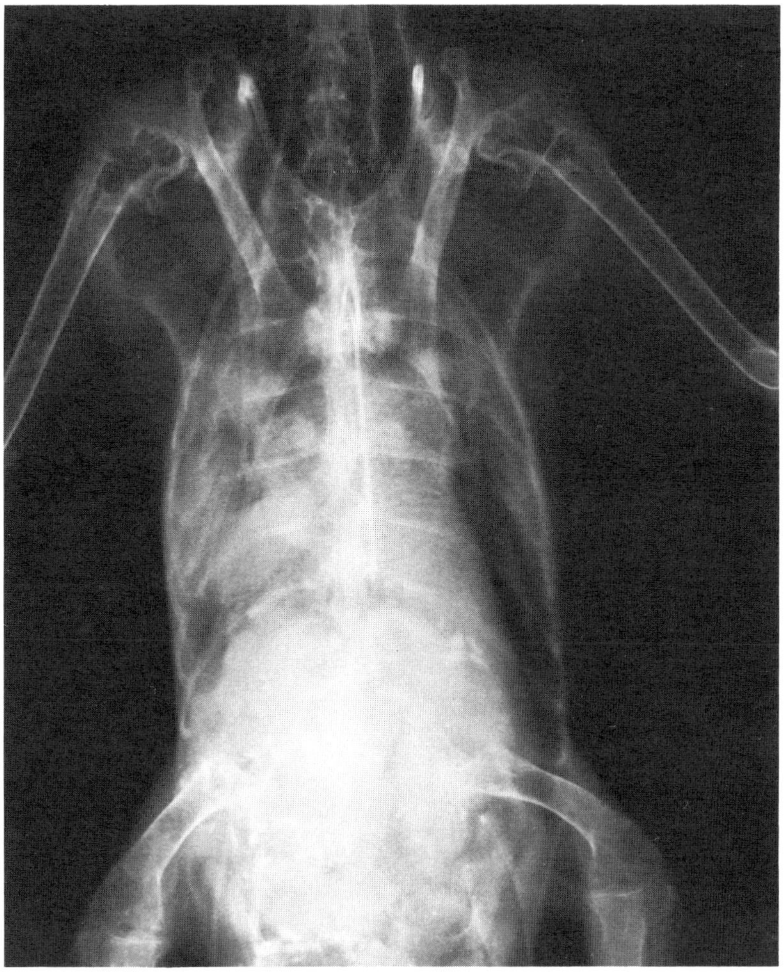

Figure 5—Consolidation present in the right lung of this mynah bird obliterated the normal reticular pattern. The lesion was caused by aspergillosis.

neopulmo contribute to the depositing of pathogens in this region. Focal areas of consolidation obliterate the parabronchial pattern so that, instead of a pronounced parabronchial wall with an air-filled center, the air is replaced by a soft tissue density. Caseous exudate or fluid, such as hemorrhage or edema, also may obliterate the parabronchi. Abscesses, fungal granulomas, or tumors also may cause discrete, well-defined, soft tissue masses that replace the normal pulmonary pattern (Figure 5). In ventrodorsal radiographs, the peripheral portions of the avian lung normally have greater density than the central portions. With the development of the neopulmo, the lateral portion of the lung increases,[7] causing increased soft tissue density. Infiltration around the bronchi results in an ability to visualize parallel walls of the air-filled bronchi. This infiltration occurs within the pulmonary parenchyma and extends into the air sacs (Figure 6).

Air sac disease may cause a barrel-shaped appearance to the avian thorax (Figure 7). Thickened and consolidated air sacs do not change in size as much as normal air sacs do during expiration, thus resulting in relatively fixed dimensions of the chest that mimic full inspiration. The abdominal air sacs become blunted, and lines across the air sacs become apparent. The normal air density becomes a subtle, gray, soft tissue density that may be homogeneous or irregular. Sharply demarcated soft tissue lines and obscured abdominal detail are present in lateral radiographs (Figure 8). Bacterial infections, hypovitaminosis A complicated by bacterial infection, and such fungal diseases as aspergillosis and mucormycosis[8] cause consolidating air sacculitis. Because viral diseases with secondary bacterial involvement play a significant role in pulmonary disease in other species, a similar situation probably exists in birds. Viruses interfere with the bactericidal action of the lung and cause direct cell damage, which may result in bacterial complications between Days 6 and 10 of infection.[9] Chlamydiosis also may cause primary air sacculitis; but it is usually a systemic disease associated with multiple-organ

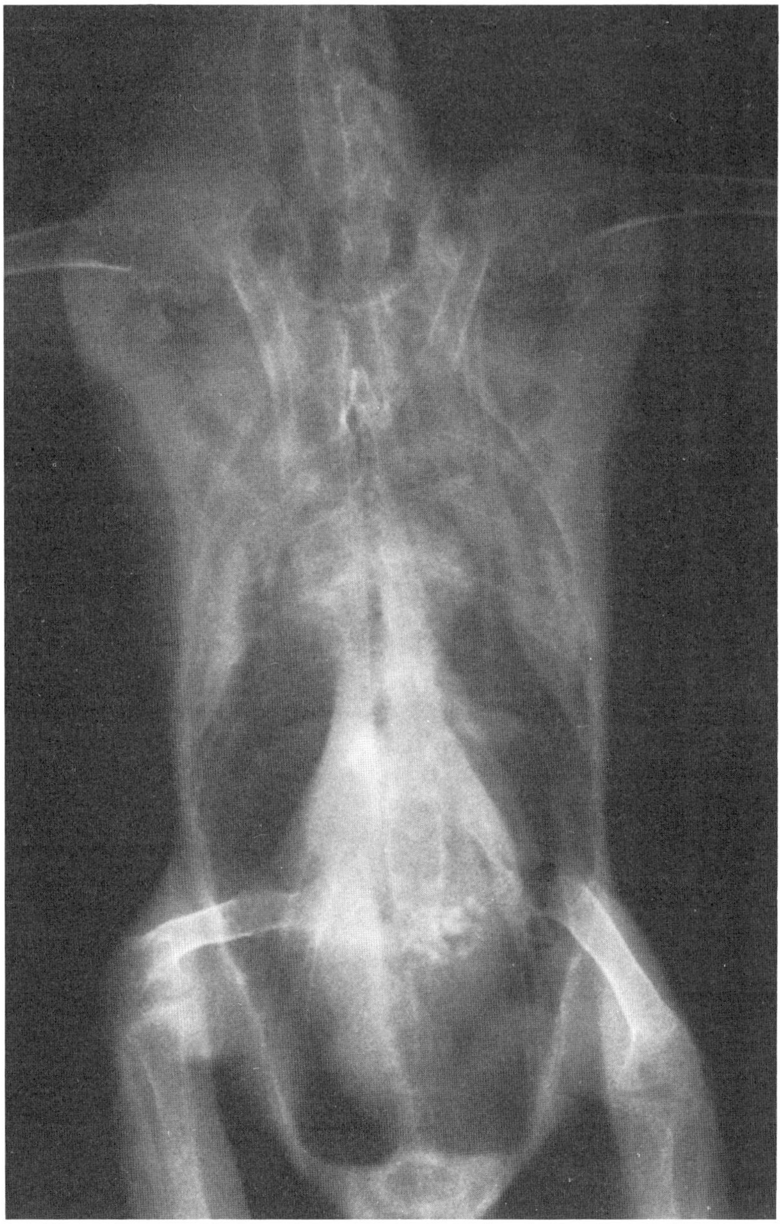

Figure 6—This view shows increased air sac density and blunting of abdominal air sacs, which were caused by air sacculitis. Prominent bronchi from wall thickening extend to clavicular air sacs.

involvement and, often, concurrent gram-negative infection.

Gas is not normally found in the gastrointestinal tract of birds. Radiographically detectable aerophagia often accompanies significant respiratory problems. In such cases, the air is uniformly distributed throughout the intestinal tract with no evidence of distention or localization (Figure 9). Subcutaneous emphysema may occur in association with traumatic air sac rupture.

Pulmonary masses are uncommon. When they do occur, they are usually abscesses or granulomas rather than neoplasms.

Summary

Radiographic changes associated with avian respiratory disorders often are subtle. The ventrodorsal view is most helpful for assessment of lung and air sac lesions. Pneumonia and air sacculitis are the most commonly encountered lower respiratory tract abnormalities. Prominence or obliteration of pulmonary reticular pattern, visualization of intrapulmonary bronchi, increased air sac density, blunted air sacs, and fixed appearance to air sacs are the radiographic changes that may be apparent. Radiographic lesions are uncommon with upper respiratory disease; but localized soft tissue masses, usually abscesses, may be apparent.

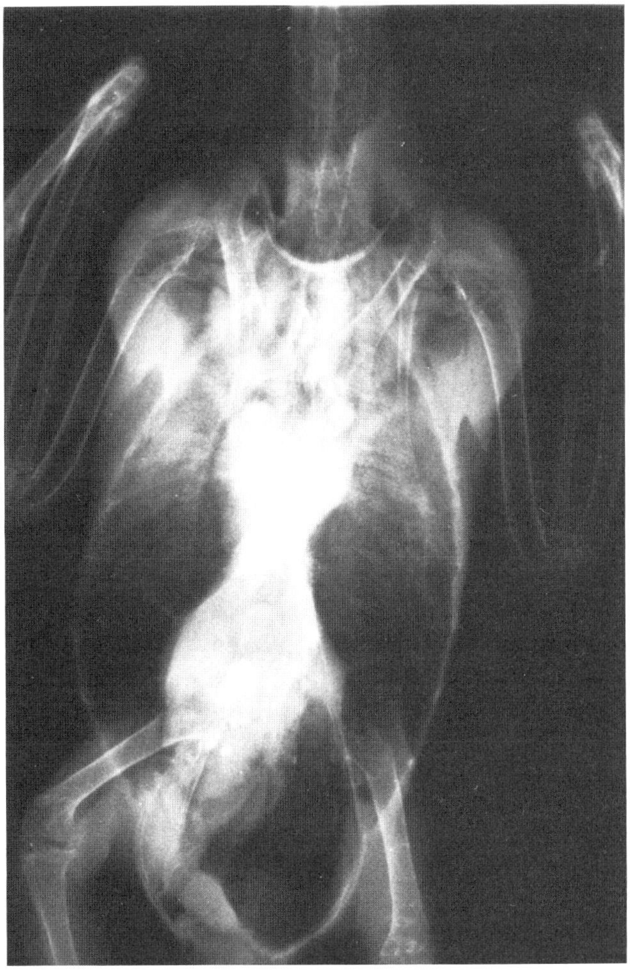

Figure 7—A barrel-shaped appearance, prominent lines across the air sacs, and increased parabronchial pattern indicate air sacculitis and pneumonia.

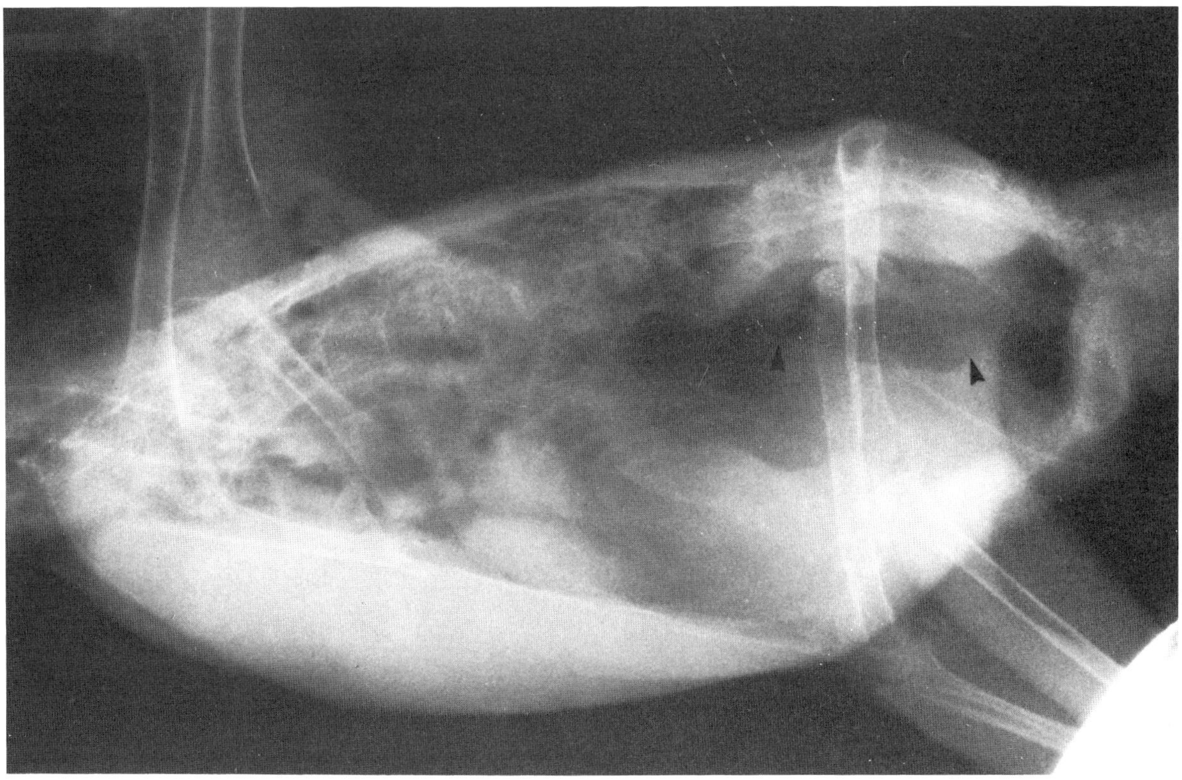

Figure 8—Ventral abdominal detail is obscured by overlying soft tissue density. Soft tissue lines in air sacs are the result of consolidating air sacculitis (*arrows*).

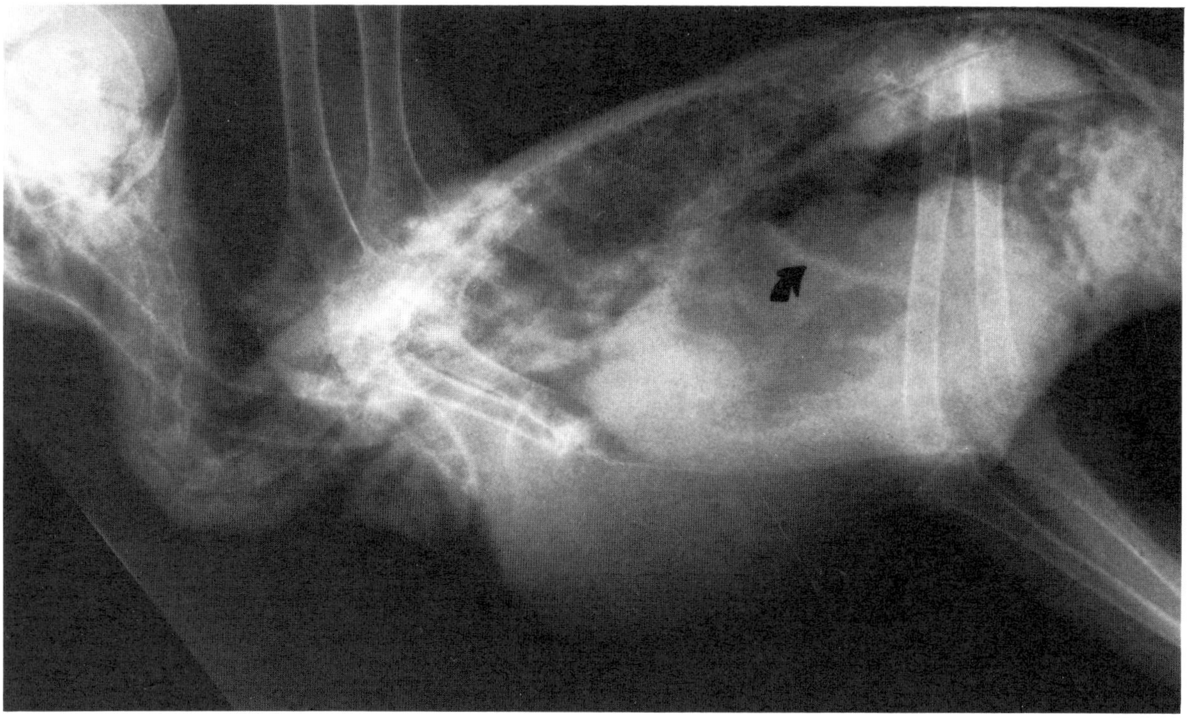

Figure 9—Gas is uniformly distributed throughout the small intestine. Air sac changes are present (*arrow*). Aerophagia is secondary to respiratory distress.

REFERENCES

1. Altman RB: Respiratory diseases of psittacine birds. *Small Anim Vet Med [Update Series]* 10:1-7, 1978.
2. Crane SW, Jacobson E, Shields RP: Cryosurgical removal of an intranasal granuloma from an African gray parrot. *VM SAC* 75(3):499-501, 1980.
3. McMillan MC: Avian radiology, in Petrak ML (ed): *Diseases of Cage and Aviary Birds*. Philadelphia, Lea & Febiger, 1982, pp 329-360.
4. Walsh MT, Mays MC: Clinical manifestations of cervicocephalic air sacs of psittacines. *Compend Contin Educ Pract Vet* 6(9):783-792, 1984.
5. McMillan MC: Unpublished radiographic studies, Angell Memorial Animal Hospital, Boston, MA, 1979.
6. Lowenstine LJ: Avian anatomy and its relation to disease processes. *Proc Annu Meet AAV*:1-9, 1984.
7. Duncker H: Structure of the avian respiratory tract. *Respir Physiol* 22:1-19, 1974.
8. Dawson CO, Wheeldon EB, McNeil PE: Air sac and renal mucormycosis in an African gray parrot (*Psittacus erimacus*). *Avian Dis* 20(3):593-600, 1976.
9. Green GM: Lung defense mechanisms. *Med Clin North Am* 57(3):547-562, 1973.

Avian Gastrointestinal Radiography

Marjorie C. McMillan, DVM
Director of Radiology
Angell Memorial Animal Hospital
Boston, Massachusetts
The Windhover Bird Clinic
Walpole, Massachusetts

Contrast studies of the avian gastrointestinal tract may be necessary for a complete evaluation of gastrointestinal disturbances.

Medical Considerations and Indications for a Gastrointestinal Barium Examination

Since infectious diseases, parasites, toxins, and metabolic disturbances associated with kidney and liver diseases are common causes of gastrointestinal signs in birds, a complete history, thorough physical examination, survey radiographs, and laboratory data are indicated prior to contrast radiography. The primary indications for a gastrointestinal barium examination in birds are acute, chronic, or nonresponsive regurgitation, vomition, or diarrhea; palpation of an abnormal crop or abnormal abdomen; hemorrhagic diarrhea; or abnormal survey radiographic findings such as an obstructive pattern or organ displacement.

When clinically evaluating avian gastrointestinal problems, differentiation between physiologic and pathologic regurgitation and between diarrhea and polyuria is important. Physiologic regurgitation is associated with courtship feeding or affection toward an owner. These birds are healthy, and sexual display often precedes the regurgitation. The regurgitated material contains undigested food and does not have a foul odor. Pathologic regurgitation is not associated with sexual behavior and often has a foul or abnormal odor. These birds regurgitate undigested food or tenacious mucus, often have weight loss, and appear unhealthy.

Polyuria is a more common cause of loose droppings than diarrhea. The fecal portion of the dropping is well formed and surrounded by a clear or opaque, watery urate (Figure 1, A and B). Determination of renal function by uric acid levels and liver involvement by serum aspartate aminotransferase (SAST; SGOT) rather than barium examination is indicated. Change in color of the fecal portion is more common than change in consistency.

Lime green or mustard green feces are associated with hepatic disease and impaired excretion of biliverdin.[1] Brown or hemorrhagic feces usually indicate enteric problems. However, determining whether bloody droppings originate from gastrointestinal or renal problems can be difficult.

Infectious diseases such as psittacosis, colibacillosis, candidiasis, and Pacheco's viral hepatitis are frequent causes of alimentary tract distur-

Originally published in Volume 5, Number 4, April 1983

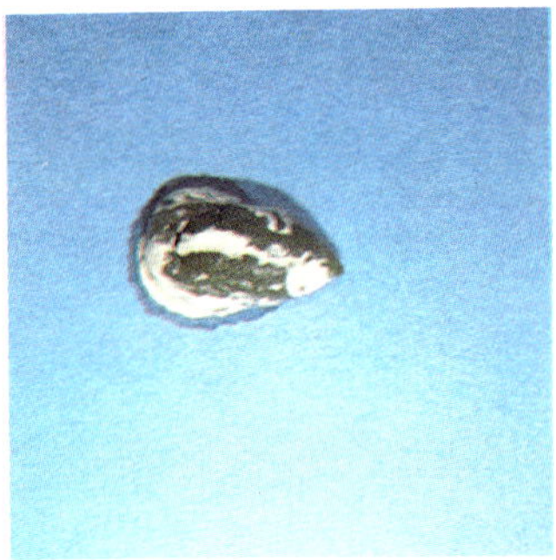

Figure 1A—Normal droppings from an Amazon parrot.

Figure 1A

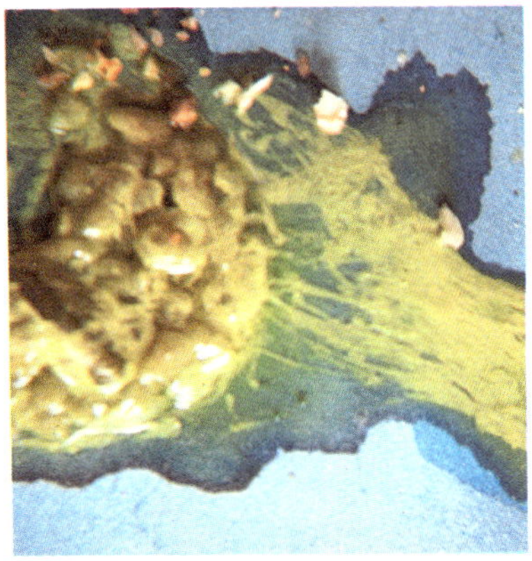

Figure 1B—Lime green droppings associated with abnormal liver and kidney functions.

Figure 1B

bances in newly acquired birds. A crop or cloacal culture helps to identify abnormal bacteria, yeast, and chlamydia. Survey radiographs in these instances show a distended, fluid-filled crop and intestines, hepatomegaly, and enlarged kidneys. Radiographs of an Amazon parrot showing enlarged kidneys and liver secondary to *Escherichia coli* infection are shown in Figure 2.

Ingestion of toxic materials such as heavy metal or plants may produce gastrointestinal signs as well as neurological signs. Lead poisoning due to ingesting paint chips from any source can cause regurgitation, diarrhea, and neurologic signs.[2] Plants, wood, and other foreign material causing local irritation can result in enteritis. Overeating grit, improper hand rearing techniques, or ingesting thread and wool from cage coverings can cause impacted crops.

Gastrointestinal parasites are uncommon in pet birds because many birds are wormed in quarantine stations or aviaries. However, since ascarids, tapeworms, and coccidia are occasionally seen, fecal examination is recommended in birds with gastrointestinal signs. Crop washings in birds with chronic regurgitation can demonstrate parasites as well as fungus and bacteria.

Kidney and liver diseases cause secondary gastrointestinal signs. Infections, neoplasia, and metabolic disorders (lipidosis[3] and hemochromatosis[4]) produce serious impairment of these organs.

Iodine deficiency resulting in thyroid enlargement, which impairs normal crop emptying, is a common cause of regurgitation in the budgerigar as a result of extrinsic crop compression (Figure 3).

Radiographic Technique

Prior to contrast examination, evaluation of survey radiographs for proper radiographic technique, location of the abdominal viscera, presence of gas and fluid, bowel distention, and foreign material is important. The presence of large amounts of gas and/or fluid in the crop often indicates gastrointestinal problems unless respiratory-induced aerophagia is present or the bird is being tube fed. Birds normally do not have gas in the intestinal tract, so that the presence of gas with or without distention is abnormal. Distended fluid-filled intestinal loops indicate gastrointestinal problems except in mynahs and toucans. Because of the high water content in their diet, these birds normally have slightly distended fluid-filled intestinal loops. Any abnormal location of the gastrointestinal tract is noted.

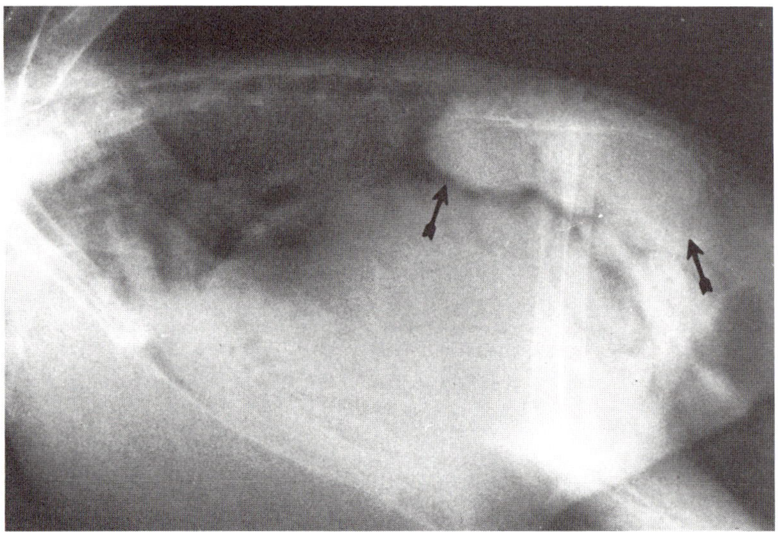

Figure 2A

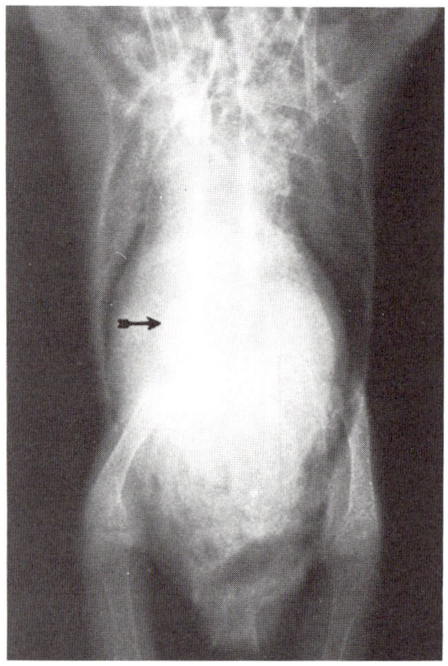

Figure 2B

Figure 2—**(A)** Lateral radiograph of an Amazon parrot showing enlarged kidneys *(arrows)* and liver secondary to *E. coli* infection. **(B)** Ventrodorsal view of the same parrot.

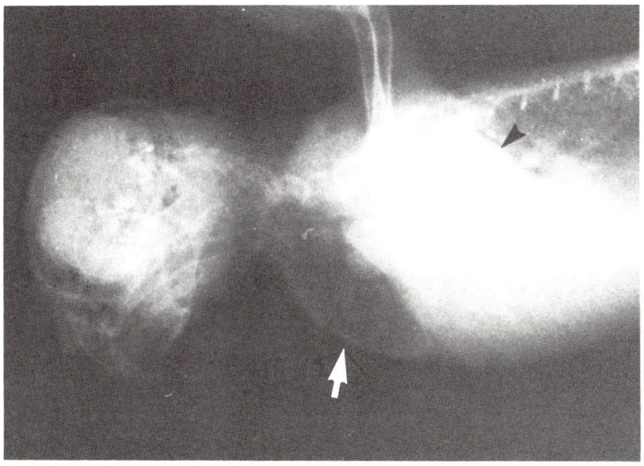

Figure 3—Lateral radiograph of the cranial thoracic area of a budgerigar showing an enlarged thyroid gland *(black arrow)* and distended crop *(white arrow)*. The soft-tissue density visualized at the thoracic inlet extending into the crop may represent an enlarged thyroid or soft tissue displaced anteriorly by a larger caudal thyroid mass.

Displacement may be due to extrinsic masses or organ enlargement. Radiopaque material is normally present in the gizzard if the bird is receiving grit. Proper positioning[5] and at least two views, lateral and ventrodorsal, are necessary for evaluation. Because exposure factors vary with the size of the bird, film-screen combinations, and radiographic equipment, it is difficult to recommend a specific kilovolt peak, milliamperage, and time. For average parrots (weighing 350 to 500 g) a technique comparable to feline radiographic studies is appropriate. Parakeets require 5 to 10 kvp less and canaries and finches need a 15 kvp decrease. Larger parrots (macaws and large cockatoos) require about the same kilovolt peak setting as cats.[6] For par speed film-screen combinations, a tabletop technique at 100 mA for 1/60 second at 40 in. provides diagnostic radiographs.

Currently, a rare-earth ultradetailed film-screen[a] combination provides the most satisfactory avian radiographs. This film-screen combination requires a fivefold increase in the milliampere seconds over the par speed combination. Single-screen mammography packs with single-emulsion film can be substituted for the cassette system.

Tranquilizers and anesthetics are usually not necessary for radiographic procedures. Since the effects of these agents on gastrointestinal motility in birds is not thoroughly known, it is better not to use such agents when evaluating the gastrointestinal tract. A Plexiglas device[b] in combination with sandbags and tape provides adequate restraint and eliminates the need for personnel in the room during an exposure.

Procedure

The barium study is often tailored to the individual bird according to the history and clinical signs. If the

[a]Kodak Lanex fine single or Kodak Ortho M-1, Eastman Kodak Co., Rochester, NY 14650.
[b]B.D. Creations, Lindenhurst, NY 11757.

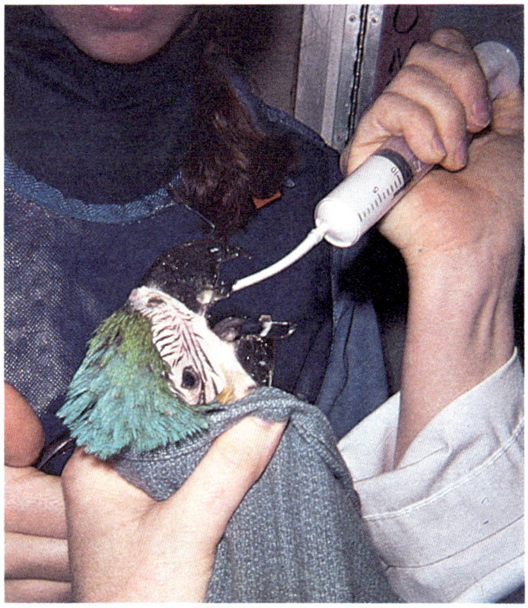

Figure 4—Administration of barium to a blue and gold macaw using a nasal speculum.

crop is the area of concern, a double-contrast examination is indicated. Food and water are withheld for about four hours. Sometimes small amounts of seeds may remain in the crop or proventriculus. If the quantity is small, the study is still undertaken, though it is best to have the gastrointestinal tract empty. Barium sulfate suspension is administered orally into the crop[d] via a stomach tube (Figure 4). The size of the bird determines the volume of barium and whether an oral speculum is necessary (Table I). When the tube is palpated in the crop, a volume of barium is slowly given to gently distend the crop. If a double-contrast study of the crop is performed, half the amount of barium is given and the remainder of the volume is given as air.

Radiographs are made in the ventrodorsal and lateral planes immediately after administration of contrast medium and 30 minutes, 60 minutes, 2 hours, 4 hours, and 24 hours later. Timing of the radiographs may vary

[c]Liquid Polibar 55% W/W, E-Z-M Co., Inc., Westbury, NY 11590.
[d]In birds without crops, such as canaries, finches, and mynahs, the barium is given into the esophagus or proventriculus.

TABLE I

VOLUME OF BARIUM SULFATE IN AVIAN GASTROINTESTINAL RADIOGRAPHY[6]

Bird	*Volume (ml)*	*Tube (French)*	*Type of Speculum*
Canary, finch	0.25–0.5	5	None
Parakeet	1.0–3.0	5	None
Cockatiel, conure, lovebird	3.0–5.0	8	Hemostat
Smaller parrots	10.0	10	Nasal
Larger parrots	15.0	12	Nasal

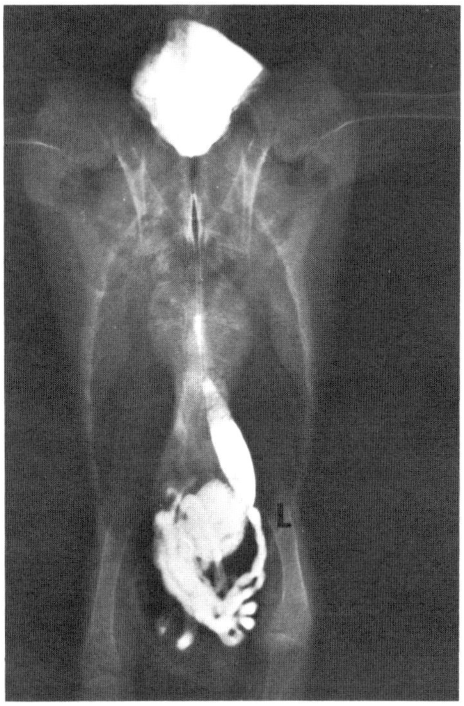

Figure 5A

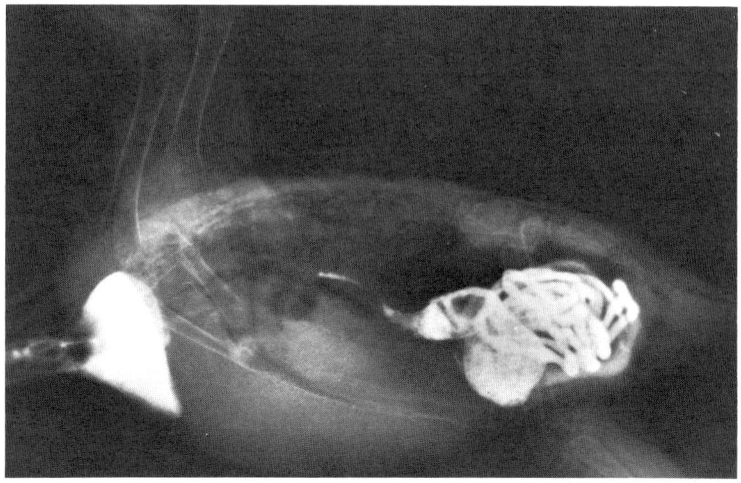

Figure 5B

Figure 5 (**A** and **B**)—A normal barium series. One-hour radiographs show filling of the crop, proventriculus, gizzard, and small intestines with barium. The radiolucent area in the proventriculus is a gas bubble.

depending on whether the upper gastrointestinal tract or lower region is of concern. Results of radiographs during the study may also alter the scheduling.

In normal studies in the immediate radiographs, the crop is filled with barium and a small amount of barium may be present in the esophagus and proventriculus (Figure 5). In 15 to 30 minutes, the proventriculus and gizzard and about half of the small intestines are filled. There is a decrease in the amount of contrast in the crop. By one hour the barium has filled the gastrointestinal tract. In four hours, the crop should be completely empty, although varying amounts of barium may remain in the proventriculus, gizzard, and intestines.

Radiographic Interpretation

Changes in transit time, thickening and/or irregularity of mucosal lining, distention, displacement of the gastrointestinal tract, and filling defects are radiographic signs associated with gastrointestinal disorders. When evaluating the significance of radiographic changes in contrast examinations, persistence of a lesion in subsequent radiographs is important. Motility in a dynamic system such as the gastrointestinal tract causes normal anatomic variation, which when visualized on only one radiograph leads to misinterpretation.

Delay in transit time results from functional or mechanical ileus. Mechanical ileus from extraluminal lesions or intraluminal masses such as foreign bodies is unusual in birds (Figure 6).

Functional ileus associated with severe gram-negative gastroenteritis is a more common cause of delayed transit of barium. Distention of the entire gastrointestinal tract is observed with severe gram-negative infections rather than obstruction (Figure 7). In addition to infection, lead toxicity, parasites, and egg peritonitis are associated with functional ileus. An increase in transit time has not been observed.

Thickening and irregularity of the crop and esophagus (Figure 8) are associated with candidiasis. Mucosal irregularity from neoplasia is difficult to distinguish from gastrointestinal fungal infections (Figures 9 and 10). Pathologic filling defects are unusual but do occur with neoplasia and fungal granuloma (Figure 11). Commonly, residual seed coated with barium is mistaken for filling defects. Thickening of the proventriculus, gizzard, and intestines has not been visualized radiographically.

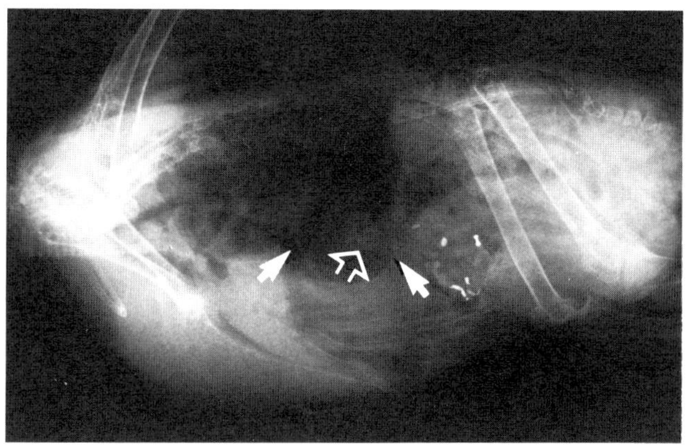

Figure 6—Distention of the proventriculus *(closed arrows)* with gas secondary to obstruction in a greater sulfur crested cockatoo. This parrot had ingested electric wire. If the type of heavy metal cannot be determined through historical information, the possibility of heavy-metal intoxication such as lead poisoning, in addition to obstruction, should also be considered. Foreign material *(open arrow)* is present in the lumen. Metallic foreign material is present in the gizzard.

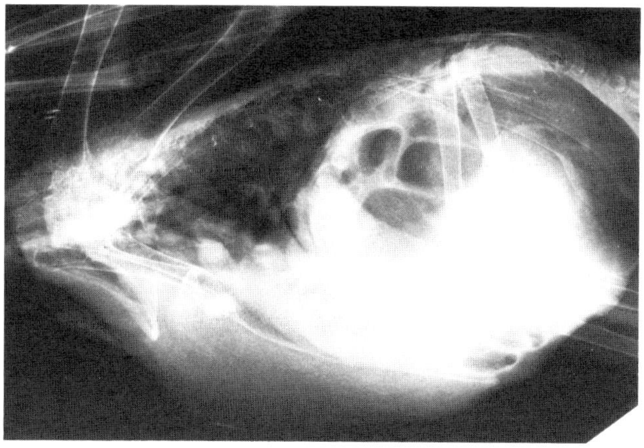

Figure 7A

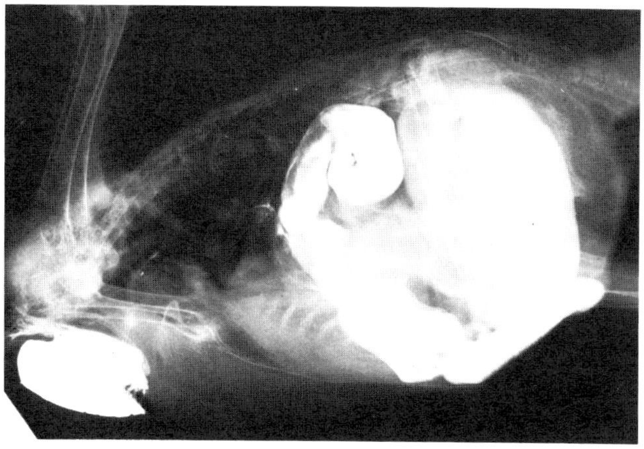

Figure 7B

Figure 7—**(A)** Survey radiographs of a blue and gold macaw showing marked distention of the gastrointestinal tract with gas. **(B)** In the one-hour radiograph, there is displacement of the duodenum and distention of the loops of intestines with barium. On autopsy, there was no evidence of obstruction. Serositis and associated gram-negative infection produced a functional ileus.

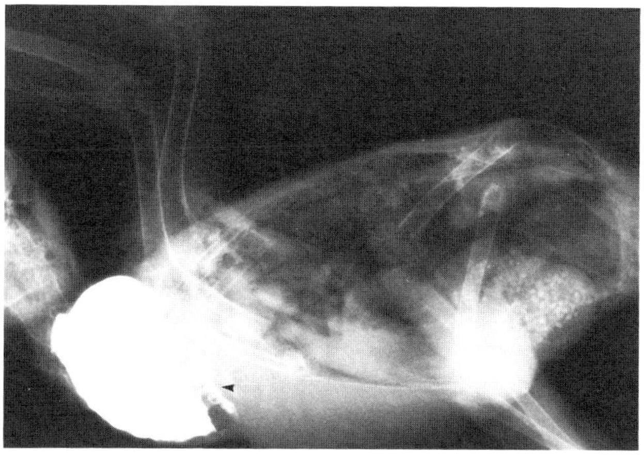

Figure 8A

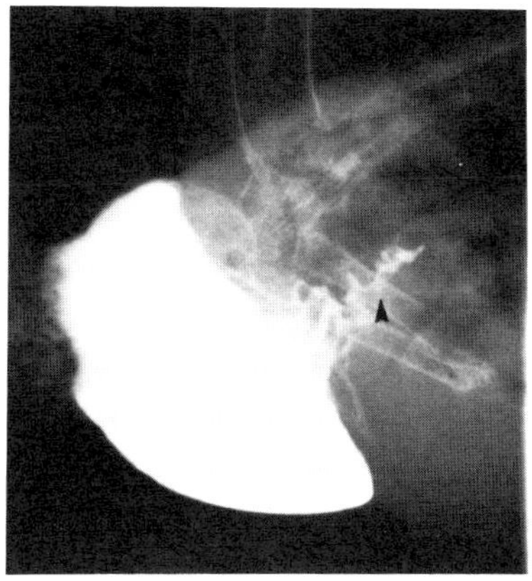

Figure 8B

Figure 8—**(A)** A double-contrast study of the crop showing thickening and irregularity of the crop wall due to candidiasis *(arrow)*. **(B)** Esophageal abnormality in same bird also due to candidiasis *(arrow)*.

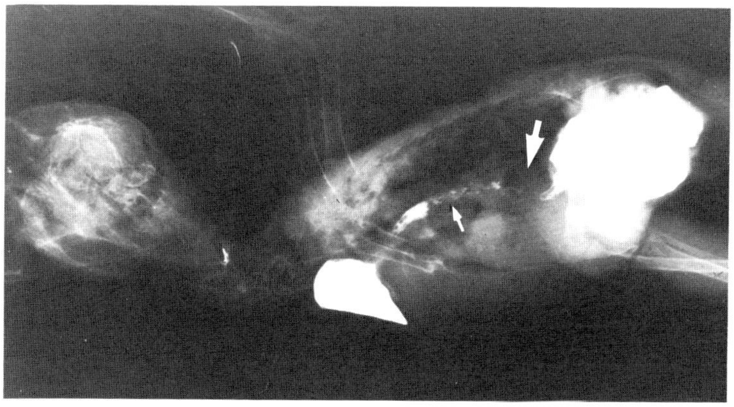

Figure 9—Squamous cell carcinoma causing a nodular mass *(large arrow)* and mucosal irregularity *(small arrow)* in the esophagus and proventriculus of a 47-year-old Amazon parrot.

Localized distention of the crop occurs secondary to enlarged thyroids, lead toxicity, and obstruction in the proventriculus, gizzard, or upper intestines. Distended atonic cloacae can occur secondary to spinal trauma and neoplastic involvement of sacral nerves.

Displacement of the gastrointestinal tract due to extrinsic mass or organ enlargement may be visualized by barium contrast examination. Viewing the direction

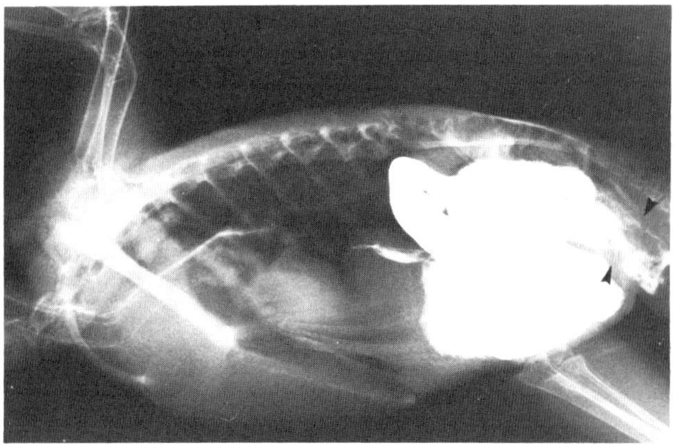

Figure 10—Filling defects and mucosal abnormality *(arrows)* in the rectum of a mynah with an adenocarcinoma.

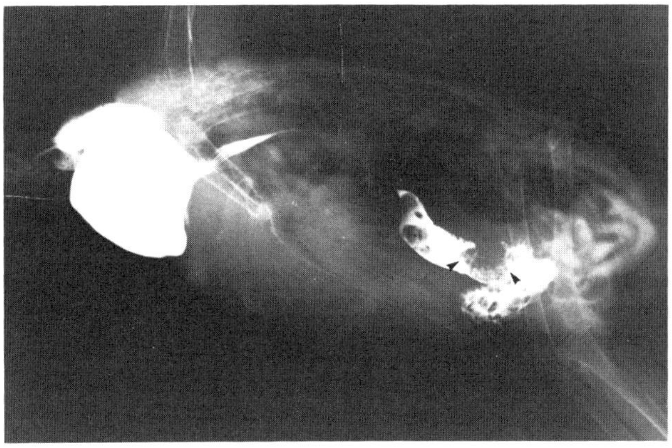

Figure 11—*Aspergillus* granuloma in an Amazon parrot *(arrows)* causing a large filling defect in the proventriculus.

in which the gastrointestinal tract is displaced will aid in determining which organ or organs may be involved (Figure 12).

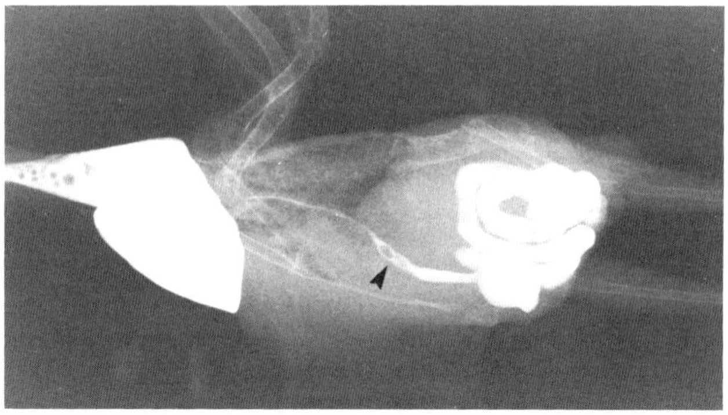

Figure 12—Ventral displacement of the esophagus and proventriculus *(arrow)* in a budgerigar from a renal tumor.

Summary

Barium contrast examination is indicated for thorough evaluation of avian gastrointestinal disturbances. An appropriate diagnostic workup should precede radiographic examination. Findings on survey radiographs suggest that gastrointestinal problems can be pursued with a barium study. In the author's experience, the most common finding on survey radiographs indicating a gastrointestinal abnormality is distention of the gastrointestinal tract with gas and fluid. Obstructive ileus causing this pattern is unusual, and other causes such as infection and toxicity should be considered. Delayed transit time, distention of intestines, and mucosal irregularities are common lesions observed during the barium series.

REFERENCES

1. McDonald SE, Bayer EV: Psittacosis in pet birds. *Calif Vet* 4:6-17, 1981.
2. Woerpel RW, Rosskopf WJ: Heavy-metal intoxication in caged birds. Part 1. *Compend Contin Educ Pract Vet* 4:729-738, 1982.
3. Leav I, et al: A naturally occupying lipidosis in shell parakeets, *Melopsittacus undulatus. Lab Invest* 18(4):433-437, 1968.
4. Lowestine LJ, Petrak ML: Iron pigment in the livers of birds, in Montali RJ, Migaki G (eds): *The Comparative Pathology of Zoo Animals.* Washington, DC, Smithsonian Institute Press, 1980, pp 127-135.
5. Evans SM: Avian radiographic diagnosis. *Compend Contin Educ Pract Vet* 3:660-666, 1981.
6. McMillan MC: Avian radiology, in Petrak ML (ed): *Diseases of Cage and Aviary Birds.* Philadelphia, Lea & Febiger, 1982, pp 329-360.

Recent Advances in Radiation Oncology*

Colorado State University
Susan M. LaRue, DVM, PhD
Edward L. Gillette, DVM, PhD

KEY FACTS

- Owners are seeking aggressive cancer therapy for their pets and expect advanced medical knowledge and technology from the veterinary profession.
- Radiation therapy is indicated if aggressive cancer treatment is appropriate and aggressive surgery may produce a significant functional deficit or cosmetic abnormality.
- If smaller doses per fraction are used, late-responding tissues can be spared relative to tumor and acutely responding tissues.
- More collaboration among surgical, medical, and radiation oncologists will result in more effective use of combined-modality treatment for tumors.

Veterinary radiation therapy began at the turn of the 20th century. In the past decade, more radiation therapy facilities have become available in private practices and facilities in veterinary institutions have improved considerably in response to the greatly increased interest in veterinary oncology. Owners are seeking aggressive cancer therapy for their pets and expect advanced medical knowledge and technology from the veterinary profession.

Recent technologic advances—including megavoltage radiation therapy machines, computerized treatment planning systems, and computed tomography scans—have dramatically influenced radiation oncology in veterinary medicine. Progress in the field of radiation biology also has affected treatment administration. This presentation considers these advances in general as well as their application to specific tumor types.

HISTORICAL PERSPECTIVE

In the 1920s, Henre Coutard, a French radiotherapist, developed what was to become conventional radiation therapy.[1] He evaluated accelerated and protracted irradiation and concluded that daily doses of approximately 2 Gy (gray) given during a six-week interval to a total of 60 Gy would provide tumor control with minimum normal tissue injury. Coutard used orthovoltage radiation, and the primary dose-limiting normal tissue was skin. Although the development of higher-energy therapy machines has reduced the incidence of skin injury, mucositis associated with the treatment of head and neck tumors remains a problem. Currently, late fibrosis and necrosis are dose-limiting responses of concern.

Veterinary radiotherapy techniques diverged from those established by Coutard because of the requirement of anesthesia for veterinary patients and the expense of protracted therapy. Alois Pommer, an Austrian veterinarian, irradiated benign and malignant diseases and established a radiation therapy protocol that was widely used for many years.[2] Today, this protocol would be considered accelerated hypofractionation (i.e., a few large fractions given in a short overall period).

ADVANCES IN RADIOBIOLOGY

Ionizing radiation can kill cells. The goal of radiation therapy is destruc-

*This publication was supported in part by grant 2 PO1-CA-29582 awarded by the National Cancer Institute. The contents of this article are solely the responsibility of the authors and do not necessarily represent the official views of the National Cancer Institute.

Originally published in Volume 15, Number 6, June 1993

tion of the tumor without loss of function of adjacent normal tissue. Research in radiobiology focuses on the achievement of therapeutic gain, that is, increasing tumor control without increasing the probability of damage to normal tissue.

Radiation sensitivity is defined by the loss of reproductive capability caused by ionizing radiation. Proliferating cells are by definition radiation sensitive. These cells include tumors and such renewing cell populations as epithelial cells. The effects of irradiation on normal rapidly proliferating tissue systems occur during or shortly after radiotherapy. These types of tissues are referred to as acutely responding tissues. More slowly dividing or nondividing cells (e.g., cells of the bone and nervous system) are also affected by irradiation, but the changes may take longer to become apparent. These types of tissues are referred to as late-responding tissues.

Changes to early-responding normal tissues occur in almost every patient undergoing irradiation; although the changes may cause discomfort, they rarely limit the dose. The adverse effects associated with irradiation in late-responding tissues can be devastating, however, and such tissues generally limit the dose. As a rule, the radiation delivered is restricted to that dose associated with a less than 5% probability of causing an adverse effect to the late-responding tissues in the region. The dose administered thus is determined not by tumor histology but by the late-responding tissue located in the treatment field. For a given dose of radiation, however, the probability of control for tumors of different histologic types will vary and can be determined. The tumor control probability helps the clinician to ascertain whether radiation is an appropriate treatment alternative.

Mammalian cells have been shown to repair part of the damage caused by radiation. This repair of sublethal damage was demonstrated via evaluation of the survival of mammalian cells in culture after irradiation.[1] A single dose of radiation caused fewer cells to survive than the same quantity of radiation divided into two fractions (if adequate time was allowed between fractions). The repair of sublethal damage during the period between fractions accounts for the improved survival.

Early- and late-responding tissues differ in their responses to irradiation. Although slowly dividing cells are apparently less sensitive to small doses of radiation than are more rapidly dividing cells, the former evidently become relatively more sensitive if radiation is delivered in larger doses per fraction. It has been suggested that because of the differences in the initial portion of survival curves between late- and early-responding tissues, the late-responding tissues might be spared relative to tumor and acutely responding tissues by administering smaller doses per fraction.[1] This phenomenon may occur because mammalian cells respond according to a linear quadratic formalism. The initial (α) portion of the survival curve is linear; this portion represents irreparable damage. The second (β) portion of the curve is continually curving and represents reparable damage (Figure 1).

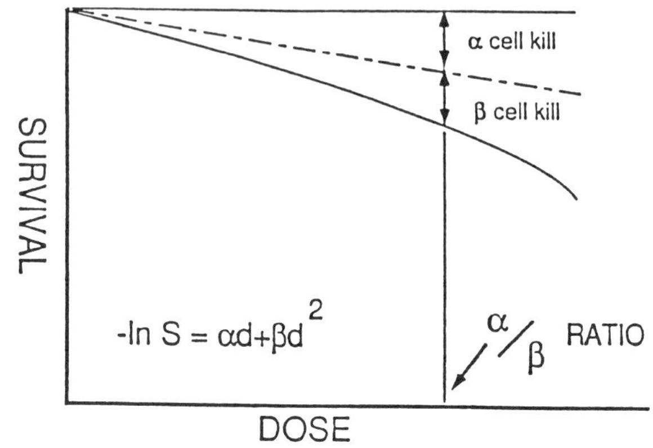

Figure 1—The α–β ratio is the dose at which the number of cells killed by the α component is equal to those killed by the β component. *-ln S* = natural log of surviving fraction, and *d* = dose.

The α–β ratio is the dose of radiation at which cell death from the α portion of the curve is equal to that from the β portion. Such ratios have been calculated from isoeffective doses for various tumors and normal tissues. The α–β ratios for late-responding tissues are generally less than 5 Gy, and those for tumor and early-responding tissues are greater than 5 Gy. In late-responding tissues, the α portion of the curve is presumed to be relatively short and the β portion is more steeply curving than in acutely responding tissues (which have a long α portion and a relatively flat β portion). This principle is increasingly used in veterinary and human medicine to allow higher total doses to be given. Such doses should result in better tumor control.

In the fractionation schedule developed by Pommer, doses of approximately 5 Gy per fraction were given to a maximum total dose of 40 or 44 Gy. The dose for a 50% probability for bone necrosis in dogs with oral carcinomas was determined to be 50 Gy (given in 10 5-Gy fractions). This approach led to an alteration in fractionation method at Colorado State University and other institutions. The alteration was made more feasible by improvements in anesthesiology. Currently, doses of 3.0 to 3.3 Gy per fraction are given in 15 daily fractions. This preserves the accelerated schedule, which is useful because it reduces the amount of time necessary for tumor cell repopulation

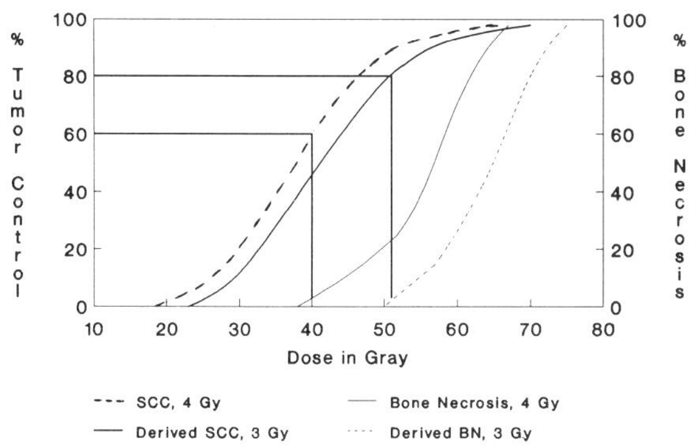

Figure 2—These curves are based on data obtained from irradiation of oral carcinomas. By reducing the fraction size from 4 to 3 Gy (gray), an increase in tumor-control probability from 60% to 80% can be achieved and the probability of bone necrosis remains less than 5%. *SCC* = squamous cell carcinomas, and *BN* = bone necrosis

during treatment and also reduces the expense of hospitalization.

The impact on tumor control and bone necrosis of reducing the dose per fraction from 4 to 3 Gy has been estimated from the linear quadratic formalism using an α–β ratio of 4 Gy for bone necrosis and 10 Gy for tumor control (Figure 2). By reducing fraction size, the total dose can be increased without increasing the probability of late effects. A higher total dose should result in increased tumor control and thus meaningful therapeutic gain.

Some tumors are more radioresponsive than others. This difference is evidently a function of tumor biology that contributes to heterogeneity of response to therapy and is not predominantly caused by a difference in radiosensitivity of tumor cells (although radiosensitivity may vary). Important factors that may contribute to heterogeneity of response include growth fraction, hypoxic fraction, and rate of cell loss.

The four *R*s of radiobiology related to radiation therapy are repair, repopulation, redistribution, and reoxygenation.[1] Acutely responding normal tissues generally repopulate such that normal tissues recover rapidly after or even during radiation therapy. Repopulation of normal tissue may be diminished when radiation therapy is delivered in a very accelerated scheme, as is used in veterinary medicine, exacerbating acute effects. Redistribution is particularly important if the growth fraction of a tumor is low. Proliferating tumor cells progress through the more sensitive portions of the cell cycle, such as mitosis as well as G1 and early S phases.

Some tumor cells may be hypoxic. By killing cells near blood vessels, cells that were distant and hypoxic possibly increase their access to oxygen. They become reoxygenated, progress through the cell cycle, and become more sensitive during the course of radiation therapy.

The processes of the four *R*s occur during radiation therapy. Fractionation of the total dose during a given period takes advantage of the repair and repopulation capabilities of normal tissues as well as reoxygenation and redistribution in the tumor. It is not yet clear how to achieve the greatest advantage from these aspects of tumor response. Smaller doses per fraction clearly spare late-responding normal tissues and allow larger total doses to be given.

An accelerated fractionation scheme reduces the opportunity for tumor cell repopulation. After radiation has begun, it should be completed as quickly as possible without long interruptions. Because the growth fraction may increase during radiation therapy, irradiation should begin early in the week; several doses can be delivered before a weekend or holiday break. For the same reason, it is probably inadvisable to allow a long delay between chemotherapy and radiation therapy used as a combined modality.

Much research is being done to more accurately predict the radioresponsiveness of tumors. Tumors should exhibit a clear dose response. This is not always the case, probably because some tumors (even of the same type, stage, and site) are very responsive to radiation therapy but others are not. If the populations could be sorted, identified, and treated as separate groups, a clear dose response could be demonstrated. Because there are several subpopulations of tumors within a specific tumor type, however, the slope of the dose-response curve resulting from a study of the entire population is less than expected.

TECHNICAL ADVANCES

Although some veterinary radiation oncology centers continue to use orthovoltage machines, megavoltage radiation (which is used almost exclusively at human centers) is becoming more accessible. Megavoltage radiation for therapy can be obtained from a linear accelerator or, more commonly, from a cobalt machine. Because megavoltage radiation has excellent penetrating capability, radiation therapy can be performed on deep-seated tumors in which orthovoltage therapy would be unsuitable.

Orthovoltage machines produce x-rays with an energy range of 150 to 400 kVp. This low-energy radiation distributes the maximum doses to the skin surface. Acute effects to the skin can be severe and cause discomfort to the patient, and late effects to the skin and subcutaneous tissue can limit the dose. Megavoltage radiation has higher energy than orthovoltage, and the photons must interact with tissue to allow the dose to build before the maximum dose can

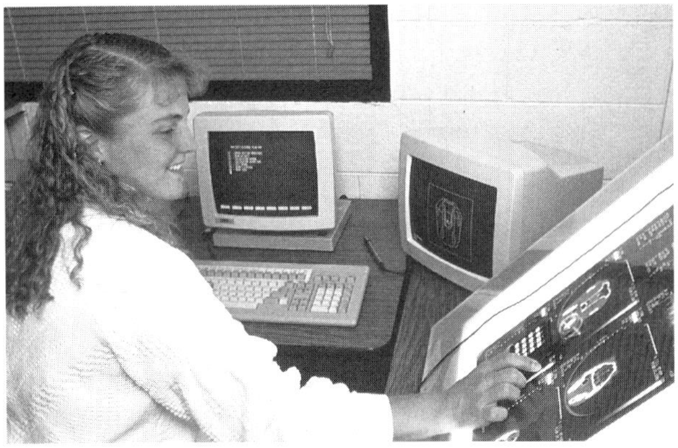

Figure 3—The dosimetrist takes information from the computed tomography scan to produce a computer-generated treatment plan. (Courtesy of William A. Cotton, Publications and Creative Services, Colorado State University)

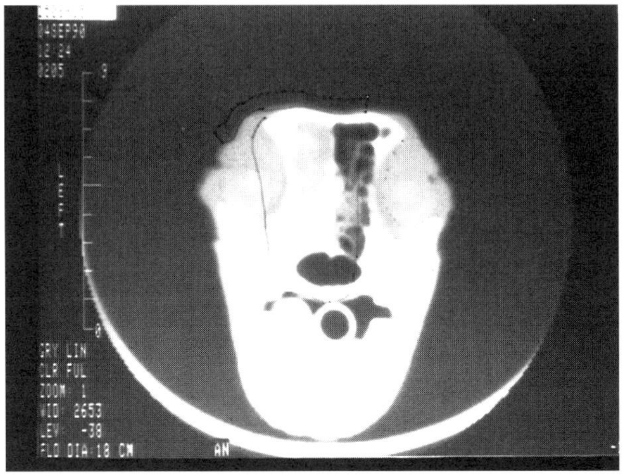

Figure 4—Computed tomography image of a nasal tumor. The radiation oncologist has circled the region that should receive the minimum tumor dose.

be delivered. The skin thus can receive a significantly smaller dose than the underlying tumor. This skin-sparing effect allows the optimum dose to be administered to the more deep-seated tumor without causing adverse reactions in the skin. When a tumor involves the skin, megavoltage radiation can be successful if a sheet of tissue-equivalent material (termed a *bolus*) is placed over the tumor. This allows dose buildup to occur before the skin is reached; the skin and associated tumor can receive the maximum dose.

The absorption of megavoltage radiation, unlike that of orthovoltage radiation, depends minimally on the density of the tissue. This permits an even distribution of radiation throughout the tissue in the field. Orthovoltage radiation is preferentially absorbed by bone. If a tumor adjacent to or overlying bone receives a significant dose of orthovoltage radiation, there is a high probability that late effects will develop in the bone.

The interaction of megavoltage radiation with tissue is predictable. This predictability has allowed the development of computerized treatment planning systems (Figures 3 and 4). These systems permit treatment of the tumor with multiple beams administered from various angles. Beam modifiers, such as wedges, can be incorporated into the treatment plan. Wedges are triangular pieces of lead placed in between the beam and patient. Less radiation penetrates the thick side of the wedge; the isodose distribution is thus modified (Figure 5).

The goals of computerized treatment planning are to ensure a desired minimum dose to a tumor in a region specified by the radiation oncologist and to spare normal tissue structures if possible. The use of treatment planning systems in veterinary medicine may lead to improved tumor control.[3]

The availability of computed tomography scans has affected radiation oncology by providing better data on the extent of disease. Images from computed tomography scans can be used by the treatment planning system to help formulate the optimum plan. Computed tomography data have improved treatment quality in general and have revolutionized the treatment of brain tumors in animals by confirming and locating masses that can then be treated.

Advances in veterinary anesthesia have permitted the implementation of improved fractionation regimens. Isoflurane and propofol in particular have allowed frequent administration of anesthesia with minimal risk to the patient. The use of ventilators makes maintenance of anesthesia safer in animals with brain tumors.

INDICATIONS FOR RADIATION THERAPY

Radiation therapy is indicated if aggressive cancer treatment is appropriate and aggressive surgery may produce significant functional deficit or cosmetic abnormality. Regional disease can frequently be treated effectively with radiation therapy. Such therapy can be used as an adjunct to surgery or chemotherapy. In veterinary medicine, radiotherapy is most often used alone or to treat residual disease after surgery.

Oral Tumors

Radiation therapy is beneficial in many oral tumors. The region is anatomically complex, and aggressive surgery often leaves functional and cosmetic abnormalities. In addition, many oral tumors are known to be responsive to radiation.

Acanthomatous epulides (previously referred to as adamantinomas) are very responsive to radiation. Tumor control with radiotherapy approaches 90%.[4] If a tumor is inoperable, radiotherapy is the preferred treatment. If the tumor is believed to be operable, the

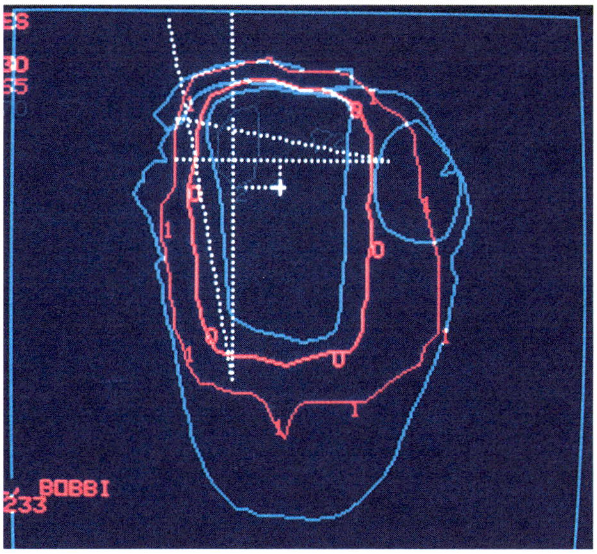

Figure 5—Computer-generated treatment plan for the tumor pictured in Figure 4. Beam-attenuating wedges were used to obtain desirable isodose distribution. Note sparing to the contralateral eye.

functional and cosmetic outcome of surgery versus radiation therapy must be considered.

Oral squamous cell carcinomas (SCC) in dogs have been studied extensively. Coarsely fractionated (10 to 11 fractions of four Gy each) radiation offers tumor control of approximately 65% at one year.[2] The use of more radiobiologically sound fractionation schedules should result in better tumor control (Figure 2). The prognosis depends on the site; rostral tumors have a better probability of being controlled.[5] Tumors of the base of the tongue and tonsils are highly metastatic and likely to recur locally or regionally. In such cases, radiation therapy has the advantage of including associated lymphatic structures in the treatment field.

Oral fibrosarcomas are unlikely to metastasize but can be difficult to control locally. The histologic appearance can be deceptive; tumors diagnosed as fibromas or low-grade fibrosarcomas can be extremely malignant in biologic behavior. The tumor should be treated aggressively if there is clinical evidence of rapid growth, invasion into bone, or tumor recurrence. En bloc surgical resection is curative but difficult because of the ubiquitous nature of the tumor. Although oral fibrosarcomas are less radioresponsive than epulides and squamous cell carcinomas, a 50% tumor control probability at one year has been reported.[6]

Conservative surgical resection of oral fibrosarcomas followed by radiotherapy is currently believed to offer the best probability of tumor control. Surgical cytoreduction improves the probability of tumor control via radiotherapy by reducing the number of clonogenic cells. The decision to follow surgery with irradiation should be made before the operation. The surgeon can then focus on removing macroscopic disease and obtaining a tension-free closure. The surgery can be less aggressive and disfiguring if microscopic disease is to be managed via radiation.

The optimum time after surgery to begin irradiation has not been determined. If difficulty in obtaining primary wound healing is possible, radiation can be delayed. Any therapeutic gain obtained from combining modalities will be lost if the tumor recurs in the interim, however. Initiating radiation therapy in the days immediately after surgery is not a problem if the suture line is free of tension. In tumors that are too large to be surgically resected to the level of microscopic disease, radiation therapy alone is indicated.

Cats with oral squamous cell carcinomas have a very poor prognosis.[7] A treatment regimen at Colorado State University improved median survival time to six months in seven cats by combining mitoxantrone with an aggressive radiotherapy protocol. A shrinking-field technique was used to deliver a total dose of nearly 60 Gy to the tumor volume. The probability of late effects caused by radiation was predictably high, but the improvement in local tumor control was encouraging. Further sparing of normal tissue by administration of the same total dose in smaller fractions may be worthwhile in such tumors.

Nasal Tumors

Nasal tumors in dogs are difficult to control locally, and surgery alone does not improve survival compared with no therapy. Radiation therapy, with or without surgery, is indicated in such tumors. Surgical cytoreduction followed by orthovoltage radiation offers the best prognosis (median survival is 16 to 23 months).[8] Megavoltage radiotherapy provides a median survival time of nearly one year.[3] Such therapy can be administered with or without prior surgery; surgery apparently does not enhance survival.[3] The role of chemotherapy in this tumor type is unclear, but some trials indicate that chemotherapy should not be administered during the course of radiotherapy.[9]

Cats with nasal tumors have a good prognosis if treated with radiotherapy.[10] Tumors of the nasal planum can be treated with such therapy.[11] When squamous cell carcinomas of the planum are excised surgically, the margins should be checked for tumor infiltration. If the margins are infiltrated, radiation therapy is indicated.

Brain Tumors

Brain tumors can be treated successfully with radiotherapy. Preliminary data analysis of 65 cases at

Colorado State University indicated a median survival time of 13.5 months for patients with brain tumors treated with radiotherapy (with or without surgery). Meningiomas and hypophysial macroadenomas were most responsive to radiotherapy, but survival was enhanced in dogs with gliomas, granulomatous meningoencephalitis, and metastatic brain tumors.

Surgery for brain tumors is clearly indicated if necessary to relieve life-threatening clinical signs. In dogs with meningiomas, surgery alone is unlikely to result in tumor control and adjuvant radiation therapy must be performed. Radiotherapy alone should be performed in dogs with surgically inaccessible meningiomas. It is currently not clear whether surgery in addition to irradiation enhances survival in dogs with meningiomas. The decision to proceed with surgery should be weighed against the potential morbidity and mortality. Meningiomas in cats (unlike dogs) can often be controlled by surgery alone. Surgical margins should be closely evaluated for tumor infiltration. If residual tumor is suspected, radiotherapy should be recommended.

Radiation alone is advocated for dogs and cats with hypophysial macroadenomas. These tumors are generally responsive to radiation, and surgical access is limited. Therapy for signs of Cushing's disease may need to be continued after radiation.

Data for other types of brain tumors are limited. Current recommendations include radiation therapy alone for inoperable tumors or after surgery if tumors are operable. In surgically accessible tumors, the morbidity associated with surgery should be weighed against the potential therapeutic gain of reducing the tumor volume.

Brain tissue is extremely sensitive to late effects of irradiation. Early delayed effects can occur from two weeks to three months after treatment and may be related to transient demyelination. Animals with early delayed effects may present with signs similar to those of the initial presentation or may be generally stuporous. The signs are often transient and respond to systemic cortisone.

Late delayed effects usually occur at least six months after treatment but can occur years later. Such effects are associated with brain necrosis. Clinical signs are like those associated with early delayed effects, but response to steroids is limited. It is often difficult to distinguish clinically between late effects and tumor recurrence.

To reduce the probability of late effects to less than 5%, the total dose should be limited to 48 Gy (or less) given in 3-Gy fractions. If surgical biopsy or excision was performed first, the dose should be limited to 45 Gy in 3-Gy fractions.

Tumors of the Body and Extremities

Many tumors that involve the body or extremities are amenable to treatment by radiotherapy. Although small tumors usually respond best, surgical excision is generally the preferred treatment in small skin tumors. Hemangiopericytomas, fibrosarcomas, and neurofibromas are classified together as soft tissue sarcomas because of similar biological behavior. Metastasis is unlikely, but local tumor control can be difficult. These tumors are locally invasive, and tumor cells may extend far beyond the bulk of the tumor. Radiation therapy can be successfully combined with surgery to gain local tumor control without amputation. Radiotherapy can be administered first to make an inoperable tumor operable.

Surgical excision of soft tissue sarcomas of the extremities can be performed first as a cytoreductive procedure, followed by radiation therapy to kill the remaining microscopic disease. Surgery alone can be curative if the tumor can be completely removed. If en bloc surgical resection is attempted, the margins should be scrutinized by a histopathologist for evidence of tumor infiltration. If tumor cells extend to the margin, radiotherapy should be recommended. The likelihood of success is much greater if the tumor is irradiated while microscopic. Soft tissue sarcomas can be treated with radiation therapy alone, but tumor control at one year is less than 50%.[6] Combining radiotherapy with surgery should provide excellent tumor control and cosmetic results.

Cutaneous mast cell tumors (grades 2.5 or less) can be successfully treated with radiotherapy. The obvious advantage is that greater margins can be obtained with radiation than with surgery. The probability of control may be improved if surgical cytoreduction is performed first.

Other Tumors

Radiation therapy is used for various tumors of the colon and urinary tract. Such therapy can follow surgery to help control microscopic tumor spread. This approach allows more conservative surgery and maintenance of better postsurgical function. There is scant information on the response of urinary tract and colon cancers to external-beam radiotherapy; based on data from human patients, the surgery and irradiation may be worthwhile.

CONCLUSION

Megavoltage radiation therapy equipment, computerized treatment planning, and computed tomography units are now available at many veterinary centers. This equipment permits far better tumor definition and dose delivery than was possible in the past. The current challenge is to use radiobiologic and tumor biology information to make the best use of radiation therapy. More effective use of combined-modality treatment for tumors should result from increased collaboration among surgical, medical, and radiation oncologists.

About the Authors

Drs. LaRue and Gillette are affiliated with the Department of Radiological Health Sciences, College of Veterinary Medicine and Biomedical Sciences, Colorado State University, Fort Collins, Colorado. Dr. LaRue is a Diplomate of the American College of Veterinary Surgeons.

REFERENCES

1. Thames HD, Hendry JH: *Fractionation in Radiotherapy.* New York, Taylor and Francis, 1987, p 297.
2. Gillette EL: Principles of radiation therapy, in Theilen GH, Madewell BR (eds): *Veterinary Cancer Medicine*, ed 2. Philadelphia, Lea & Febiger, 1987, pp 137–143.
3. McEntee MC, Page RL, Heidner GL, et al: A retrospective study of 27 dogs with intranasal neoplasms treated with cobalt radiation. *Vet Radiol* 32:135–139, 1991.
4. Thrall DE: Orthovoltage radiotherapy of acanthomatous epulides in 39 dogs. *JAVMA* 184:826–829, 1984.
5. Evans SM, Shofer F: Canine oral nontonsillar squamous cell carcinomas: Prognostic factors for recurrence and survival following orthovoltage radiation therapy. *Vet Radiol* 29: 133–137, 1988.
6. McChesney SL, Withrow SJ, Gillette EL, et al: Radiotherapy of soft tissue sarcomas in dogs. *JAVMA* 194:60–63, 1989.
7. Withrow SJ, MacEwen EG: *Clinical Veterinary Oncology.* Philadelphia, JB Lippincott Co, 1989, p 183.
8. Thrall DE, Harvey CE: Radiotherapy of malignant nasal tumors in 21 dogs. *JAVMA* 183:663–666, 1983.
9. LaRue SM, Gillette EL, Ogilvie G, et al: Irradiation plus mitoxantrone for treatment of canine nasal tumors. *Proc Annu Meet ACVR*:38, 1990.
10. Straw RC, Withrow SJ, Gillette EL, McChesney AE: Use of radiotherapy for the treatment of intranasal tumors in cats: Six cases (1980–1985). *JAVMA* 189:927–929, 1986.
11. Cox NR, Brawner WR, Powers RD, Wright JC: Tumors of the nose and paranasal sinuses in cats: 32 cases with comparison to a national database (1977 through 1987). *JAAHA* 27:339–347, 1991.

Veterinary Radiation Therapy

University of Wisconsin-Madison
W. M. Adams, DVM

KEY FACTS

- **Radiotherapy should be considered in the treatment of any solid tumor not known to be systemic.**
- **The rationale for combining radiation and surgery is based on two facts: radiation alone does not control large tumors, and surgery often fails to control local tumors.**
- **As with chemotherapy, the success of radiation therapy is limited by the toxic side effects that necessarily accompany it.**

Radiation therapy has been available at some veterinary institutions for more than 20 years.[1–4] Today at least 26 centers in North America offer veterinary radiation therapy (Table I). This presentation gives a brief overview of radiation therapy and provides a quick reference table of radiation therapy response by tumor type (Table II). The Supplement beginning on page 230 lists some reported results of radiation treatment for cancer in dogs and cats by tumor type.

CONCEPT

Ionizing radiation from gamma rays or x-rays is toxic to living tissue. Use of radiation in the control of cancer is based on the knowledge that many tumors are more sensitive than surrounding normal tissue to the toxic effects of radiation. Some histologic tumor types generally fall into this category, whereas other types are known to be radioresistant.

MAXIMS

- The histologic tumor type is only a rough predictor of response to therapy. Predicting the clinical response of an individual tumor to radiotherapy is strictly an educated guess (i.e., a tumor of a radioresistant histologic type may in fact be radiocurable).[5]
- For most tumors, there is a narrow safety margin between a curative radiation dose and a radiation dose that causes unacceptable side effects to normal tissue (i.e., if no normal tissue injury is observed following radiotherapy, a curative radiation dose probably has *not* been delivered to the tumor).
- Radiation toxicity is both repairable and cumulative (i.e., normal tissue can repair a certain amount of radiation injury within a given time frame; the longer the time frame of total dose delivery, the higher the tolerable dose).
- Response to radiotherapy depends on four interrelated factors: rate of radiation delivery, total dose of radiation given, tumor type and location, and unique biologic relationship between the host and its neoplasm.
- Radiosensitivity varies markedly between normal tissue types (e.g., bone marrow is very radiosensitive, while tendons are very radioresistant).

WHEN TO CONSIDER RADIOTHERAPY?

Radiotherapy with curative intent should be considered in the treatment of any solid tumor that is not known to be systemic. This excludes tumors

Originally published in Volume 13, Number 2, February 1991

TABLE I

Some U.S. and Canadian Veterinary Centers That Offer Radiotherapy Services

Centers (by region)	*Contact Person and Phone Number*	*Type of Radiotherapy Available*
NORTHEAST		
New England Veterinary Medical Center Grafton, MA	Dr. Larry Kleine 617-769-9574	Orthovoltage
The Animal Medical Center New York City	Dr. Neal Mauldin 212-838-8100	Cobalt
University of Pennsylvania Philadelphia, PA	Dr. Sydney Evans 215-898-3303	Orthovoltage
Ontario Veterinary College Guelph, Canada	Dr. Paul Pennock 519-824-4120	Cobalt
Henry Ford Hospital Detroit, MI	Dr. Elsa Beck 313-876-2590	Cobalt
The Ohio State University Columbus, OH	Dr. Wendy Myer 614-292-1040	Cobalt, orthovoltage
Michigan State University East Lansing, MI	Dr. U. V. Mostosky 517-355-2163	Orthovoltage
Purdue University West Lafayette, IN	Dr. William Blevins 317-494-1107	Orthovoltage, iodine
SOUTHEAST		
North Carolina State University Raleigh, NC	Dr. Donald Thrall 919-829-4200	Cobalt
NORTHCENTRAL		
University of Wisconsin Madison, WI	Drs. Chess Adams and Lisa Forrest 608-263-7600	Cobalt, orthovoltage
University of Illinois Urbana, IL	Drs. Jean Cloran and John Losonsky 217-333-2000	Cobalt
University of Minnesota St. Paul, MN	Drs. Dan Feeney and Patricia Walter 612-625-1200	Cobalt, orthovoltage
SOUTHCENTRAL		
University of Tennessee Knoxville, TN	Drs. William Adams and Robert Toal 615-974-5809	Cesium, interstitial, iodine
Auburn University Auburn, AL	Drs. Jan Bartels and William Brawner 205-826-5045	Cobalt, interstitial
Animal Radiology Clinic Dallas, TX	Dr. Catherine Lustgarten 214-484-5637	Cesium, iodine
Veterinary Cancer Associates Houston, TX	Dr. Glen King 713-666-4414	Cobalt
Texas A&M University College Station, TX	Dr. Michael Walker 409-845-9143	Cobalt, interstitial
MOUNTAIN AND WEST		
Colorado State University Fort Collins, CO	Dr. Ed Gillette 303-491-1276	Linear accelerator
Washington State University Pullman, WA	Dr. David Barbee 509-335-0754	Cobalt, orthovoltage
Southwest Veterinary Oncology Tucson, AZ	Dr. M. K. Klein 602-327-8131	Cobalt

(continues next page)

TABLE I (continued)

Centers (by region)	*Contact Person and Phone Number*	*Type of Radiotherapy Available*
University of California Davis, CA	Dr. Alain Theon 916-752-2517	Cobalt
Special Veterinary Services Berkeley, CA	Drs. Jerry Owens and Jeanine Fidel 415-848-5150	Orthovoltage
Veterinary Oncology Specialties Pacifica, CA	Dr. Jane Turrell 415-359-9870	Injectable radioisotope, orthovoltage
Santa Cruz Veterinary Hospital Santa Cruz, CA	Drs. Jay Stone and Margaret McEntee 408-475-5400	Cobalt, iodine
Animal Cancer Center Hermosa Beach, CA	Dr. Alice Villalobos 310-372-8881	Orthovoltage
All Care Animal Referral Center Fountain Valley, CA	Dr. Robert Rooks 714-963-0909	Cobalt

that have distant metastases and most lymphosarcomas. Involvement of regional lymph nodes does not preclude radiotherapy (regional lymph nodes would be irradiated as well as the primary tumor). Palliative radiotherapy should be considered when extent of disease or client factors preclude curative therapy. Because palliation requires only three or four treatments, is less expensive than curative radiotherapy, and results in few or no side effects, client satisfaction is generally assured. Temporary relief from pain and dysfunction is expected and may last for months following palliative radiotherapy.

In addition to histologic type, practitioners should consider the site of the tumor, extent of disease (including metastatic potential), and overall condition of the patient when discussing prognosis. Because of cost, extended nature of the treatment schedule (typically two to four weeks), and a likelihood of mild to moderate side effects, some owners may not wish to pursue radiotherapy.

It is vital that the owner has a clear understanding of the expected and likely outcome. Marked or minimal response may be noted in the tumor size following radiation therapy. A neoplasm may be inactivated but change little in size if there is either slow proliferation or a large amount of stromal support. The primary goal of radiation therapy is to stop continuing growth of the tumor while preserving normal tissue function. Failure should be defined on the basis of persistent tumor growth or regrowth of a tumor that initially decreased in size.

It is generally agreed that perianal adenomas, perianal adenocarcinomas, squamous cell carcinomas, acanthomatous epulides of periodontal origin, mast cell tumors, and transmissible venereal tumors are radioresponsive. Quantitating that response, however, has been difficult. This is because of the various ways in which response data have been reported, variety of treatment protocols used, and the individual variability of tumors within each histologic type. Table II and the Supplement cite the response of various tumor types to radiation therapy. As suggested in Table II, response of each tumor type may need to be considered according to anatomic site.

RADIOTHERAPY AND SURGERY

Two facts provide rationale for the combination of radiation and surgery in the treatment of cancer[6]:

1. Radiation alone usually fails to control large tumors.
2. Surgery often fails to result in local tumor control, even if all grossly visible tumor is removed.

When Should Radiation Be Given Relative to Surgery?

Preoperative Irradiation. Preoperative irradiation is usually completed three to four weeks before surgery. Blood supply to subclinical tumor margins is not disturbed by surgery; tumor cells may therefore be more radiosensitive (better oxygenated) than they would be after surgery. The volume of tissue treated can be more conservative, as surgically manipulated tissue is not a factor. Tumor cells subsequently disseminated at surgery are less likely to be viable (less likely to cause metastasis). Also, following radiotherapy, the tumor is often smaller, thereby allowing a more conservative surgical resection.

A disadvantage of preoperative irradiation is the increased potential for postoperative complications. This potential is minimized by allowing three to four weeks between irradiation and surgery.

Intraoperative Irradiation. Intraoperative irradiation can be combined with preoperative radiotherapy for lesions that are nonresectable. Following a course of

(continues on page 234)

TABLE II
Radiation Therapy Response

Type of Tumor	Response to Radiotherapy	Metastatic Potential[a] and Site	Comments
Oral Tumors			
Acanthomatous epulis[7,9]	Excellent	0	Radical surgery also curative; second malignancy reported within radiation site
Fibrosarcoma[1,2]	Poor to fair	1; regional lymph node	Combine with surgery and/or hyperthermia or do wide surgical resection only
Melanoma[10]	Fair to good	3; regional lymph node, lung	Combine with systemic therapy or hyperthermia
Squamous cell carcinoma[3,11,27,28]	Poor to good	1; regional lymph node	Tongue and tonsilar—poor; caudal mandible and maxilla—fair; rostral mandible and maxilla—good
Nasal Tumors			
Adenocarcinoma[12–14,29]	Fair to good	1; regional lymph node	If using orthovoltage, combine with rhinotomy
Poorly differentiated and squamous cell carcinoma[12]	Poor to fair	2; regional lymph node, lung	If using orthovoltage, combine with rhinotomy and systemic therapy
Sarcoma[13,29]	Fair to good	1; regional lymph node	If using orthovoltage, combine with rhinotomy
Other Head and Neck Tumors			
Salivary gland adenocarcinoma[15]	Excellent	Unknown	Few cases but very responsive
Squamous cell carcinoma[4,16]	Poor to good	1; regional lymph node	Prognosis worse if deeply invading or canine nasal plane
Thyroid carcinoma[17]	Poor to fair	3; mediastinum, lung	Use I_{131} if functional tumor
Multilobular osteochondrosarcoma[18]	Fair (?)	3 (late); lung	Aggressive surgery may provide long-term control; role of radiotherapy unclear
Brain tumors[20,30,31]	Poor to good	1; may be secondary	Generally poor prognosis but some are very responsive
Tumors of the Trunk			
Mast cell[19]	Fair to good	2; regional lymph node	Irradiate positive regional lymph node; some require systemic therapy
Perianal gland adenoma[3]	Excellent	0	Castration may be curative
Perianal gland adenocarcinoma[3]	Fair to good	3; sublumbar lymph node, lung	Often deeply invading; irradiate regional lymph node
Transmissible venereal tumor[21]	Excellent	1; regional lymph node, contact sites	Respond to chemotherapy; may regress spontaneously
Extremity Tumors			
Hemangiopericytoma[22]	Fair to good	1; regional lymph node	Metastatic potential increases with number of times excised; early amputation curative
Mast cell tumor[19]	Good to excellent if localized	1; regional lymph node	Irradiate positive regional lymph node; some require systemic therapy
Osteosarcoma[23,32]	Good; palliative	3; lung	Effective temporary pain relief; may be combined with limb-sparing surgery
Soft tissue sarcoma[24]	Fair to good	2; lung	Combine with surgery and systemic therapy
Abdominal Tumors			
Prostatic adenocarcinoma[25,26]	Poor to fair	3; regional lymph node, spine, lung	Often advanced on presentation; combine with intraoperative radiotherapy
Transitional cell carcinoma[26]	Poor to fair	2; regional lymph node, lung	Trigone often involved; combine with intraoperative radiotherapy

[a]Metastatic potential at initial presentation on a scale of 0 = little or no chance; 1 = <15%; 2 = 15% to 30%; 3 = >30%. If metastasis is classed as 2 or 3 and regional lymph node is indicated, then aspirate the regional lymph node as part of workup.

SUPPLEMENT
Abstracts of Veterinary Radiotherapy Literature

GENERAL GUIDELINES

- Thrall DE: **Radiation therapy**. *Proc 10th Kal Kan Symp*:53–63, 1986.

  This chapter examines rationale, patient evaluation, combination of radiation therapy and surgery, technical factors, tumor response, complications, and **causes of radiotherapy failure.**

- McLeod DA, Thrall DE: **Combination of surgery and radiation** in the treatment of cancer—A review. *Vet Surg* 18(1):1–6, 1989.

  This presentation reviews the rationale for combining radiation and surgery and the ways in which the two modalities can be combined, with emphasis on the **advantages and disadvantages of preoperative and postoperative radiotherapy.**

- Turrell JM, Theon AP: **Reirradiation** of tumors in cats and dogs. *JAVMA* 193(4):465–469, 1988.

  Fifty-one cats and dogs with tumor recurrence after irradiation were treated with a second course of radiotherapy using either teletherapy or brachytherapy. **Thirty-six percent of the tumors had partial or complete response at two months after reirradiation.** Predictors of local tumor control were reirradiation field size less than 10 cm^2 and reirradiation dose greater than 40 Gray. Animals with cutaneous tumors had the longest survival times, while animals with oral tumors had the shortest survival times. Acute effects of reirradiation on normal tissue were acceptable; but 43% had moderate late complications, and 12% had severe late complications. A significant risk of complications was associated with squamous cell carcinoma and reirradiated field size greater than 30 cm^2. When the interval between irradiations was longer than five months, the risk of complications was significantly lower. The doses required for recurrent tumor control should be similar to those required for initial control; this theory held true. No increase in complications occurred in animals reirradiated at longer than five-month intervals; therefore, high doses can be given safely for recurrent tumors. Late complications are, however, observed more frequently and the potential for life-threatening complications is increased.

ORAL TUMORS

- Thrall DE: Orthovoltage **radiotherapy of acanthomatous epulides** in 39 dogs. *JAVMA* 184(7): 826–829, 1984.

  The tumors were treated with a wide range of doses. Thirty dogs received between 35 and 50 Gray. The tumor recurred in only three dogs, two of which were successfully retreated with radiation. **Development of a malignant tumor at the site of the irradiated epulis was confirmed in seven (18%) of the dogs.** The median time to this occurrence in the seven dogs was 47 months. **The median survival time for all dogs was 37 months.** One- and two-year survivals were 85% and 67%, respectively. The cause of death was infrequently related to the acanthomatous epulis.

- White RA, Gorman NT: Wide local **excision of acanthomatous epulides** in the dog. *Vet Surg* 18(1): 12–14, 1989.

  Twenty-five dogs underwent tumor resection by wide local excision. Procedures included rostral mandibulectomy, removal of the mandibular body, premaxillectomy, and partial maxillectomy. **Postoperative complications were rare, and local recurrence was not encountered** in any dogs from one to six years (median of 22 months) later. The high incidence of local recurrence after simple excision and the potential for malignant transformation after radiation indicate that wide surgical resection is the technique of choice for management of this tumor. Resection involving incisor arcades often resulted in marginally impaired prehension but normal masticatory function. Those with resection of the mandibular body retained normal prehension but occasionally suffered variably impaired mastication. Complications of wound healing were encountered in one case of partial maxillectomy.

- Thrall DE: Orthovoltage radiotherapy of **oral fibrosarcomas in dogs.** *JAVMA* 179(2):159–162, 1981.

  Thirteen dogs received orthovoltage of 4000 to 5450 rads surface dose in a 10-fraction Monday–Wednesday–Friday schedule. One dog (8%) remained tumor free at 27 months. **The average time to regrowth for the other 12 dogs was 3.9 months, and the average survival time was 6.8 months** (longest survival was 14 months).

- Brewer W, Turrell JM: Radiotherapy and hyperthermia of **fibrosarcomas** in the dog. *JAVMA* 181(2): 246–250, 1982.

  Six dogs with oral fibrosarcoma and three dogs with external nasomaxillary fibrosarcoma received orthovoltage (3200 to 4800 rad). Seven of the dogs also received local hyperthermia. **Three dogs were alive with no evidence of tumor 20 months after treatment,** and a fourth was tumor free at 12 months. The survival rate at one year was 45%.

SUPPLEMENT (continued)

- Dewhirst MW, Sim DA, et al: Primary canine **malignant melanomas** treated with hyperthermia and/or radiotherapy. *Int J Hypertherm* 1(3):219–234, 1985.

  Forty-three dogs were randomized into two treatment groups. **The frequency of complete response and of a one-year disease-free interval was 21% and 8%, respectively, for radiation alone.** A trend in improved disease-free interval was noted in dogs given both hyperthermia and radiotherapy.

- McMillan M, Gillette E, et al: Surgery and regional irradiation for treatment of canine **tonsillar squamous cell carcinoma:** Retrospective review of 8 cases. *JAAHA* 18(2):311–314, 1982.

  Eight dogs received cobalt 60 teletherapy in 10 fractions on a Monday–Wednesday–Friday schedule for a total of 3500 to 4250 rads. The investigators reported six of the eight dogs had local control after one month. One dog died of other causes after 631 days. The remaining seven dogs died or were **euthanatized because of local recurrence or distant metastasis after 44 to 180 days (average of 96 days and median of 101 days).**

- Hutson CA, Willauer CC, et al: Treatment of **mandibular squamous cell carcinoma in cats** by use of mandibulectomy and radiotherapy. *JAVMA* 201(5):777–781, 1992.

  Seven cats with mandibular squamous cell carcinoma received 32 to 54 Gray (five cats received 45 Gray) of **orthovoltage or cobalt radiation 10 to 14 days after surgery. Survival after surgery was a mean and median of 15 and 14 months, respectively (range 3 to 36 months).** Six cats were euthanatized because of disease recurrence. In comparison, other studies reported median survival times of 2.5 to 6 months in cats receiving mandibulectomy.

- Evans SM, LaCreta F, et al: Technique, pharmacokinetics, toxicity and efficacy of intratumoral etanidazole and radiotherapy for treatment of spontaneous **feline oral squamous cell carcinoma.** *Int J Radiat Oncol Biol Phys* 20:703–708, 1991.

  All 11 cats in the study died as a result of tumor recurrence or tumor-related complications. **Median survival was 116 days.** Etanidazole and radiation therapy caused rapid regression, but not cure, of feline squamous cell carcinoma at a dose of 52 Gray delivered on a Monday–Wednesday–Friday schedule of 4.3 Gray × 12 fractions, using 3 mm Cu HVL orthovoltage to the primary tumor and associated submandibular lymph nodes. Tumors included two of the maxilla, one of the mandible, four of the frenulum, and four of the tongue and/or floor of the mouth. **Survivals ranged from 19 to 389 days.**

NASAL TUMORS

- Theon AP, Madewell BR, et al: Megavoltage irradiation of **neoplasms of the nasal and paranasal cavities in 77 dogs.** *JAVMA* 202(9):1469–1475, 1993.

  Tumors included **58 carcinomas and 19 sarcomas.** Fifty-six dogs were treated with radiation alone and 21 had partial tumor resection prior to radiotherapy. Treatment dose was 48 Gray on a Monday–Wednesday–Friday schedule at 4 Gray/fraction. **One- and two-year overall survival rates were 60.3% and 25%, respectively. One- and two-year relapse-free survival rates were 38.2% and 17.6%, respectively.** Their modified staging scheme was a significant prognostic indicator. Dogs with carcinoma had a poorer prognosis than dogs with sarcoma (predominantly chondrosarcoma). **Chronic ocular complications were seen in 45% of the dogs.**

- Evans SM, Goldschmidt M, et al: Prognostic factors and survival after radiotherapy for **intranasal neoplasms** in dogs: Seventy cases. *JAVMA* 194(10):1460–1463, 1989.

  Of 70 dogs undergoing radiotherapy, 34 died of tumor recurrence and 12 were lost to follow-up. Twenty-three percent of the dogs had facial masses. **The presence of a facial mass was not significant to the prognosis,** thereby suggesting that extensive disease should not preclude treatment. Four dogs with squamous cell carcinoma and 49 dogs with other types of carcinoma were treated. Sixteen dogs with sarcoma were treated. **The median survival time for all tumor types was 16.5 months with one-, two-, and three-year survival rates of 54%, 43%, and 35%, respectively.** The median survival time for dogs with carcinoma was 13.5 months. All dogs were treated after surgical debulking. Two significant posttreatment factors that affected survival and prognosis following radiotherapy were recurrence of epistaxis and confirmed recurrence of disease. Histologic grading of tumors was not significantly related to survival.

- Beck ER, Gillette EL, et al: Tumor stage and radiation dose as predictors of survival in **canine nasal carcinomas.** *Proc 7th Annu Vet Cancer Soc Conf:*15, 1987.

  Sixty-six dogs were treated with megavoltage. Histologic diagnosis included adenocarcinoma (40%), solid epidermoid carcinoma (31%), mixed carcinoma (17%), and acinous carcinoma (11%). The median age of the dogs was 8.3 years. Tumors recurred in 78% of the patients. Of these, 47% had local and regional failure, 38% had local failure

SUPPLEMENT (continued)

only, 5% had regional lymph node recurrence only, and 10% had distant metastases without failure at the primary site. The most common sites other than regional lymph nodes were the lung, bone, and kidney. Extension to the brain or eye occurred in 38% of the cases. Ninety percent of treatment failures were detected within nine months and 95% within two years.

Tumor recurrence rates correlated with the tumor stage: three dogs in T_1 stage were controlled at both nine months and two years; 50% and 36% of dogs in T_2 stage at nine months and two years, respectively; 22% and 11% of dogs in T_3 stage at nine months and two years, respectively; and 10% of dogs in T_4 stage at both nine months and two years. Twelve percent of the dogs had detectable lymphatic involvement at the time of treatment. All of these had metastasis at necropsy compared with 31% of dogs with no detectable lymphatic involvement.

Local tumor control correlated with dose. **Those receiving 48 Gray or more had 67% local control at nine months and 44% at two years. Dogs receiving 40 Gray had 22% and 10% local control at nine months and two years, respectively.** No dogs receiving less than 40 Gray survived nine months.

The causes for failure of nasal tumor treatment in this study were (1) inadequate dose, (2) geographic miss, and (3) tumor stage.

OTHER TUMORS OF THE HEAD AND NECK

- Evans SM, Thrall DE: Radiation therapy of **parotid salivary gland adenocarcinoma** in three dogs. *JAVMA* 182(9):993–994, 1983.

Three dogs were given 45 Gray of orthovoltage radiation in 10 fractions. **Two were alive after 12 and 25 months, and the third died of other causes at 40 months.**

- Carlisle CH, Gould S: Response of **squamous cell carcinoma of the nose of the cat** to treatment with x-rays. *Vet Rad* 23(5):186–192, 1982.

Sixty-two cats received orthovoltage of half-value layer 2.5-mm aluminum in 1 to 12 fractions on a once-monthly as-needed basis (median total dose of 4000 rad). The investigator reported 37% total remission for two years and 26% total remission for three years. An additional 26 cats received orthovoltage (half-value layer 2.5-mm aluminum) in 3 fractions on a Monday–Wednesday–Friday schedule for a total of 3000 rads. The investigator reported **57% total remission for two years** in this group.

- Thrall DE, Adams WM: Radiotherapy of **squamous cell carcinomas** of the canine nasal plane. *Vet Rad* 23(5):193–196, 1982.

Six dogs received orthovoltage in 7 to 10 fractions on a Monday–Wednesday–Friday schedule for a total dose of 3500 to 5000 rads. **Recurrence occurred at an average of 2.9 months, with the longest tumor control being eight months.**

- Turrell JM, Feldman EC, et al: **Thyroid carcinoma** causing hyperthyroidism in cats: 14 cases. *JAVMA* 193(3):359–364, 1988.

Twelve cats were treated with iodine 131, which is reported to be the best therapy for functioning thyroid carcinoma. Postoperative cobalt 60 teletherapy was used on one cat with a nonfunctional thyroid carcinoma. Nine cats were necropsied, all of which had local tumors with or without metastasis. The survival times ranged from one week to 39 months; **the mean and median were 11.7 and 9.2 months, respectively.** The rate of metastasis at the time of death was 71% (higher than the 40% previously recorded for cats but similar to that of dogs with thyroid carcinoma).

- Straw RC, Lecouteur RA, et al: **Multilobular osteochondrosarcoma** of the canine skull: 16 cases. *JAVMA* 195:1764–1769, 1989.

This condition, also called chondroma rodens (calcifying aponeurotic fibroma, multilobular osteoma, etc.) occurred in large dogs (mean body weight of 29 kg). **Eleven dogs were treated by excision only**; two had excision plus radiation; and one had radiotherapy, chemotherapy, and excision. Seven of 12 dogs had local recurrence, and seven developed metastasis. **The median survival time of the 12 dogs was 21 months, with a mean disease-free interval of 12 months.** For the two dogs receiving postoperative radiotherapy, one had recurrence at 26 months and the other died at 27 months because of metastasis. The role of radiotherapy in treating this tumor remains unclear; however, slow growth would suggest it to be radioresistant.

- Evans SM, Dayrell-Hart B, et al: **Radiation therapy of canine brain masses.** *J Vet Intern Med* 7(4):216–219, 1993.

Fourteen dogs were treated with orthovoltage radiation following computed tomography for treatment planning. Total doses of 39 Gray (nine dogs) or 45 Gray (five dogs) were administered over 25 to 41 days. Two or three portals were used. Histopathologic diagnoses were available in nine dogs. There were four dogs with meningiomas, one with lymphosarcoma, one with pituitary adenoma, one with metastatic anaplastic carcinoma, one with anaplastic oligodendroglioma, and one with granulomatous meningoencephalitis. Ten dogs could be

SUPPLEMENT (continued)

evaluated for progression of clinical signs following therapy—three dogs deteriorated or failed to improve and seven dogs improved. **Mean and median survival times from the beginning of radiation therapy were 345 and 489 days, respectively.** This compares to mean survival times of 30 to 81 days for dogs with brain tumors that did not receive treatment. Orthovoltage radiation can be given in total dose of 45 Gray and 3.75 Gray fractions over 28 days without adverse effects.

- Heidner GL, Kornegay JN, et al: Analysis of survival in a retrospective study of **86 dogs with brain tumors.** *J Vet Intern Med* 5(4):219–226, 1991.

  Forty-one dogs received definitive treatment in addition to medical management. Treatment included surgery, cobalt-60 radiation, whole body hyperthermia, iodine-125 implants, and chemotherapy alone or in combination. **Twenty-five dogs treated with cobalt-60 radiation,** with or without other combinations of therapy, **lived significantly longer than dogs who received surgery or received symptomatic treatment. Median survival times of dogs receiving cobalt-60 radiation,** surgery, or no therapy (or symptomatic therapy only) were **4.9,** 0.9 and 0.2 **months,** respectively. The five survivors at the end of this study all received cobalt-60 therapy. Irradiation appears to be the most successful therapy. Brain tumors carry a poor prognosis for long-term survival.

TUMORS OF THE TRUNK

- Turrell JM, Kitro BE, et al: Prognostic factors for radiation treatment of **mast cell tumor** in 85 dogs. *JAVMA* 193(8):936–940, 1988.

  Ninety-five mast cell tumors in 85 dogs were irradiated. **The median and mean survival times were 19 and 61 months, respectively. Survival rates after one and two years were 76% and 73%, respectively.** Prognostic factors that significantly affected survival rates were the clinical stage and the grade and location of neoplasms. Dogs with neoplasms on their extremities had a significantly higher tumor-free rate than those with neoplasms on the trunk. The histologic grade and presence of metastatic disease (usually to regional lymph nodes) at the time of treatment were not significant variables. Regional lymph nodes were irradiated if aspirates were considered positive for metastasis. Tumor-free and survival rates at one year compared favorably with the results of surgical excision from other reports. No tumor-related deaths occurred within 7.5 months in a surgical report and within 8 months in this study. Survival to one year is probably a good proximation of cure.

  Orthovoltage or cobalt was used, depending on the depth of the lesion. Total doses of 36 to 48 Gray were given in 9 to 12 equal fractions for a period of 19 to 27 days. Irradiation port included a margin of two centimeters of normal tissue.

- Thrall DE: Orthovoltage radiotherapy of canine **transmissible venereal tumors.** *Vet Rad* 23(5):217–219, 1982.

  Eighteen dogs received orthovoltage in 1 to 3 fractions for a total dose of 1000 to 3000 rads. The investigator reported no recurrence after a single dose of 1000 rads. **All 18 dogs had no recurrence within one year after completion of radiotherapy.**

- Gillette EL: Radiation therapy of canine and feline tumors. *JAAHA* 12(3):359–362, 1976.

  Of 101 canine **perianal adenomas and adenocarcinomas,** 47% were controlled at one year. Fifty-two of these tumors received at least 30 Gray; **58% of these were controlled at one year.**

  Of 44 canine and 8 feline **squamous cell carcinomas,** 34% were controlled at one year. Twenty-six of these tumors received at least 40 Gray; **46% of these were controlled at one year.**

EXTREMITY TUMORS

- Evans SM: Canine **hemangiopericytoma.** *Vet Rad* 28(1):13–16, 1987.

  Twenty-two dogs were given postoperative orthovoltage radiotherapy. Factors significantly related to survival were that dogs with hindlimb tumors had longer tumor-free intervals and dogs with less than 50 cm^2 portals had longer tumor-free intervals. Tumor-free intervals ranged from 1.5 to 55 months, with **41% of the dogs tumor free at 24 months.** Survival ranged from 2.5 to 55 months, with 40% of the dogs dead because of the tumor. Available published reports of postsurgical recurrence rates (no radiotherapy) range from 7.5% to 56% in the literature.

- Larue SM, Withrow SJ, et al: Limb sparing treatment for **osteosarcoma** in dogs. *JAVMA* 195:1734–1744, 1989.

  Twenty dogs with osteosarcoma of extremities were treated with cisplatin and radiation. Radiation therapy involved 25 or 40 Gray in 10 fractions on a Monday–Wednesday–Friday schedule. Three weeks after final treatment, the tumors were excised and orthopedic reconstruction was done.

  Forelimb procedures had better results. Local tumor control was obtained in 79% (11 of 14). Fifteen dogs developed metastasis at a median time of eight months from the time of diagnosis. **The mean**

SUPPLEMENT (continued)

and median survival times for all dogs were 11.7 and 8 months, respectively. Five dogs (31%) developed infections at the surgical site.

- McEntee MC, Page RL, et al: **Palliative radiotherapy for canine appendicular osteosarcoma.** *Vet Radiol and Ultrasound* 34(5):367–370, 1993.

  Fifteen dogs were treated with three 10 Gray fractions of cobalt radiation on a 0-, 7-, and 21-day protocol for a total dose of 30 Gray. Twelve dogs had improved limb function. Long-term follow-up was available for nine of the twelve responders. **Duration of response was 17–288 days (mean and median survivals were 116 and 130 days, respectively).** Response duration did not appear to be related to initial tumor size. Palliative radiotherapy can result in improved limb function in dogs with appendicular osteosarcoma.

- McChesney SL, Gillette EL, et al: Influence of WR 2721 on radiation response of canine **soft tissue sarcomas.** *Int J Rad Oncol Biol Phys* 12:1957–1963, 1986.

  Randomization of 73 dogs with soft tissue sarcomas was divided into two treatment groups: irradiation alone or with WR 2721. The tumor control dose for 50% of the dogs at one year was 52 Gray. **Of 52 dogs treated, 13 had tumor control for one year (25%).** This tumor control time is an improvement over a previous report of 4 of 25 (16%) controlled at one year (Hilmas and Gillette, *J Natl Cancer Inst* 56(2):365–368, 1976).

- Turrell JM, Kitro BE, et al: Prognostic factors for radiation treatment of **mast cell tumor** in 85 dogs. *JAVMA* 193(8):936–940, 1988.

  Refer to the section on Tumors of the Trunk for the accompanying abstract.

- Dewhirst MW, Sim DA, et al: Primary canine **malignant melanomas** treated with hyperthermia and/or radiotherapy. *Int J Hypertherm* 1(3):219–234, 1985.

  Refer to the section on Oral Tumors for the accompanying abstract.

ABDOMINAL TUMORS

- Turrell JM: Intraoperative radiotherapy of **carcinoma of the prostate gland** in ten dogs. *JAVMA* 190(1):48–52, 1987.

  Seven dogs had tumors confined to the prostate and urethra, and three dogs had regional lymph node involvement. The total doses delivered via orthovoltage ranged from 20 to 30 Gray. One dog was treated during surgery with 15 Gray, followed by a boost of 40 Gray using cobalt 60 teletherapy. Survival ranged from 41 to 750 days. **The median and mean survival times were 114 and 196 days, respectively.** The median survival for seven dogs with localized tumor was 180 days versus 80 days for three dogs with metastasis (difference not significant). Surgical complications occurring in two dogs resulted in their deaths.

- Withrow SJ, Gillette EL, et al: **Intraoperative irradiation** of sixteen spontaneously occurring canine neoplasms. *Vet Surg* 18(1):7–11, 1989.

  Intraoperative radiation therapy was given immediately after surgical debulking. Fractionated external-beam radiation was given to 11 dogs after surgery. Healing of surgical incisions was uncomplicated in 14 of 16 cases. Tumors were debulked to a depth of less than 1.5 centimeters. Five dogs received a total dose of 60 Gray or more, eight dogs received 30 Gray or more during surgery, and one third had no postoperative radiotherapy. It was anticipated by the authors that 25 Gray would result in approximately 50% incidence of skin necrosis. **Tumor control was poor.** Fourteen animals were necropsied; 13 had evidence of viable tumor at the radiotherapy site. Half of the potential candidates for intraoperative radiation were disqualified at the time of exploratory surgery because of metastasis beyond regional lymphatics or tumors that could not be reduced to 1.5 centimeters or less in thickness.

(continued from page 228)

preoperative irradiation and three to four weeks of rest, the patient can undergo surgery with resection of all gross tumor possible. The surgeon and radiotherapist then identify any remaining gross or suspected residual tumor for treatment with a boost dose of irradiation at the time of surgery. This technique is used for abdominal and retroperitoneal neoplasms. The advantage is to be able to deliver a high dose of radiation to a very localized area without risking damage to adjacent normal tissue (e.g., bowel or kidney).

Two potential disadvantages of intraoperative irradiation are irreversible damage to such vital structures as ureters and the urinary bladder and increased risk of infection during the longer surgical exposure.

Postoperative Irradiation. Postoperative irradiation is begun on Day 0 or delayed until 10 to 14 days after surgery. Radiotherapy should be delayed if the surgical wound is extensive or complications with healing are anticipated.

The advantages of primary surgical therapy include

the psychologic benefit to the owner of having the mass removed as soon as possible. Also, the full extent of the tumor may be more completely understood following surgery.

The disadvantages of postoperative radiation include the need to enlarge the radiation field to include all tissue handled during surgery. Also, there is an increase in the number of circulating cancer cells after surgical manipulation of the tumor, with the potential of inducing metastasis. Surgery also disturbs the blood supply in the area of a tumor, creating areas of hypoxia and thereby increased radioresistance around residual tumor.

Dealing with Side Effects from Radiotherapy

As with chemotherapy, the success of radiation therapy is limited by its attendant toxicity. Acceptable side effects are related to normally renewing tissue and are frequently seen during or shortly following therapy. Acceptable side effects include mucositis and moist desquamation. These problems resolve with time because some stem cells remain to regenerate following therapy. Supportive measures, such as gentle cleaning and application of mild ointments, may be helpful during the usual 10- to 14-day healing phase. Prevention of self-trauma (e.g., use of an Elizabethan collar) is critical to early healing of the inflamed site. Hair loss within the radiation field is expected and will probably be permanent, although hair may regrow (often a different color or texture). Keratoconjunctivitis sicca, corneal ulceration, and cataracts are bothersome potential side effects when the eye is within the radiation field. Because they are not life-threatening and do not materially diminish the quality of life, these effects should be acceptable to most owners, although some may find the potential of such effects objectionable and decline therapy accordingly.

In tissue that is not undergoing constant renewal, side effects from overdosing may not be noted for months to years after therapy is completed. Muscles, bones, and nerves are potentially affected with late fibrosis, necrosis, and nonhealing ulcerations. Such side effects are unacceptable. Another reported late effect that occurs two or more years after radiotherapy is development of a second primary tumor within the radiation field.[7] When a curative radiation dose is given to the original tumor site, subsequent development of a secondary tumor is rare.

Reirradiation of tumor recurrence after giving a full dose of radiation has been reported.[8] Late complications may be severe in these cases, especially if the interval between radiotherapy courses is fewer than five months. With care, this can be an effective method of dealing with recurrence.

About the Author

Dr. Adams, who is a Diplomate of the American College of Veterinary Radiology, is Associate Professor and Radiology Section Head, Department of Surgical Sciences, School of Veterinary Medicine, University of Wisconsin-Madison, Madison, Wisconsin.

REFERENCES

1. Thrall DE: Orthovoltage radiotherapy of oral fibrosarcomas in dogs. *JAVMA* 179(2):159–162, 1981.
2. Brewer W, Turrell JM: Radiotherapy and hyperthermia of fibrosarcomas in the dog. *JAVMA* 181(2):246–250, 1982.
3. Gillette EL: Radiation therapy of canine and feline tumors. *JAAHA* 12(3):359–362, 1976.
4. Carlisle CH, Gould S: Response of squamous cell carcinoma of the nose of the cat to treatment with x-rays. *Vet Rad* 23(5): 186–192, 1982.
5. Thrall DE: Radiation therapy. *Proc 10th Kal Kan Symp*: 53–63, 1986.
6. McLeod DA, Thrall DE: Combination of surgery and radiation in the treatment of cancer—A review. *Vet Surg* 18(1):1–6, 1989.
7. Thrall DE: Orthovoltage radiotherapy of acanthomatous epulides in 39 dogs. *JAVMA* 184(7):826–829, 1984.
8. Turrell JM, Theon AP: Reirradiation of tumors in cats and dogs. *JAVMA* 193(4):465–469, 1988.
9. White RA, Gorman NT: Wide local excision of acanthomatous epulides in the dog. *Vet Surg* 18(1):12–14, 1989.
10. Dewhirst MW, Sim DA, et al: Primary canine malignant melanomas treated with hyperthermia and/or radiotherapy. *Int J Hypertherm* 1(3):219–234, 1985.
11. McMillan M, Gillette E, et al: Surgery and regional irradiation for treatment of canine tonsillar squamous cell carcinoma: Retrospective review of 8 cases. *JAAHA* 18(2):311–314, 1982.
12. Adams WM, Withrow SJ, et al: Radiotherapy of malignant nasal tumors in sixty-seven dogs. *JAVMA* 191(3):311–315, 1987.
13. Evans SM, Goldschmidt M, et al: Prognostic factors and survival after radiotherapy for intranasal neoplasms in dogs: Seventy cases. *JAVMA* 194(10):1460–1463, 1989.
14. Beck ER, Gillette SL, et al: Tumor stage and radiation dose as predictors of survival in canine nasal carcinomas. *Proc 7th Annu Vet Cancer Soc Conf*:15, 1987.
15. Evans SM, Thrall DE: Radiation therapy of parotid salivary gland adenocarcinoma in three dogs. *JAVMA* 182(9):993–994, 1983.
16. Thrall DE, Adams WM: Radiotherapy of squamous cell carcinomas of the canine nasal plane. *Vet Rad* 23(5):193–196, 1982.
17. Turrell JM, Feldman EC, et al: Thyroid carcinoma causing hyperthyroidism in cats: 14 cases. *JAVMA* 193(3):359–364, 1988.
18. Straw RC, Lecouteur RA, et al: Multilobular osteochondrosarcoma of the canine skull: 16 cases. *JAVMA* 195:1764–1769, 1989.
19. Turrell JM, Kitro BE, et al: Prognostic factors for radiation treatment of mast cell tumor in 85 dogs. *JAVMA* 193(8): 936–940, 1988.
20. Turrell JM, Fike JR, et al: Radiotherapy of brain tumors in dogs. *JAVMA* 184:82–86, 1984.
21. Thrall DE: Orthovoltage radiotherapy of canine transmissible venereal tumors. *Vet Rad* 23(5):217–219, 1982.

22. Evans SM: Canine hemangiopericytoma. *Vet Rad* 28(1):13–16, 1987.
23. Larue SM, Withrow SJ, et al: Limb sparing treatment for osteosarcoma in dogs. *JAVMA* 195:1734–1744, 1989.
24. McChesney SL, Gillette EL, et al: Influence of WR 2721 on radiation response of canine soft tissue sarcomas. *Int J Rad Oncol Biol Phys* 12:1957–1963, 1986.
25. Turrell JM: Intraoperative radiotherapy of carcinoma of the prostate gland in ten dogs. *JAVMA* 190(1):48–52, 1987.
26. Withrow SJ, Gillette EL, et al: Intraoperative irradiation of sixteen spontaneously occurring canine neoplasms. *Vet Surg* 18(1):7–11, 1989.
27. Hutson CA, Willauer CC, et al: Treatment of mandibular squamous cell carcinoma in cats by use of mandibulectomy and radiotherapy. *JAVMA* 201(5):777–781, 1992.
28. Evans SM, LaCreta F, et al: Technique, pharmacokinetics, toxicity and efficacy of intratumoral etanidazole and radiotherapy for treatment of spontaneous feline oral squamous cell carcinoma. *Int J Radiat Oncol Biol Phys* 20:703–708, 1991.
29. Theon AP, Madewell BR, et al: Megavoltage irradiation of neoplasms of the nasal and paranasal cavities in 77 dogs. *JAVMA* 202(9):1469–1475, 1993.
30. Evans SM, Dayrell-Hart B, et al: Radiation therapy of canine brain masses. *J Vet Intern Med* 7(4):216–219, 1993.
31. McEntee MC, Page RL, et al: Palliative radiotherapy for canine appendicular osteosarcoma. *Vet Radiol and Ultrasound* 34(5):367–370, 1993.
32. Heidner GL, Kornegay JN, et al: Analysis of survival in a retrospective study of 86 dogs with brain tumors. *J Vet Intern Med* 5(4): 219–226, 1991.

Radiation Biology and Radiation Safety

KEY FACTS

- Radiation damage to living tissue is caused by alteration of biologic macromolecules.
- In considering the harmful effects of radiation on body systems, a distinction should be made between exposure, absorbed dose, and dose equivalent of ionizing radiation.
- It is difficult to distinguish changes induced by low-level radiation (e.g., shortened life span and cancer induction) from changes that are spontaneous or not induced by radiation.
- According to the current philosophy of radiation protection, all radiation is harmful.

Purdue University
William R. Widmer, DVM, MS
H. Dan Cantwell, DVM, MS
Stanley M. Shaw, PhD
Kimberly M. Vogel, RVT
Cheryl D. Hurd, RVT
Connie M. Han, RVT
William E. Blevins, DVM, MS

RADIOLOGY is a commonly used diagnostic modality in veterinary medicine. The safe use of diagnostic x-rays is the responsibility of veterinarians and veterinary technicians.[1-4] Training programs that emphasize radiation safety are not widely available or are not routinely sought. This article outlines the fundamental procedures that are beneficial to veterinary professionals who use ionizing radiation.

Radiation safety, or health physics, is concerned with protecting living systems from the harmful effects of ionizing radiation while allowing the beneficial use of such radiation.[5-8] Ionizing radiation is radiation that has enough energy to produce ion pairs in living tissue.[5] Alpha and beta particles, gamma rays, x-rays, and neutrons are forms of ionizing radiation that are important in medicine. Nonionizing radiation includes microwaves, ultraviolet radiation, and visible light. Although nonionizing radiation can injure living tissue, such radiation does not create ion pairs and thus is excluded from this discussion.

In veterinary medicine, radiation safety mainly involves x-rays and gamma rays. X-rays are used for diagnostic and therapeutic purposes. Gamma-emitting radionuclides are used in nuclear medicine and radiotherapy. The principles of radiation protection are similar for x-ray and gamma radiation. The only difference between x-ray and gamma radiation is the origin. X-rays are produced by changes in the orbital electron energy levels of an atom; gamma rays are created by changes in nuclear energy levels.[5,9] Gamma rays and x-rays are forms of electromagnetic radiation, have no mass or charge, and travel at the speed of light (3.0×10^8 m/sec).

RADIOBIOLOGY OF CELL DAMAGE

Radiation damages living tissue by altering biologic macromolecules.[3,5,6,10-12] Critical targets that have been proposed within the mammalian cell include nucleic acids, enzymes, lipoproteins, structural proteins, polysaccharides, membranes, and intracellular organelles.

Current evidence suggests that DNA is the most sensitive cellular component.[9,11,12] DNA is ultimately responsible for all cellular functions via the mechanisms of intracellular protein synthesis, DNA replication, and cell division. Considering DNA to be the critical target for radiation injury is thus reasonable and explains how relatively low doses of radiation can damage many cells. DNA damage is the most significant change produced by irradiation of living cells; such damage can produce cell dysfunction (somatic effects) or mutations (genetic damage).

Originally published in Volume 11, Number 10, October 1989

Cell Death

There are three possible outcomes when radiation strikes a living cell: radiation can pass through the cell with no effect, it can be scattered, or it can be absorbed and thus cause damage. Cell damage can be either sublethal and reparable or lethal. Cell death after irradiation can occur in cells undergoing mitosis (reproductive death) or in nondividing cells (interphase death).[6,11]

Reproductive death occurs only in cells that are capable of undergoing mitosis during their lifetime. In reproductive death, cells irradiated during mitosis will be killed and cells not undergoing mitosis will die during a future mitotic cycle. Low to moderate doses of radiation cause reproductive death in proliferative cells. Unlike reproductive death, interphase death is not restricted to proliferative cells and can be duplicated in any cell type. Interphase death requires relatively large doses of ionizing radiation. The mechanism of such death is unknown.[11]

Direct Action

When radiation interacts directly with the molecules of a living cell, ionization is the most significant change. Ionization is characterized by structural changes in critical target molecules of the cell (Figure 1). Ionization of DNA molecules causes single- and double-strand breaks, base deletions, base substitutions, and DNA cross-linking.[10-12] DNA changes can alter the function of irradiated parent cells or can produce mutations in daughter cells.

Some damage is reparable by natural cellular mechanisms. Excision repair, postreplication repair (recombination), and possibly double-strand break repair can occur. Error-free repair is the removal of damaged DNA and its replacement with normal nucleotides; normal DNA base sequence is thus restored.[11,12] Error-prone repair can also occur; the damage is bypassed rather than repaired.

INCOMPLETE REPAIR or nonrepair results when the continuity of DNA strands cannot be reestablished. Nonrepair is usually lethal, but it is not always mutagenic if the cell lives.[11,12] Double-strand breakage is a serious consequence of radiation injury because the DNA repair mechanism is less capable of repairing such injury.[12] Excitation also occurs but causes slight damage because energy is quickly dissipated among the many bonds in biologic macromolecules. The direct action of radiation on target molecules (a direct hit) is more commonly associated with radiations of higher linear energy transfer (LET), such as alpha particles, beta particles, and neutrons (Table I).

High linear energy transfer radiation is also referred to as densely ionizing radiation because dense areas or tracks of ionization are produced as radiation passes through tissue.[9,10] This phenomenon is contrasted with sparsely ionizing radiation, which is characterized by sparse areas of ionization within tissue. X-rays and gamma rays are examples of low linear energy transfer radiation and are considered sparsely ionizing radiations.

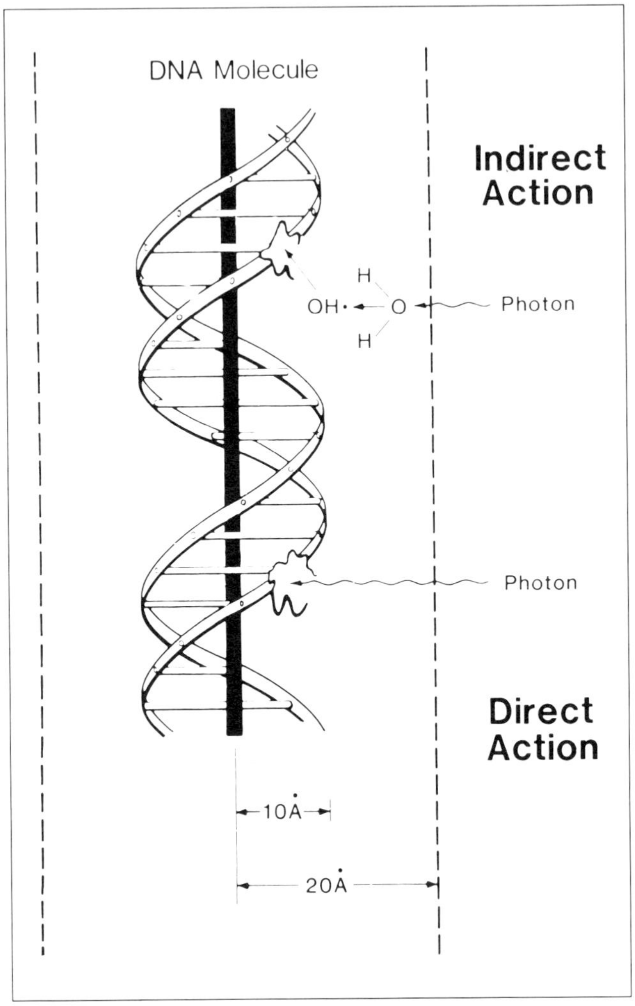

Figure 1—Indirect and direct action of x-ray radiation or gamma radiation on a DNA molecule. Direct action results when the incident photon strikes the molecule and causes damage by ionization and excitation. Indirect action results when the incident photon first ionizes intracellular water molecules, thus creating reactive free radicals that damage the DNA. (From Hall EJ: *Radiobiology for the Radiologist*, ed 2. Hagerstown, MD, Harper & Row, 1978, p 10. Modified with permission.)

Indirect Action

When cells are irradiated, some of the radiation strikes molecules other than critical targets. Within a cell, the interaction of radiation with atoms and molecules (especially water) forms unstable ion pairs that rapidly become free radicals. A free radical is an atom with an unshared, or odd-spin, electron.[6,10] Free radicals are reactive and can alter organic macromolecules within living tissue.

The interaction of free radicals (produced by ionizing radiation) with target molecules is referred to as an indirect hit or as indirect action of radiation[9] (Figure 1). Free radical damage to the DNA molecule consists of base changes and deletions, breakage of the DNA double helix, and DNA cross-linking; such damage is similar to that with direct action by ionizing radiation. Some of the damage can be repaired by naturally occurring DNA repair mechanisms. Repair depends on the type of radiation, the rate of exposure (dose rate), and the phase of the cell cycle at the time of irradiation.[6,11,12]

Because biologic tissues have a high water content, there is a high probability of interaction of sparsely ionizing radiations (e.g., x-rays and gamma rays) with water molecules rather than with enzymes, carbohydrates, or DNA.[9,11] Irradiation of water, or radiolysis, is represented by the following general formulas:

$$\text{radiation} \rightsquigarrow \text{HOH} \rightarrow \cdot\text{H} + \cdot\text{OH (hydrogen and hydroxyl free radical)}$$

$$\cdot\text{H} + \text{O}_2 \rightarrow \cdot\text{HO}_2 \text{ (peroxyl free radical)}$$

The hydroxyl and peroxyl free radicals are chemically active and damage molecular structure by reduction and oxidation reactions.[9-11] Radiolysis occurs approximately 10^{-18} seconds after photon interaction, and reactive free radicals cause biologic damage in the next 10^{-6} seconds.

FREE RADICALS can diffuse over distances of 20 angstroms (Å) before interacting with target molecules.[9] Depending on the particular biologic effect, expression can take days, months, or years.[9,11,12] If cell killing occurs, the biologic effect becomes evident in hours or days, cancer induction can require years, and genetic damage (e.g., mutation) can occur in future generations. The type of biologic effect is influenced by the tissue or organ involved, radiation dose, dose rate, quality of the radiation, distribution of the dose in tissue, and age.

CLASSIFICATION OF EFFECTS OF RADIATION BY BODY SYSTEM

Radiation Units

Distinctions should be made between exposure, absorbed dose, and dose equivalent of ionizing radiation (see Units and Definitions). Exposure pertains to exposure of an object to x-ray or gamma radiation in air but does not indicate the amount of radiation absorbed. The unit of exposure is the roentgen (R). Absorbed dose (rad) is used to measure the dose of radiation absorbed and represents an energy deposition of 100 erg/g of soft tissue. Dose equivalent (rem) is the absorbed dose in rads multiplied by the quality factor (QF) for the type of radiation (Table I).

The dose equivalent standardizes the degree of biologic damage so that the effects of various types of radiation can be compared. Because 1 R of x-ray or gamma radiation causes an energy deposition of approximately 98 erg/g in soft tissues, 1 R nearly equals 1 rad. Similarly, 1 rad of diagnostic x-ray or gamma radiation is equal to 1 rem because the quality factor for x-ray and gamma radiation is 1. Therefore, for diagnostic x-rays or gamma rays, 1 R $\simeq$ 1 rad = 1 rem. New nomenclature, which uses the SI system (Système International d'Unités), substitutes the gray (Gy) for the rad (1 Gy = 100 rad) and the seivert (Sv) for the rem (1 Sv = 100 rem).

TABLE I

Quality Factors for Various Types of Radiation

Type of Radiation	*Value*
X-ray and gamma	1
Beta	1 to 1.7
Proton	5
Neutron	3 to 10
Alpha	20

Acute Effects

Acute effects result from local or whole-body exposure to a large dose of ionizing radiation and are mediated by functional (parenchymal) cell damage of the affected organs.[3,6,9,10] Changes in the skin include erythema, dry desquamation, moist desquamation, and sloughing.[13] Local exposure to other radiosensitive organs (e.g., the thyroid gland, lymphoid organs, intestines, and kidneys) can cause parenchymal cell loss, which leads to organ failure and loss of function. The outcome of acute whole-body radiation exposure is more serious and can be terminal. Whole-body effects are classified in three acute radiation syndromes:

- Bone Marrow (hematopoietic) Syndrome—250 to 500 rads of whole-body exposure. If the patient is untreated, death occurs in 15 to 30 days. Bone marrow failure results in infection, immune deficiency, and hemorrhagic diathesis. The functional cells of the gastrointestinal system are also damaged. Vomiting, diarrhea, fluid loss, and breakdown of the mucosal barrier to infection contribute to death.
- Gastrointestinal Syndrome—500 to 1200 rads of whole-body exposure. If the patient is untreated, death occurs in 3 to 10 days. There is a loss of functional and stromal cells of the gastrointestinal tract. The bone marrow is irreparably damaged, but death occurs before clinical signs of marrow failure are evident.
- Cerebrovascular Syndrome—10,000 (or more) rads of whole-body exposure. Death occurs in a few hours. Cerebrovascular damage is probably the primary alteration. The exact pathogenesis is unknown, but whole-body irradiation is necessary. The syndrome is not produced by doses of 10,000 (or more) rads to the head only.

The $LD_{50\text{-}30}$ dose (which causes death in 50% of patients at 30 days) for whole-body x-ray and gamma radiation varies according to species. For most mammals, the dose ranges from 250 to 700 rads.[10] The $LD_{50\text{-}30}$ for humans is approximately 450 rads. Phylogenically lower animals (e.g., laboratory animals, reptiles, and fish) have a higher $LD_{50\text{-}30}$.[3,6,14]

Late Effects

Late, or delayed, effects of radiation damage include

loss of organ stroma, cancer induction, shortening of life span, and genetic injury. These effects can result from a single acute dose or from chronic low-level exposure. Late effects are preceded by a latent period, the length of which depends on the dose and the nature of the effect.[10,15,16]

Bone necrosis, fibrosis, skin ulceration, cataracts, keratoconjunctivitis sicca, and neuropathy are late changes that can follow local radiation exposure in animals.[13,17,18] In humans, thyroid tumors, squamous cell carcinoma of the hands, mammary gland carcinomas, and hematopoietic neoplasia have been linked to x-ray and gamma radiation exposure.[6,15] The incubation (latent) period in humans can be 10 to 30 years after a single dose of ionizing radiation. In dogs, osteosarcoma has occurred three to five years after orthovoltage radiotherapy.[19] Malignant tumor transformation was reported in four dogs at the site of previously irradiated acanthomatous epulides.[20]

GENETIC EFFECTS include gene mutations and chromosomal aberrations.[6,10,11,15] Gene mutations involve a small, permanent change in the DNA of reproductive cells; the change affects future generations. Radiation-induced mutations can be dominant or recessive. Rather than producing bizarre mutations or monsters, radiation increases the frequency of the mutations that spontaneously occur in a given population.[15]

The mutations accumulate in the precursor cells of reproductive tissues and increase the risk, over time, of new mutations transmitted by the individual chronically exposed to radiation. Chromosomal aberrations, including aneuploidy and polyploidy, can produce death or altered function of daughter cells. The importance of other chromosomal alterations caused by radiation injury is unclear. Radiation is among the most potent mutagens known.[10,21,22]

Radiation is known to be teratogenic. Embryos and fetuses are sensitive to relatively low doses of radiation.[11,21] Mammalian embryos are at greatest risk of radiation damage during the period of organogenesis in the first trimester. After differentiation of the various types of tissue, fetuses are less sensitive to radiation injury. Near the end of gestation, the sensitivity of fetal tissue is similar to that of adult tissue. The fetal central nervous system is an exception because neural development is incomplete at birth.

Radiosensitivity Versus Radioresponsiveness

Radiosensitivity is the susceptibility of a particular cell type to lethal radiation damage.[23] Such damage is usually recognized in vitro as loss of reproductive capability (reproductive death). Radioresponsiveness is the gross response of tissue to irradiation. The response to a given dose of radiation is affected by the inherent radiosensitivity of the cells and by such tissue factors as the rate of cell division and the level of tissue oxygenation.

The radioresponse of tissue to a dose of ionizing radiation is characterized by the Bergonie-Tribondeau law.[10,24] According to this law, the radioresponse is inversely proportional to the degree of cellular differentiation and is directly proportional to cell turnover rate. Cells that are rapidly replaced, such as small intestinal crypt cells and germinal cells of the epidermis, are thus likely to be damaged by a given dose of radiation. Neurons and erythrocytes, which are highly differentiated and do not divide, are unlikely to be damaged by a given dose of radiation.

It is probable that all mammalian cells are equally radiosensitive when the observed end point is loss of reproductive capability. With the x-ray and gamma radiation used in diagnostic radiology and radiotherapy, tissue must be proliferating or differentiating in order to express radiation damage (radioresponse).[8,23,25] An exception is the mature lymphocyte, which is inherently more radiosensitive than other mature cells. Radiation doses that are commonly used in radiotherapy can cause rapid disappearance of circulating lymphocytes.[15]

PRINCIPLES OF RADIATION PROTECTION

Low-Level Exposure

Radiation workers are primarily concerned with low-level radiation exposure. The actual effects of chronic low-level exposure are unknown. It is difficult to distinguish changes induced by low-level radiation (e.g., shortened life span and cancer induction) from changes that are spontaneous or not induced by radiation.[10,11,26]

Spontaneous mutations are indistinguishable from mutations caused by radiation. Because the effects of low-level radiation follow long-term, fractionated exposure, it is difficult to determine the dose received by an individual. Extremely large population samples are necessary to acquire statistically significant data because low-dose radiation causes only a slight increase in the incidence of a given effect.[26]

RADIATION EFFECTS are difficult to document if the same effect is caused by multiple factors, including biologic variation. The issue is also clouded by the capability of mammalian species to repair DNA damage induced by low-level radiation.[11]

The dose-response relationship for low-level exposure has been established by extrapolation of data obtained from atomic bomb survivors, peacetime nuclear accidents, and experimental animals. In these situations, various types of radiation (high and low linear energy transfer), high doses, and high dose rates were used. It thus might be incorrect to extrapolate the response to low linear energy transfer, low dose, and low-dose-rate radiation based on these data.

The shape of the initial (low-dose) segment of dose-response curves for somatic and genetic effects is unknown and is a source of debate among radiobiologists.[6,8,26] Linear and linear-quadratic (curvilinear) dose-response models are illustrated in Figure 2. Current data indicate that the risk of genetic damage and cancer induction is most accurately represented by a linear-quadratic model with no threshold dose.[6,26]

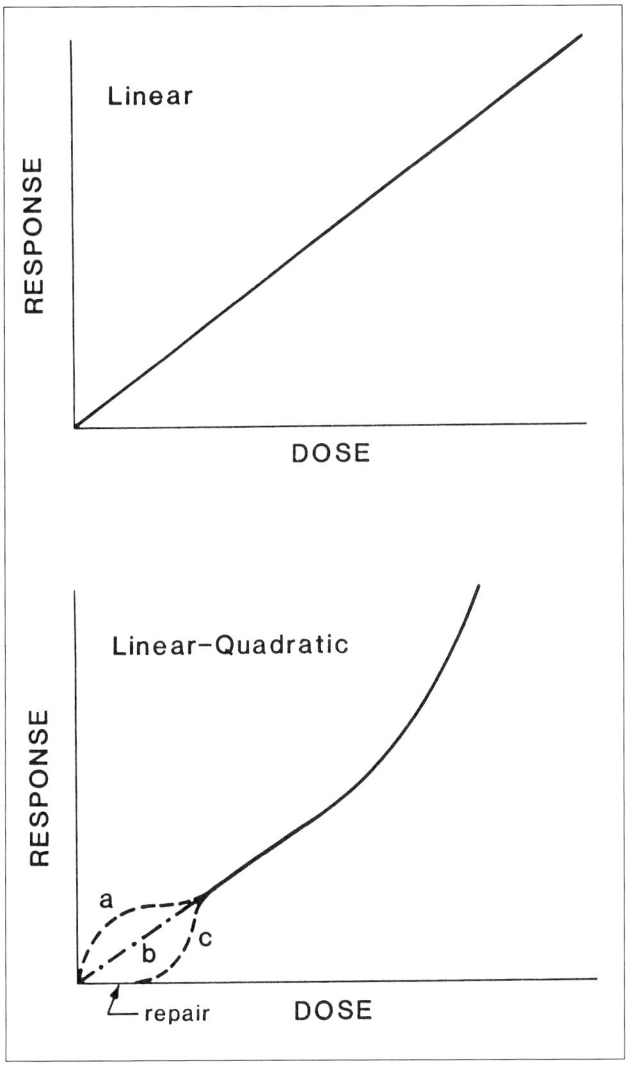

Figure 2—Two radiation dose-response models. The linear model of the dose-response curve was used to determine the maximum permissible dose and was originally preferred for describing genetic effects and some radiation-induced cancers. Linearity implies (1) no repair mechanism and (2) an increasing probability of effect in proportion to dose. The linear-quadratic dose-response curve has been proposed to define the somatic and genetic effects of ionizing radiation (including most cancers). The shape of the low-dose (less than 10-rad) portion of the curve is unknown. Line *a* suggests enhancement of somatic effects at low levels of ionizing radiation exposure. Line *b* is curvilinear and is currently used to describe the risk of cancer induction and genetic effects. Line c represents data that indicate a threshold dose below which radiation-induced effects are not detectable.

For most somatic effects, including cataracts, radiodermatitis, and infertility, the dose-response curve is also curvilinear; however, data strongly support the existence of a threshold dose below which repair can occur. The linear model, or linear hypothesis, has been refuted by several investigators. The linear-quadratic model best represents present dose-response data.[6,26] A unique dose-response curve probably exists for most radiation-induced genetic and somatic effects.[26]

Philosophy of Protection

Because any exposure to ionizing radiation can be harmful, the potential risk of medically used radiation must be weighed against the benefit derived. The diagnostic or therapeutic benefits of radiation exposure of the patient usually outweigh the risks. For radiation workers, the benefit of employment is believed to exceed the risk.[8,27-29] This philosophy is based on two hypotheses, which are expressed as acronyms:

- ALARA—Exposure must be kept as low as reasonably achievable.
- MPD (maximum permissible dose)—During a career, a person can acquire certain quarterly and annual whole-body and organ doses of radiation without a significant risk of harmful effects (Table II). The maximum permissible dose is cumulative. Whole-body exposure is expressed by the following formula:

whole-body MPD (in rems) = 5 (age in years − 18)

Maximum Permissible Dose

According to the formula for whole-body maximum permissible dose, the maximum permissible cumulative dose at a given time is 5 rem multiplied by the age of the individual minus 18. Eighteen is subtracted from the age because individuals younger than 18 years of age should not engage in the occupational use of ionizing radiation.

For educational and training purposes, it might be necessary for students younger than 18 to accept occasional exposure to ionizing radiation. In such instances, the recommended dose equivalent is 0.1 rem per year (Table II). The maximum permissible dose formula can also be used to determine the cumulative doses for specific organs; the appropriate annual rem doses listed in Table II are substituted. State governmental regulations might prohibit persons younger than 18 years of age from assisting in veterinary radiographic procedures.

THE MAXIMUM permissible dose limits have been established by considering the probability of genetic effects and cancer induction caused by ionizing radiation for which there might be no threshold dose or biologic repair.[5,6,26-28] Maximum permissible doses were derived from data extrapolated from the linear segment of experimental dose-response curves. The maximum permissible doses are low but can cause a few genetic or somatic effects. The probability of occurrence is low enough to be considered acceptable.

The question of acceptable levels of radiation exposure (dose) has been discussed.[5,6,26,27] There is no consensus on a safe dose. Most health physicists agree that maximum permissible doses are significantly below levels likely to cause injury during the career of a radiation worker.[6,8,28]

According to the current philosophy of radiation protection, all radiation is harmful. Although the risk of damage

(continues on page 246)

The Four Factors of Radiation Protection for Workers Using Veterinary Diagnostic X-Ray Equipment

- Common Sense—Avoid the primary beam (Figures 3 through 5). Keep the head and hands as far as possible from the beam. To protect the lenses of the eyes, look away during exposure (Figure 6). Never hold a portable x-ray machine during exposure; all machines are legally permitted to leak a minimal amount of radiation. The lead apron should be positioned between the beam and the body during exposure.

- Time—Use film-screen systems and technique charts that minimize the time of exposure. Rotate available personnel so that no worker spends a disproportionate amount of time producing radiographs.

- Distance—Maximize the distance between the x-ray beam and the worker. The radiation incident (exposure) on an absorber is inversely proportional to the square of the distance from the source (Figure 7). This is referred as the inverse square law. Although the law is defined for radiation from a point source, the relationship is also approximately valid for the broad-beam radiation sources used in diagnostic radiology. The inverse square law (which pertains to primary and scatter radiation) is represented by the following formula:

$$I = k \times \frac{1}{D^2}$$

I = intensity (or exposure), k = constant, and D = distance from the source.

- Shielding—Use protective barriers, lead aprons, lead gloves, and protective eyeglasses (see Figure 6). Report No. 36 of the National Council on Radiation Protection and Measurements (NCRP) describes construction methods and specifications for primary and secondary barriers in veterinary hospitals. Primary barriers shield against primary and scatter radiation; secondary barriers, lead aprons, and lead gloves only inhibit scatter radiation (Figure 8). Lead-impregnated plastic shields between the patient and the worker reduce the exposure of personnel to scatter radiation.[30,31]

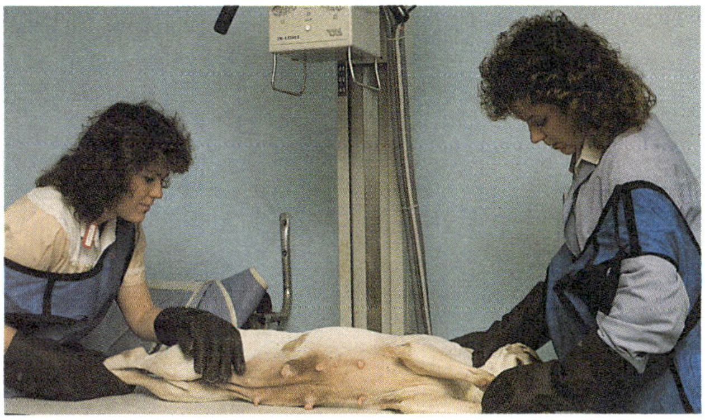

Figure 3—An example of poor technique in small animal radiography. A common error is leaning or looking into the beam during manual positioning of the patient. The gloved hand of the technician on the left is positioned in the primary beam; 0.5-mm lead gloves do not protect against the high-energy x-rays of the beam. Note the improper use of lead aprons, exposing the upper body to scatter radiation.

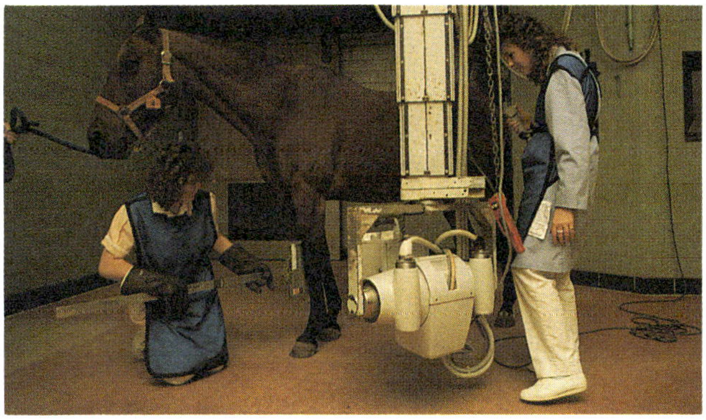

Figure 4—An example of poor technique in large animal radiography. The cassette handle is not being held properly. The length of the handle should be used to maximize the distance from the primary beam. The workers are too close to the primary beam. One worker is also too close to the forelimb of the patient (compare with Figure 7).

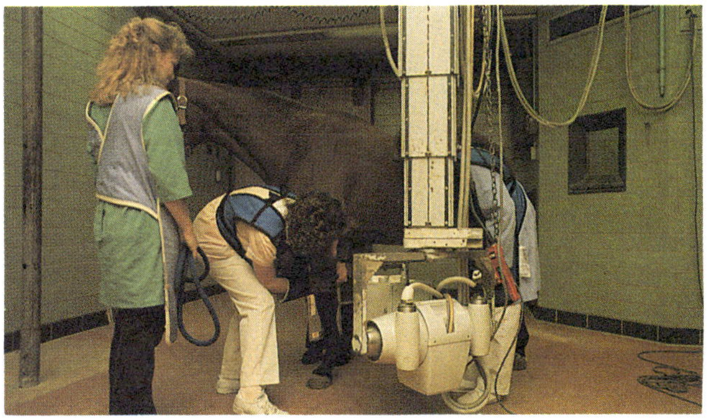

Figure 5—An example of poor technique in large animal radiography. The technicians are leaning into the primary beam. The cassette is being held with a gloved hand, placing the hand in the primary beam. The worker holding the patient is too close to the patient and to the head of the x-ray tube. Personnel making radiographic exposures should be positioned away from the primary beam or behind a protective barrier (compare with Figure 7).

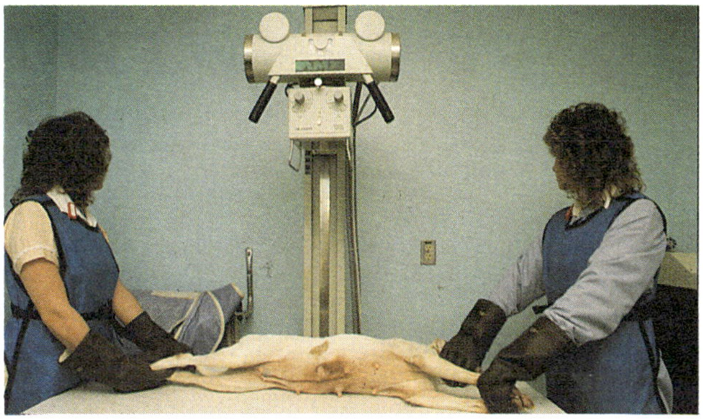

Figure 6—An example of good technique in small animal radiography. The use of lead gloves and aprons is mandatory during manual positioning of a patient. Note that the technicians are maintaining maximum distance from the patient and the primary beam and are looking away to minimize whole-body and eye exposure. Lead gloves (equivalent to 0.5 mm) and lead-impregnated eyeglasses are used to shield the hands and eyes from scatter radiation. Dosimetry methods include monitoring whole-body surface exposure, deep exposure (clip-on film badge), and hand exposure (thermoluminescent dosimeter).

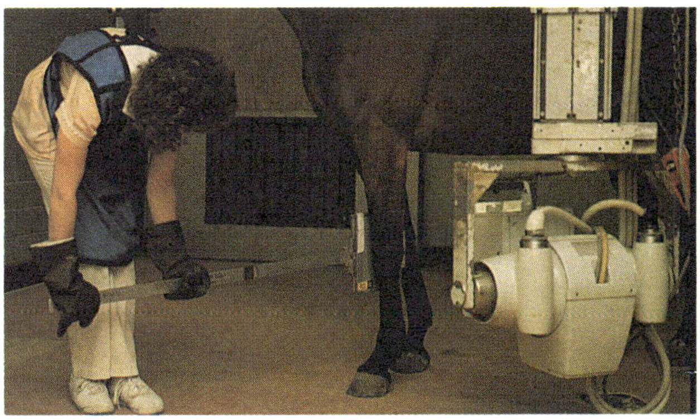

Figure 7—An example of good technique in large animal radiography. Protective garments and distance are properly used to reduce exposure of personnel. Note that the technician holding the patient has positioned herself away from the primary beam. Patient thickness and low-output equipment can increase exposure of personnel during radiography of large animals.

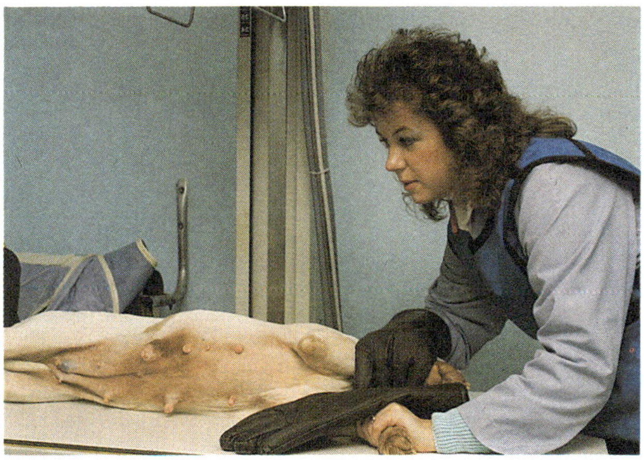

Figure 8—A glove or a lead shield is ineffective if placed over the hand; radiation scattered back from the cassette and table is absorbed by the underside of the hand.

General Radiation Safety Rules

The following rules benefit all radiation workers by minimizing exposure to ionizing radiation.[3,4,7,32] State and local regulations should be consulted for more specific information. Radiation safety and control programs for veterinary hospitals have been described in the literature.[1,2,4] In addition, the National Council on Radiation Protection and Measurements, an advisory group chartered by the U.S. Congress, collects scientific information and makes recommendations on radiation protection for the health sciences. These recommendations are generally incorporated by federal, state, and local governments. The council's Report No. 36 pertains to the use of diagnostic x-rays in veterinary medicine. The use of diagnostic radiation in most veterinary practices is regulated by state or provincial governments.

- Remove all nonessential personnel from the room during an x-ray exposure.
- Do not allow pregnant women or personnel younger than 18 years of age in the diagnostic x-ray room.
- Use tape, sandbags, plastic positioners, and restraining devices to eliminate the need for personnel in the x-ray room during an exposure.
- Use chemical restraint if possible.
- Never permit any part of the worker's body to be in the primary beam, including a gloved hand. An 80-kVp x-ray beam can penetrate 0.5-mm lead gloves (see Figure 8).
- Do not place any part of the body behind the cassette during an exposure. Never hold a cassette, even with a gloved hand.
- Always wear protective aprons when positioning a patient, and always wear lead gloves when the hands are placed next to the primary beam. Remember that these devices protect against scatter radiation only (Figure 9).
- To reduce scatter radiation, collimate and cone down as much as possible.
- Position a 2-mm aluminum filter between the x-ray tube and the patient in order to reduce the number of less energetic, soft x-rays emitted in the primary beam.
- Wear a film badge outside the protective apron, at neck level, to monitor radiation dose (Figure 6).
- Use protective eyeglasses and thyroid shields.
- Plan the radiographic procedure carefully in order to avoid repeated filming. Use a technique chart and proper darkroom processing.
- Use intermittent exposure during fluoroscopy. An intermittent exposure technique (with the fluoroscope on one second and then off one second) provides the same visual information but requires half the radiation dose.

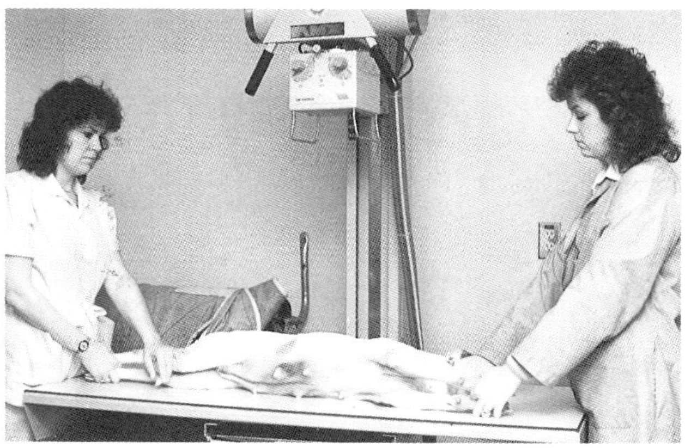

Figure 9—An example of poor radiographic technique. Failure to use lead gloves and protective aprons needlessly exposes personnel to scatter radiation. The technicians are also not wearing radiation-monitoring devices. If film badges are not continuously worn in controlled radiation areas, occupational exposure cannot be effectively monitored.

Units and Definitions

***alpha (α) particle*:** A high-speed particle, consisting of two protons and two neutrons, with a unit charge of 2+. Identical to a helium nucleus. Alpha particles are damaging (high QF). Because of relatively large mass and charge, the particles travel short distances in an absorber.

***beta (β) particle*:** A high-speed particle with the mass of one electron and a unit charge of 1. A positron has a positive charge, and a negatron has a negative charge. High-energy electrons travel near the speed of light.

***coulomb per kilogram (C/kg)*:** SI unit of radiation exposure. The amount of x-ray or gamma radiation that produces a charge of 1 coulomb in air.

***gray (Gy)*:** SI unit of absorbed dose. Equal to the amount of energy absorbed in joules per kilogram (J/kg) of mass. 1 Gy = 100 rad.

***linear energy transfer (LET)*:** The amount of energy deposited by radiation per unit length of travel in an absorber. Expressed in kiloelectron volts per micron (KeV/μm).

***quality factor (QF)*:** A unitless value that compares the relative damage (risk) caused by specific types of radiation. Defined without reference to a particular end point. Quality factor is relevant to low dose, low-dose-rate radiation, and late effects. Quality factor is proportional to the linear energy transfer (KeV/μm) of a given type of radiation as it passes through an absorber.

***rad*:** Radiation absorbed dose. The unit of absorbed dose. One rad is equal to energy deposition of 100 erg/g of absorber. Applies to all types of radiation.

***rem*:** Roentgen (or rad) equivalent mammal (or man). The unit of dose equivalent. Equal to the absorbed dose multiplied by the quality factor (rem = rad × QF). A measure of radiation-induced biologic damage that allows comparison of types of radiation.

***roentgen (R)*:** The unit of radiation exposure that causes enough ionization of air to liberate a charge of 2.58×10^4 C/kg. Roentgen pertains to gamma and x-ray radiation in air only.

***seivert (Sv)*:** SI unit of dose equivalent. 1 Sv = 100 rem.

TABLE II

Maximum Permissible Dose Recommendations[a]

Body Part or Type of Person	*Average per Week (mrem)*	*Maximum per Quarter (rem)*	*Maximum per Year (rem)*
Occupational Exposure (workers)			
Whole body, gonads, blood-forming organs, lenses of eyes	1	3	5
Skin of whole body	—	10	30
Hands, forearms, head, neck, feet, ankles	1.5	25	75
Fertile women (entire gestational period for fetuses)	—	—	0.5
Nonoccupational or Occasional Exposure (general public)			
Whole body	0.1		0.50
Students[b]	—		0.10
Population[c]	—		0.17

[a]Exposure of patients to radiation for medical and dental purposes is not included in the maximum permissible dose equivalent.
[b]The dose limit for students is a guideline for nonoccupational personnel occasionally exposed to ionizing radiation for training or educational purposes. This dose limit does not imply that all students and persons younger than 18 years of age should routinely engage in such activities. The limit does suggest that the risk of low-level radiation exposure is acceptable in these instances in light of the benefits of education.
[c]Population dose limits are intended to define the risk of genetic and somatic effects in the general public. The population dose limit is one third the nonoccupational dose limit.

(continued from page 241)

increases with the dose, radiation workers are considered to be at an acceptable risk level if maximum permissible dose values are not exceeded. The maximum permissible dose guidelines should be used in concert with the ALARA hypothesis; doses are used as ceilings, not as desired exposure levels.

ACKNOWLEDGMENTS

The authors thank David Pekarek and Rose Beghtol-Hunt, of the Medical Illustration Unit, School of Veterinary Medicine, Purdue University, for their technical assistance in preparing this article.

About the Authors

Drs. Widmer, Cantwell, and Blevins are Diplomates of the American College of Veterinary Radiology. Dr. Widmer, Dr. Cantwell, Ms. Vogel, Ms. Hurd, Ms. Han, and Dr. Blevins are affiliated with the Department of Veterinary Clinical Sciences, Diagnostic Imaging Section, School of Veterinary Medicine, Purdue University, West Lafayette, Indiana. Dr. Shaw is affiliated with the Department of Medicinal Chemistry, School of Pharmacy, Purdue University.

REFERENCES

1. Morgan JP, Silverman S, Zontine WJ: Radiation safety. *Mod Vet Pract* 59(10):739–746, 1978.
2. Kleine LJ: Radiation control program. *AHT* 4(3):172–177, 1983.
3. Morgan JP, Silverman S: *Techniques in Veterinary Radiography*, ed 3. Davis, CA, Veterinary Radiology Associates, 1980, pp 121–149.
4. Rendano VT, Watrous BJ: Radiation safety. *Mod Vet Pract* 61(9):730–731, 1980.
5. Noz MN, Maguire GQ: *Radiation Protection in the Health Sciences*, ed 2. Philadelphia, Lea & Febiger, 1985, pp 3–23.
6. Pizzarello DJ, Witkofski RL: *Medical Radiation Biology*, ed 2. Philadelphia, Lea & Febiger, 1986.
7. NCRP Report 36: *Radiation Protection in Veterinary Medicine*. Bethesda, MD, National Council on Radiation Protection and Measurements, 1975.
8. Hall EJ: *Radiobiology for the Radiologist*, ed 2. Hagerstown, MD, Harper & Row, 1978, pp 413–441.
9. Hall EJ: *Radiobiology for the Radiologist*, ed 2. Hagerstown, MD, Harper & Row, 1978, pp 3–12.
10. Pizzarello DJ, Witkofski RL: *Basic Radiation Biology*, ed 2. Philadelphia, Lea & Febiger, 1975.
11. Sutherland RM, Mulcahy RT: Basic principles of radiation biology, in *Clinical Oncology for Medical Students and Physicians: A Multiple Disciplinary Approach*. Rochester, NY, American Cancer Society, 1983, pp 40–57.
12. Coggle JE: *Biological Effects of Radiation*, ed 2. New York, International Publications Service, 1983, pp 29–51.
13. Johnston GR, Feeney DA: Radiotherapy of the extremities. *Vet Radiol* 24(3):130–137, 1983.
14. Hall EJ: *Radiobiology for the Radiologist*, ed 2. Hagerstown, MD, Harper & Row, 1978, pp 205–215.
15. Hall EJ: *Radiobiology for the Radiologist*, ed 2. Hagerstown, MD, Harper & Row, 1978, pp 297–410.
16. Withers HR, Peters LJ, Kogelnik HD: The pathobiology of late effects of irradiation, in Myen ER, Withers HR (eds): *Radiation Biology in Cancer Research*. New York, Raven Press, 1980, pp 439–448.
17. Roberts SM, Lavach JD, Severin GA, et al: Ophthalmic complications following megavoltage irradiation of the nasal and paranasal cavities of dogs. *JAVMA* 190(1):43–47, 1987.
18. LaRue SM, Wrigley RH, Powers BE: A review of effects of radiation therapy on bone. *Vet Radiol* 28(1):17–22, 1987.
19. Thrall DE, Goldschmidt MH, Evans SM, et al: Bone sarcoma following orthovoltage radiotherapy in two dogs. *Vet Radiol* 24(4):169–173, 1983.
20. Thrall DE, Goldschmidt MH, Biery DN: Malignant tumor formation at the site of previously irradiated acanthomatous epulides in four dogs. *JAVMA* 178(2):127–132, 1981.
21. Glauden ME, Murry RC: Medical radiation and possible adverse effects on the human embryo, in Myen ER, Withers HR (eds): *Radiation Biology in Cancer Research*. New York, Raven Press, 1980, pp 277–294.
22. Goodhead DT: Models of radiation inactivation and mutagenesis, in Myen ER, Withers HR (eds): *Radiation Biology in Cancer Research*. New York, Raven Press, 1980, pp 231–247.
23. Thrall DE: Principles of radiation therapy in cancer, in Ettinger SJ (ed): *Textbook of Veterinary Internal Medicine*, ed 2. Philadelphia, WB Saunders Co, 1983, pp 393–405.
24. Bergonie J, Tribondeau L: Interpretation de quelques resulats, de la radiotherapie et de fixation d' une technique rational. *Can R Acad Sci* 143:983–985, 1906.
25. Thrall DE, Dewhirst MW: Application of radiotherapy in the control of neoplasia, in Gorman NT (ed): *Contemporary Issues in Veterinary Medicine*. New York, Churchill Livingstone, 1986, pp 71–87.
26. NRC Report: *Biological Effects of Ionizing Radiation*. Washington, DC, National Academy of Science, National Research Council, 1980.
27. NCRP Report 43: *Review of the Current State of Radiation Protection Philosophy*. Bethesda, MD, National Council on Radiation Protection and Measurements, 1975.
28. Curry TS, Dowdey JE, Murry RC: *Christensen's Introduction to the Physics of Diagnostic Radiology*, ed 3. Philadelphia, Lea & Febiger, 1986, pp 401–419.
29. Coggle JE: *Biological Effects of Radiation*, ed 2. New York, International Publications Service, 1983, pp 188–205.
30. Hise JR, Schuchman SM: Lead-impregnated acrylic shielding for a diagnostic x-ray unit. *JAVMA* 184(1):95–96, 1984.
31. Rendano VT, Ryan GD, Bassano DA: Radiation safety—Transparent leaded-plastic panels: A product evaluation. *JAAHA* 23(2):141–144, 1987.
32. Ticer JE: *Radiographic Technique in Veterinary Practice*, ed 2. Philadelphia, WB Saunders Co, 1984, pp 70–77.

Radiation Protection in Veterinary Hospitals

John Watters, DVM, MS
Veterinary Clinical Sciences
School of Veterinary Medicine
Louisiana State University
Baton Rouge, Louisiana

An awareness of the importance of radiation safety has come to the forefront in recent years and it is necessary that the veterinary profession be cognizant of the hazards of x-rays. Also, one must be practical when considering the quantity of shielding required in a veterinary hospital. Therefore it is necessary to know the levels of radiation present at various points adjacent to the x-ray room when the x-ray machine is activated. In addition, personnel monitoring by use of a film-badge service is absolutely essential.

A survey published in 1953 stated that of 134 practicing veterinarians, 19% did not use lead gloves and 20% did not use lead aprons. Of those performing fluoroscopy, 76% hand-held the patients and 52% used hand-held fluoroscopes. Lead-lined walls were thought to be necessary by 13% and 72% thought some type of lead shield was necessary.

If the same questionnaire was distributed now, the results might be very similar to those of 25 years ago. Many veterinarians have had little training in radiology and even fewer understand the relationship of x-ray energies, penetration and shielding requirements. Therefore, it is understandable that there is confusion as to when and why shielding or radiation protection is necessary.

The use of shielding has been discounted by some who say that veterinarians do not take enough radiographs to warrant its use. On the other hand some veterinarians have added excessive lead to the walls where additional shielding was not necessary. Some architects rely on the veterinarian to tell them how much shielding is required in the x-ray room, or they refer to values that have been established for busy human hospitals. The purpose of this paper is to present a typical veterinary x-ray facility and the expected radiation exposure to the personnel and to the areas adjacent to the x-ray room.

Radiation Units—The *roentgen* (R) is the unit of radiation used to express the radiation *exposure* at a given point in air or at the surface of an absorber, (mR = 1/1000R).

Radiation absorbed dose (RAD) is the unit used to indicate the quantity of radiation *absorbed* in tissue or other material.

Radiation Equivalent Man (REM) is the unit used by radiobiologists and health physicists to express the quantity of radiation that will produce a given biologic response regardless of the type of radiation.

Originally published in Volume 1, Number 6, June 1979

The REM dose is numerically equal to the absorbed dose (RAD) multiplied by a quality factor. For the radiation energies used in diagnostic radiology the RAD and REM can be considered equal. (mREM = 1/1000 REM).

Radiation Shielding—Most states have Radiation Control Agencies that spot-check x-ray facilities. Some agencies request that plans for hospitals be submitted for inspection prior to construction. It is the responsibility of these agencies to determine if the x-ray room shielding is adequate but they cannot give information as to the most economic means of accomplishing the necessary degree of protection.

In order to meet the minimum protection standards without investing in more shielding than is required, it is recommended that a qualified person be consulted prior to building or remodeling. It is best to discuss the floor plan and other information in detail with the consultant who must be furnished the following information, in addition to the floor plan:

1. Maximum KVP and mA of the x-ray machine.
2. Average number of exposures per week.
3. Average mA per exposure.
4. Location of the machine within the room.
5. Rotational capability of the tube head.
6. Percentage of time tube head will be in each position.
7. Wall material and thickness if not indicated on the floor plan.

The following example is presented to illustrate a typical shielding analysis for a busy veterinary facility that might be radiographing as many as 7 patients per day, 5 days per week with an average of 3 exposures per patient:

1. X-ray Machine
   a. KVP—125
   b. mA—300
   c. Total Filtration—3.0 mm Aluminum
2. Radiation Exposures
   a. Average number of exposures/week—100
   b. Average time/exposure—1/15 second
   c. Average mAs/exposure—20
   d. Number of exposures/week with beam in horizontal position—1
3. Construction Material
   a. Concrete block—density of 147 lb/ft^3
   b. Thickness of concrete in 4″ and 8″ blocks—2 inches
   c. Gypsum wallboard—3/8″ thick x 2

The following information is measured or calculated by the radiological physicist based on the above information.

1. Primary Beam Exposure—14mR/mAs at 91 cm
2. Scatter Exposure—0.01mR/mAs, 90° angle at 91 cm, 20 cm x 20 cm field.
3. Average Exposure Time/week—6.6 seconds (0.11 minutes)
4. mA-minutes/week—33
5. mR/week—25,600 at 1 meter

Calculation of shielding required for an x-ray room is based on the *workload* (W, mA-minutes), *use factor* (U, percentage of time the primary beam is pointed in a given direction), *occupancy factor* (T, the percentage of time a location might be occupied by personnel), and the *distance* from the x-ray machine to the point of interest (D, measured in meters). These factors are used to determine from available charts the barrier thickness (B) required at each point of interest.

Figure 1 illustrates an x-ray room with points of interest one foot beyond the walls. Exposure rates were calculated for these points. Table I lists the exposure dose at each point from the primary beam, scattered radiation, and the total exposure for the stated distances without considering attenuation by wall material. The actual doses without wall attenuation were calculated for each point in this case to illustrate the shielding provided by both types of wall materials. The radiation protection guide (RPG) specifies that for the hallway, darkroom, surgery and storage areas the exposure dose will not exceed 100 mREM per week because these are considered *controlled areas*. A controlled area is one that requires control of access, occupancy and working conditions for radiation protection purposes.

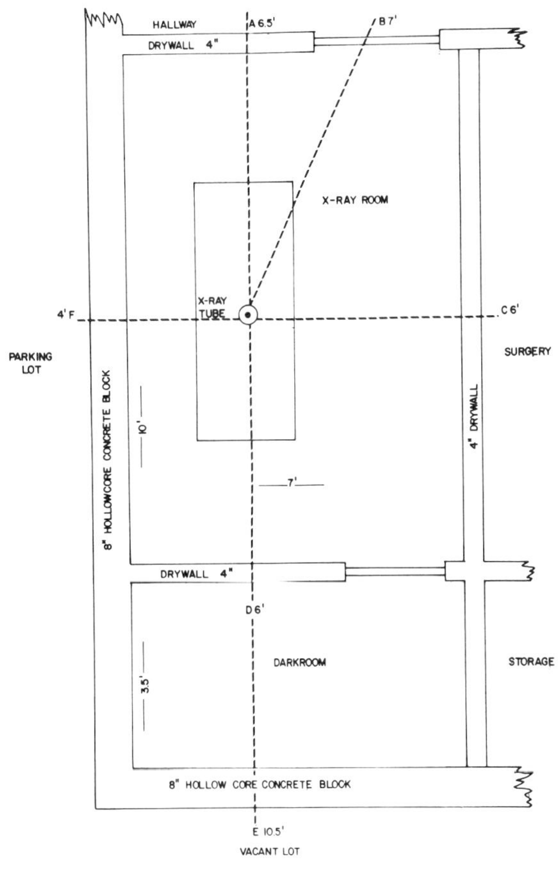

Fig 1

A vacant lot or parking lot are noncontrolled areas and the RPG specifies a maximum exposure of 10 mREM per week for these areas. A non-

TABLE I

CALCULATED RADIATION EXPOSURE AT SPECIFIC POINTS OUTSIDE THE X-RAY ROOM

Exposure Dose (mR/wk)

Location	Distance (meters)	*No Wall Shielding* Primary	Scattered	Total	*With Wall Shielding* Total
A	2.0	70	13	83	39
B	2.1	64	12	76	76
C	1.8	—	14	14	7
D	1.8	86	14	100	47
E	3.2	27	8	35	4
F	1.2	—	21	21	3

controlled area is one that requires no control of access, occupancy or working conditions and therefore is accessable to the general public.

The calculations for this case were based on all exposures being made at 125 KVP and 20 mAs, representing the highest radiation energy possible with the available x-ray machine. Even under these extreme conditions the room would be adequate without any additional shielding. Points A, B and D are higher radiation areas based on the assumption that horizontal radiography would be performed one percent of the total exposure time and the tube would be directed at either point A or D.

The exposure levels in the darkroom would be 47 mR/wk if the horizontal beam (HB) was directed towards point D. Therefore, it would be recommended that the HB exposures be directed toward point A, which would reduce the darkroom exposure to 7mREM/week. This radiation level in the darkroom would produce a film-fog density of 0.5 optical density units in 4 weeks with maximum exposure techniques of 125 KVP and 20 mAs. With a nominal technique of 75 KVP and 20 mAs the film could be stored for 10 weeks before accumulating a film density of 0.5 optical density units which is about twice that of the normal fog value. It is recommended that extra film be stored in another room or in a lead-lined box because any extra fog will reduce the diagnostic quality of radiographs.

Radiation Exposure—Another consideration is exposure of personnel who are positioning and holding patients during radiographic procedures. Table II lists the *maximum permissible dose* (MPD) for certain areas of the body over given periods of time.[2] It can be seen from the table that the whole body (blood forming organs), gonads and the lens of the eyes are the most sensitive organs and the radiation to those tissues should be limited to 3 REM/quarter. The limits for shorter periods of time are no more than 2 mREM/hour or 100 mREM/week. It is also important that no one under 18 years of age be occupationally exposed. The maximum permissible accumulated dose for an individual is 5 REM x (Age-18 yrs.).

Table III lists the radiation doses which one could be exposed to under the given conditions of: 75 KVP, 30 mAs, a focus-to-film distance (FFD) of 90 cm, 3 mm of aluminum filtration, 20 x 20 cm exposure field and 100 exposures per week. The shielding for the hands and body is considered to be gloves and aprons containing the equivalent of 0.5 mm of lead. Less expensive protective clothing is available which has 0.25 mm of lead. If the less expensive items are used, then the shielded weekly exposure doses in Table III should be doubled.

If the distance of the hands to the primary beam is reduced then the exposure dose from scatter will be much higher; for example, if the hands are located 5 cm from the beam the dose will be 1120

TABLE II

MAXIMUM PERMISSIBLE DOSE FOR OCCUPATIONALLY EXPOSED PERSONNEL

Type of Exposure	*REMS/Week*	*REMS/Quarter*	*REMS/Year*
Whole Body, Gonads Lens of the Eyes	0.1	3	5
Skin of the Whole Body	*	10	30
Extremities	1.5	25	75

*No weekly guidelines are specified in tables.

TABLE III

EXPOSURE OF BODY PARTS (MR/WK) FOR 75 KVP, 30 MAS, FFD OF 90 CM, 3MM ALUMINUM FILTRATION, 20 x 20 CM EXPOSURE FIELD, 100 EXPOSURES PER WEEK. LEAD EQUIVALENT SHIELDING OF 0.5MM IN GLOVES AND APRON.

	Hands		*Eyes*	*Sternum*	*Gonads*
	In Beam	10 cm From Beam	35 cm	45 cm	50 cm
Unshielded	15,000	1,240	35	50	61
Shielded	3,400	280	—	11	14

MR/wk instead of 280 MR/wk at 10 cm because the dose is inversely proportional to the square of the distance. A dose of 15 REM to the hands is 10 times the weekly MPD as listed in Table II, and is more than twice the MPD even if the hands are protected by gloves. This should stress the point that the hands should never be exposed to the primary beam even with gloves. The dose to bare hands 10 cm from the beam is approaching the weekly MPD of 1.5 REM. The sternum and gonads would receive approximately one half of the weekly MPD without any lead shielding and about 10% of the MPD if a lead apron was worn during all radiographic procedures.

The next important exposure dose is that to the eyes. If the eyes are at a distance of 35 cm from the point where the beam strikes the patient as proposed in the example, then that is no problem; but if the holder's eyes are only 15 cm from the point then the dose would be 190 MR/wk which is almost twice the recommended permissable dose.

Radiation exposure can be greatly reduced by wearing eyeglasses. Protective glasses are commercially available which will reduce the radiation exposure to approximately 2% at a 65 KVP energy level. However, these glasses cost approximately $50 to $200 depending on the type of glass and style configuration. Photochromic glasses which change color with changes in light intensity will reduce x-ray transmission to about 23% of the incident radiation, whereas plain eyeglasses reduce the exposure only to about 47%.

Personnel Exposure—While it is important to know what the theoretical exposure is to the various body parts, it is essential to know what is the absorbed dose for the personnel who are holding the patients during radiography. All individuals in a practice who may be responsible for positioning patients or who are working adjacent to the x-ray equipment should be monitored with film badges. Several firms provide this service at a cost of about $2 to $3 per month per film badge. Information as to the availability of such a service can be gained from the local hospital administrator or radiological technologist in the area. The veterinary employer is legally responsible for providing this monitoring service. Details are available in the NCRP Report, no. 36.

REFERENCES

1. Radiation protection in veterinary medicine, NCRP Report No. 36, National Council on Radiation Protection and Measurements, Washington, D.C., 20008.
2. National Bureau of Standards, Handbook No. 59 with addendum of April 15, 1958. National Bureau of Standards Washington, D.C., 20008.

X-ray Production

John W. Watters, DVM, MS
Associate Professor of Radiology
School of Veterinary Medicine
Louisiana State University
Baton Rouge, Louisiana

Radiology is an important tool in the diagnosis, prognosis, and follow-up of many cases. However, the tool loses its usefulness if good-quality radiographs are unobtainable. The purpose of this series of articles on radiology is to present the basic information necessary for the veterinarian to understand how to produce high-quality radiographs. Once he has this understanding, he must attempt to get the most information possible from a radiographic examination. It is also important that he understand the functioning of the equipment so that proper adjustments can be made to achieve the desired end product.

X-ray Production

The basic components necessary for x-ray production are (1) an x-ray tube, (2) a step-up transformer for high-voltage potential, (3) a step-down transformer for filament current and (4) an on-off switch. Other essentials are control devices that permit regulation of the high-voltage (kilovoltage peak [kVp]), tube current (milliamperes [mA]), and time (seconds).

X-rays are a type of electromagnetic radiation that has no charge and no mass and that travels at the speed of light. The energy of x-rays in the diagnostic range extends from 12.4 kiloelectron volts (keV) to 124 keV. An electron volt represents the energy possessed by an electron traveling through a potential of 1 volt. kVp is a unit of measurement of the peak voltage applied to the x-ray tube; it should not be confused with keV. *Kilovoltage (kV)* is the term used with x-ray machines that operate with constant voltage applied to the tube rather than fluctuating voltage.

Figure 1 is an illustration of the basic components of an x-ray tube. The filament must be heated by current from the step-down transformer. The heat in the filament causes a cloud of free electrons to form around the tungsten filament. The electrons are drawn to the anode side of the tube when high voltage from the step-up transformer is applied across the tube. The number of filament electrons available and thus the number of x-rays produced is controlled by the mA knob on the control panel. The kVp knob controls the voltage potential applied to the tube. As kVp increases, the speed with which the electrons are drawn to the target (anode) and thus the energy of the x-rays produced,

Originally published in Volume 3, Number 2, February 1981

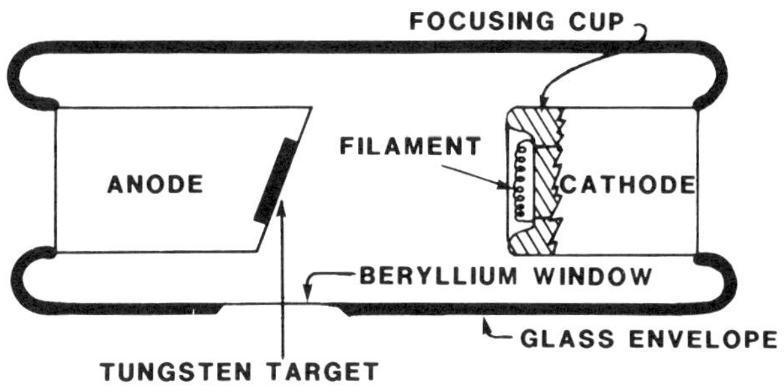

Figure 1—Components of a stationary anode x-ray tube.

increases. The number of x-rays produced also increases as the kVp is raised, because more energetic electrons have more interactions with the target material, producing more x-rays. However, kVp affects the x-ray energy more than the number of x-rays produced.

Two types of tubes used in diagnostic radiography are stationary anode tubes and rotating anode tubes. Figure 1 is an illustration of a stationary anode tube in which the electrons bombard an area of the target that corresponds to the filament size. The electrons are focused electronically by the focusing cup which has the same negative charge as the electrons. The glass housing of the tube is evacuated of gas; this can cause reduction in electron speed between the cathode and anode.

The rotating-anode tube (Fig 2) has an anode that rotates at 3000 to 3600 RPM. The rotating action provides a large area over which the electron bombardment can occur. The advantage of a large striking surface is better heat distribution, which prolongs tube life and the utilization of higher voltage and current.

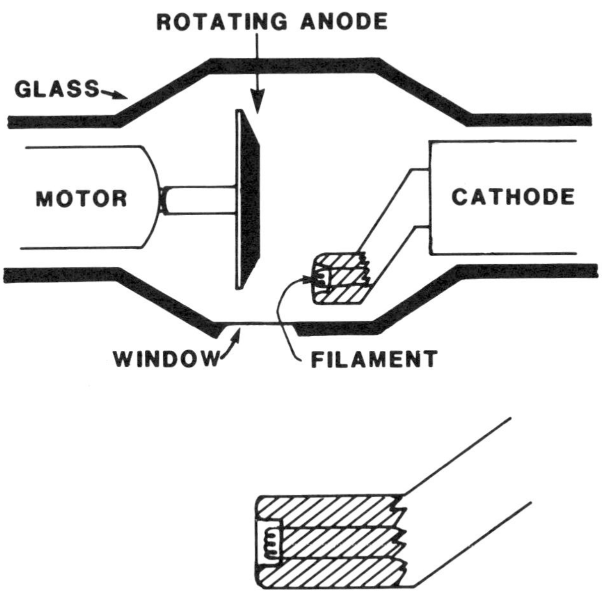

Figure 2—Components of a rotating-anode x-ray tube.

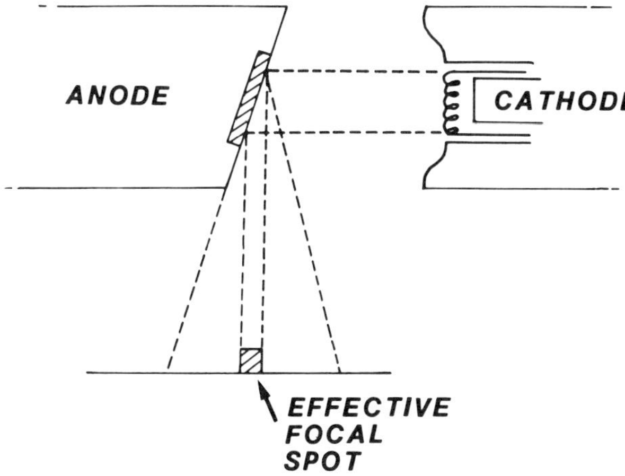

Figure 3—Effective focal spot from a 20° stationary anode.

Focal Spot

The best detail is achieved with a small focal spot. The *effective* focal spot size is controlled by filament size and anode angle. The width of the spot is determined by the filament width, and the effective spot length is determined by the anode angle and the filament length. Some tubes have two or three filaments for variable spot control. The effective spot size of 2 × 2 mm in Fig 3 is produced by a 20° anode and a filament that measures 2 × 5.5 mm.

The distribution of x-rays is not uniform from the anode side to the cathode side of the tube. Figure 4 illustrates that a larger percentage of x-rays is emitted on the cathode side of the tube than on the anode side. This characteristic is referred to as the *heel effect.* The effect is negligible when using film sizes smaller than 14 x 17 inches and with

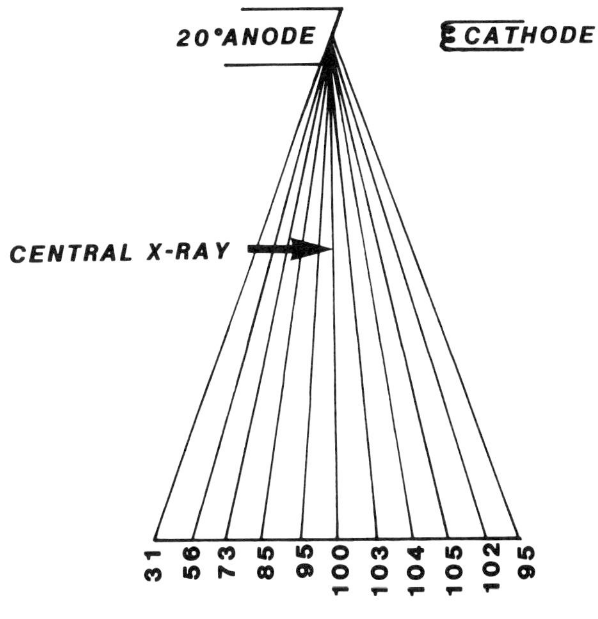

Figure 4—Heel effect. There is a reduced number of x-rays on the anode side of the tube.

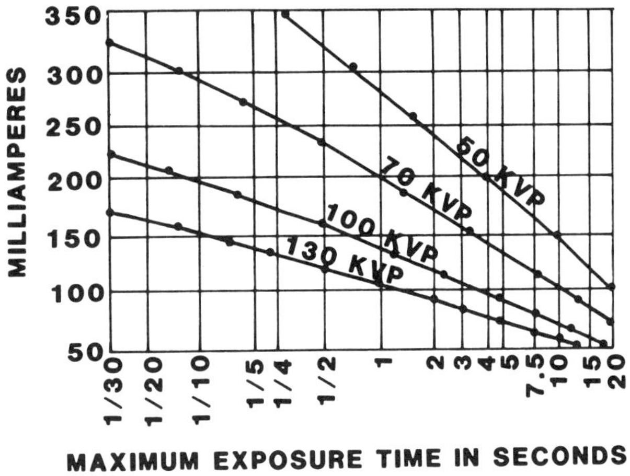

Figure 5—Tube-rating chart to illustrate maximum permissible exposure techniques.

anode angles greater than 15°. However, it can be used to advantage when radiographing the chest and abdomen of a large patient.

Thermal Buildup

A great deal of heat is generated in the x-ray tube and tube housing during the production of x-rays. Only 1% of the electron energy results in the production of useful x-rays—the remainder is converted to heat. Most tubes are surrounded with oil in the tube housing, and this helps to dissipate the heat buildup during x-ray production.

Manufacturers provide tube-rating charts that indicate the safe working limits for each tube type; these should be closely followed. Each tube-rating chart is for one tube type only; therefore the charts cannot be used interchangeably. Figure 5 is a tube-rating chart for a single-phase, full-wave rectified machine with an effective focal spot size of 1 mm. From this chart it can be determined that, using a tube with 100 kVp and 200 mAs, ⅒ second is the longest exposure that can be safely made.

Another factor that must be considered when making multiple exposures is the maximum heat-storage capacity of the tube. For example, the thermal rating for a tube might be 100,000 heat units (HU). kVp × mA × seconds = HU; thus, 70 kVp, 200 mA, ⅒ second = 1400 HU/exposure. In such a case, 70 exposures (70 × 1,400 = 98,000) could be made in a short period of time, whereas only seven exposures should be made with 70 kVp, 200 mA, 1 second (14,000 HU).

Damage to the anode can result from using high kVp and mA exposures with a cold anode. Therefore, it is advisable to warm the tube up prior to placing heavy loads on it. A typical warm-up procedure for a 300 mA machine is to make a 2-second exposure at 70 kVp and 200 mA. Then two more exposures should be made with a 5-second interval between them. This procedure will only keep the tube warmed up for about 30 minutes. The procedure is not necessary if the use of the machine will be less than the warm-up procedure.

Pulse Rectification

X-ray machines can be classified as having circuits that are self-rectified, half-wave rectified, or full-wave rectified. This classification refers to the manner in which the 60 cycle/second (Hz) alternating current is electronically conditioned on its way to the x-ray tube. Machines are also classified as being single phase, three-phase, constant potential, or capacitive discharge. The majority of veterinary machines use 60 Hz, single-phase current. This is generated as one cycle of electricity 60 times per second. In self-rectified machines, this results in x-rays being produced only during the positive half of each cycle when the current flow is from the cathode to the anode (Fig 6). During the negative half of the cycle, electrons from a hot anode can be attracted toward the cathode, and this reduces the filament life. This undesired alternating current flow is called *self-rectification.* Effects of the negative cycle can be prevented by the use of rectifying diodes, sometimes called *valve tubes,* that stop negative current flow. This is termed *half-wave rectification.* Additional circuitry modifications can be made that not only stop the negative part of the cycle but invert and direct it to the cathode so that two pulses of x-rays can be produced during each cycle. This is full-wave rectification with 120 pulses/second (Fig 6, *bottom*). If the machine is set up for three-phase electricity and the power company can supply it, 360 pulses/second are produced with full-wave rectification. Constant-potential x-ray machines have direct current (DC) applied to the tube, and the voltage to the tube is expressed in kilovolts since

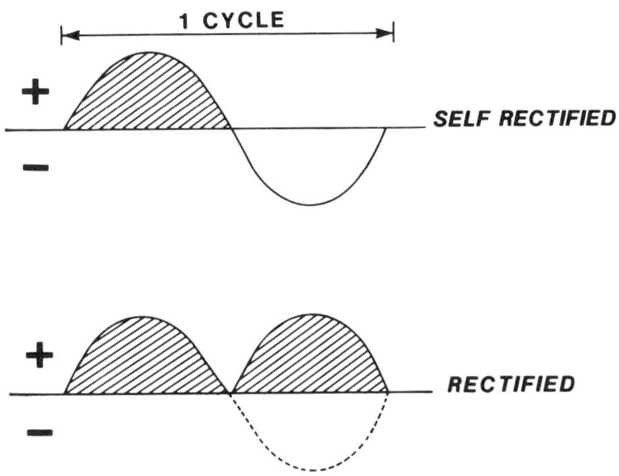

Figure 6—Self-rectified electrical cycle illustrating x-ray production during the positive half of the cycle (*top*). Full-wave rectified cycle illustrating production of two x-ray pulses/cycle (*bottom*).

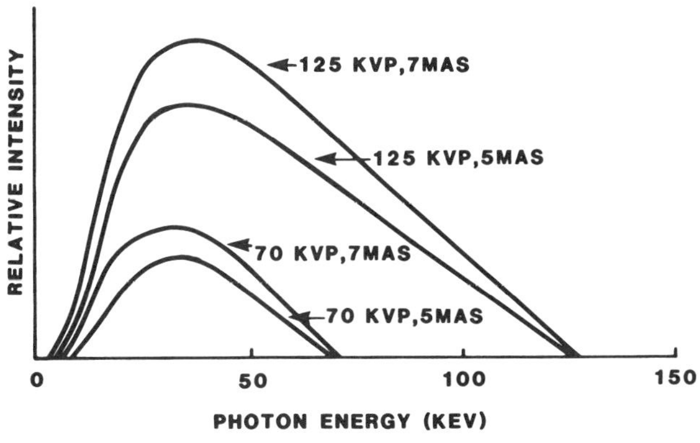

Figure 7—Relative x-ray production with two different kVp and mAs settings.

there is no kVp. Machines are manufactured that use large capacitors to produce DC power to the tube when the switch is closed. These machines can produce one exposure even without being plugged in, because the energy has been stored in the capacitors.

X-ray Spectrum

The individual x-rays produced during an exposure are not all of the same energy; there is a spectrum ranging from low energy (long wavelength) to high energy (short wavelength). The proportion of high-energy x-rays in the spectrum increases as the kVp is increased. A larger number of x-rays is produced as the mAs is increased, but the relative proportion of x-ray energies remains the same. Therefore, the kVp controls the *penetration quality* of the x-ray beam and the mAs controls the *number* of x-rays produced. Figure 7 is an illustration of the photon energy spectra produced with 70 kVp, 5 mAs compared to 70 kVp, 7 mAs and 125 kVp, 5 mAs compared to 125 kVp, 7mAs.

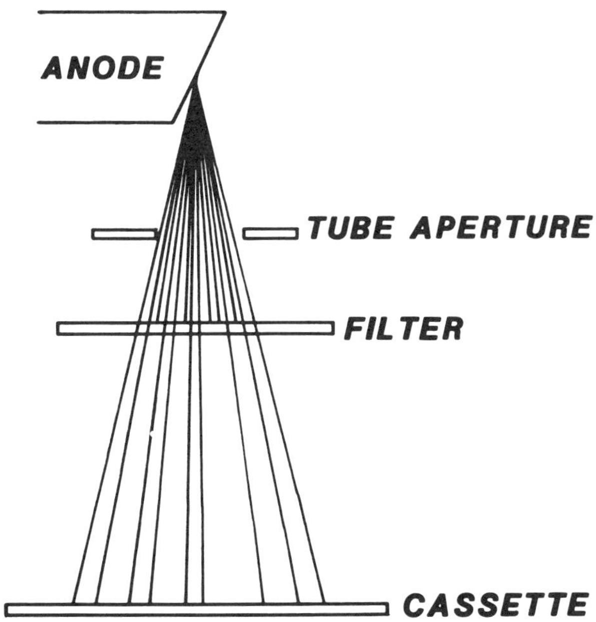

Figure 8—Soft x-rays absorbed by the aluminum filter.

Low-energy x-rays (soft radiation) are not useful for diagnostic radiography but do contribute to patient and personnel exposure. Therefore, the soft component of the beam is filtered out, as illustrated in Fig 8. All x-ray machines are required by law to have a certain amount of beam filtration, the amount depending on the maximum kVp. Some machines also have a removable filter that permits variation of the beam *hardness* by adding more aluminum (this is in addition to the required filtration).

Beam Collimation

Since x-rays are emitted in all directions from the anode, it is necessary that the tube housing be shielded to prevent excessive radiation of personnel. The x-ray beam is directed to the desired location through an aperture in the tube housing. The x-rays coming through the aperture are shaped to a given dimension by a beam-limiting device. This can be accomplished with a cylindrical cone or with a diaphragm type of collimation that has variability of size and shape. A collimator, as shown in Fig 9, permits variation of the beam size and shape by means of lead *blades* that are moved closer together or further apart. Cones or cylindrical devices (Fig 10) form a circular pattern, and the field size can be changed by varying the cone-to-film distance. Some cylindrical cones are telescopic, and this permits the end of the cone to be positioned closer to the film without moving the tube head.

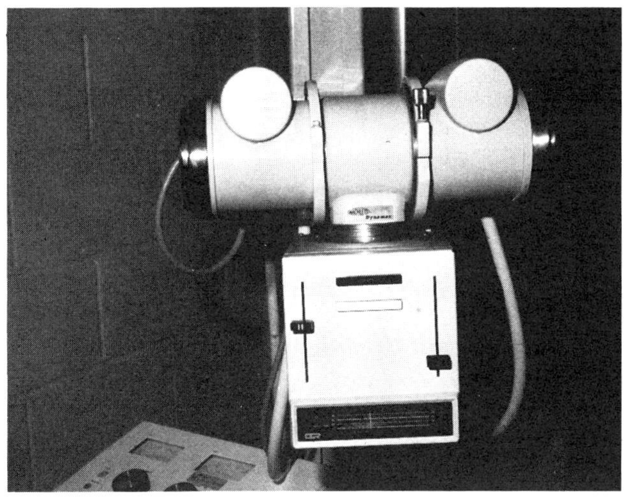

Figure 9—Adjustable diaphragm-type collimator.

Sheet-lead apertures are available with square, circular, and rectangular patterns of various sizes. They must be used with special cones that have a slot for insertion of the aperture. Some of the older

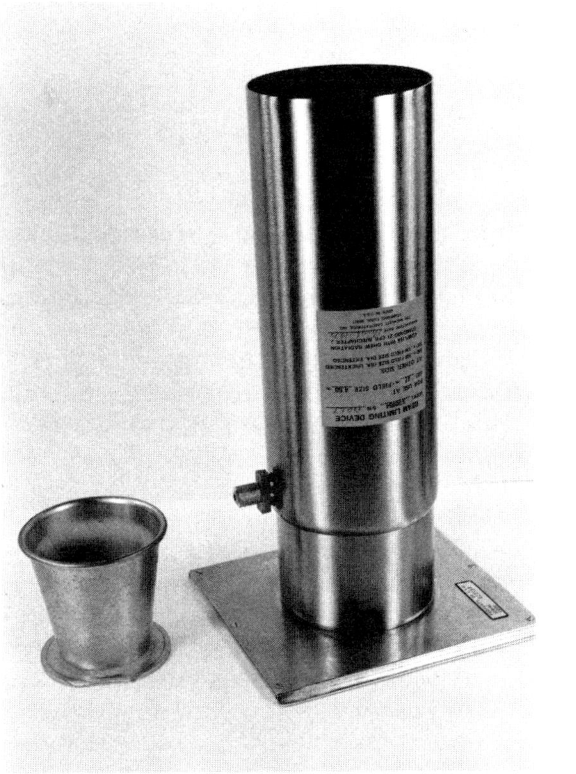

Figure 10—Flared-cone attachment (*left*), and extendable type of cylindrical cone (*right*).

machines have wide-flared cones which should be modified to accept fixed-size apertures to meet federal and state safety standards.

X-rays follow the same laws that govern visible light rays. The photon intensity (number of x-rays) increases as the distance to the source decreases. This is an inverse square relationship, meaning that the intensity will increase by four times if the distance is reduced by one-half. If a proper radiographic density is produced at 36 inches, the film will be overexposed by four times if the distance is reduced to 18 inches. The formula for this calculation is

$$\frac{In}{Io} = \frac{18^2}{36^2} \qquad In = \frac{Io}{0.25}$$

where I_n = new intensity and I_o = original intensity.

Timers

A timing device is necessary to control the duration of an x-ray exposure. Most of the old machines have mechanical, spring-loaded timers. These are not very accurate as to the exact time of exposure but are fairly reproducible when functioning properly and when used carefully. Most of the mechanical timers have minimum settings of 1/10 or 1/4 second, but some can be set at one or two *clicks* below that. Modern x-ray machines have timers that are electronically controlled and that can be set as low as 1/1000 second.

Rotating anodes must be brought up to speed prior to the exposure. The lag time between activation of the timer and the beginning of the exposure can be 0.5 to 1.0 second. This delay can be a problem when trying to obtain an inspiratory radiograph of the thorax. A *boost* switch incorporated in the exposure switch may be of help. With this mechanism, the rotating anode can be started prior to the exposure. The boost switch should not be kept on longer than necessary because the filament is maintained at full current while in the boost mode, and this will shorten the tube life.

REFERENCES

1. Goodwin PN, Quimby EH, Morgan RH: *Physical Foundations of Radiology*, ed 4. New York, Harper & Row, 1970.
2. Johns HE, Cunningham JR: *The Physics of Radiology*, ed 3. Springfield, IL, Charles C Thomas, 1969.
3. *Radiological Health Handbook*, revised ed. Rockville, MD, USDA, PHS, US Government Printing Office, 1970.
4. *Technical Data Bulletin, Dynamax 42-40*. Stamford, CN, the Machlett Laboratories, Inc, 1978.
5. *The Fundamentals of Radiography*, ed 11. Rochester, NY, Eastman Kodak Co, 1968.
6. Ticer JW: *Radiographic Technique in Small Animal Practice*. Philadelphia, WB Saunders Co, 1975.

The Radiographic Darkroom and Film Processing

John W. Watters, DVM, MS
Associate Professor of Radiology
School of Veterinary Medicine
Louisiana State University
Baton Rouge, Louisiana

Achieving quality radiographs requires not only a good x-ray machine but proper darkroom and film-processing techniques. Potentially good radiographs can be reduced to nondiagnostic quality by improper processing techniques. As much attention should be given to processing and handling of radiographs as that given to techniques of film exposure. A very high percentage of radiographic artifacts are caused in the darkroom.

The Darkroom

The following basic principles concerning the darkroom should be considered when remodeling or building a new facility. The darkroom must be lighttight and located near the x-ray room, especially if a film transfer box is to be used to store cassettes. Electrical outlets should be installed for safelights, illuminators, and a film drying cabinet. Additional outlets and water supply should be included in the plans if an automatic processor is to be installed at a later date. In addition to being lighttight for film handling and processing, there must also be a white light to illuminate the room for making repairs, changing solutions, and cleaning. Although some recommend that the inside of the darkroom be painted black, visibility is greatly improved if the walls and ceiling are painted white. Reflection of the safelight from the white walls and ceiling is not detrimental to handling and processing x-ray film. Giving counter tops a light-colored finish is also helpful for visibility.

The layout of a darkroom should be based on the necessity of having a dry area separated from a wet area (Figure 1). The room should probably be at least 6 × 8 ft to allow this separation. The dry side of the room has places for film and hanger storage and a counter top on which to load and unload cassettes and is where film is inserted and removed from the hangers. Film hangers can be stored on boards extending from the wall beneath the dry counter (Figure 2). Storage of hangers above the dry counter is discouraged because of possible film and intensifying-screen damage if a hanger falls from an upper rack. If a photoflashing film identification system is used, it too should be on the counter on the dry side of the room. The wet side of the room should accommodate processing tanks (Figure 3), a drip counter, drying racks, and a drying cabinet. The drying cabinet can be located outside the darkroom if desired; this will also reduce excess heat buildup in the darkroom. If drip drying rather than a drying cabinet is used, it is necessary to have a catch pan beneath the drying rack.

Originally published in Volume 4, Number 4, April 1982

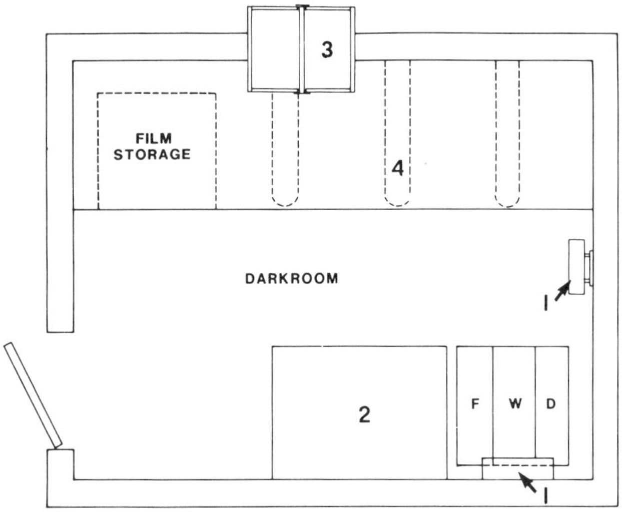

Figure 1—Floor plan of a darkroom illustrating the separation of wet (*bottom*) and dry (*top*) areas. *F* = fixer, *W* = water, *D* = developer (processing tanks); *1* = safelights; *2* = hot-air dryer; *3* = film transfer box; and *4* (*dotted lines* beneath the dry-counter top) = under-the-counter hanger racks.

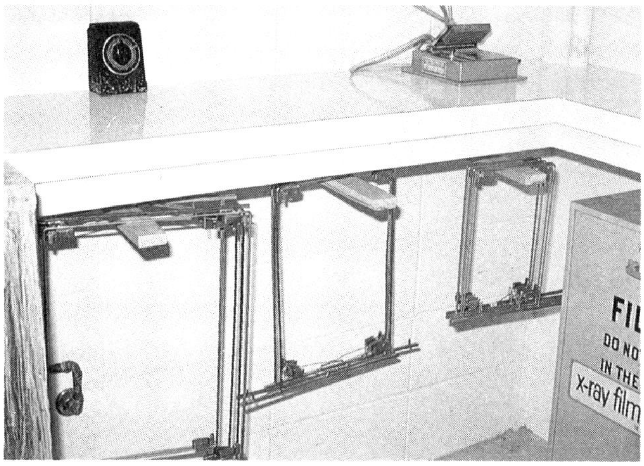

Figure 2—Film-hanger storage beneath the counter top. A film identification photoflasher and a spring-loaded timer on the working surface. (Courtesy of the Jefferson Animal Hospital, Baton Route, LA)

It is usually not necessary to have additional shielding in the walls of the darkroom, even when it is adjacent to the x-ray room, because in most situations the personnel responsible for processing the films are also the ones helping to restrain the patients during radiography. (However, some states have laws forbidding manual restraint of patients during radiography.) The average weekly dose rate from scatter radiation at a distance of 5 ft and with a workload of 62.5 milliamperage-minutes/week (approximately twice that expected in a very busy veterinary practice) at 100 kVp does not require any shielding according to NCRP Report No. 36.[1] However, consideration should be given to shielding film in the darkroom to prevent film fogging. This can be accomplished by using a steel film storage cabinet, a lead-lined cassette transfer box, a mobile lead-lined cassette storage box, or a storage box lined with lead purchased from a plumbing supply company. When using a film storage cabinet, the tops of the x-ray film boxes should be kept in place to prevent film fogging if the storage cabinet is accidentally opened while the room lights are on or the darkroom door is open. It is recommended that unopened boxes of film be stored in a refrigerator to extend their shelf life; film fog can be produced by high ambient temperature and chemical fumes in the darkroom. To prevent the formation of condensation on the film, boxes stored in a refrigerator should be removed at least 12 hours prior to being opened.

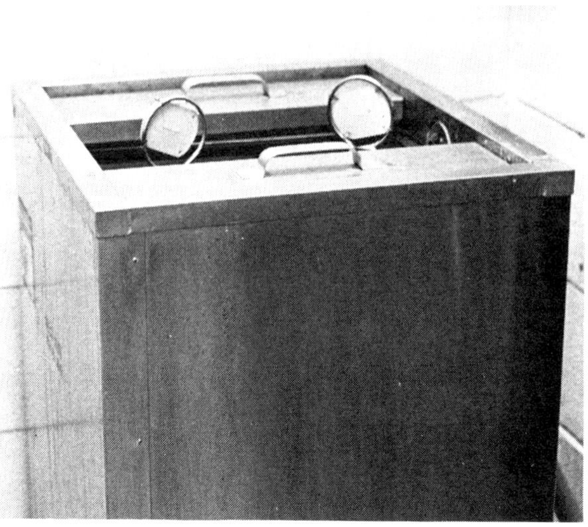

Figure 3—Photograph of a portion of a darkroom showing processing tank with stirring rods.

Darkroom safelights with 15-watt bulbs should not be closer than 4 ft to the surface where film is handled.[2] Overhead safelights and ceiling white lights are recommended. The use of indirect lighting (Figure 4), light directed away from the processing tanks, is also beneficial. A combination illuminator and safelight is useful over the tank areas. Safelights are only safe if the proper filter is used for the type of film being handled and processed. A Wratten series 6B filter should be used with blue-sensitive film. One should consult the film manufacturer's information sheet (packed with the film) for filters to be used with other types of film such as orthochromatic (*rare-earth*) film. Some rare-earth systems require film that is primarily sensitive to blue and ultraviolet light; film sensitive to blue, green, and ultraviolet light can be used with other rare-earth systems. The light fixture and filter should be closely examined for leaks and cracks. A 15-watt bulb can be used safely if the recommended distance (4 ft) to the film surface is maintained. Blue-sensitive film can be safely handled and processed with filters that are safe for green-light–sensitive film.[a]

There is a new type of safelight available that uses a special fluorescent tube with a filter which fits over the tube and has seals at each end to prevent unfiltered light from escaping into the darkroom. These are somewhat

[a]Kodak GBX filter, Eastman Kodak Co., Rochester, NY 14650.

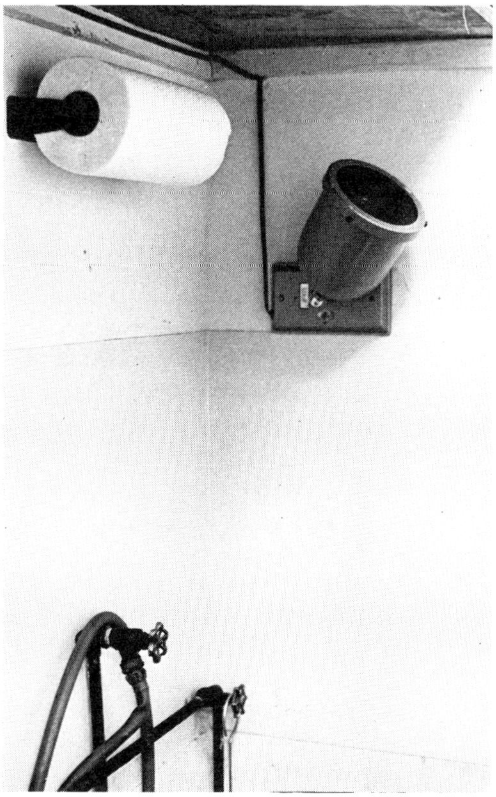

Figure 4—A safelight used for indirect lighting over the processing tanks.

more expensive than the conventional types, but they provide a wider distribution of light.

The effect of safelight illumination and possible light leaks can be checked by using the following procedure.

1. One-half of a loaded cassette is exposed to 5 mAs and 40 kVp at 40 in. with two magazines on top of the cassette to absorb some of the soft x-rays. This will sensitize the film and result in film that has received a normal diagnostic exposure.
2. All lights in the darkroom are turned off.
3. The film is removed from the cassette and placed on the dry work counter.
4. All except 1 in. of the film is covered with a piece of black cardboard (cut from the inside of a film box).
5. The safelights are turned on.
6. The cardboard cover is moved to expose approximately 1 in. of the film every minute for a total of seven times.
7. The safelights are turned off and the film is processed in total darkness.
8. The film is dried.
9. Step 6 is repeated with the safelights off to check for darkroom light leaks.

Figure 5 is an illustration of a film used during a safelight and darkroom light leak test. It can be seen that fogging was produced when the unprotected part of the film was exposed for as little as one minute. It was determined that the film fog was produced by darkroom

Figure 5—Radiograph made during a darkroom safelight test. The *left* portion of the film was preexposed to a low dose of radiation to hypersensitize the film. The *right* side was not exposed to x-irradiation. A piece of black cardboard was used to cover all of the film except for the narrow strip at the top of the film (7). Additional strips of film were uncovered at one-minute intervals and exposed to darkroom safelights for a total of seven minutes. The top strip therefore received seven minutes of exposure and the bottom portion of the film was totally protected from the safelights. There is an increased film density even at the one-minute exposure time.

light leaks because similar results were obtained when the test was repeated with the safelights turned off. Another test was performed with the safelights on after the light leaks around the door had been sealed; the film did not have any fog (above background) after seven minutes of exposure.

If the safelights are producing film fog, it is important to check for cracked filters, oversized bulbs, leaks around the filter and bulb housing, leaks around the filter, old filters that have faded with time, and the distance from the safelight to the work surface. It is necessary to become adapted to the dark to adequately check for safelight and darkroom light leaks. Adaptation requires staying in the darkroom for 15 to 20 minutes to allow for the buildup of rhodopsin (visual purple) in the retinal rods.

Other items that should be in the darkroom include a timer, a thermometer, and an illuminator for viewing wet radiographs. Illuminators used in the darkroom should have incandescent bulbs, because fluorescent bulbs can have an afterglow for a short time after they are turned off and this can produce film fog. It is also important that the illuminator be corrosion resistant and specially wired to prevent electrical shock. Installing a foot switch for the illuminator can avoid having to place a wet hand on the electrical switch, but care must be taken not to accidentally step on the switch while handling and processing film.

Another important item is a paper towel dispenser. A terry cloth towel can be used, but it should be replaced daily to prevent contamination of the hands. Hands should be clean and thoroughly dry prior to handling exposed or unexposed film to prevent fingerprint artifacts.

Processing Chemicals

X-rays and light exposure from the intensifying screens form a latent image on the film. This is produced by small physical changes in the silver halide (usually silver bromide) crystals which make them developable. When this film is placed in the developer solution the silver halide crystals that have been exposed are converted to metallic silver grains. The developer does not react with normal silver halide crystals that have not been exposed if the proper developing time is used. Developer solution (usually a compound of hydroquinone) also contains accelerators (sodium or potassium carbonate and sodium or potassium hydroxide), preservatives (sodium or potassium sulfite) to reduce oxidation, and restrainers (potassium bromide and potassium iodide) to prevent development of unexposed silver halide crystals.

Developing solution becomes exhausted through the process of converting silver halide to metallic silver. The alkaline solution is slowly neutralized and the released bromide ions have a restraining action on development. Developer oxidizes and becomes weak even when no films are processed. Therefore, the tanks should be covered when not in use. Some developer adheres to the film and hanger when they are transferred from the developer tank to the wash compartment, and thus developer volume becomes reduced. There is also a small amount lost as a result of evaporation. The level and activity of the solution must be maintained if adequate film development is to be achieved. This should be done with a replenishment solution. Water should never be used to maintain the proper fluid level because it reduces the developer activity. Replenisher can be purchased ready-made or as chemicals that can be compounded according to the manufacturer's directions, which are supplied with the chemicals. The replenisher solution is stronger than the original developer solutions. The term *seasoned* is used to describe a developer that has been in use for a while. Original solution is artificially seasoned by use of a restrainer in freshly mixed developer, but restrainers are not incorporated in replenisher solutions. Radiographs will be underdeveloped and will appear underexposed if proper replenishment is not maintained. It is economically not wise to adjust the exposure variables to offset inadequate development; it is difficult and time-consuming to attempt to incrementally increase the developing time to increase film density, and this procedure affects film quality by altering contrast and film speed.

The emulsion of developed film contains silver halide crystals which must be removed to produce the clear portion of the radiograph. Clearing is one of the actions of the fixer solution. In addition to clearing agents (sodium or ammonium thiosulfate), the fixer contains a hardener (an aluminum salt) which prevents excessive swelling of the gelatin during washing and allows faster drying of the films; a preservative (sodium sulfite) to retard decomposition of the fixer solution; acidifiers (acetic acid) to maintain proper chemical action; and buffer compounds to stabilize the acidity of the solution against the addition of alkaline developer that occurs when films are transferred from the developer tank. Some buffers also help to reduce sludge formation in the fixer tank.[3]

The fixer tank level does not lower as rapidly as that of the developer tank because some water is carried into the fixer solution on the film and hanger from the wash tank. Therefore, the fixer is being constantly diluted as well as being exhausted by chemical activity. Replenishment of the fixer often requires that some of the solution be removed so there will be room to add replenisher. The volume to remove is approximately the same as that used to replenish the developer tank. Replenishment can be accomplished by using the same concentration of fixer that was used for the original solution. Maintaining fixer concentration allows maximum fixing in a minimal period of time.

Processing chemicals are toxic hazards and should be handled with caution and preferably mixed in a room that has good ventilation. It is also recommended that the darkroom be vented to prevent the accumulation of toxic fumes.

The recommended frequency for changing developer and fixer depends on many variables: the number and size of films processed, film density, amount of replenisher added, evaporation, and the age of the solutions. The tanks should be covered when not in use to prevent or reduce evaporation and oxidation. The chemicals undergo chemical decay with time even when no films are being processed. A rule of thumb is to replace the solutions each month, but this can be extended to once every two months if the number of films processed is sufficient to require daily replenishment of solutions. Under no circumstances should the solutions be used for more than three months, because of the accumulation of sludge, gelatin, and impurities as well as aerial oxidation. Film quality cannot be maintained with exhausted and contaminated solutions. It is advisable that a chart be kept in the darkroom on which to record the dates when the solutions are changed. It is easy to lose track of the age of the solutions if a record of the changing dates is not kept. The tanks should be thoroughly drained and cleaned prior to refilling with new solutions. It is not recommended that any "economic additives" be used in an effort to extend the life of the solutions because they usually do not produce good results.

Film Processing

Prior to processing film, the developer and fixer solutions should be stirred (with separate paddles) and the water temperature should be checked. Floating thermometers can be left in the wash water, but these can interfere with film processing. Most medical x-ray film is recommended to be developed at 20°C (68°F) for five minutes.

If temperature control is not maintained with water-temperature mixing valves or refrigeration units, a time-temperature chart should be available. It is suggested that the temperature be checked daily with a reliable thermometer even if temperature control devices are used. The film information brochure should be checked for proper developing times. Development time-temperature relationships for x-ray film intended for ideal temperature development at 20°C (68°F) are shown in Table I. It can be seen from the table that a change of one degree requires a change in development time of approximately 0.5 minute in the lower temperature range and about 0.25 minute in the upper range. The author has found that XL film,[b] which is recommended to be developed for 7 minutes at 21°C (70°F), can be developed for 3 minutes at 26°C (80°F), which is the temperature of tap water in the author's facility.

Development time should be measured with an accurate timer, because errors in estimated times are easy to make and can produce serious reduction in radiographic quality. If the time-temperature relationship is not adhered to, it is difficult to determine whether certain film artifacts are due to darkroom error or x-ray machine malfunction. Therefore, the inspection technique or *sight developing* is highly discouraged.

Before turning the white lights off and the safelights on, it is advisable to check the work surface to be sure it is clean and dry. After the white lights are turned off, the cassette is opened and the film is gently removed, with care taken not to damage the intensifying screens. One way of doing this is to place a finger on the inside of the back cover of the cassette and turn the cassette upside down, allowing the film to fall against the finger. The tube side of the cassette is then opened and the film is removed. The cassette should be closed to prevent accidental damage to the screens. Only the outermost edges of the film should be touched and care should be taken not to bend the film while it is being removed from the cassette or placed into the hanger. With the film hanging in a vertical plane, the corners of the film are secured by the bottom hanger clips. The clips should perforate the film edge. The film and hanger are inverted while the top of the film is held in the same plane as the hanger. The spring clips are then placed on the remaining corners (Figure 6). If more than one film is to be processed, the film and hanger of each should be placed in an upright position leaning against the wall until all films are ready to be put in the developer. The timer is then set for the proper time and all of the loaded hangers are placed into the developer and spaced so the films are not touching. The timer is started after all films are in the developer tank. The hangers are raised and lowered several times to remove the air bells (bubbles) from the film surface. The raising and lowering process is repeated once every minute. It is important that rapid-process film not be agitated in the developer solution or severe streaking might result. The cassettes can be reloaded while waiting for the film to develop. Some people recommend covering the developer tank so they can leave the darkroom during the developing time. However, films are often overdeveloped because they are not removed promptly at the proper time. Therefore,

TABLE I
Time-Temperature Relationships for Medical X-ray Film*

Temperature	*Time (minutes)*
16°C (60°F)	8.50
18°C (65°F)	6.00
20°C (68°F)	5.00
21°C (70°F)	4.50
24°C (75°F)	3.25

*This film is intended to be developed (ideally) at 20°C (68°F).

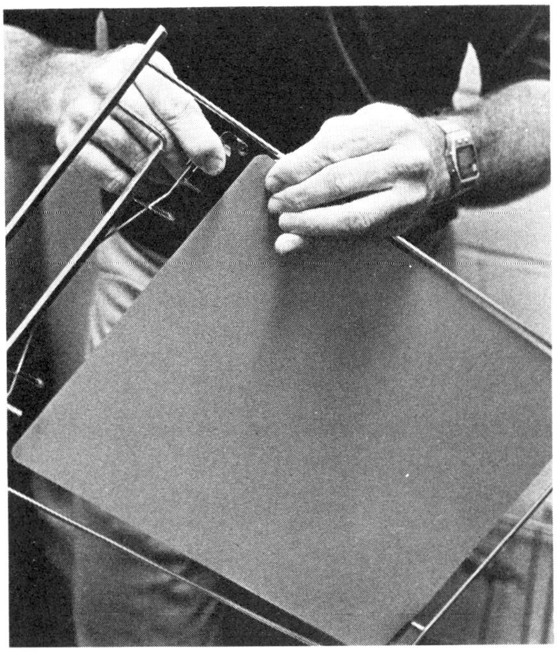

Figure 6—Film loading. Only the outer margins of the film are handled and the spring-loaded clips are attached last.

[b]Eastman Kodak Co., Rochester, NY 14650.

the author recommends that the darkroom not be left until the films are placed into the fixer solution.

Film should be removed slowly from the box, especially in low-humidity climates, to prevent static discharge which can produce tree-shaped black patterns on the film. Antistatic sprays can be used to reduce electrostatic discharge, but caution should be taken not to spray areas which could contaminate x-ray film. Touching a grounded surface prior to film handling is also recommended for reducing electrostatic discharge artifacts. The film should be lifted vertically from the film box and placed in the cassette without excessive bending. The film must be properly positioned before the cassette is closed and locked. Protruding film acts as a light pipe that can transmit light an inch or farther into the film.

When the timer bell rings, the film hangers are lifted and moved to the wash water without allowing the solution to drip back into the developer tank.[3] The solution that drains off is partially exhausted and does not significantly contribute to the developer strength. The volume of solution removed with a 14- × 17-inch film and hanger is about 2.75 oz (approximately 1 oz for an 8- × 10-inch film), and this will be replaced later with fresh replenisher. The film should be agitated in the rinse compartment for 25 to 30 seconds for most screen types of film, and 30 to 60 seconds is usually required for nonscreen types of film. The film is drained for a few seconds prior to being placed in the fixer solution.

Adequate fixing requires about twice as much time as it takes for the film to clear. Clearing can be difficult to determine; a rule of thumb is to fix the film twice as long as the developing time. The film should be agitated when placed in the fixer solution and periodically thereafter. Simply because the film is cleared adequately for viewing of the image does not mean that the dissolved silver halide crystals have been washed from the emulsion. The image will deteriorate severely over a period of time if adequate fixing is not accomplished. The films are removed from the fixer, without permitting drainage back into the fixer tank, and placed into the wash compartment.[3] Because some of the exhausted fixer is carried out with the film and hanger, fixer replenisher can be added to the fixer tank for more consistent results.

It is during the wash phase that films are most often abused. During this time the films are washed for a few seconds and then viewed for radiographic quality, and too often for interpretation. If the film is allowed to partially dry during this time, distortion of the emulsion results in permanent streaking. More diagnostic information can be seen on dry films. Therefore, one should resist the temptation to make a final diagnosis from wet films. Films should be left in the wash tank for about 20 to 30 minutes for most types of film, but five minutes is adequate for manual processing of rapid-process film. It is not advisable to leave films in the wash tank for more than 30 to 60 minutes because the emulsion becomes waterlogged and requires a longer drying time. The wash-water flow rate should be about 8 volumes/hour to adequately remove the developer and fixer contaminants. A final rinse of approximately 30 seconds in a solution containing a surface-tension reducing agent such as Photo-flow[b] will reduce drying time and help reduce streaking.

Rapid-process film can be developed manually, but it is recommended that the film not be agitated in the developer. Rapid-process film should be vigorously agitated when the film is first placed in the fixer and every two minutes thereafter. It should be continuously agitated for 30 seconds at the start of the wash phase.

The ideal method of drying films is with a warm-air drying cabinet (Figure 7). The air temperature in such a cabinet should not be above 49°C (120°F), and film should not be left in it for more than one hour while the dryer is running or the films might become brittle. The most commonly used drying technique is to hang the films in a vertical position, allowing them to drip and air dry. It is important that the films not be moved while partially dried or film streaking will result. The film-holding clip area is always the last part to dry.

The corners of the films should be cut when the films are removed from the hangers to prevent the perforations from scratching the emulsion of other films. Corners can be cut with a device specifically made for this purpose or with scissors. Another method is to remove the perforations with a hand-held hole punch.

Automatic Film Processing

The alternative to manual processing is the use of a machine into which an exposed film is placed and a dry radiograph emerges 1.5 to 5 minutes later. The disad-

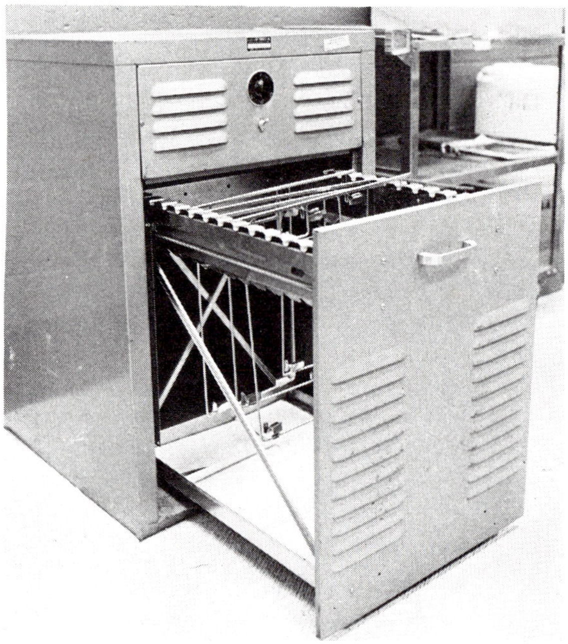

Figure 7—An electric hot-air film dryer.

vantages are (1) high initial cost, (2) required periodic maintenance, and (3) higher chemical cost. These disadvantages should be weighed against the advantages, which are (1) greatly reduced processing time for a dry film, (2) reduced personnel time, and (3) reduction of many darkroom artifacts. The decision to buy an automatic processor is not always based on economic feasibility. Before a decision is made about such a purchase, it is recommended that opinions be sought from other veterinarians who own various types of processors. It is also wise to check whether one-day service is possible in case of mechanical failure. It is recommended that manual processing capability be maintained so that radiography can be continued if the automatic processor has to be down for a long period awaiting parts or service.

Silver Recovery

One hundred sheets of 14- × 17-inch green film contain about 5 troy oz of silver. Approximately one-half of this ends up in the fixer solution. Veterinarians should consider recovering silver for three reasons: (1) silver is a limited natural resource; (2) there are regulations concerning disposal of corrosive chemicals through public systems, and (3) it is economically wise. Recovery can be accomplished in a variety of ways.

Electrolytic recovery units can be placed on an automatic processor or a container of used solution which has been removed from the fixer tank. These units cost at least $300 and are not feasible for veterinary facilities unless more than 500 films are processed per month. The recovery rate for such units is about 85 to 90% on a flow-through system and close to 100% when used with a batch method.

Metallic replacement is used to recover silver by flowing fixer solution through a specially prepared recovery cartridge available from most x-ray supply distributors. This type of system is efficient if the flow of solution is regulated and the system is used on a daily basis.

There are other methods of silver recovery, but the most practical one for veterinarians is to sell the used fixer solution to a recovery company. If this method is chosen, the silver content should be measured or estimated with test strips and not sold strictly on a per gallon basis.

Silver that is not removed from the film during the fixing process is of course still on the radiograph. Therefore radiographs that are no longer needed can be sold at a price based on the current value of silver bullion. This not only is economical but it reduces storage problems.

Radiographic Storage and Retrieval

For radiographs to be of value, as with any record, they must be filed according to a system that permits rapid retrieval. They should be conveniently located and marked for easy identification. The terminal digit filing system used with case records can be applied to radiograph filing. Numeric filing systems have advantages over alphabetic systems since each patient is given a unique identification regardless of the number of pets owned by the client. It is advisable to have some form of color coding on the envelope edge to alleviate the need for pulling out several cases to find the proper file.

The radiograph envelope should have a place in which to record case information including the date of each examination, region examined, and the radiographic impression. A code number containing the anatomic part and the pathologic condition can also be recorded. The code number and case number make retrieval easy for writing up case reports covering particular conditions. This information can be kept on a card file, or a simple mailing-list type of computer program can be easily modified for case search and retrieval in veterinary facilities that use a computer.

The length of time radiographs should be kept for legal purposes depends on state statutes and requirements imposed by veterinary examining boards. In Louisiana, for example, there are no statutory requirements, but the examining board recommends that case reports be kept for five years and radiographs be kept for three years. The statutes of limitation regarding the type of possible litigation could also be a determining factor.

REFERENCES

1. *NCRP Report No. 36, Radiation Protection in Veterinary Medicine.* Washington, DC, National Council on Radiation Protection and Measurements, 1970, Appendix B, p 34.
2. Information brochure packed with Kodak Film. Rochester, NY, Eastman Kodak Co, 1979.
3. *The Fundamentals of Radiography*, ed 12. Rochester, NY, Eastman Kodak Co, 1980.
4. Ticer JW: *Radiographic Technique in Small Animal Practice.* Philadelphia, WB Saunders Co, 1975, pp 37-57.
5. Gillete EL, Thrall DE, Lebel JL (eds): *Carlson's Veterinary Radiology*, ed 3. Philadelphia, Lea & Febiger, 1979.

An Approach to Interpretation of Radiographs

KEY FACTS

- Systematic review of radiographs is necessary to extract the maximum amount of available information.
- An organized, stepwise approach to film interpretation is recommended.
- The recommended steps are (1) identify film artifacts, (2) identify patient's signalment, (3) locate radiographic abnormalities, (4) describe lesions, (5) make the radiographic diagnosis, (6) construct and rank a list of diagnostic differentials, and (7) make a final clinical diagnosis using ancillary information.

University of Pennsylvania
Sydney M. Evans, VMD, MS

SYSTEMATIC REVIEW of radiographs is necessary to extract the maximum amount of available information. This article is intended to help the veterinary practitioner avoid the pitfalls[1] associated with a random approach to evaluation of radiographs. The information in this article pertains to the interpretation of radiographs of excellent quality. Radiographs should be viewed in a dark or dimly lit room, and a high-intensity light (bright light) should be used to examine black or overexposed areas.

The recommended approach to studying radiographs consists of the following seven steps:

1. Identify the artifacts of radiographic technique, positioning, and processing as well as the normal variants
2. Identify the patient's species, age, breed, and sex
3. Locate any radiographic abnormalities
4. Describe the lesions
5. Make a radiographic diagnosis
6. Construct and rank a list of diagnostic differentials
7. Choose the most likely diagnostic differential based on history, clinical findings, and ancillary tests.

Initially, a conscious effort must be made to perform each step for every radiograph. With practice, however, the routine becomes automatic and the evaluation becomes less time-consuming.

ARTIFACTS AND NORMAL VARIANTS

Normal anatomic variants and technical artifacts must be identified to avoid interpreting them as signs of disease. If a chest radiograph is underexposed or the patient is in an expiratory phase of respiration, the pulmonary parenchyma will have an apparently interstitial pattern that could be misinterpreted as a sign of interstitial pulmonary disease. Rotation of the thorax can make a normal heart appear enlarged[2]; asymmetrical skull positioning may create the illusion of disease. Mechanical devices (e.g., catheters or electrocardiographic leads) may mimic or hide evidence of disease. Artifacts may also be caused by the cassette, intensifying screen, film, and processing (Figure 1).

Normal variants for a given breed and species must also be noted and not misinterpreted. For example, the trachea of bulldogs is normally more narrow than that of other breeds[3]; the heart of barrel-chested dogs normally appears somewhat enlarged on radiographs; and curved, short legs are normal for chondrodystrophoid breeds.

SIGNALMENT

The viewer must attempt to identify the patient's species, age, breed, and sex from radiographic signs. Identifying the patient's signalment helps ensure that the correct radiograph is being evaluated. For example, if the radiograph is supposed to represent the pelvis of a six-month-old, male Great Dane, the physes should be open, a baculum and prepuce should be visible, and the dog should be large. In addition, the clinician must ensure that the radiographic findings are consistent with the patient's signalment. Many diseases characteristically occur in particular patient

Originally published in Volume 11, Number 7, July 1989

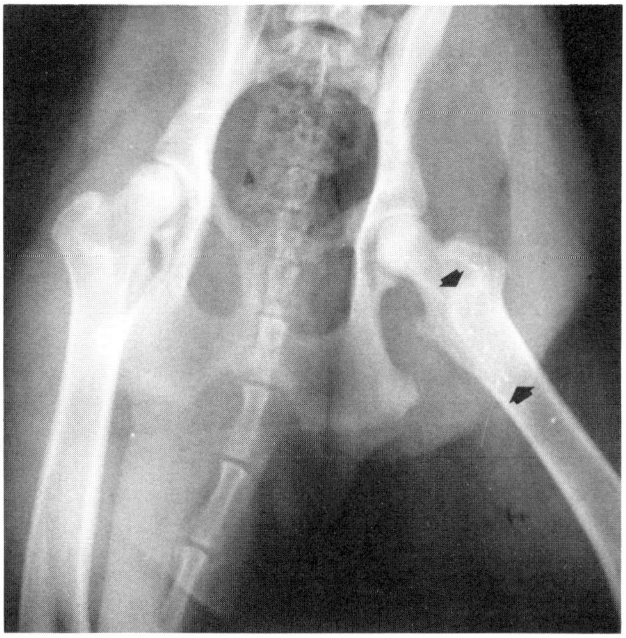

Figure 1A

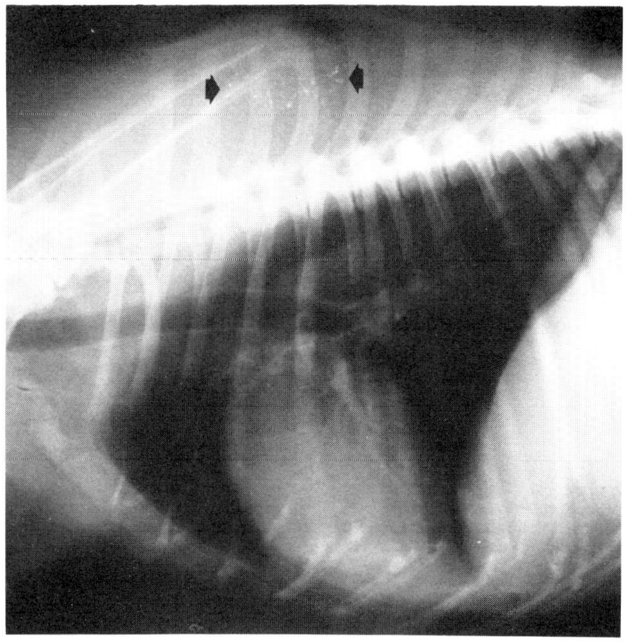

Figure 1B

Figure 1—(**A**) Pelvic radiograph of an adult female dog with a history of left hindlimb lameness. Metallic opacities are associated with the proximal femur (*arrows*). (**B**) Right lateral thoracic radiograph of an adult dog made using the same cassette. Metallic opacities associated with spinous processes have the same pattern of distribution and were in the same location on the sheet of film as in **A** (*arrows*). Screen artifacts were concluded to be the source of the opacities.

groups. Panosteitis occurs only in dogs, prostate disease can only occur in males, and cancer is more common in old patients.

ANATOMIC ABNORMALITIES

Identification of anatomic abnormalities is the next step in interpreting radiographs. An organized approach to reviewing the entire radiograph is critical in ensuring that no abnormalities are missed. Ideally, this step should be performed without knowledge or consideration of the clinical history, thus assuring that the viewer is neither biased nor using the radiographs to confirm a preconceived notion.

The entire radiograph can be reviewed using either a pattern or anatomic approach. In the pattern approach, a geometric pattern is superimposed on the radiograph. The viewer uses the pattern to ensure that all areas of the radiograph are studied. With the pattern approach, the viewer is less likely to abbreviate the radiographic examination when a particular disease process is suspected.

In the anatomic approach, the reader examines organs or areas in a predetermined sequence, noting whether the size, shape, density, and location of each structure are normal. The specific sequence depends on the body part being imaged and the preferences of the reader. Tables I and II list suggested sequences of review for thoracic, abdominal, and musculoskeletal radiographs.

LESIONS

It is often helpful to describe lesions according to their opacity and location. Such descriptions force the clinician to define the radiographic changes. The following are listed in descending order of radiographic opacity: metal, bone, soft tissue, fat, and air.

The radiographic changes may be sufficient to define the differential diagnosis. A poorly demarcated lytic lesion in the distal radial metaphysis of a Great Dane may represent a primary bone tumor or a site of infection. In the northeastern United States, neoplasia (probably a primary bone tumor) would be the most likely diagnostic differential. If the Great Dane's lesion is diaphyseal, a metastatic tumor would be a more likely differential.

RADIOGRAPHIC DIAGNOSIS

Radiographic diagnoses (e.g., abdominal mass, alveolar lung disease, aggressive bone lesion, or loss of intraperitoneal detail) are descriptions of the radiographic changes. Unlike many clinical diagnoses, radiographic diagnoses do not state the cause of the disease. After the radiographic diagnosis is made, the reader must consider all of the clinical diagnostic differentials that the radiographic diagnosis may represent.

RANKING THE DIAGNOSTIC DIFFERENTIALS

The so-called gamut approach is used in considering the differential diagnosis; the whole range of possible causes for the radiographic diagnosis is considered. The mnemonic *DAMN ITCH* represents the categories of disease. The patient's history, clinical signs, and laboratory data are used to rank the diagnostic differentials.

CASE 1: MUSCULOSKELETAL SYSTEM

A 10-year-old, spayed female Golden Retriever (Figure

TABLE I
Review Pattern for Chest and Abdominal Radiographs

General Category	*Chest*	*Abdomen*
External structures	Body wall and associated structures	Body wall and associated structures
Bony structures	Ribs (cervical and thoracic), front legs, sternum	Spine (thoracic, lumbar, and sacral), pelvis, hindlimbs, ribs
Surface of diaphragm	Thoracic surface of diaphragm	Abdominal surface of diaphragm
Organ systems	*Cardiovascular:* heart and blood vessels *Pulmonary:* lungs, trachea, and bronchi	*Gastrointestinal:* liver, spleen, stomach, small intestine, gallbladder, pancreas, mesentary, colon *Genitourinary:* kidneys, prostate, gonads, ureters, bladder, urethra, uterus *Other:* adrenal glands, lymph nodes
Serosa-lined and potential spaces	Pleural and extrapleural spaces, mediastinum, pericardial sac	Peritoneal and extraperitoneal spaces

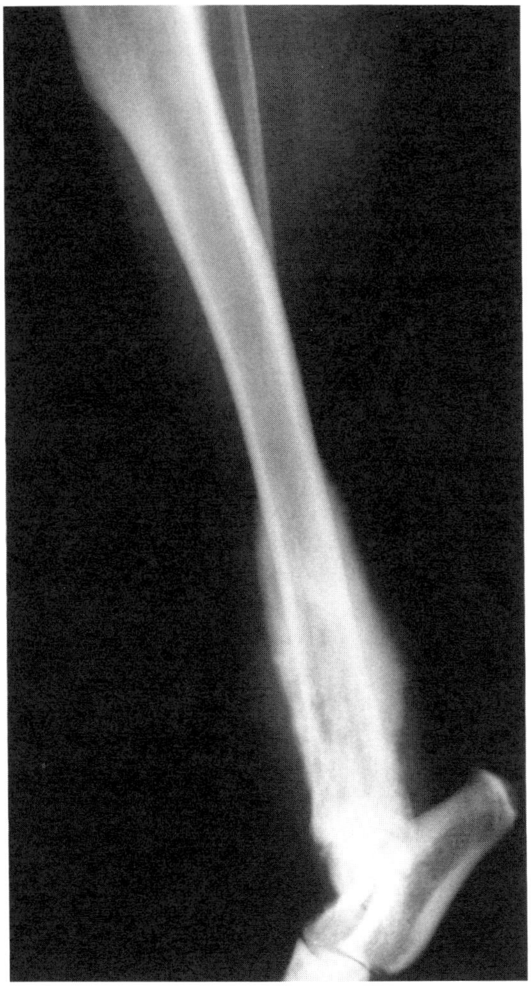

Figure 2A

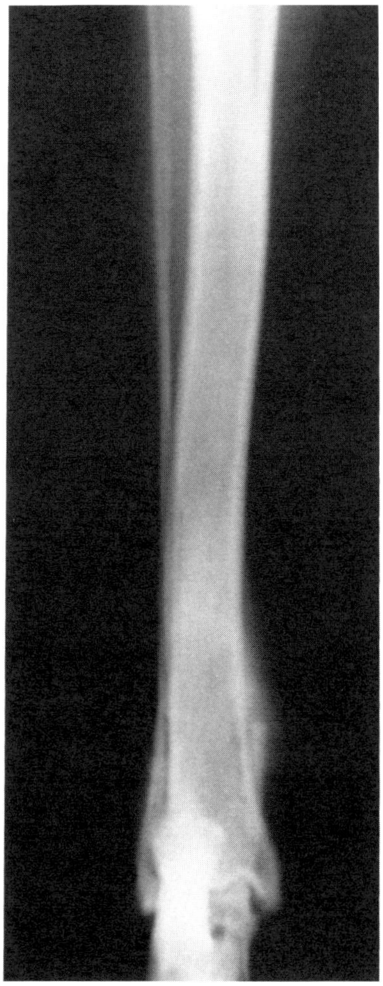

Figure 2B

Figure 2—(A) Lateral and **(B)** craniocaudal radiographs of the tibia of a 10-year-old spayed female Golden Retriever with a six-week history of right hindlimb lameness. Note the lytic and proliferative lesion involving the distal third of the right tibia and centered at the metaphysis. Soft tissue swelling, cortical destruction, sunburst periosteal reaction, and poor margination are also visible. The minimal degenerative joint changes in the cranial aspect of the tarsocrural joint are an incidental finding.

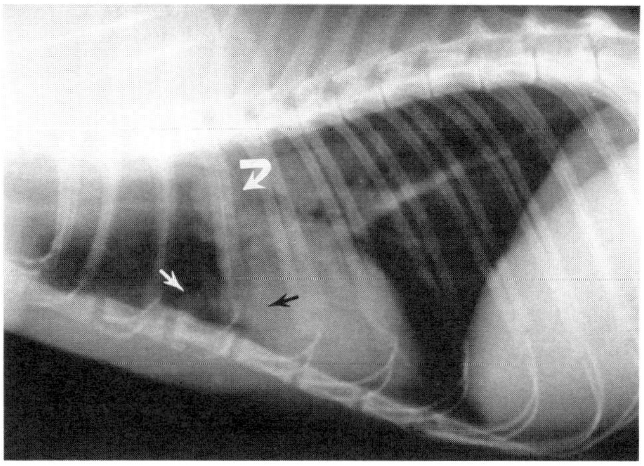

Figure 3A

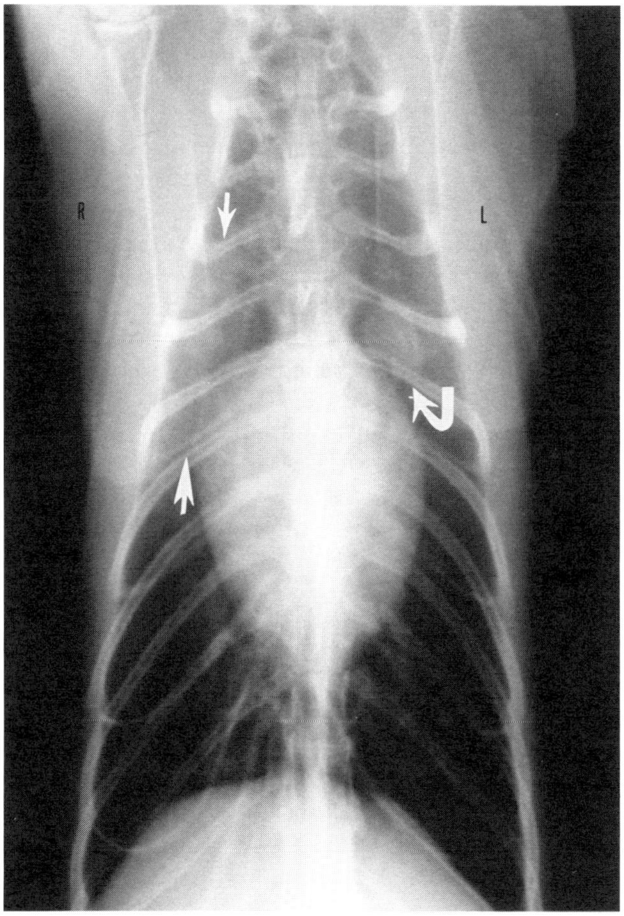

Figure 3B

Figure 3—(**A**) Lateral and (**B**) ventrodorsal radiographs of a two-year-old Manx cat with chronic cough, depression, and anorexia. Note the round and well-demarcated soft tissue mass (*curved arrow*) on the dorsal aspect of the left cranial lobe. Note also the poorly defined soft tissue opacity (*straight arrows*) in the right cranial thoracic cavity.

2) with a six-week history of progressive right hindlimb lameness was examined at the Veterinary Hospital of the University of Pennsylvania. Table III presents the radiographic findings.

TABLE II

ABCS Review Pattern for Musculoskeletal Radiographs

Area	*Considerations*
Arthrosis	Alignment
Bone	Medullary cavity versus cortex; diaphysis, metaphysis, epiphysis, apophysis; continuity and shape
Cartilaginous areas	Physes, articular cartilage
Soft tissues	Joint soft tissues, periarticular fascia and fat pads, muscles, tendons, lymph nodes, ligaments

TABLE III

Radiographic Findings: Case 1

Step	*Finding*
Artifacts and variants	None
Signalment	Canine, mature, large-breed, sex not identifiable
Lesion location	Distal third of right tibia, centered at metaphysis
Lesion description	Lytic and proliferative lesion involving the distal third of the right tibia and centered at the metaphysis; soft tissue swelling, cortical destruction, sunburst periosteal reaction, poor margination; minimal degenerative joint changes in the cranial aspect of the tarsocrural joint
Radiographic diagnosis	Aggressive bone lesion
Clinical diagnostic differentials	Primary bone tumor; infection, most likely fungal
Rank of differentials	1. Primary bone tumor 2. Infection, most likely fungal

In an old, otherwise healthy dog living in the northeastern United States, the most likely diagnosis is a primary bone tumor; however, fungal titers should be performed if the dog has traveled outside the northeastern United States. Because the location of the lesion is uncharacteristic for osteosarcoma, other primary bone tumors, such as fibrosarcoma, chondrosarcoma, hemangiosarcoma, and liposarcoma, could be considered. Biopsy of this lesion confirmed a primary osteosarcoma.

CASE 2: THORAX

The patient, a two-year-old Manx cat (Figure 3) with a history of chronic cough, depression, and anorexia, had previously resided in the southeastern United States. A test for feline leukemia virus was negative, and the cat had eosinophilia. Radiographs of the cat in right lateral recum-

TABLE IV
Radiographic Findings: Case 2

Step	*Finding*
Artifacts and variants	None
Signalment	Feline, mature, sex not identifiable
Lesion location	a. Dorsal aspect, left cranial lobe b. Ventral aspect, right cranial thoracic cavity
Lesion description	*Dorsal aspect, left cranial lobe:* round and well-demarcated soft tissue mass (*curved arrow*, Figure 3) *Ventral aspect, right cranial thoracic cavity:* poorly defined soft tissue opacity, may contain air (*straight arrows*, Figure 3), possible pulmonary or (less likely) pleural origin.
Radiographic diagnosis	a. Left cranial lung lobe: interstitial pulmonary nodule b. Right cranial thorax: soft tissue mass with possible cavitation
Clinical diagnostic	
Right cranial thoracic lesion	a. Pneumonia, abscesses b. Cysts (traumatic, parasitic, congenital) c. Granulomas d. Neoplasia (primary or secondary) e. Infarction
Left cranial thoracic lesion	a. Neoplasm b. Fluid-filled cyst c. Granuloma, abscess
Rank of differentials	a. Parasitic cysts b. Abscesses c. Granulomatous inflammation

bent and ventrodorsal positions were obtained. Table IV presents the findings.

In a young cat with systemic clinical signs, the most likely diagnostic differentials are abscesses, granulomatous inflammation, and parasitic cysts. Because the patient had lived in the southeastern United States and had eosinophilia, parasitic disease was a concern. Because a fecal examination is noninvasive and inexpensive, it was performed early in the examination. *Paragonimus kellikotti* infection was diagnosed.

Acronym for Categories of Disease

- **D** Degenerative, developmental
- **A** Anatomic, anomalous, allergic
- **M** Metabolic, metastatic
- **N** Neoplastic, nutritional, normal

- **I** Immunologic, infectious, idiopathic, inflammatory, iatrogenic
- **T** Traumatic, toxic
- **C** Congenital
- **H** Hereditary

DISCUSSION

The described approach or variants of it are frequently time-consuming and frustrating to novices. With time and practice, however, all aspects of a series of radiographs can be reviewed quickly. By using an organized method of radiograph review, the practitioner is less likely to miss or misinterpret radiographic lesions.

About the Author

Dr. Evans is an Assistant Professor in the Section of Radiology, School of Veterinary Medicine, University of Pennsylvania, Philadelphia, Pennsylvania.

REFERENCES

1. Thrall DE: *Textbook of Veterinary Diagnostic Radiology*. Philadelphia, WB Saunders Co, 1986, p 11.
2. Holmes RA, Smith FG, Lewis RE, Kern DM: The effects of rotation on the radiographic appearance of the canine cardiac silhouette in dorsal recumbency. *Vet Radiol* 26:98–101, 1985.
3. Harvey CE: Tracheal diameter: Analysis of radiographic measurements in brachycephalic and nonbrachycephalic dogs. *JAAHA* 18:570–576, 1982. □

Problems in Radiographic Interpretation: An Exercise Using Cases with Multiple Diagnoses

Michael R. Metcalf, DVM
Resident in Radiology and
Nuclear Medicine

S. K. Kneller, DVM, MS
Diplomate, ACVR
Associate Professor of Radiology

College of Veterinary Medicine
University of Illinois
Urbana, Illinois

The interpretation of radiographs should be based on a comprehensive and systematic approach, which enables the viewer to find and evaluate all of the radiographic abnormalities present. Such an approach allows the viewer to find the primary as well as secondary problems. It is important to notice the radiographic signs that have little or nothing to do with the primary finding but which contribute to the total clinical presentation. Different methods are used to systematically appraise geomorphic and density changes on a radiograph, such as viewing from the periphery to the center or evaluating each organ system in order. No matter what approach is taken, consistency is the key to using any system for the perception of any and all radiographic abnormalities. This article illustrates some of the problems in radiographic interpretation to help the practitioner avoid incomplete and incorrect diagnoses.

There are many ways in which significant radiographic abnormalities are overlooked or misread. Distractions from clients, coworkers, telephones, and impending cases can affect the level of concentration or the time allowed for evaluating the radiograph. In evaluating the radiograph itself, there are other pitfalls the viewer should be aware of and should avoid. The most common of these is to recognize an obvious lesion on a radiograph while overlooking a second less obvious abnormality that either may be contributing to the clinical problem or may be an entirely separate disease. The obvious abnormality that can be directly linked to the clinical signs tends to satisfy the need for making the radiograph. An unrelated or separate problem evident on the radiograph goes unnoticed because an obvious abnormality has already been revealed.

Preconceived notions of what will be seen on the radiograph cause another pitfall. If the viewer finds what was suspected, the tendency is to go no further in evaluation of the film. An example is a trauma case in which a fracture is palpated and a radiograph is only made to evaluate the fracture, and underlying pathologic bone is not seen.

There is also the mental problem of jumping to conclusions without thorough and logical evaluation of the radiographic findings. Once found, abnormalities must be completely evaluated. At first glance, the pattern of the radiographic abnormalities may give the impression of one disease process, and other possible diagnoses may not even be considered. A complete radiographic evaluation should enable a list of

Originally published in Volume 4, Number 9, September 1982

differential diagnoses to be made, from which the most likely diagnosis can be determined according to all available clinical data.

The above pitfalls can be classified as mental processes that inhibit complete evaluation of the radiograph and are often loosely called *tunnel* or *telescope vision*. Added to these are the peculiarities of the physical aspects of a radiographic study. For example, many radiographic studies such as those for an equine extremity and gastrointestinal contrast study may consist of many views. Finding an abnormality that may be visible on only one of the set of radiographs can be difficult. Another pitfall is to view radiographs in an unsuitable physical environment. Radiographic abnormalities can be masked by improper background lighting; the absence of a hotlight can prevent visualization of a lesion on an overexposed portion of a radiograph; or an abnormality can be obscured under the clips holding the film to the x-ray viewer.

This article presents various examples of related or unrelated radiographic abnormalities which test the reader's method of radiographic appraisal, and some pitfalls that can beset the evaluator. The reader of this article has the advantage of knowing that the following cases are not straightforward.

Case 1

A five-year-old female Doberman-shepherd mixed-breed dog was presented with a progressive left rear lameness of three years duration. The dog began to carry the leg six to nine months previous to presentation, at which time the stifle became swollen. There was no history of trauma, although the dog lives on a farm and could free run. On physical examination, the dog appeared underweight with atrophy of the left rear leg. The left stifle was enlarged, very firm, and fixed in a semiflexed position. The joint was not painful. No other joint involvement was discovered. The heart and lungs were normal on auscultation except for an end-diastolic click. The white blood cell count was 5100, of which 64% were segmented neutrophils, 14% were eosinophils, 18% were lymphocytes, and 4% were monocytes. Radiographs were made of the left stifle and the thorax (Figure 1).

Radiographic Signs

On a lateral radiograph of the stifle there is periosteal new bone on the distal femur and proximal tibia. There is also erosion and irregularity of all articular surfaces, obliteration of the infrapatellar fat pad, and exuberant osteophyte formation. On a lateral radiograph of the thorax there are numerous circumscribed increased densities throughout the lungs and irregular mineralized densities in the hilus.

At first glance, this might appear to be a case of a primary bone tumor with lung metastases. However, upon closer evaluation of the stifle radiograph, the periosteal and periarticular new bone has a very smooth border and organized appearance. There are radiographic signs of inactivity and chronicity.[1] In addition, the radiographic abnormalities in the stifle are centered in the joint rather than being in only one bone. These changes in the stifle are most compatible with a severe, chronic, inactive, hypertrophic degenerative joint disease, and not a bone tumor.[1]

The lung changes may also be deceptive. The small nodules in the pulmonary interstitium are mineralized rather than soft tissue densities. These densities are of a uniform size (2 to 3 mm in diameter) and, although

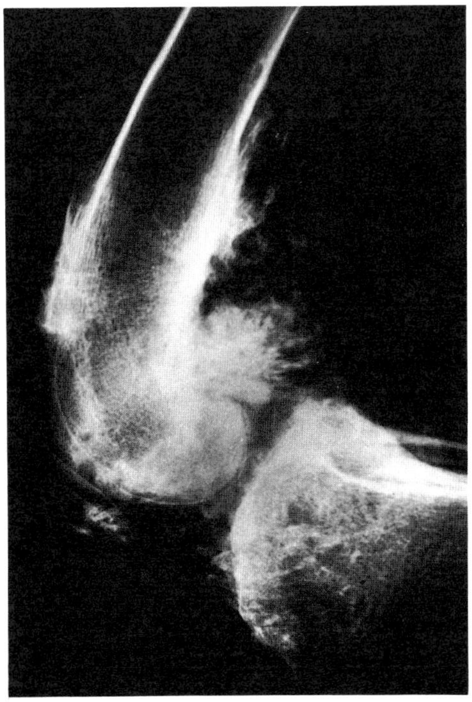

Figure 1A

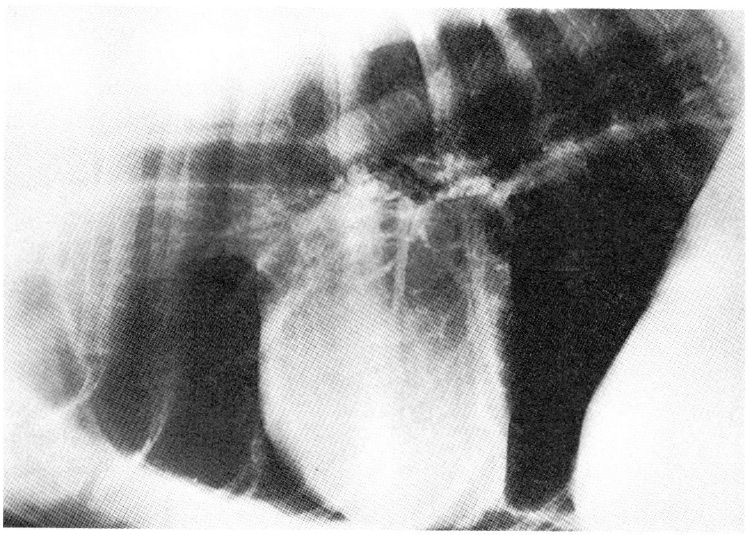

Figure 1B

Figure 1—(**A**) Lateral radiograph of the left stifle of a five-year-old female Doberman-shepherd mixed-breed dog. (**B**) Lateral radiograph of the thorax of same animal.

circumscribed, they have angular borders. These mineralized densities contrast sharply with the surrounding air-filled lung and appear well delineated. In comparison, metastatic nodules usually vary from 3 mm to several centimeters in diameter, are circumscribed, and contrast less well with the lung because they are usually made up of soft tissue.[2] The mineralized densities in the hilus are in the area of the tracheobronchial lymph nodes. The radiographic abnormalities are most consistent with dystrophic mineralization of multiple pulmonary nodules and of the tracheobronchial lymph nodes and are indicative of chronic or previous histoplasmosis.[3]

Subsequently, skeletal and lung perfusion scintigraphy was performed which indicated extensive soft tissue mineralization, none of which, however, appeared abnormally active, and no perfusion defects in the lungs consistent with pulmonary metastasis were found. The leg was amputated and a biopsy was taken which confirmed degenerative disease of the stifle joint.

In this case, instead of a primary disease process with secondary ramifications, there are two separate disease entities. This is an example of how an incomplete evaluation of the radiographic findings could have led to an erroneous conclusion and a much poorer prognosis for the patient.

Case 2

A six-month-old male St. Bernard was presented with a one week history of fever and reluctance to move. On physical examination, both carpal and tarsal areas were swollen, hot, and painful. Other joints were swollen in all four limbs. The lab work was unremarkable. Radiographs were made (Figure 2, A and B).

Radiographic Signs

The distal metaphyses of the radius, ulna, and tibia have an irregular decreased density. Associated with this is a cufflike periosteal reaction. These radiographic abnormalities represent hypertrophic osteodystrophy.[1] Since the radiographic diagnosis of hypertrophic osteodystrophy also correlates well with the clinical signs, there might be a tendency for a veterinarian to end the evaluation of these radiographs at this point. However, if the stifle is examined closely, a bony defect can be seen in one condyle of the femur. The cranial-caudal view of the stifle (Figure 2C) shows that the defect is on the medial aspect of the lateral condyle and represents osteochondritis.[1] This is an example of one disease with good clinical and radiographic correlation and a second disease involving the same joint. The second disease may or may not have contributed to this dog's lameness.

Case 3

A seven-year-old standardbred gelding was presented with a sore right front fetlock which developed after training approximately one month previously. Radiographs were made (Figure 3, A and B).

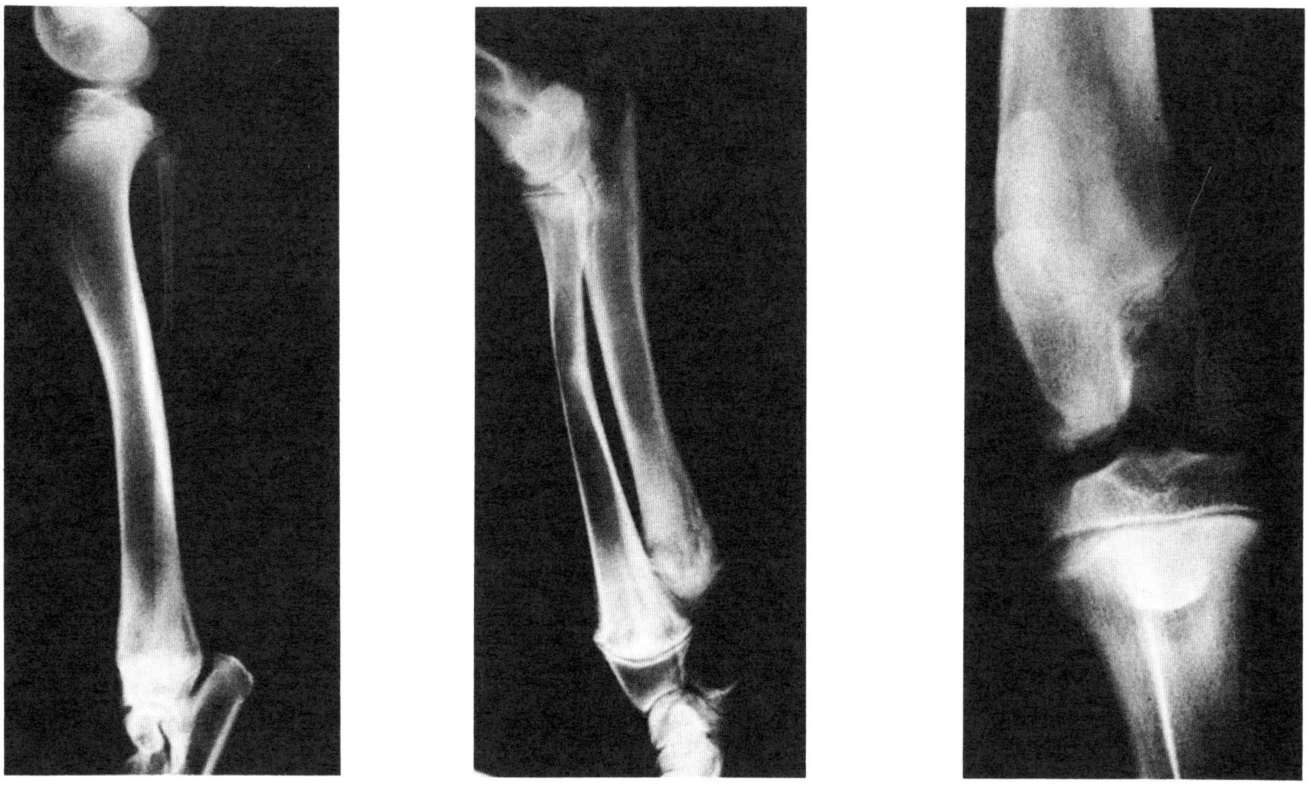

Figure 2A **Figure 2B** **Figure 2C**

Figure 2—(**A**) Lateral radiograph of the left tibia of a six-month-old St. Bernard. (**B**) Lateral radiograph of the left radius and ulna of the same dog. (**C**) Cranial-caudal radiograph of the left stifle of the dog.

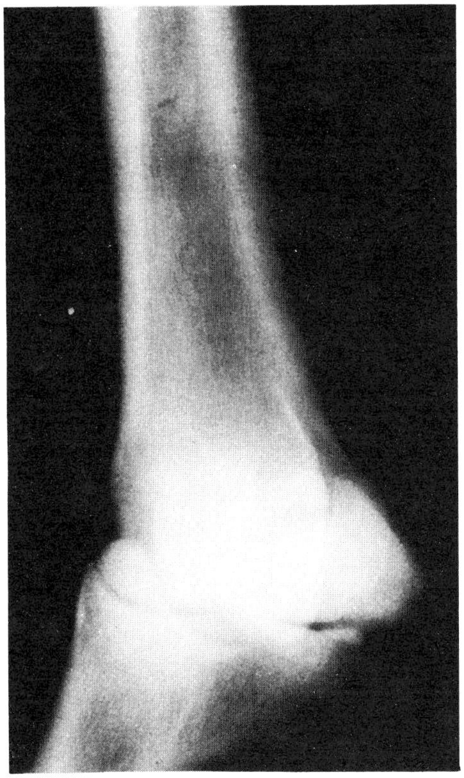

Figure 3A

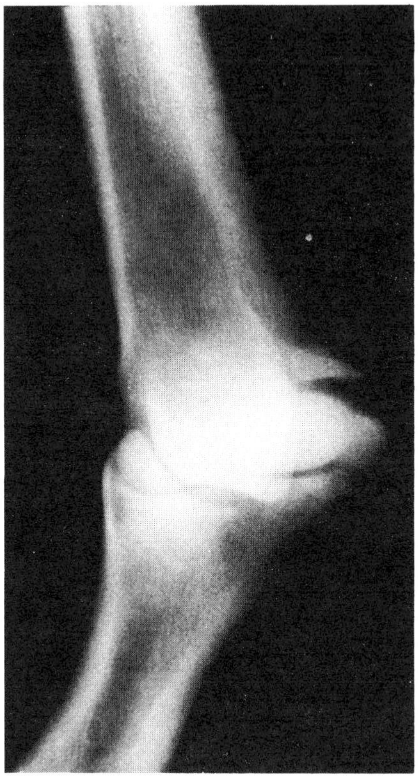

Figure 3B

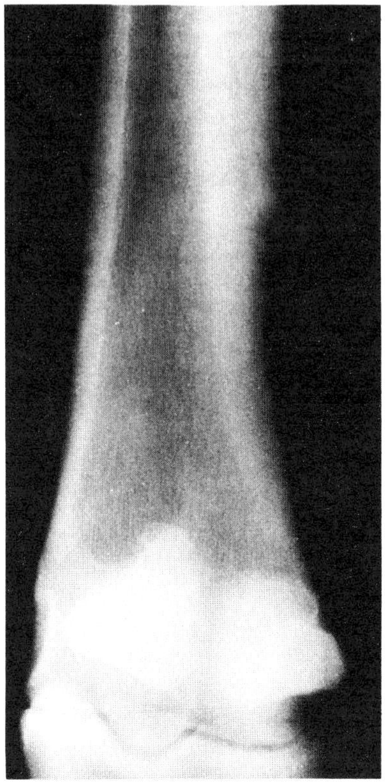

Figure 3C

Figure 3—(**A**) Dorsoventral lateral to medial oblique radiograph of the right front fetlock of a seven-year-old standardbred gelding. (**B**) Dorsoventral medial to lateral oblique radiograph of the right front fetlock of the same gelding. (**C**) Dorsoventral medial to lateral oblique radiograph of the right front fetlock of the same animal on two-month reexamination.

Radiographic Signs

There is a large apical fracture of the medial proximal sesamoid bone with enlarged vascular channels of both medial and lateral proximal sesamoid bones. This is compatible with sesamoiditis and a fracture of the sesamoid bone.[4] The apical fracture fragment was removed surgically. Two months later, the horse developed a hard, painful swelling proximal to the sesamoid bones and radiographs were again made (Figure 3C). At this time there is a nonunion fracture of the second metacarpal bone with a thick, well-marginated bony proliferation present. In retrospect, the distal second metacarpal fracture can be seen superimposed on the medullary cavity of the third metacarpal bone on the dorsoventral lateral to medial oblique view (Figure 3A). The fracture is also seen on the dorsoventral medial to lateral oblique view (Figure 3B) on the periphery of the radiograph. It is interesting to note that, when the dorsoventral medial to lateral oblique radiograph is placed on an x-ray viewer, the metacarpal fracture is hidden from view by the viewbox clip.[a]

Case 4

A two-month-old male Doberman mixed-breed dog was presented with a two-day history of straining while defecating. The stool was solid. On the day of presentation, the puppy was not eating or drinking. On physical examination, the dog was depressed, stood with a tucked-up abdomen, and would grunt softly when his abdomen was palpated. A hard, golf-ball–sized mass was palpated cranial to the urinary bladder. The hematocrit was 32, the white blood cell count was 21,400, of which 65% were segmented neutrophils, 9% were nonsegmented neutrophils, 24% were lymphocytes, and 2% were monocytes. At this time, radiographs were made for further evaluation of the abdomen (Figure 4).

Radiographic Signs

The abdomen is distended, with the colon displaced ventrally and to the left by a large homogeneous soft tissue density in the retroperitoneal space. The urinary bladder is not distinctly visualized. A tentative diagnosis of a mass of or near the kidneys was made. The observer's eye is drawn to the center of the abdomen in this dog because of the obvious abnormal appearance, but on the periphery of the lateral radiograph, two small mineralized densities are present in the area of the urethra between the ischial arch and penile urethra.

Bilateral hydronephrosis was confirmed by excretory urography. Urethral obstruction by calculi and stricture were confirmed by urethrography. This is an example of a cause and effect where the effect (hydronephrosis) is

[a]*Editor's Note*: The two fractures (sesamoid and metacarpal) are two of the triad of clinical and radiographic indicators (the third being suspensory ligament swelling) of suspensory ligament disease. One should always look for the triad.

Darryl Biery, DVM

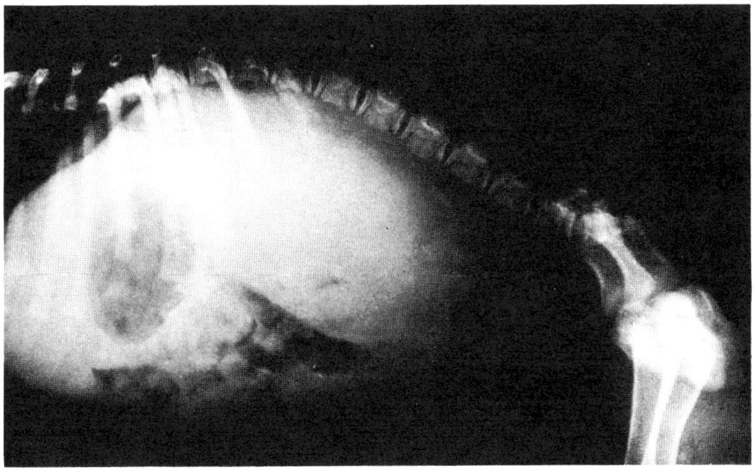

Figure 4A

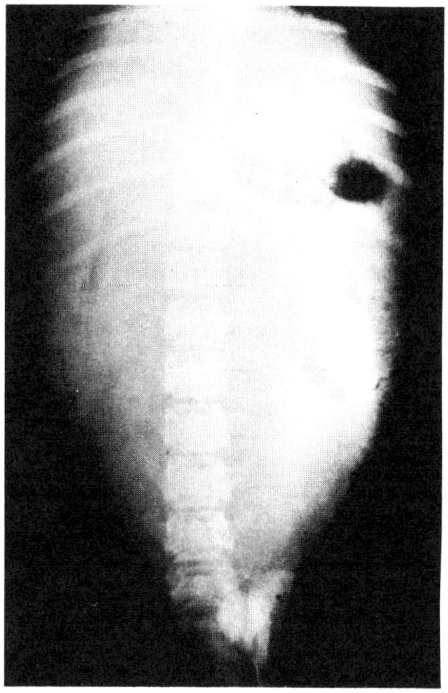

Figure 4B

Figure 4—(**A**) Lateral radiograph of the abdomen of a two-month-old male Doberman mixed-breed dog. (**B**) Ventrodorsal radiograph of the abdomen of the same dog.

the most obvious radiographic abnormality, but the cause (urethral obstruction due to calculi) is much less obvious, although present on the same radiograph.

Case 5

A five-year-old female mixed-breed dog was presented with a history of being a diabetic. For the past three days the dog had become progressively depressed and anorectic. Radiographs were made to assess the abdomen which was tense and difficult to palpate (Figure 5).

Radiographic Signs

The liver appears markedly enlarged. There is also free gas within the urinary bladder wall and lumen. These radiographic abnormalities are compatible with diabetes mellitis. Sugar-splitting, gas-forming organisms in the urinary bladder have created the free gas in the wall and lumen of the bladder, creating the halo effect.[5] In addition to these striking, related radiographic abnormalities of the liver and urinary bladder, there is a third abnormality present. Bilateral, convoluted, tubular, soft tissue densities are present in the ventral abdomen, indicative of an enlarged uterus. Other tubular densities normally visualized in the abdomen include

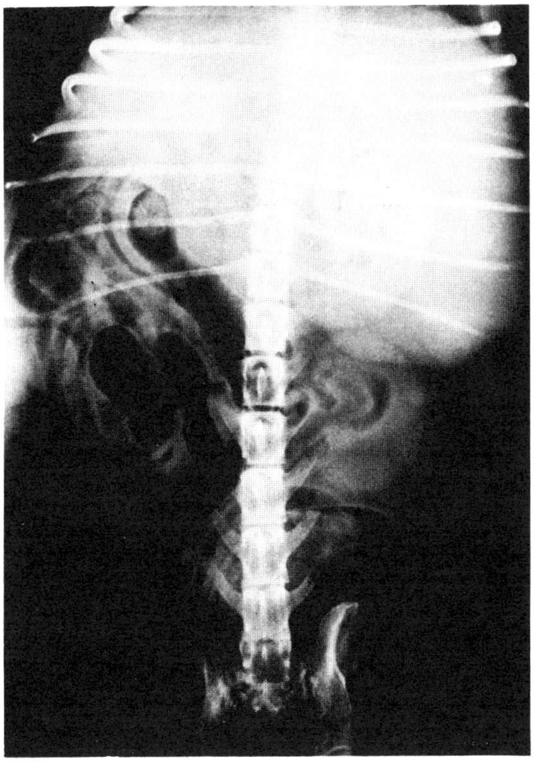

Figure 5A

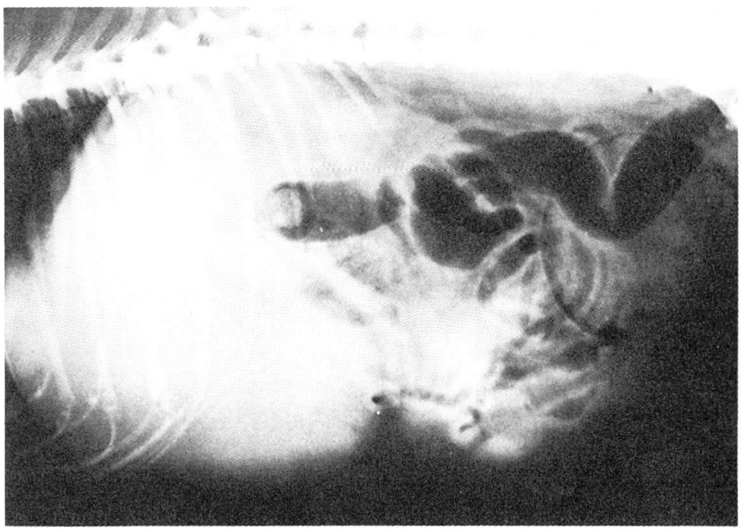

Figure 5B

Figure 5—(**A**) Ventrodorsal radiograph of the abdomen of a five-year-old female mixed-breed dog. (**B**) Lateral radiograph of the abdomen of the same dog.

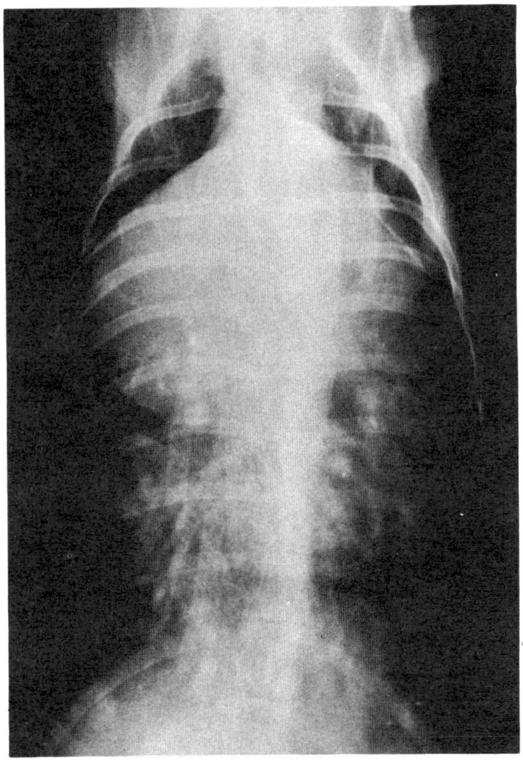

Figure 6A

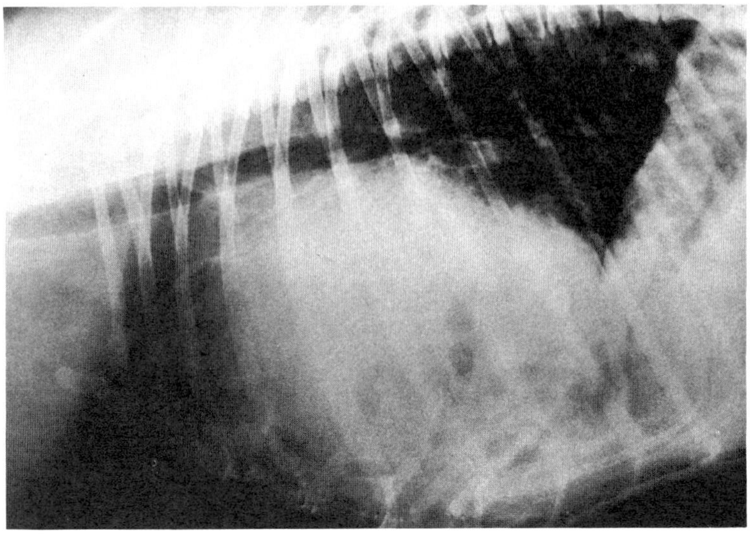

Figure 6B

Figure 6—(**A**) Dorsoventral radiograph of the thorax of a five-year-old female spayed Irish setter dog. (**B**) Lateral radiograph of the thorax of the same dog.

the small and large bowel. The colon is identified by its contents of gas and fecal matter. The small intestine is readily identified by its smaller normal diameter. If abnormally enlarged, small intestine is usually distended by gas rather than appearing as a homogeneous soft tissue density. The diagnoses of hepatomegaly, emphysematous cystitis, and pyometra were confirmed by laparotomy. This last abnormality may be particularly difficult to detect because of superimposition of other structures such as small bowel, colon, and the diseased urinary bladder. Thus, it is important to not stop evaluation of the radiographs because one abnormality that can explain the clinical signs is found. There may be other causes.

Case 6

A five-year-old female spayed Irish setter was presented with a history of being hit by a car 17 months previously. The dog had not been treated and had made an uneventful recovery. The dog was presented because of vomiting and weight loss, and a referring veterinarian had diagnosed a diaphragmatic hernia. On the current physical examination, the dog appeared icteric and there was a lack of abdominal contents on palpation. On auscultation, the heart sounds were muffled, and there were moist and dry rales. Bilirubin, serum alanine aminotransferase (SALT, or SGPT), and serum alkaline phosphatase values were elevated, and a complete blood count indicated a stress leukogram. Radiographs of the chest were made for further evaluation (Figure 6).

Radiographic Signs

The cardiac silhouette is greatly enlarged and contains multiple tubular gas densities. The ventral mid-diaphragmatic shadow is also obscured. The radiographic signs are most compatible with a pericardial diaphragmatic hernia. It was thought that the hernia was either congenital or that the trauma of being hit by a car caused a congenitally weakened area of the diaphragm to open and allow abdominal contents into the pericardial space. In either case, the hernia was considered surgically correctable. However, additional radiographic abnormalities are present. There are multiple, circumscribed, soft tissue nodules of various sizes present in the lungs which are highly suggestive of metastatic disease.[2] On postmortem examination after euthanasia, a congenital, pericardial diaphragmatic hernia was confirmed. A mass of 7 cm diameter, an undifferentiated sarcoma, adhered to the proximal duodenum and common bile duct. Multiple 1- to 6-mm metastatic lung nodules were present throughout the lung.

This case is another example of an obvious radiographic abnormality (hernia) superimposed over another abnormality (metastatic lung disease) which, in this case, proved to be the more serious and clinically significant lesion. If the metastases had not been noticed radiographically, surgical treatment for the hernia would probably have inappropriately been done.

Case 7

A two-year-old female spayed malamute dog was presented with a history of having hit its right hindleg on a step four months previously. This resulted in a lameness which resolved after six weeks. The lameness recurred within two months and the dog was taken to a veterinarian.

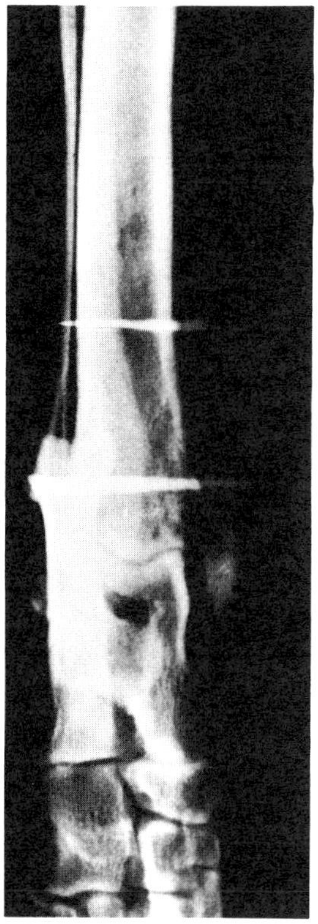

Figure 7A

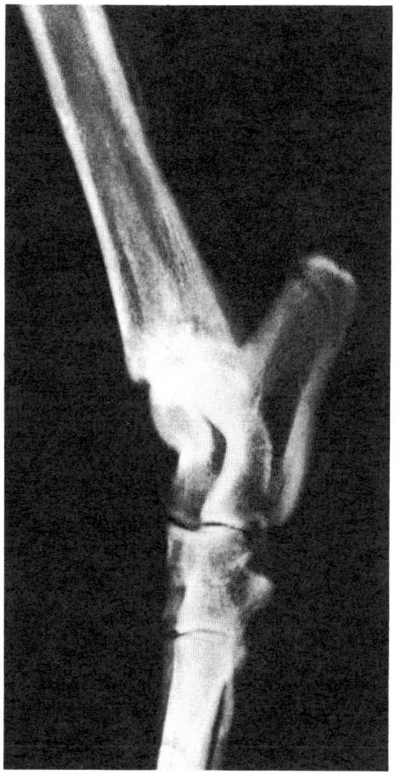

Figure 7B

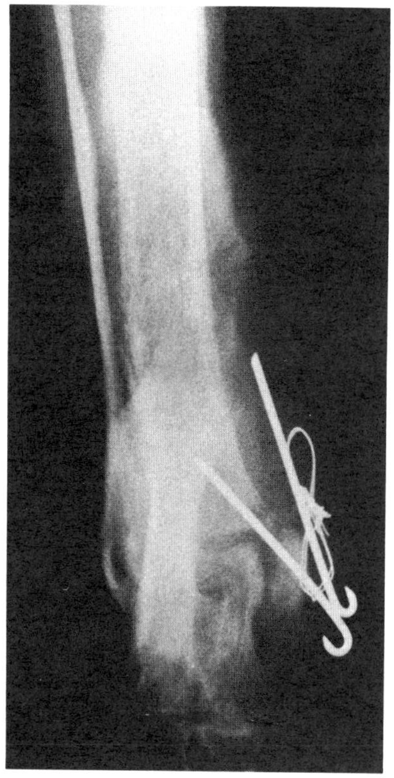

Figure 7C

Figure 7—(**A**) Cranial-caudal radiograph of the right tarsus of a two-year-old female spayed malamute dog (white streaks on the film are artifacts). (**B**) Lateral radiograph of the right tarsus of the same dog. (**C**) Cranial-caudal radiograph of the right tarsus of the same dog on one-month reexamination.

Radiographic Signs

Radiographs of the right tarsal area were made which showed a medial malleolar fracture (Figure 7, A and B). During the follow-up after fracture fixation, the lameness became progressively worse and a progressive swelling over the distal tibia developed. On a postfixation radiograph (Figure 7C), the internal fixation devices have migrated out of the distal tibia into the soft tissue mass medially. There is permeative lysis throughout the distal tibia with periosteal new bone proximal to and surrounding the lytic area. These radiographic abnormalities are compatible with a malignant tumor involving the distal tibia.[1]

On the initial radiographs, periosteal new bone can be seen on the caudal and caudomedial aspect of the tibia proximal to the fracture site. Because the periosteal reaction had smooth borders, it was considered benign and clinically insignificant.

This case is an example of an obvious abnormality (malleolar fracture) that could explain the lameness and thus satisfied the need for the radiograph. Once the fracture is noted, other radiographic abnormalities may often be missed or considered insignificant because a diagnosis has already been made. During follow-up, the fracture site is the focus of attention; the radiograph is used as a confirmatory tool and not used with the idea that additional diagnoses might be found.

Discussion

These cases illustrate by example some of the mental and physical pitfalls of viewing and evaluating radiographs. These pitfalls should be kept in mind when viewing any radiograph. The following list may help the practitioner avoid the common pitfalls.

Mental Processes That Inhibit Complete Evaluation[6]

1. An obvious lesion near to or superimposed on a second lesion and distracting the evaluator's attention.
2. An obvious lesion that distracts the evaluator's attention from a second lesion distant to the obvious lesion or on the periphery of the radiograph.
3. An obvious lesion that answers a clinical question, thereby stopping further evaluation of the radiograph.
4. Preconception of what will be found on the radiograph, so that when the preconception is confirmed, the viewing of the radiograph ends.
5. Jumping to conclusions, which leads to incomplete evaluation of findings on the radiograph.

Physical Aspects That Inhibit Complete Evaluation

1. Large numbers of radiographs, e.g., contrast studies, equine extremity studies, skull series.

2. Improper environment for reading films, such as improper background lighting, the absence of a hotlight, and the masking of lesions by film clips on the viewer.
3. Improper radiographic technique (not covered in this article).

Many important factors that can interfere with the detection of a lesion in a radiograph have been discussed. Additional information can be found in published articles.[7]

REFERENCES

1. Morgan JP: *Radiology in Veterinary Orthopedics.* Philadelphia, Lea & Febiger, 1972, pp 76; 122-138; 345-350.
2. Suter PF, Carrig CB, O'Brien TR, Koller D: Radiographic recognition of primary and metastatic pulmonary neoplasms of dogs and cats. *Vet Radiol* 15:3-25, 1974.
3. Burk RL, Corley EA, Corwin LA: The radiographic appearance of pulmonary histoplasmosis in the dog and cat: A review of 37 case histories. *Vet Radiol* 19:2-7, 1978.
4. O'Brien TR, Morgan JP, Wheat JD, Suter PF: Sesamoiditis in the thoroughbred: A radiographic study. *Vet Radiol* 12:75-87, 1971.
5. Root CR, Scott RC: Emphysematous cystitis and other radiographic manifestations of diabetes mellitus in dogs and cats. *JAVMA* 158:721-728, 1971.
6. Suter PF, Gomez JA: *Diseases of the Thorax—Radiographic Diagnosis.* Davis, CA, Venture Press, 1981, pp 7-10.
7. Kundel HL, Revesz L: Lesion conspicuity, structured noise and film reader error. *AJR* 126(6):1233-1238, 1976.

The Radiology of Aging: Its Clinical Applications

C. S. Farrow, DVM
Professor of Radiology
Department of Veterinary Anesthesiology,
Radiology and Surgery
Western College of Veterinary Medicine
University of Saskatchewan
Saskatoon, Saskatchewan, Canada

Most dogs and cats have begun to show signs of aging by the conclusion of their first decade. These visible aging signs progress according to a combination of biologic and environmental factors.

Age-associated tissue and organ changes may also be seen on radiographs, usually found incidentally. Such signs can simulate disease, so one must be able to recognize age-related radiographic changes so that a rational differential diagnosis can be made. It is also important to search the films of older animals for disorders that are apt to be encountered in this age group, recognizing that the potential for positive radiographic diagnosis is enhanced considerably when specific signs are sought.

A catalogue of radiologic findings that may be anticipated in older dogs and cats as well as their clinical applications are presented. A regional anatomic approach is employed to simplify classification and to facilitate future reference.

Head

The teeth of older dogs and cats normally show radiographic signs of aging. These may include a closure of the apical foramen, narrowing of the pulp cavity, reduced definition of the alveolar margin (lamina dura), and varying degrees of regression of the alveolar crest (Figure 1).[1] Crown wear is also a frequent finding in older pets, although it is probably more a function of the amount and nature of what is being chewed than it is of aging per se.

Periodontal disease often accompanied by a loss of teeth is very common in older animals. The radiographic signs of periodontal disease include flattening of the normally angled junction between the dental crown and its associated root structures (cemento-enamel junction), increased periodontal space, loss of a distinct alveolar margin, and a moderate to severe alteration to the alveolar crest.[1] Root resorption may occur in more advanced cases of periodontal disease (Figure 2). Periapical disease, usually in the form of focal abscessation, is a common finding in older dogs with or without associated clinical signs. The maxillary carnassial tooth is most commonly involved, but other teeth may be affected as well. This disorder typically shows as a focal, circular lucency surrounding the apex of one or more dental roots and extending variable distances into the surrounding bone. When it is associated with the maxillary

Originally published in Volume 6, Number 12, December 1984

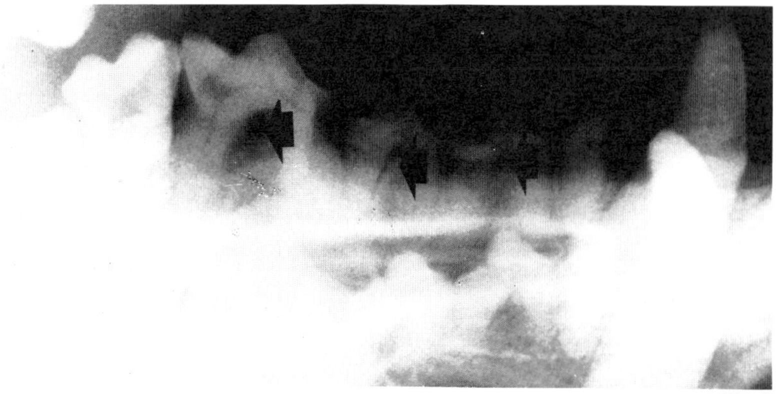

Figure 1—This lateral oblique view of the mandible shows resorption of the alveolar crest (*arrows*) in a 14-year-old cat.

carnassial teeth, there may be focal swelling just below the eye along with drainage in more advanced cases (Figure 3). Cavities (caries) are rare and appear to be a function of diet rather than aging.[2]

Jaws

The maxilla and mandible of older dogs and cats often appear osteoporotic, probably as part of a generalized age-related osteoporosis.[3] Radiographic density variations are often more easily appreciated in flat bones, such as the jaws, because of their relative radiographic accessibility and thinness. A localized or regional reduction in bone density is sometimes seen following dental extractions, probably resulting from occlusal loss and associated stress-related changes in the supporting bone.[1]

Skull

Older dogs and cats are not subject to the extensive structural changes seen in humans, but they often exhibit a loss of trabecula within the cancellous bone of the skull (diploë) (Figure 4).[1]

Neck

Throat

Pharyngeal calcification almost always occurs in older pets and has not been associated with functional abnormality.

Trachea

Calcification of the tracheal rings is a common finding in older dogs and cats. Although theoretically calcification could alter the tracheal dynamics, this has not been demonstrated.

Tracheal collapse is often seen in older dogs, although it is not confined to this age group.[5] Radiographically, tracheal collapse may be regional or generalized, and the degree of narrowing varies. Radiographic assessment of such disorders is improved considerably by making lateral thoracic radiographs on both inspiration and expiration, thereby changing the relative influences of the intrapleural and extrapleural pressures on the tracheal lumen. This inspiratory/expiratory sequence may document the range of tracheal caliber, giving the observer an idea of the luminal dynamics. This infor-

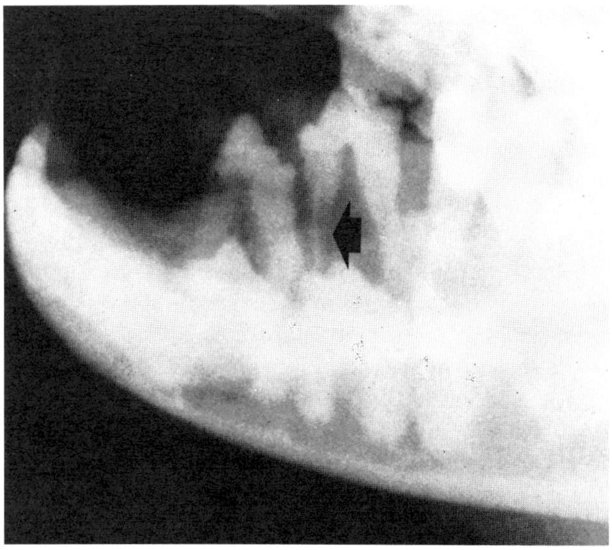

Figure 2—This lateral oblique view of the mandible shows root resorption (*arrow*) in a 12-year-old dog with advanced periodontal disease.

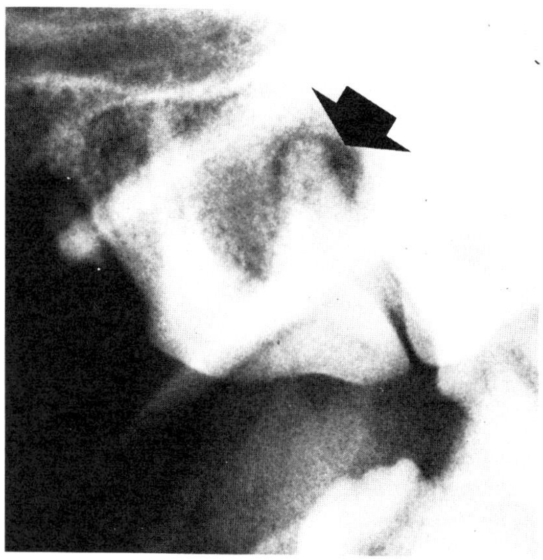

Figure 3—This lateral oblique view of the maxilla shows a periapical abscess (*arrow*) in a 15-year-old dog.

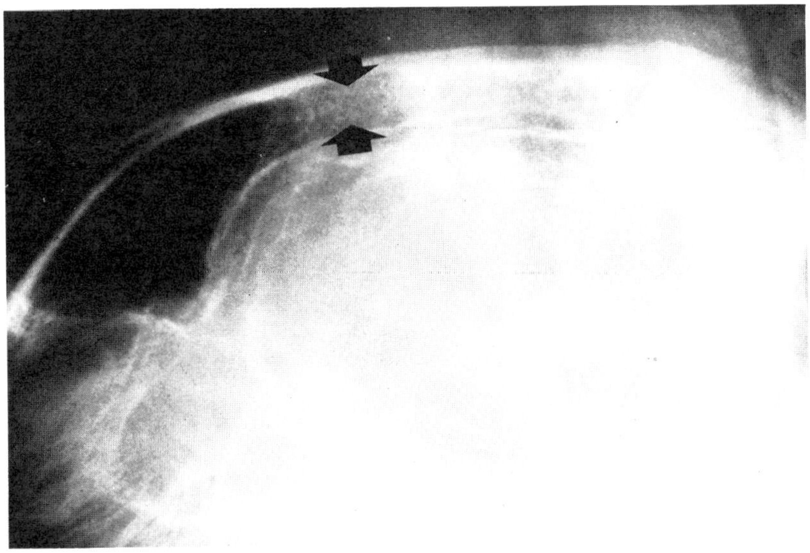

Figure 4—Lateral view of a skull. Mottling of the diploë (*arrows*), reflecting age-related osteoporosis, can be seen in this 14-year-old dog.

mation is most useful if surgery is contemplated, because not all areas of collapse are readily operable. This is particularly true of the proximal main-stem bronchi, which may also be involved in the collapse (carinal collapse).

Regional and, rarely, diffuse ballooning of the trachea is sometimes seen. The trachea is often irregular or undulent. This finding may be identified in the thoracic portion of the trachea during inspiration, and in the cervical portion of the trachea during expiration, particularly during coughing.[6]

Cervical Spine

Many older dogs and cats exhibit a unique density pattern in the dorsal spinal process of the second cervical vertebra. This pattern is composed of multiple small spherical or oval lucencies, some of which are surrounded by sclerotic margins. A number of these shadows appear to coalesce, depending on their size and to a lesser degree on the amount of radiographic penetration (Figure 5). This pattern extends throughout the spinal column but is less evident elsewhere because of the smaller size and the superimposition resulting from the multifaceted structure of the vertebrae. Histologic investigation at the author's institution has failed to reveal disease in affected individuals. This pattern represents an age-related osteoporosis with no more than a theoretic concern for potential structural weakness.[1] The condition loosely resembles the spinal lesions of multiple myeloma as well as other spinal neoplasms, but the diffuse nature of these changes should indicate that these diagnoses are incorrect. Other radiographic considerations for the cervical spine follow.

Back

Posture

Many older dogs exhibit a swayback posture resulting from ventral convexity of the lumbar spine. Although not described as a distinct entity in the veterinary literature, this curvature probably results from a combination of degenerative changes in the intervertebral disks, axial ligaments, and axial musculature.

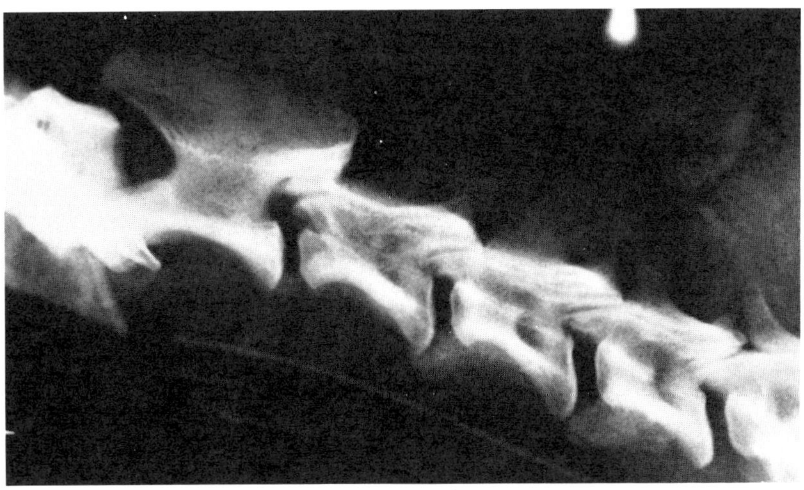

Figure 5—This lateral view of a cervical spine shows a density pattern typical of age-related osteoporosis. Changes in the first cervical vertebra are the most obvious.

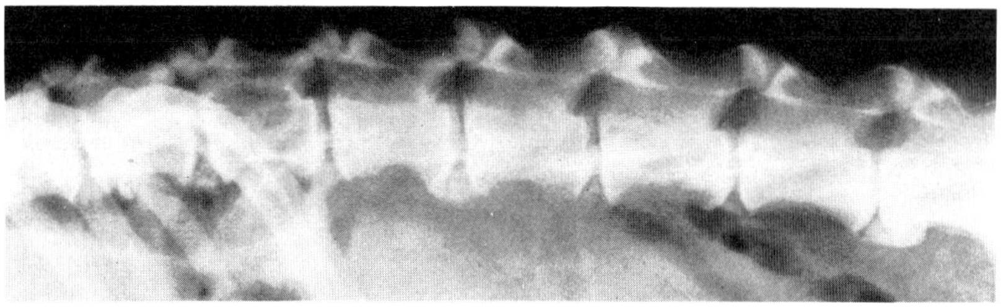

Figure 6—Lateral view of the lumbar spine. Widespread spondylosis is seen in this 10-year-old dog.

Osteoporosis is often seen in older pets, particularly cats. It has no practical clinical implications.

Spondylosis, although not confined to older dogs and cats, is generally more extensive when it occurs in this age group (Figure 6). The condition is usually considered to be benign or, at the most, a subclinical entity.[7] Recently, this view has been challenged with the suggestion that some of the osteophytic configurations previously described as *spondylosis deformans* are in fact clinical entities resembling ankylosing hyperostosis in people.[8]

A spondyloticlike condition affecting the lumbosacral junction has recently been described. It is called *spinal stenosis*. The signs are large ventral and lateral osteophytes, end-plate sclerosis, and facetal joint arthritis. The condition can be confirmed only by using intraosseous vertebral venography.[7] It is considered relatively rare in the author's clinic, and the majority of animals exhibiting these radiographic changes fail to show related clinical signs.

Facetal Joint Arthritis

Arthritis of the facetal joints is often seen in older dogs, and this author believes it may be a significant clinical entity. Some dogs that exhibit arthritic radiographic changes, though, fail to show related clinical signs.

Dural Mineralization

Dural mineralization, known by a number of synonyms, is characterized by the presence of bony plaque on the inner surface of the dura. These plaques occur in over 60% of both large- and small-breed dogs older than two years of age and are found most commonly in the most movable areas of the spine, the cervical and lumbar areas. Radiographically, these plaques appear as thin radiopaque linear shadows and are seen most easily at the site of the intervertebral foramina.[7] The clinical significance of this condition is currently unknown.[7] The author has not encountered a clinical case in his hospital.

Disk Degeneration

Degenerative intervertebral disk disease is a disease of middle-aged and older, chondrodystropic breeds, producing varying degrees of spinal cord compression and sensory and motor dysfunction.[7] The spines of older dogs should be examined closely for signs referable to this disorder to establish the presence of disease as well as its potential. Such findings may vary from subtle to obvious, depending on the visibility of the disk material and the degree of narrowing of disk space.

Hips

Older dogs and cats frequently show radiographic signs of degenerative joint disease. Clinically, and in light of human data, some of these patients are probably suffering from the primary form of degenerative joint disease in which it appears that the articular cartilage is unable to maintain itself as aging occurs.[9] Other animals—particularly dogs—have past medical histories that indicate that their arthritic conditions are subsequent to previous developmental or acquired disorders. An example of the former is hip dysplasia, which produces arthritis early in life but often worsens substantially with age. It is important to recognize the often progressive nature of this condition because it frequently explains why some older dogs are reluctant to exercise. Older cats exhibit what this author believes to be primary arthritis of the hips, which is usually less severe than that seen subsequent to dysplasia or trauma.[1] It must be emphasized that radiographic appearances of primary and secondary degenerative joint disease do not differ.[10] These conditions thus must be differentiated either circumstantially or inferentially.

Chest

Chest Wall

Many older dogs and cats fatten as they age as a result of exercising less and continuing to eat at preaging levels. This increased fat burden has at least two major influences on thoracic radiography. First, there is fat deposition surrounding the chest wall that usually results in some reduction in pulmonary image quality (Figure 7). It appears that an excessive amount of perithoracic fat is capable of influencing respiration.[a] This possibly results in a relative hypoxia in some individuals—it is called the *Pickwickian syndrome* in humans. Secondly, fat is also deposited in the mediastinum, resulting in a marked widening. This mass effect may be mistaken for an actual mass or infiltrative disease process (Figure 8).

[a]Suter P: Personal communication, University of Zurich, 1973.

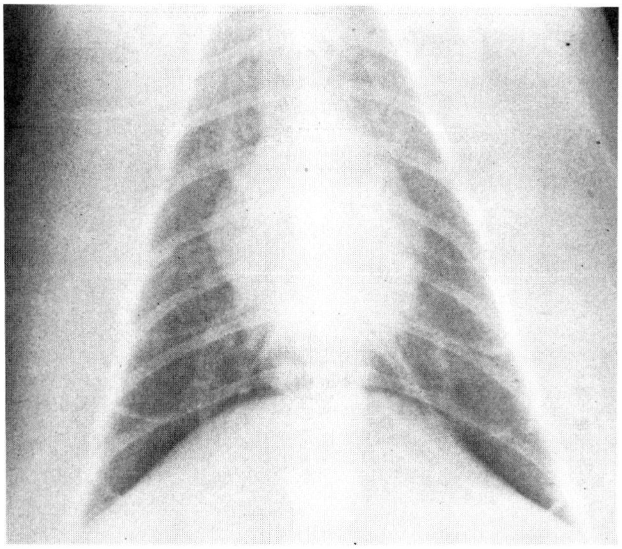

Figure 7—Ventrodorsal view of the thorax of a 13-year-old cat. Massive perithoracic fat is decreasing the pulmonary contrast and detail.

Ribs

The ribs are subject to extensive metaplastic changes as a result of aging, including calcification of cartilaginous ribs and costochondral junctions. The latter, often spherical in shape and heterogeneous in density, may resemble lung masses, particularly in the dorsoventral or ventrodorsal views (Figure 9). Rib mineralization in the lateral view is often mottled in appearance. Thus it may be mistaken for early pneumonia, particularly if there is strong clinical bias as a result of the preradiographic examination (Figure 9). There is no evidence that rib calcification is clinically significant.[11]

Sternum

Although spondylotic changes are not widely recognized, especially in the sternebrae of older dogs, they appear to vary as greatly as those in the spine. Unlike in the spine, though, these spondylotic changes rarely produce clinical signs. Their greatest importance probably lies in potential misdiagnoses in which trauma and infection are often invoked to explain their presence. Changes in sternal configuration, which are particularly common in cats, often provoke dire clinical predictions and/or are the basis for inaccurate causative speculations (Figure 10). In the author's experience, very few of these sternal variations can be related to past or present trauma or disease. Congenital deformities in the feline sternum appear to be more common than those in dogs.[4]

Trachea

Alterations in tracheal caliber and course may be anticipated when viewing thoracic films of older animals. As mentioned previously, these findings usually necessitate additional films to fully evaluate the extent of the condition. Tracheal calcification is common.

Pleura

Pleural thickening has been noted radiographically in most dogs older than five years. It is seen best in the dorsoventral view as a thickened, scalloped line of radiopacity at the lateral margins of the lung. The line often can be traced medially as it forms the fissure between the middle and caudal lobes. In the lateral view, the middle-caudal lobe lung fissure is seen superimposed on the caudal aspect of the cardiac silhouette as a fine, nonbranching linear density. The cranial-middle lobe lung fissure is less commonly seen.[12] Densities of this nature usually require end-on projection to be identified radiographically. They must be differentiated from alternative sources of increased pleural densities such as small volumes of pleural fluid and fibrinous pleuritis.

Lung

The lungs of aged dogs have been described in terms

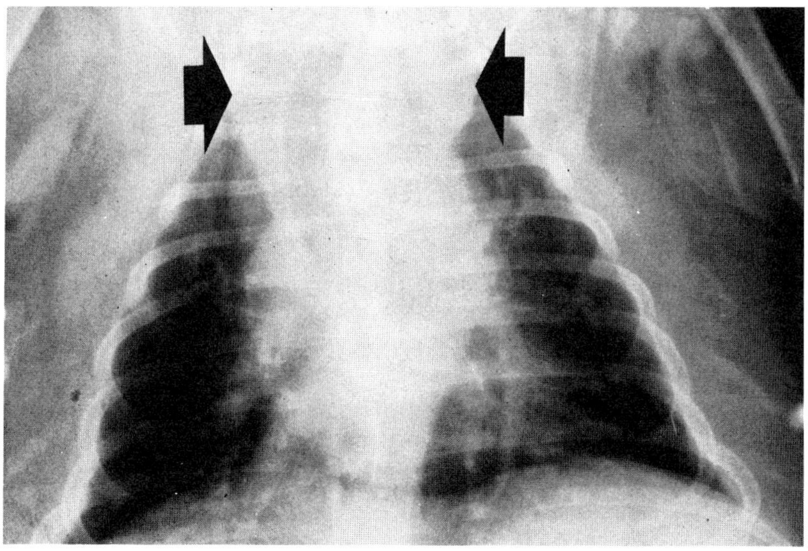

Figure 8—This dorsoventral view of the thorax shows mediastinal fat creating a mass effect (*arrows*) in a 15-year-old dog.

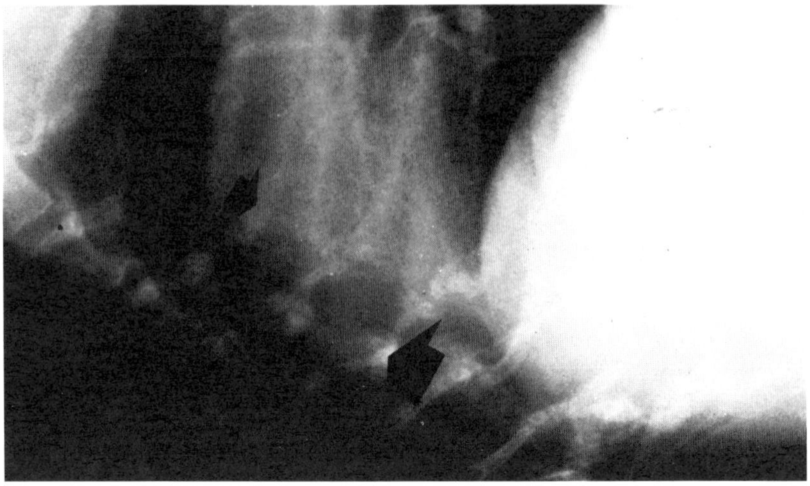

Figure 9—Lateral view of the thorax of a 12-year-old dog. Calcification of the chondral ribs (*small arrow*) and costochondral junctions (*large arrow*) as well as hypertrophic changes in the sternum are seen.

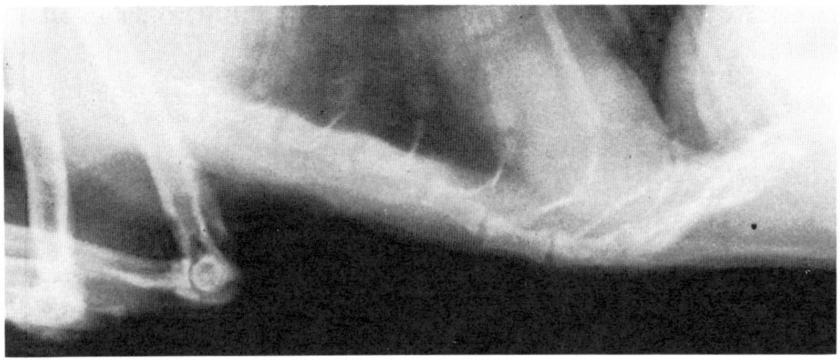

Figure 10—Lateral view of the sternum of a 16-year-old cat with no history of congenital deformity or trauma. Marked convexity of the middle segments with dorsal deflection of the caudal part, as well as arthritic elbows, are seen.

of their radiographic-morphologic correlation.[12] A radiographic pattern consisting of pleural thickening and an increase in nonvascular linear markings was observed regularly with no clinical evidence of current pulmonary or cardiovascular disease. Discrete nodular densities and evidence of tracheal and bronchial calcification also were seen. Histologic analysis revealed foci or interstitial fibrosis often associated with the presence of focal areas of emphysema. These latter changes were not appreciated radiographically. Pleural fibrosis, heterotopic bone formation, bronchial cartilage calcification (Figure 11), and anthracosis were also noted with varying frequency.[12] No such study has been carried out on the lungs of aged cats.

The author and co-workers believe increased interstitial lung density to be a significant finding in the preoperative screening of older dogs even if there are no referable clinical signs. Specifically, there is at least a theoretic reduction in lung compliance with a resultant loss in ventilatory capacity. Consequently, the author manages these patients differently during anesthesia.[4]

Pulmonary osteomas are an occasional finding in the lungs of older dogs. They are probably a benign condition and the author treats them as such, although the patient's medical background is routinely investigated for evidence of previous mycotic lung disease that may result in a similar lung pattern following resolution.

Heart

Cardiac assessment is the most frequent radiographic examination performed in the author's geriatric patients. This examination is requested for diagnosis, therapeutic assessment, progress evaluation, and presurgical screening. The heart and associated pulmonary vascul-

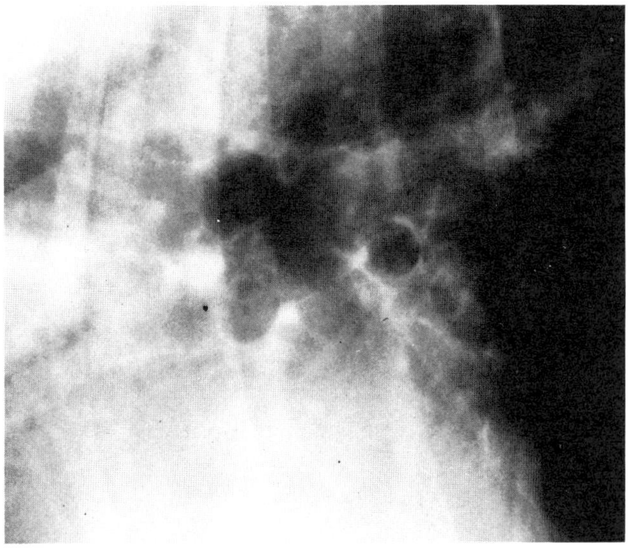

Figure 11—This lateral view of the thorax shows calcification of the tracheal and bronchial walls in a 12-year-old dog.

ature (great and small vessels) are routinely evaluated as an anatomic as well as functional unit. In suspected cases of heart failure, the author renders a positive diagnosis based on the presence or absence of lung edema, increased vascular size and number, and cardiomegaly. The presence of pleural and/or abdominal fluid is considered in addition to liver size. The assessment of these potential radiographic findings often results in a diagnosis of pending failure, which may then form the basis of prophylactic treatment.[1]

The size of the left atrium is of paramount importance in assessing the hearts of older animals because it is a reliable inferential indicator of pulmonary venous hypertension (Figure 12). Of the four cardiac chambers, enlargement of the left atrium is most often detected early in humans, and in the author's experience, in dogs too.[1,13]

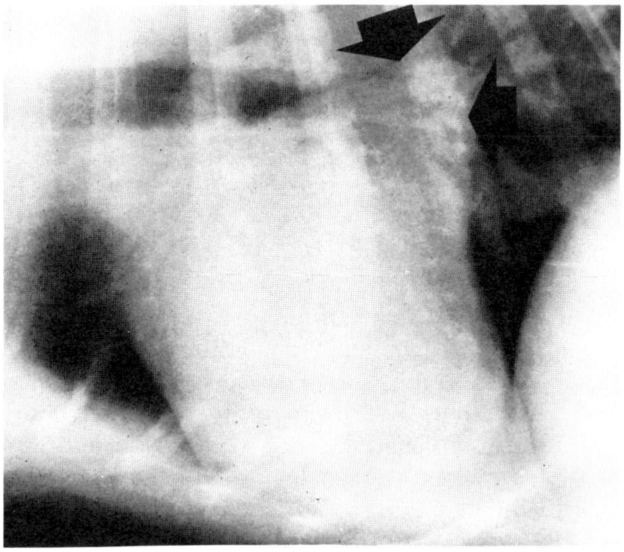

Figure 12—Lateral view of the thorax of a 13-year-old dog. Marked left-atrial enlargement (*arrows*), indicating pulmonary venous hypertension, can be seen.

Pulmonary Vasculature

The pulmonary vasculature varies widely in detail, size, and number in both old and young dogs. The major concern is its relationship to heart disease in the older pet, in which it may precede overt failure, as mentioned previously. In such circumstances the heart and pulmonary vessels are assessed as a functional unit. The pulmonary vessels are also very useful in differentiating cardiac and noncardiac sources of pleural fluid. The vessels are usually normal in size and number in fluid formations unassociated with failure. Many older cats exhibit an irregular vascular course compared with younger animals.[1] The reason for this appearance has not been determined.

Abdomen

Abdominal Wall

The abdominal wall of many older animals loses tone, resulting in a distinctive potbellied appearance. Radiographically this is associated with a relative redistribution of the abdominal contents into the ventral aspect of the abdomen (Figure 13). Combined with increased intraabdominal fat accumulation, such positional changes may be mistaken for organomegaly.

Liver

The liver in older dogs has been reported to decrease in weight with advancing years.[3] The experience at the author's clinic, however, has been contrary, with the majority of older dogs and cats exhibiting normal or somewhat enlarged livers. In cases in which histologic analysis has been performed, the author has found the majority of the liver enlargements to result from varying degrees of fatty infiltration.[1] Endocrine disease has also been a reported source of hepatomegaly.[11]

Spleen

The spleen undergoes involution with advancing age.[3,1] Radiographic interpretation of splenomegaly,

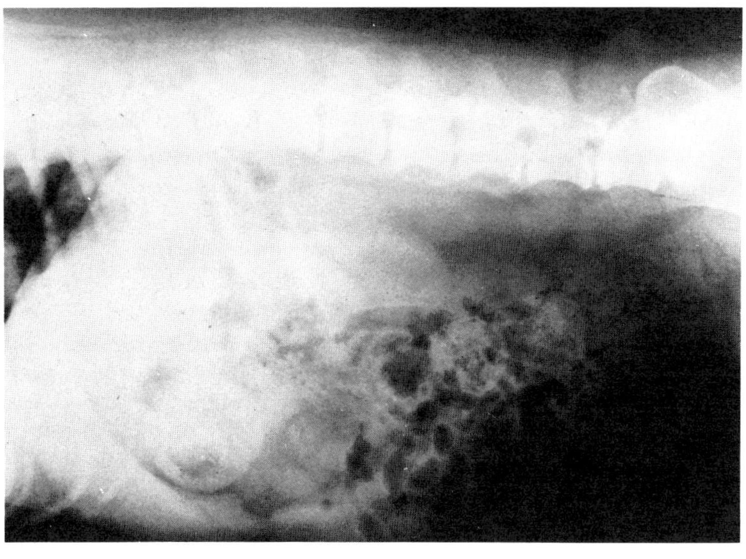

Figure 13—This lateral view of the abdomen of a 14-year-old dog shows generalized ventral displacement of the viscera.

focusing on the extent of enlargement and marginal characteristics, has been reported previously.[15]

Intestine

The bowel tends to move ventrally in older dogs because of a combination of decreased abdominal tone, ligamentous laxity, and increased intraabdominal fat content both within the abdomen generally and within the mesenteric walls. Mesenteric fat may also increase periintestinal contrast, which can result in a better appreciation of bowel detail.

Kidneys

Like many of the organs mentioned previously, the kidneys become radiographically more visible in older animals because of an increase in retroperitoneal fat content. This, along with generalized visceral laxity, often results in the kidneys being visualized in a more central location than normal. The summation of the renal shadows, particularly in this location and with lighter radiographic techniques, may create the impression of a mass. Because of this possibility, masses in this area should be closely scrutinized.

Prostate

Prostatic enlargement is present to some extent in most older dogs, usually as a result of benign prostatic hyperplasia. This condition may result in clinical signs, such as constipation and tenesmus, or it may produce no detectable abnormality.[16]

Hind Limbs and Forelimbs

General Considerations

The posture of the forelimbs and hind limbs in older dogs and to some extent in cats often changes dramatically with advancing years. This may take the form of either varus or valgus conformations. The specifics of these postures have not been reported, but they are likely related to altered joint structures, especially the supporting soft tissues. Age-associated reduction in muscle mass is probably a secondary contributor.

Osteoporosis of the aged results in a generalized reduction in bone mass, specifically atrophy of the interior of the bone. Notably, the overall external dimensions of the skeleton do not change. This decrease in bone mass is the result of increased resorption of bone, which begins at a relatively early age in both humans and animals.[17,18]

Corticomedullary ratios have been described for humans and are often used to objectively assess bone for the presence of osteoporosis. Similar measurements have been a problem in veterinary medicine because of the considerable breed variation among dogs. Theoretically, such measurements are better suited to cats, in which little morphological difference exists. This has yet to be investigated.

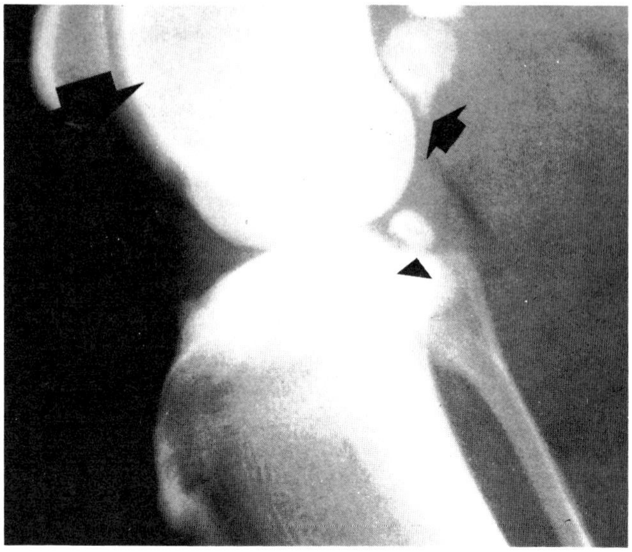

Figure 14—Lateral view of the stifle of a 14-year-old dog. Mild hypertrophic changes in the patella, fabella, and popliteal sesamoid (*arrows*) are visualized.

Joints

The joints constitute the primary radiographic focus in the aged dog and cat. Both these species frequently exhibit arthritic changes, although it is often difficult to establish whether or not these conditions are primary or secondary (Figure 14). The cat seems especially prone to arthritic changes, which may be severest in the elbow and stifle joints. Many such affected animals have been observed closely throughout their lifetimes and have no history of illness or trauma. This suggests the possibility of primary osteoarthritis in the cat as well as infectious or etiologic disorders of a subclinical nature. The reader is referred to a recent discussion of this subject for additional clinical information.[18]

Conclusions

The radiographic changes of aging present in the majority of dogs and cats at the conclusion of their first decade are many and varied. Some are subtle, and others are easily identified. The significance of such radiographic findings ranges from clinically important to merely intellectual curiosities.

The primary importance of this radiologic data lies in its differentiation from non-age-related findings.

One must be constantly cognizant of the disorders, such as heart failure, that mostly affect the geriatric population. Increased awareness and anticipation of such entities will enhance radiodiagnosis.

REFERENCES

1. Zontine WJ: Dental radiographic technique and interpretation. *Vet Clin North Am (Small Anim Pract)* 4:741-762, 1974.
2. Harvey CE, et al: Oral, dental, pharyngeal, and salivary gland disorders, in Ettinger, SJ (ed): *Veterinary Internal Medicine*. Philadelphia, WB Saunders Co, 1983, pp 1126-1160.
3. Bloom F: Geriatrics, in Catcott EJ (ed): *Canine Medicine*. Santa Barbara, American Veterinary Publications, Inc, 1968, pp 822-841.
4. Farrow CS: Unpublished material, University of Saskatchewan, 1981-1983.
5. Ettinger SJ, Ticer JW: Diseases of the trachea, in Ettinger SJ (ed): *Veterinary Internal Medicine*. Philadelphia, WB Saunders Co, 1983, pp 723-747.
6. McKiernan B: Diseases of the canine and feline tracheobronchial tract, in Kirk RW (ed): *Current Veterinary Therapy VII*. Philadelphia, WB Saunders Co, 1980, pp 229-235.
7. Bailey CS, Morgan JP: Diseases of the spinal cord, in Ettinger SJ (ed): *Veterinary Internal Medicine*. Philadelphia, WB Saunders Co, 1983, pp 532-608.
8. Wright JA: A study of vertebral osteophyte formation in the canine spine. II. Radiographic surgery. *J Small Anim Pract* 23:747-761, 1982.
9. Pederson NC, Pool R: Canine joint disease. *Vet Clin North Am (Small Anim Pract)* 8:465-493, 1978.
10. Owens JM, Ackerman N: Roentgenology of arteritis. *Vet Clin North Am (Small Anim Pract)* 8:453-464, 1978.
11. Mitten RW: Radiographic examination of the ribs and sternum in the dog and cat. *Compend Contin Educ Pract Vet* 2(9):738-744, 1980.
12. Reif JS, Rhodes WH: The lungs of aged dogs. *J Am Vet Rad* 7:5-11, 1966.
13. Elliott LP, Schiebler GL: *The X-ray Diagnosis of Congenital Heart Disease in Infants, Children, and Adults*. ed 2. Springfield, IL, Charles C Thomas, 1979, pp 3-114.
14. Ticer JW: Roentgen signs of endocrine disease. *Vet Clin North Am (Small Anim Pract)* 7:465-486, 1977.
15. O'Brien TR: *Radiographic Diagnosis of Abdominal Disorders in the Dog and Cat*. Philadelphia, WB Saunders Co, 1978, pp 450-459.
16. Greiner TP, Johnson RG: Diseases of the prostate gland, in Ettinger SJ (ed): *Veterinary Internal Medicine*. Philadelphia, WB Saunders Co, 1983, pp 1459-1493.
17. Steinbach HL: Roentgenology of the skeleton in the aged. *Rad Clin North Am* 2:277-292, 1965.
18. Weigel J, Alexander JW: Aging and the musculoskeletal system. *Vet Clin North Am (Small Anim Pract)* 11:749-764, 1981.

Lumbosacral Disease *(continued from page 175)*

The axial images are also helpful in detecting lateralization of disc protrusions. We have used coronal images to detect lateral displacement of the cauda equina arising from a lateralized disc protrusion.

MRI is in its infancy as a diagnostic tool in veterinary medicine. At present, there is a strong need for descriptions of normal MRI anatomy in the dog. With respect to lumbosacral disease, description of the lumbosacral anatomy in clinically normal (asymptomatic) middle- to old-aged large breed dogs would help us become more adept at detecting and describing pathology.

Acknowledgment

Our sincere gratitude is extended to Murray A. Solomon, MD, and the staff at Los Gatos MRI for their clinical service and training.

REFERENCE

1. de Hann JJ, Shelton SB, Ackerman N: Magnetic resonance imaging in the diagnosis of degenerative lumbosacral stenosis in four dogs. *Vet Surg* 22:1–4, 1993.